NARCOTIC ANTAGONISTS

Advances in Biochemical Psychopharmacology

Volume 8

Advances in Biochemical Psychopharmacology

Series Editors

Erminio Costa, M.D.
Chief, Laboratory of Preclinical Pharmacology
National Institute of Mental Health
Washington, D.C., U.S.A.

Paul Greengard, Ph.D.
Professor of Pharmacology
Yale University School of Medicine
New Haven, Conn., U.S.A.

NARCOTIC ANTAGONISTS

Advances in Biochemical Psychopharmacology
Volume 8

Sponsored by the
National Institute of Mental Health
Center for Studies of Narcotic and Drug Abuse
Special Action Office for Drug Abuse Prevention

EDITORS:

Monique C. Braude
Acting Chief,
Preclinical Drug Study Section
Center for Studies of Narcotic and Drug Abuse
National Institute of Mental Health
Rockville, Maryland, U.S.A.

Louis S. Harris
Chairman,
Department of Pharmacology
Medical College of Virginia
Richmond, Virginia, U.S.A.

Everette L. May
Chief,
Section on Medicinal Chemistry
National Institute of Arthritis and
*   Metabolic Diseases*
National Institutes of Health
Bethesda, Maryland, U.S.A.

Jean Paul Smith
Assistant Chief,
Center for Studies of Narcotic
*   and Drug Abuse*
National Institute of Mental Health
Rockville, Maryland, U.S.A.

Julian E. Villarreal
Director,
Behavioral Pharmacology
Instituto Miles de Terapeutica
*   Experimental*
Laboratorios Miles de Mexico
Mexico City, Mexico

Raven Press, Publishers ∎ New York

International Standard Book Number 0-911216-55-3
Library of Congress Catalog Card Number 73-84113
International Standard Serial Number 0065-2229

The work upon which this publication is based was performed pursuant to Contract No. HSM-42-73-172(ND) with the National Institute of Mental Health, Health Services and Mental Health Administration, Department of Health, Education and Welfare.

In recognition of the fact that materials prepared by the following individuals were prepared by them as part of their official duties as United States Government employees, these materials are not covered by the above-mentioned copyright statement: Monique C. Braude, William E. Bunney, Jr., Erminio Costa, Charles Gorodetzky, Alan I. Green, Charles Haertzen, Jerome H. Jaffe, Everette L. May, Jo Ann Nuite, Jorge Perez-Cruett, and Jean Paul Smith.

Preface

The view that antagonists may be socially important and clinically necessary in treating or preventing opiate dependence is of relatively recent origin, although there has long been scientific interest in these compounds. Throughout the 1960's, optimism for the potential contribution of antagonists gained support from the work of Martin and associates (1), after early clinical exploration in the 1950's by Eckenhoff et al. (2) and by Wikler et al. (3).

With the increase in heroin use in the U.S. in the drug decade of the 1960's, treatment tools were needed in addition to the major modalities then available: methadone substitution and drug-free therapies. Several pharmaceutical firms, the Addiction Research Center at Lexington, Kentucky, and a small number of university-based investigators were then conducting initial studies on antagonists. In the early 1970's, the Government accelerated its sponsored research program by adding several million dollars to support additional research on narcotic antagonists. As part of the Federal Government's efforts to stimulate work in this field, the First International Conference on Narcotic Antagonists was held at Airlie House in Warrenton, Virginia, in November 1972.

Co-sponsored by the National Institute of Mental Health's Division of Narcotic Addiction and Drug Abuse and the White House Special Action Office for Drug Abuse Prevention, the purpose of the Conference was to bring together a select group of chemists and preclinical pharmacologists who were actively working in the antagonist field. Clinical aspects of antagonist evaluation were not included since it was felt that insufficient experimental data were then available for detailed discussion. To describe what we know about antagonists before man enters the picture was the main purpose of the Conference. A group of people was selected to serve as the combined Planning Committee and Editorial Board. They were Drs. Everette May (Chief of Medicinal Chemistry, National Institutes of Health), Louis Harris (Chairman, Department of Pharmacology, the Medical College of Virginia), and Julian Villarreal (then of the Department of Pharmacology, University of Michigan), along with the two co-project officers, Dr. Monique Braude and myself (NIMH). The task of the Planning Committee was to develop a conceptual organization of the major areas of chemical and preclinical research in the antagonist field and to identify individuals to prepare papers and make presentations at the Conference on their topics. The papers invited for discussion at the Conference were oriented toward promising drugs and techniques of evaluation. This Conference focused on antagonist actions of compounds including classes of chemicals which are not analgesics, thus distinguishing it from the *Aberdeen Conference on Agonist and Antagonist Actions of Narcotic Analgesic Drugs,* held 16 months earlier in Scotland. The Committee on the Problems of Drug Dependence of the National Academy of Sciences–National Research Council assisted in planning this antagonist Conference. At the 1972 meeting of the Committee in Ann Arbor, Michigan, a discussion session was held to obtain the opinions of many of the scientists working in this field as to recommended contents and timing.

The Planning Committee did not include in the substantive discussions of the Conference many broad issues such as the potential utility of these compounds, questions of patients' rights, epidemiological aspects of opiate use and abuse, and important philosophical and value questions. The number and breadth of topics to be covered and the limitations of time and funds resulted in a strategic decision to concentrate on evaluations of drugs, review of methods of research, and presentation of available data.

In the initial planning stages, the Planning and Editorial Committee identified five goals of the Conference as follows:

- establish the state of the art in chemical and preclinical pharmacological research on narcotic antagonists;
- provide a forum for the exchange of information and ideas on narcotic antagonists;
- evaluate the most promising antagonists;
- evaluate preclinical testing methods used to determine antagonists' potentials;
- suggest lines of development for future research for both government and nongovernment programs.

Two parallel purposes were defined for the Conference. The first was to establish a forum for direct interchange of ideas by scientists actively working with antagonists so that new data, articles not in the open literature, unreported observations, and spontaneous discussion would take place. The second was to produce the published proceedings of the Conference containing prepared papers and discussions.

A challenge to every major scientific conference, the integration and balancing of forum and archival purposes, was planned as follows: first, each presentation at Airlie House contained the major ideas of the paper authored by each scientist or team. The spontaneous discussion afterward reflected the reaction of the participants to these ideas and the data presented. Second, the introductory remarks made at the Conference and included here in somewhat altered version tied the content of the Conference to the social context in which research on antagonists takes place. Third, the evaluation of the project casts an analytical eye at both the Conference process and the content of the presentations.

The structure of the Conference is clear from the Contents which closely follows the program outline. Three members of the Planning Committee (May, Harris, and Villarreal) served in key roles as Section Chairmen. Individual papers were grouped under significant topics and Topic Chairmen were selected to guide the discussion afterward and to ensure reasonable adherence to the plan. The main fare at the Conference was the presentation of data and discussions by selected individuals. The open discussion which followed has been transcribed, partially edited, and is available separately in mimeographed form.*

Jean Paul Smith, Ph.D.
September 1973

Acknowledgments: We acknowledge with thanks the contributions of many individuals — authors, discussants, administrators, contractors, consultants, and staff — whose efforts made this book possible. Support for the project is courtesy of the U.S. taxpayer, the NIMH budget, and contracts HSM 42-73-172 and HSM 42-72-184.

REFERENCES

1. Martin, W. R.: Opioid antagonists. *Pharmacological Reviews*, 19:463–521, 1967.
2. Eckenhoff, J. E., Elder, J. D., and King, B. D.: The effect of N-allyl-normorphine in treatment of opiate overdose. *American Journal of Medical Science*, 222:115–117, 1951.
3. Wikler, A., Fraser, H. F., and Isbell, H.: N-Allylnormorphine: Effects of single doses and precipitation of acute "abstinence syndromes" during addiction to morphine, methadone or heroin in man (postaddicts). *Journal of Pharmacology and Experimental Therapeudics*, 109:8–20, 1953.

---

* The detailed evaluation and transcriptions of the discussions are available on request from the Center for Studies of Narcotic and Drug Abuse, NIMH, 5600 Fishers Lane, Rockville, Maryland 20852.

Contents

III. PHARMACOLOGY

A. Pharmacological Assay Procedures

1. Assays of Analgesic Activity

2. Assays of Antagonist Activity

3. Special Tests and Procedures

NATHAN BROWNE EDDY
1890–1973

A towering figure has passed from us. Truly a pioneer in the research on drugs, Dr. Eddy held many important positions in his lifetime and won many high honors.

He grew up in upstate New York and was educated at Cornell. For more than 20 years he was a leading figure at NIH, and for many more he advised high government officials, international bodies, pharmaceutical firms, scientific societies, and colleagues. Dr. Eddy carried on his work long past retirement in 1960. He died peacefully in his sleep March 27, shortly after finishing a history of the National Research Council's Involvement in the Opiate Problem.

Dr. Eddy's contributions to the science of analgesia and narcotic dependence are countless; his authoritative publications and compendia number over 200. His acumen and research, particularly in structure-activity relationships and with the narcotic antagonists, have helped pave the way for the development of improved pain-relieving drugs and methods for combating narcotic abuse.

It is a tribute to his vitality and dedication that to help wrap up the First International Conference on Narcotic Antagonists, he proceeded directly to Airlie House from a 10-day United Nations meeting in Geneva for the concluding day of this Conference.

Dr. Eddy was a formidable man of immense intellectual vigor. His opinions were direct, his dedication strong, and his heart warm. None of us today remembers a time before him. For his many friends and colleagues, the time after will not be the same. We cherish his memory.

Everette L. May   Jean Paul Smith

Narcotic Antagonists, edited by M. C. Braude, L. S. Harris, E. L. May, J. P. Smith, and J. E. Villarreal. *Advances in Biochemical Psychopharmacology, Vol. 8.* Raven Press, New York © 1974.

Introduction

William E. Bunney, Jr.

Division of Narcotic Addiction and Drug Abuse, National Institute of Mental Health, Rockville, Maryland 20852

Narcotic addiction affects the lives of hundreds of thousands of individuals in this country. Fortunately, progress has been accelerated in recent months toward developing and making available treatment services for a large portion of that population, utilizing a number of different treatment modalities.

The goal of this Conference is to push forward the day when a long-acting narcotic antagonist will be widely available as an effective additional treatment alternative for addicts. Through in-depth evaluation of the chemistry, pharmacology, and pharmacokinetics of antagonists, the Conference participants will define the state of the art on antagonist research, and set the stage for further rapid advancement in understanding these compounds and their benefit for treating opiate addiction.

The potential value of narcotic antagonists in helping addicts overcome compulsive heroin use has been clearly indicated. Cyclazocine is already being used on a limited basis in controlled settings, including several National Institute of Mental Health grant- and contract-supported facilities. Preliminary studies on other antagonists such as EN 1639A have shown them to offer even more promise.

This Conference is part of an intensive program which the NIMH Division of Narcotic Addiction and Drug Abuse has underway, in cooperation with the White House Special Action Office for Drug Abuse Prevention and with the pharmaceutical industry, to accelerate progress in this area. Components of this comprehensive research program include identification of compounds with antagonist potential, testing of selected compounds in the laboratory, and evaluation of promising antagonists for short-term and long-term safety and efficacy in patients. The ideal compound would have a long duration of action, few agonistic side effects, and be an inexpensive oral preparation which is accepted by the addict.

At present, our three million dollar program includes 10 major research contracts from NIMH and 27 grant-supported investigations. The NIMH Addiction Research Center in Lexington, Kentucky, which had a pioneering

1

role in research on narcotic antagonists, continues to make major contributions to this area. The number of pharmaceutical firms that are associated with the Conference clearly indicates the leading role that industry also has assumed in the development of antagonists.

The development of long-acting narcotic antagonists which neutralize the effects of opiates without producing undesirable side effects will add an important chemotherapeutic adjunct to the current armamentarium of modalities with which to reach addicts.

Effective antagonists will also represent a valuable treatment approach to specific population groups, such as youths, for whom some current methods such as methadone maintenance are not suitable. We are also interested in the use of antagonists in prevention of addiction in known experimenters, and in their potential as a prophylactic measure for possible use in the future among high-risk populations.

The research program on antagonists will, of course, have other benefits of major importance. The knowledge gained in this effort will undoubtedly make a contribution to a broader understanding of brain metabolism and the nature of the neuronal receptor sites. The narcotic antagonist thus offers a very exciting research tool.

The participants in this Conference represent the major contributors to our present information on the chemistry and animal pharmacology of narcotic antagonists, and the presentations to be made indicate this meeting will be a benchmark in the development of increased understanding toward these goals.

Narcotic Antagonists, edited by M. C. Braude, L. S. Harris, E. L. May, J. P. Smith, and J. E. Villarreal. *Advances in Biochemical Psychopharmacology, Vol. 8.* Raven Press, New York © 1974.

Pharmacological and Societal Factors in the Management of Drug Dependence

Jerome Jaffe

Special Action Office for Drug Abuse Prevention, Washington, D.C.

If you try to link drugs with antagonists, you begin with the observation that all societies respond to the fact that psychoactive drugs and their citizens coexist in a number of ways. They range from the control of the availability of psychoactive substances and treating the victims of drug dependence all the way through to actually licensing and distributing the substances. These various kinds of responses interact with each other. In order to know how to manipulate them you have to know these interactions.

In a sense it does no good to talk about knowing the interactions or manipulating them unless you first know the goals you want to achieve. How does a society set its goals for problems of drug dependence? The goals of the society are not simply dependent on the pharmacological actions of the substances they are concerned with. They are also dependent on the beliefs, attitudes, and the values of the society. Our society, as most societies, is going through a phase of value change, belief change, and attitude change and, in effect, you have an uncontrolled variable. It's very difficult to set goals now. And so you try to concentrate, therefore, on those goals about which we can at least have some consensus. I think we can probably agree that a reasonable goal would be at least to reduce the incidence of drug dependence and/or its social cost. It's not clear on which of these we should put our emphasis. Our efforts to reach these goals will be rational only to the extent that our assumptions about the nature of the problem are valid.

The general approach that this country takes to the problem of drug dependence is built on a number of assumptions and among them are the following: Primarily, drug dependence is itself an abstraction that takes in a wide variety of behaviors related to the use of a number of substances. Secondly, any approach to reducing the use of these substances or the social costs must involve a consideration not only of the pharmacological actions but also the values, attitudes, and beliefs of the society in which that use occurs. Thirdly, among the various substances used for these objective

3

effects, there is such a diversity of pharmacological effect related behaviors and social attitudes and beliefs, that there can be no single policy toward the problem as a whole. Rather for each substance or class there must be a specifically designed strategy that considers the specific effects and the social and historical context in which its use and abuse occur.

At the same time it is essential to recognize that the relationships between patterns of drug use are such that by reducing the social cost of one pattern, the social costs of other patterns may be increased. The net effect then could be to increase the overall social cost. What we are talking about are specific approaches to one of a range of problems, and that range of problems is the use of opioid substances by people in this particular society.

Any cursory survey of the state of our knowledge about this problem reveals that there are few islands of uncontested fact. Indeed every viewpoint about the motives for initial use, the etiology of compulsive abuse, and the optimum approach to intervention both on the individual and societal levels has its vigorous proponents and equally vigorous critics. Fortunately it's not necessary to have universal consensus on all issues to reach substantial agreement on a few.

This First International Conference on Antagonists arises from only partial agreement in the following area. First, once compulsive opioid use develops, there is no single intervention approach that is likely to be effective for all compulsive users, no matter how we define the term effective. We can all agree, therefore, that it would be useful to explore additional approaches to reducing the social costs of the opioid dependent syndrome. In addition most of us would agree that effective methods of preventing its development are a problem that deserves high priority.

I will reiterate what Dr. Bunney said. There are perhaps four clinical areas where antagonists might prove to be of some use. First, there is an experimental approach to prevention. There are a number of viewpoints as to the etiology of opioid dependence. They range from viewpoints of how people get started to how they move from experimentation to compulsive drug use. I won't go into the details of the various views, but obviously there are some who believe that basically, in the initial stages, people experiment as a result of peer pressure. There is a kind of contagion process, such that it is the early user who introduces nonusers to the process of drug use. There is also the view that if the process goes on long enough at least two things may happen. The user becomes the subject of a process of operant and classical conditioning such that relapse is dependent upon this process. Another factor might be that the user acquires a life style that relates to drug use more than it does to anything else.

Whether you believe in any of these strongly, there is at least some validity to the argument that if you could get the early user to give up the use of drugs you might be able to prevent progression from use to dependence. You might also interrupt the process of contagion based on the idea that someone who does not use the drug himself might not induce others to use it.

The idea, therefore, of antagonists in this syndrome stems from the notion that antagonists could, in a very crudely analogous way, be thought of as temporary immunizing agents. If you had an antagonist that was sufficiently free of side effects and sufficiently nontoxic, you could think of it almost in the way you think of gamma globulin in a hepatitis epidemic. It would confer a kind of temporary immunity on those who are experimenting. The experimenter who is taking an antagonist would perhaps perceive little effect of the opiate and would not progress to drug dependency. There would be no reinforcement and very few biochemical changes, and because there is very little gratification from the drug itself, there would perhaps be less motivation to encourage others to get involved with drug-using behavior.

A second major area, and all of this is of course theoretical, would be an alternative to the treatment of those already dependent. We have a number of major approaches to opioid dependence in this country: civil commitment or supervisory deterrent approaches, maintenance approaches with oral drugs such as methadone, and therapeutic communities. For a number of drug users, these various major options do not seem suitable or appropriate. The use of antagonists might in fact provide an alternative.

The use of antagonists can be thought of as an ancillary approach to other treatments or as a later phase in other treatments. For example, there is no reason why the antagonist could not be added to a regimen which, up to this time, has been primarily based upon a supervisory deterrent situation. As you know, a civil commitment program is largely based on the idea that drug use is optional. People who have been institutionalized and then released to a situation in which they are closely supervised, will avoid relapsing to opiate use, if carefully supervised, because relapse is generally tantamount to a period of reinstitutionalization.

Generally these programs have met with only modest success at best. The question is, would the rate of success be increased to any extent if the people being supervised were ingesting a long-acting narcotic antagonist? That's obviously a question to which we have no answers at the present time.

A third use for narcotic antagonists might be with those people maintained on methadone for months or years who feel ready to discontinue that drug. Thus far the results of withdrawing people from methadone have not been overwhelmingly successful. There are a lot of reasons for this. It has been found that in the withdrawal of people from methadone, there are some successes, but there are probably more people who relapse over a period of time to opiate use.

The next question is, would antagonists used in that context help prevent relapse for those people who have been withdrawn from opiates? Dr. Bunney has already outlined the desirable characteristics of clinically useful antagonists. Obviously they have to be nontoxic and safe. Hopefully they should be so free of agonistic activity that they cause virtually no side effects, and therefore could be suitable for use in people who are only experimenting. This is a situation where I think most of us would agree that imposing a drug with severe side effects would be inappropriate. Obviously for drugs that have to be used chronically the cost of the drug is a factor.

I think we ought to point out one other aspect about the need for long-acting drugs in which ingestion can be supervised. There is a small ethical issue which we must consider. We now have in this country somewhere in the range of 60,000 people maintained on drugs such as methadone. Given the fact that we are dealing with people who tend to share medications of all varieties, we have to ask what will be the impact of people maintained on methadone ingesting a potent long-acting or orally effective antagonist? What is the severity of the syndrome? What kinds of additional effects are we likely to run into and how can we handle them? Obviously this would not be a factor if there were no diversion of antagonists. This can be achieved only with sufficiently long-acting antagonists that can be given under supervision. These kinds of adverse consequences are not often considered because at the time we began thinking about diversion of antagonists, we didn't have the same population dependent on drugs such as methadone.

In closing, I would like to emphasize that at the present time we should admit that the promise of the antagonist is largely a promise unfulfilled. At this point their value is primarily theoretical. In spite of the fact that Martin, Wikler, and their co-workers suggested some of these clinical applications about seven years ago, there have been few adequately controlled clinical studies testing the basic proposition that narcotic antagonists could in any way ameliorate the narcotics problem either at the clinical or societal level. I know a few studies have been done. I would like to emphasize again that few of them have been adequately controlled.

There are probably a number of reasons for this lag in controlled studies on narcotic antagonists. The major reason is probably related to the properties and quantities of the compounds that were available for clinical testing. This brings us to the primary purpose of this meeting and demonstrates that these things are in fact integrally related. You can't do adequate clinical tests if you don't have adequate compounds. You can't test the theoretical applicability unless you can do adequate clinical tests. In effect we have a sequence problem. We are hopeful, therefore, that these factors will be eliminated.

Furthermore, as Dr. Bunney pointed out, the funding of toxicity testing and early clinical trials has already been arranged in anticipation of the development of suitable compounds, and funds are presently available for adequately controlled clinical trials in various situations. Whether or not we will ever again be in so favorable a position to develop new approaches is not clear. It is clear that it is not enough to proclaim the theoretical value of compounds indefinitely; we must take the steps to put those theories to the test. I'm confident that the appropriate clinical studies will be initiated and that in the near future we shall at least have a preliminary notion of whether antagonists will fulfill their promise.

Narcotic Antagonists, edited by M. C. Braude, L. S. Harris, E. L. May, J. P. Smith, and J. E. Villarreal. *Advances in Biochemical Psychopharmacology, Vol. 8.* Raven Press, New York © 1974.

Origin and History of Antagonists

Nathan B. Eddy and Everette L. May

National Institute of Arthritis and Metabolic Diseases, National Institutes of Health, Bethesda, Maryland 20014

The first recorded specific narcotic antagonist, N-allylnorcodeine, was synthesized by J. Pohl about 1914. This finding lay dormant until 1940 when McCawley, Hart, and Marsh, with the aim of producing an analgesic essentially without respiratory-depressant effects, attempted to prepare N-allylnormorphine. They reported slightly stronger (than N-allylnor-codeine) antagonism to morphine's actions with their preparation which apparently was a mixture containing principally 3(O),N-diallylnormorphine. A year or two later, Weijlard and Erickson provided a pure, authentic specimen of N-allylnormorphine (nalorphine) which was found by several investigators to antagonize most of the pharmacologic effects of morphine. Since then, nalorphine has become important in the diagnosis of and research on narcotic dependence. Properties of analgesia have also been demonstrated for nalorphine. Thus, it has provided the stimulus toward development not only of new and improved antagonists but also of compounds with a mixture of agonist and antagonist properties in the morphine, morphinan, and 6,7-benzomorphan series. Among these are naloxone, a pure antagonist, and cyclazocine and pentazocine, antagonist-analgesics.

N-Allylnorcodeine

As is often the case in a development of major consequence, the initial discovery regarding narcotic antagonism came about serendipitously. Thus, Pohl (12) in 1915, in an attempt to improve the analgesic properties of codeine, synthesized N-allylnorcodeine and observed that it would mildly antagonize the *respiratory depression* and *sleep* induced by morphine. Large doses produced an excitatory effect. Between 1915 and 1926 von Braun and co-workers (1a) synthesized a fair number of N-substituted norco-deines (ethyl to heptyl; cyclopropylmethyl to cyclohexylmethyl; cinnamyl;

propargyl; etc.). Weak antagonist action was shown by the cyclopropyl-methyl compound.

Some 25 years after Pohl's discovery, McCawley et al. (9) attempted to prepare N-allyl-normorphine, the phenolic congener of N-allylnorcodeine, but not as a specific narcotic antagonist, if history, in this instance, is accurately recorded. The reasoning was that replacement of the N-methyl group of morphine with allyl might reduce respiratory depressant and other adverse effects without causing a marked change of the analgesic action of this much stronger (than codeine) narcotic. In other words, they sought a strong analgesic with a "built-in" antagonist action to depressant effects. These investigators (6, 9) reported antagonism stronger than that of N-allylnorcodeine for their preparation which, it developed later, apparently was a mixture containing principally 3(O),N-diallylnormorphine (7). Using an authentic specimen of N-allylnormorphine (nalorphine), prepared by Weijlard and Erickson about 1942 (15), Unna (14) and Hart and McCawley (9) observed strong antagonism to almost all of the actions of morphine.

Early studies with nalorphine also indicated some *morphine*-like effects, and, indeed, as is well known, this drug ultimately proved to be a fairly strong analgesic in man (3) and in certain animals (10, 11). But, obviously more germane to our present discussions are nalorphine's properties as a specific narcotic antagonist which were later confirmed and exploited. Following series of careful studies by Eckenhoff (2a) and at the Addiction Research Center, Lexington, Kentucky by Fraser et al. (3), nalorphine became a valuable drug for use in narcotic overdosage, and for *research* on drug dependence of the morphine type. It also largely provided the stimulus for the discovery of a host of antagonists with varying degrees of antagonistic and agonistic potency and perhaps for much of the progress that has been made since 1955 toward development of a strong, pain-relieving agent without abuse potential.

For example, an identical structural change, replacement of N-methyl by allyl, has given stronger antagonists in the morphinan, benzomorphan and 14-hydroxy-dihydromorphinone series. Thus, levallorphan [(−)-N-allyl-3-hydroxymorphinan], first synthesized by Schnider and Hellerbach (13), N-allyl-normetazocine by Gordon et al. (5), and naloxone (N-allyl-14-hydroxydihydro-morphinone) by Lewenstein and Fishman (8) bear about the same potency relationships to each other (as antagonists) as do their N-methyl counterparts as agonists. These compounds also possess somewhat less agonist property than nalorphine. In fact, naloxone is relatively inert in all other CNS effects and is regarded as a "pure" antagonist.

Systematic studies in the morphine series by Clark et al. (2) in the early 1950's have shown that groups other than allyl (on nitrogen), e.g., propyl, isobutyl, methallyl, also confer antagonist characteristics to morphine-type molecules. Application and extension of these findings have been made in other parent series. More recently, cycloalkylmethyl (particularly cyclopropylmethyl) radicals have been introduced as N-substituents in the morphinan series by Gates and Montzka (4), in the benzomorphan series, by Archer et al. (1), and in still other series.

Finally, powerful antagonist-agonists and relatively "pure" antagonists have been developed lately, from thebaine, the 6,7-benzomorphans and 14-hydroxymorphinans in a number of brilliant investigations. But this is simply a brief historical review, and your attention is invited to detailed accounts of all these topics and of novel types of potent, long-acting antagonists elsewhere in this volume.

REFERENCES

1. Archer, S., Albertson, N. F., Harris, L. S., Pierson, A. K., and Bird, J. G.: Pentazocine. Strong analgesics and analgesic antagonists in the benzomorphan series. J. Med. Chem. 7:123–127, 1964.
1a. von Braun, J., Kuhn, M., and Siddiqui, S.: Ungesattige reste in chemische und pharmakologische beziehung (V). Ber. 59B:1081–1090, 1926.
2. Clark, R. L., Pessolano, A. A., Weijlard, J., and Pfister, III, K.: N-Substituted epoxymorphinans. J. Amer. Chem. Soc. 75:4974–4967, 1953.
2a. Echenhoff, J. E., and Elder, J. D.: N-Allylnormorphine in the treatment of morphine or demerol narcosis. Am. J. Med. Sci. 223:191–197, 1952.
3. Eddy, N. B.: Agonist-Antagonists. A Historical Overview
4. Gates, M., and Montzka, T. A.: Some potent morphine antagonists possessing high analgesic activity. J. Med. Chem. 7:127–131, 1964.
5. Gordon, M., Lafferty, J. J., Tedeschi, D. H., Eddy, N. B., and May, E. L.: A new potent analgesic antagonist. Nature (London) 192:1089–1090, 1961.
6. Hart, E. R.: N-Allylnorcodeine and N-allylnormorphine, two antagonists of morphine. J. Pharmacol. Exp. Ther. 72:19, 1941.
7. Hart, E. R., and McCawley, E. L.: The pharmacology of N-allylnormorphine as compared with morphine. J. Pharmacol. Exp. Ther. 82:339–348, 1944.
8. Lewenstein, M. J., and Fishman, J.: Morphine Derivatives. U.S. Patent, 3,254,088. 1966.
9. McCawley, W. L., Hart, E. R., and Marsh, D. F.: The preparation of N-allylnormorphine. J. Amer. Chem. Soc. 63:314, 1941.
10. Pearl, J., Stander, H., and McKean, D. B.: Effects of analgesics and other drugs on mice in phenylquinone and rotarod tests. J. Pharmacol. Exp. Ther. 167:9–13, 1969.
11. Perrine, T. D., Atwell, L., Tice, I. B., Jacobson, A. E., and May, E. L.: Analgesic activity as determined by the Nilsen method. J. Pharm. Sci. 61:86–88, 1972.
12. Pohl, J.: Ueber das N-allylnorcodeine, einen antagonisten des morphins. Z. Exp. Path. Ther. 17:370–378, 1915.
13. Schnider, O., and Hellerback, J.: Synthese von morphinanen. Helv. Chim. Acta 33:1437–1448, 1950.
14. Unna, K.: Antagonistic effect of N-allylnormorphine upon morphine. J. Pharmacol. Exp. Ther. 79:27–31, 1943.
15. Weijlard, J. and Erickson, A. E.: N-Allylnormorphine. J. Amer. Chem. Soc. 64:869–890, 1942.

Narcotic Antagonists, edited by M. C. Braude, L. S. Harris, E. L. May, J. P. Smith, and J. E. Villarreal. *Advances in Biochemical Psychopharmacology, Vol. 8.* Raven Press, New York © 1974.

Narcotic Antagonists — Structure-Activity Relationships

Louis S. Harris

Department of Pharmacology, Medical College of Virginia, Virginia Commonwealth University, Richmond, Virginia 23219

Over the past few decades one of the most fascinating areas of narcotic research has involved the narcotic antagonists (4, 13, 20, 37). These compounds, which represent only minor molecular modifications of the parent narcotic, are capable of preventing or reversing most of the pharmacological properties of the narcotics. Indeed, they will precipitate an abrupt abstinence syndrome in morphine-dependent animals or man. This class of compounds has found an important place in medicine: as antidotes for narcotic overdosage, as analgesics with a lessened abuse potential, and recently in the treatment of narcotic dependence.

This review of the structure-activity relationships of the antagonists is not intended to be exhaustive. It will concentrate on the broad structural features and will be presented in an eclectic nonchronological fashion.

I. MORPHINE ANALOGUES

Morphine (IA) has a number of important structural features. It has five rings, a phenolic and an alcoholic hydroxyl, an aromatic planar ring, and a basic tertiary nitrogen. Actually, the first narcotic antagonist, N-allylnorcodeine (IB), was first reported in 1915 (43, 47). As so often happens in this field, the finding lay dormant for 25 years until the properties of N-allylnormorphine (IC), nalorphine, were described (25, 26, 49).

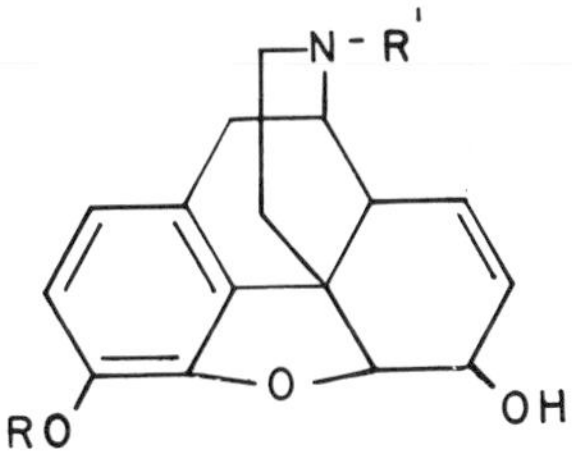

A. $R = H$, $R' = CH_3$
B. $R = CH_3$, $R' = CH_2CH{=}CH_2$
C. $R = H$, $R' = CH_2CH{=}CH_2$
D. $R = CH_3$, $R' = CH_2\triangle$

I

The structural feature most important for antagonistic activity is that of the piperdine nitrogen. Thus, alkylation of normorphine with a three-carbon side chain, with or without branching, leads to antagonistic activity. These substituents include propyl, allyl, propargyl, isopropyl, 2-methylallyl, etc. Increasing the chain length to amyl restores agonistic activity.

In 1926 von Braun and his colleagues (48) also reported that replacement of the N-methyl of codeine by a variety of cycloalkyl-methyl groups resulted in antagonistic activity. Unfortunately, the material they described did not represent homogenous compounds but later work did reveal N-cyclopropylmethylnormorphine (ID) to be a potent antagonist. This is also true for the oxymorphone analogue IIA (12). It is from this series that naloxone, N-allylnoroxymorphone (IIB), is derived (36). Naloxone holds a pivotal place in the field since it was the first relatively "pure" antagonist to be discovered. Naloxone is a potent antagonist in a variety of systems (9, 22, 31) and is essentially inactive as an agonist in animals (10, 42) and man (30).

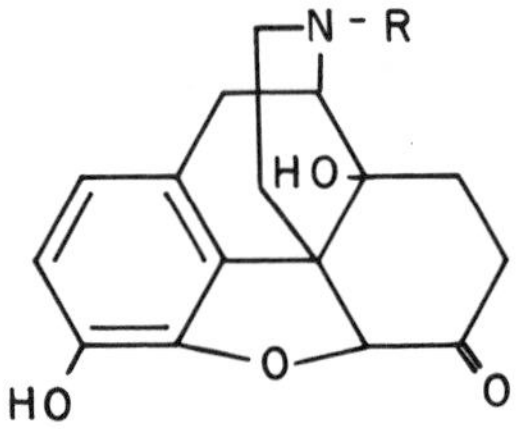

A. $R = CH_2\triangle$
B. $R = CH_2CH{=}CH_2$

II

All of the morphine antagonists are derived from natural morphine and are thus pure optical (levorotatory) isomers. Gates and Tschudi (16) did synthesize racemic morphine which has been resolved. The dextrorotatory form of morphine is inactive as an agonist. No other racemic or dextrorotatory N-alkyl-normorphine derivatives have been reported. The importance of optical isomerism and conformation will become more evident in the other series discussed below.

II. MORPHINAN ANALOGUES

The removal of the furan ring of morphine provides the four-ring mor-phinan structure (III). As in the morphine series, activity resides in the levorotatory isomers with the parent N-methyl compound, levorphanol (IIIA), being some four times more potent than morphine. The morphinan system was first synthesized and explored by Grewe and his colleagues (18, 19) and Schnider and Grüssner (44). As in the morphine series, replacement of the N-methyl group by an allyl function gives a potent antagonist, levallorphan (IIIB), (27). Other three-carbon side chains, e.g., propargyl (compound IIIC) also confer potent antagonistic activity. A series of cycloalkylmethyl derivatives has been prepared by Gates and Montzka (15), and one of these, cyclorphan (IIID), is a potent antagonist in animals (24) with potent agonistic activity in animals and man (35). Cyclorphan did not prove to be a useful therapeutic agent because of the high incidence of psychotomimetic activity associated with its use.

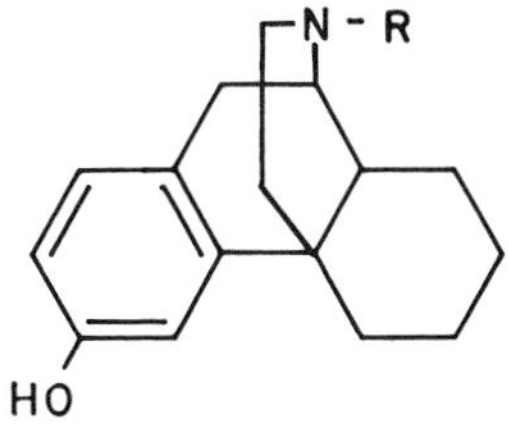

A. $R = CH_3$
B. $R = CH_2CH{=}CH_2$
C. $R = CH_2C{\equiv}CH$
D. $R = CH_2\triangle$

III

A variety of other structural modifications have recently been introduced into the morphinan series of antagonists. These are detailed in the chemical sections of this volume by Drs. Leimgruber, Gates, and Pachter.

III. BENZOMORPHAN ANALOGUES

As we know from the agonist series, the morphine ring system can be further simplified to the triannular benzomorphan series (IV) with no loss of activity. This is perhaps the most extensive antagonist series, thanks to the pioneering work of Dr. May and his colleagues (1, 40, 41), whose elegant synthetic methods opened the field for exploration by Archer and his colleagues (2, 3, 5, 45) and others (8, 17).

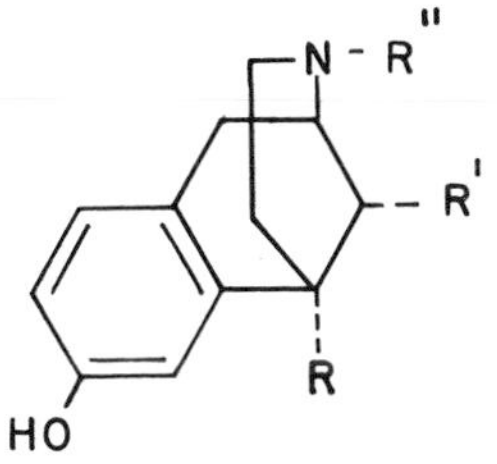

A. $R = R' = CH_3$, $R'' = CH_2CH{=}C(CH_3)_2$
B. $R = R' = CH_3$, $R'' = CH_2\triangle$
C. $R = R' = C_2H_5$ $R'' = CH_3$

IV

Again, replacement of the N-methyl substituent by propyl, allyl, propargyl, methylallyl, cyclopropylmethyl, etc. leads to potent antagonists. The N-dimethylallyl compound, pentazocine (IVA), is a weak antagonist (23) and has become a useful, strong analgesic (29) with a lessened abuse potential (14). Cyclazocine (IVB) is a potent narcotic antagonist (23), which also has potent agonistic activity, being some 40 times more potent than morphine as an analgesic in man (34). It was while studying the abuse potential of this compound that Martin and his colleagues (38) first postulated the potential use of narcotic antagonists in the therapy of narcotic addiction.

Again, as in the agonist series, antagonistic activity in the 5,9-dimethyl series lies in the levorotatory isomers (5, 45). In addition, geometric isomerization around the 5,9-positions can easily be explored. The situation, however, becomes quite complex, especially when the substitutions at the 5- and 9-positions are larger and different. This work is thoroughly discussed in the chemical sections presented by Drs. Albertson, Clarke, Merz, Janssen, and Takeda. Of particular interest, however, are some isomers in the N-methyl series prepared in May's laboratory (39). For instance, L-*cis*-2-methyl-5,9-diethyl 2'-hydroxy-6,7-benzomorphan (IVC) is a potent agonist in the mouse hot-plate test, yet behaves like an antagonist in morphine-dependent monkeys (46). This represents the first example of antagonistic activity being associated with an N-methyl substituent and may provide some clue to the drug-receptor interaction at the molecular level.

IV. MEPERIDINE ANALOGUES

The morphine ring structure can be further divided into the two-ring meperidine series (V). Although there is a considerable loss of agonistic activity, this is due, in part, to the absence of a phenolic hydroxyl group in the appropriate position.

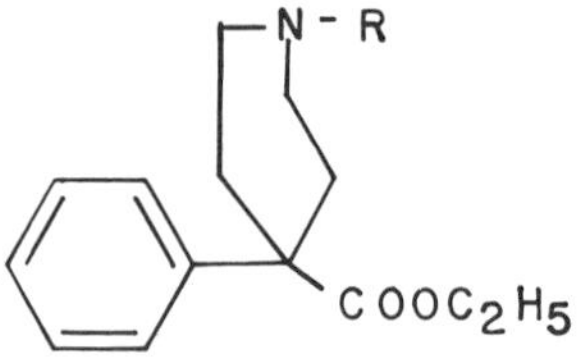

A. $R = CH_2CH{=}CH_2$
B. $R = CH_2\triangle$

V

Replacement of the N-methyl group of meperidine by the usual alkyl groups which lead to antagonists in the other series gave only agonists.

Thus, N-allylnormeperidine (VA) behaves like a typical narcotic analgesic (11, 51). This is also true for the N-cyclopropylmethyl derivative (VB). Archer and Harris (4) postulated that this lack of antagonistic activity might be related to the absence of a phenethylamine fragment in the structure. Evidence supporting this hypothesis comes from the work of Kugita and his colleagues (32, 33), who have described the antagonistic properties of the N-allyl-3-phenylpiperidine structure VI. In this regard, mention should be made of the pyrrolidine derivative, profadol (VII).

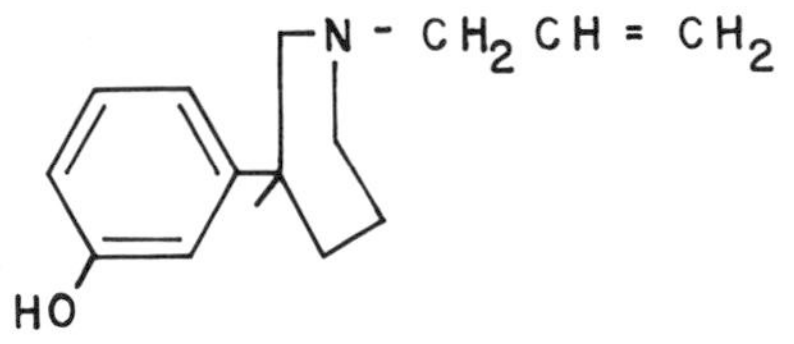

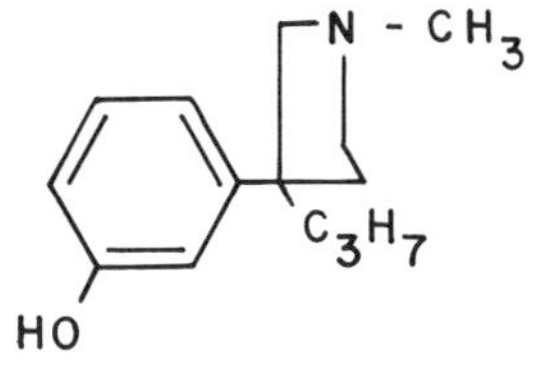

This compound has the phenethylamine structure and, like the N-methyl-benzomorphan IVC, has both agonist and antagonist activity (28, 46, 50). This pyrrolidine series is covered more fully by Dr. McCarthy in the chemical section.

It should be noted, however, that Langbein and his colleagues have recently prepared antagonists in the 4-phenylpiperidine series by the introduction of structural features such as a phenolic *m*-hydroxyl group. This is discussed in detail in the chemical portion of this volume.

V. ORIPAVINE DERIVATIVES

In addition to ring contraction of the basic morphine structure, Bentley and his group (7) have recently described a ring expansion to the six-ring oripavine or 6,14-*endo*-ethenotetrahydrorooripavine series (VIII). The N-methyl derivatives have provided agonists of extremely high potency.

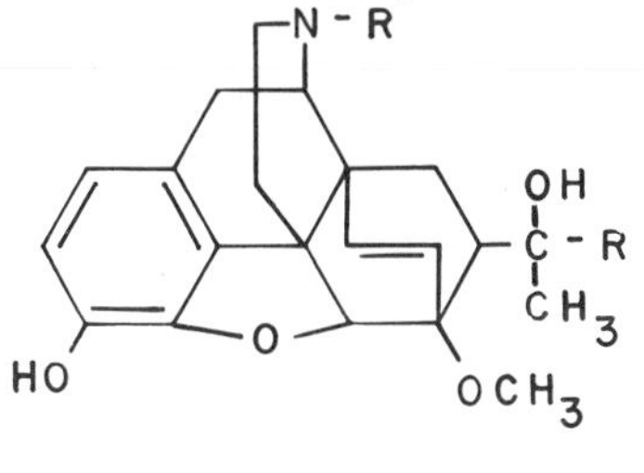

A. R = isoamyl, R' = CH_3
B. R = isoamyl, R' = $CH_2CH{=}CH_2$
C. R = isoamyl, R' = CH_2
D. R = CH_3, R' = $CH_2CH{=}CH_2$
E. R = CH_3, R' = $CH_2\triangle$

For instance, VIIIA is 5,000 to 10,000 times more potent than morphine. N-allyl and N-cyclopropylmethyl substituents have been introduced into this series. As a general rule, until this time, the antagonistic potency of a series paralleled the agonistic potency of the parent N-methyl compound. However, when the usual antagonistic substituents were introduced in the most potent series, the compounds were not antagonists. They appear to possess an atypical morphine-like analgesic activity. For instance, when the substituent in the carbon side chain is isoamyl, the N-allyl (VIIIB) and N-cyclopropylmethyl (VIIIC) derivatives show potent agonistic activity in the tail-flick tests. On the other hand, although they do not antagonize the actions of morphine in this test, they do not add to them (21).

When a smaller alkyl group is introduced into the carbon side chain, typical antagonists (VIIID and E) can be obtained (6). The N-cyclopropyl-methyl compound (VIIIE) is approximately 35 times more potent than nalorphine. The extensive recent work in this series is detailed by Lewis in the chemical section.

I trust that this brief overview provides some perspective to this fascinating field. I am continually amazed by the profound pharmacological changes which can be achieved in this area by relatively trivial chemical modifications. It is my hope that some understanding of this at the molecular and biochemical level will lead to a greater understanding of the puzzling phenomena of analgesia, tolerance, and physical dependence.

ACKNOWLEDGMENTS

The work from the author's laboratory, described in this report, was supported, in part, by grants from the National Institute of Mental Health (MH-19759) and the National Academy of Sciences-National Research Council Committee on Problems of Drug Dependence (D-72-7).

REFERENCES

1. Ager, J. H., and May, E. L.: Structures related to morphine. XIX. Benzomorphans from 3,4-diethylpyridine. J. Org. Chem. 27:245–247, 1962.
2. Archer, S., Albertson, N. F., Harris, L. S., Pierson, A. K., and Bird, J. G.: Pentazocine. Strong analgesics and analgesic antagonists in the benzomorphan series. J. Med. Chem 7:123–127, 1964.
3. Archer, S., Albertson, N. F., Harris, L. S., Pierson, A. K., Bird, J. G., Keats, A. S., Telford, J., and Papadopoulos, C.: Narcotic antagonists as analgesics. Science 137:541–543, 1962.
4. Archer, S., and Harris, L. S.: Narcotic antagonists. Progr. Drug Res. 8:261–320, 1965.
5. Archer, S., Harris, L. S., Albertson, N. F., Tullar, B. F., and Pierson, A. K.: Narcotic antagonist analgesics; laboratory aspects. Advan. Chem. Ser. 45:162–169, 1964.
6. Bentley, K. W., Boura, A. L. A., Fitzgerald, A. E., Hardy, D. G., McCoubrey, A., Aikman,

M. L., and Lister, R. E.: Compounds possessing morphine-antagonizing or powerful analgesic properties. Nature *206*:102–103, 1965.

7. Bentley, K. W., and Hardy, D. G.: Novel analgesics and molecular rearrangements in the morphine-thebaine group. I. Ketones derived from 6,14-*endo*-ethenotetrahydrothebaine. J. Amer. Chem. Soc. *89*:3267–3273, 1967.

8. Block, F. B., and Clarke, F. H.: 1,2,3,4,5,6-Hexahydro-6-phenyl-2,6-methano-3-benza-zocines. I. The 3- carboxamido-8-hydroxy derivative as an orally effective analgetic. J. Med. Chem. *12*:845–847, 1969.

9. Blumberg, H., Dayton, H. B., George, M., and Rapaport, D. N.: N-Allylnoroxymor-phone: A potent narcotic antagonist. Fed. Proc. *20*:311, 1961.

10. Blumberg, H., Wolf, P. S., and Dayton, H. B.: Use of writhing-test for evaluating anal-gesic activity of narcotic antagonists. Proc. Soc. Exp. Biol. Med. *118*:763–766, 1965.

11. Costa, P. J., and Bonnycastle, D. D.: The effect of levallorphan tartrate, nalorphine HCl, Win 7681 (1-allyl-4-phenyl-4-carbethoxypiperidine) on respiratory depression and anal-gesia induced by some active analgesics. J. Pharmacol. Exp. Ther. *113*:310–318, 1955.

12. Deneau, G. A., and Seevers, M. H.: Evaluation of new compounds for morphine-like physical dependence in the rhesus monkey. Addendum I, Comm. Drug. Addiction Nar-cotics, 1967.

13. Fraser, H. F., and Harris, L. S.: Narcotic and narcotic antagonist analgesics. Ann. Rev. Pharmacol. *7*:277–300, 1967.

14. Fraser, H. F., and Rosenberg, D. E.: Studies on the human addiction liability of 2'-hydroxy-5.9-dimethyl-2-(3.3-dimethylallyl)-6,7-benzomorphan (Win 20,228): A weak narcotic antagonist. J. Pharmacol. Exp. Ther. *143*:149, 1964.

15. Gates, M. D., and Montzka, T.: Some potent morphine antagonists possessing high analgesic activity. J. Med. Chem. *7*:127–131, 1964.

16. Gates, M., and Tschudi, G.: The synthesis of morphine. J. Amer. Chem. Soc. *74*:1109–1110, 1952.

17. Gordon, M., Lafferty, J. J., Tedeschi, D. H., Eddy, N. B., and May, E. L.: A new potent analgetic antagonist. Nature *192*:1089, 1961.

18. Grewe, R., and Mondon, A.: Syntheses in the phenanthrene series. VI. Synthesis of morphinane. Ber. Deut. Chem. Ges. *81*:279–286, 1948.

19. Grewe, R., Mondon, A., and Nolte, E.: Total synthesis of tetrahydrodesoxycodeine. Ann. Chem. *564*:161–198, 1949.

20. Harris, L. S.: Structure-activity relationships in narcotic drugs. *In:* Biochemical Pharma-cology, edited by D. H. Clouet, pp. 89–98. Plenum Press, New York–London, 1971.

21. Harris, L. S.: *Unpublished observations.*

22. Harris, L. S., Dewey, W. L., Howes, J. F., Kennedy, J. S., and Pars, H.: Brain acetyl-choline levels and inhibition of the tail-flick reflex in mice. J. Pharmacol. Exp. Ther. *169*:17–22, 1969.

23. Harris, L. S., and Pierson, A. K.: Some narcotic antagonists in the benzomorphan series. J. Pharmacol. Exp. Ther. *143*:141–148, 1964.

24. Harris, L. S., Pierson, A. K., Dembinski, J. R., and Dewey, W. L.: The pharmacology of (-)-3-hydroxy-N-cyclopropylmethylmorphinan (cyclorphan). Arch. Int. Pharmacodyn. *165*:112–126, 1967.

25. Hart, E. R.: N-Allyl-norcodeine and N-allyl-normorphine, two antagonists to morphine. J. Pharmacol. Exp. Ther. *72*:19, 1941.

26. Hart, E. R., and McCawley, E. L.: The pharmacology of N-allyl-normorphine as com-pared with morphine. J. Pharmacol. Exp. Ther. *82*:339–348, 1944.

27. Hellerbach, J., Grüssner, A., and Schnider, O.: Hydroxymorphinans (VII) (-)-3-hydroxy-N-allylmorphinan and related compounds. Helv. Chim. Acta. *39*:429–440, 1956.

28. Jaskinski, D. R., Martin, W. R., and Sapira, J. D.: *Personal communication.*

29. Keats, A. S., and Telford, J.: Studies of analgesic drugs. VIII. A narcotic antagonist analgesic without psychotomimetic effects. J. Pharmacol. Exp. Ther. *143*:157–164, 1964.

30. Keats, A. S., and Telford, J.: *Personal communication.*

31. Kosterlitz, H. W., and Watt, A. J.: Kinetic parameters of narcotic agonists and antago-

nists, with particular reference to N-allyl-noroxymorphone (naloxone). Brit. J. Pharmacol. *33*:266–276, 1968.

32. Kugita, H., Inoue, H., Oine, T., Hayashi, G., and Nurimoto, S.: 3-Alkyl-3-phenylpiperidine derivatives as analgesics. J. Med. Chem. *7*:298–301, 1964.
33. Kugita, H., Oine, T., Inoue, H., and Hayashi, G.: 3-Alkyl-3-phenylpiperidine derivatives as analgesics. II. J. Med. Chem. *8*:313–316, 1965.
34. Lasagna, L., DeKornfeld, T. J., and Pearson, J. W.: The analgesic efficacy and respiratory effects in man of a benzomorphan "narcotic antagonist." J. Pharmacol. Exp. Ther. *144*:12–16, 1964.
35. Lasagna, L., Pearson, J. W., and DeKornfeld, T.: *Personal communication.*
36. Lewenstein, M. J. and Fishman, J.: U.S. Patent 3,254,088.
37. Martin, W. R.: Opioid antagonists. Pharmacol. Rev. *19*:463–521, 1967.
38. Martin, W. R., Gorodetzky, C. W., and McClane, T. K.: An experimental study in the treatment of narcotic addicts with cyclazocine. Clin. Pharmacol. Ther. *7*:455–465, 1966.
39. May, E. L., and Eddy, N. B.: Interesting pharmacological properties of the optical isomers of α-5,9-diethyl-2′-hydroxy-2-methyl-6,7-benzomorphan. J. Med. Chem. *9*:851–852, 1966.
40. May, E. L., and Fry, E. M.: Structures related to morphine. VIII. Further syntheses in the benzomorphan series. J. Org. Chem. *22*:1366–1369, 1957.
41. May, E. L., and Kugita, H.: Structures related to morphine. XV. Stereochemical control of methyl-metallo additions to 9-oxobenzomorphans. J. Org. Chem. *26*:188–193, 1961.
42. Pearl, J., and Harris, L. S.: Inhibition of writhing by narcotic antagonists. J. Pharmacol. Exp. Ther. *154*:319–323, 1966.
43. Pohl, J.: Uber das N-allylnorcodein, einen antagonisten des morphins. Z. Exp. Pathol. Ther. *17*:370–382, 1915.
44. Schnider, O., and Grüssner, A.: Synthesis of hydroxymorphinans. Helv. Chim. Acta. *32*:821–828, 1949.
45. Tullar, B. F., Harris, L. S., Perry, R. L., Pierson, A. K., Soria, A. E., Wétterau, W. F., and Albertson, N. F.: Benzomorphans. Optically active and *trans* isomers. J. Med. Chem. *10*:383–386, 1967.
46. Villarreal, J. E., and Seevers, M. A.: *Personal communication.*
47. von Braun, J.: Untersuchungen uber morphium-alkaloide. III. Metteilung. Ber. Deut. Chem. Ges. *49*:977–989, 1916.
48. von Braun, J., Kuhn, M., and Siddiqui, S.: Chemical and pharmacological relationships of unsaturated residues. Ber. Deut. Chem. Ges. *59*:1081–1089, 1926.
49. Weijlard, J., and Erickson, A. E.: N-allylnormorphine. J. Amer. Chem. Soc. *64*:869–870, 1942.
50. Winder, C. V., Welford, M., Wax, J., and Kaump, D. H.: Pharmacologic and toxicologic studies of *m*-(1-methyl-3-propyl-3-pyrrolidenyl) phenol (CI-572), an analgetic and antitussive agent. J. Pharmacol. Exp. Ther. *154*:161–175, 1966.
51. Winter, C. A., Orahovats, P. D., and Lehman, E. G.: Analgesic activity and morphine antagonism of compounds related to nalorphine. Arch. Int. Pharmacodyn. *110*:186–202, 1957.

Narcotic Antagonists, edited by M. C. Braude, L. S. Harris, E. L. May, J. P. Smith, and J. E. Villarreal. *Advances in Biochemical Psychopharmacology, Vol. 8.* Raven Press, New York © 1974.

Chemistry of Narcotic Antagonists of the Nalorphine Type

Franklin M. Robinson

Medicinal Chemistry Department, Merck Sharp and Dohme Research Laboratories, West Point, Pennsylvania 19486

Replacement of the N-methyl group of morphine with substituents containing from three to five carbon atoms is the only structural change which has produced narcotic antagonists. Modifications of other portions of the molecule (e.g., acylation, etherification, hydroxylation, reduction of the double bond, and oxidation or removal of the alcoholic hydroxyl), however, strongly influence the antagonist potency and side effects of the N-substituted analogues. The N-substituents which produce the greatest antagonism are cyclopropylmethyl, propyl, and allyl. Slightly larger groups (e.g., methallyl, crotyl, isobutyl, cyclobutylmethyl) reduce antagonist potency. Analogues with N-substituents larger than hexyl are usually morphine-like analgesics. N-Allylnormorphine (nalorphine) retains the analgesic potency of morphine but has only minimal capacity to produce a physical dependence of a type unlike that of narcotics. Test data on a limited number of other analogues indicate that these properties are common to most but not all of them. In particular, the N-*n*-propyl analogues show little or no analgesic activity. Nalorphine and related antagonists which have been studied clinically produced psychotomimetic effects, and, as a result, their potential utility for purposes other than as opiate antidotes and for detection of opiate dependence is limited.

INTRODUCTION

Nalorphine (N-allylnormorphine, Nalline*) was the first narcotic antagonist made available for medical use, and for the last 20 years has been in standard use as an antidote for narcotic overdosage. It was also the first compound found to have potent analgesic action in man without the capacity to produce significant physical dependence, although side effects prevented its practical use as an analgesic.

The study of nalorphine analogues established certain basic structural

---

* Reg. Trademark, Merck and Co., Inc.

requirements for narcotic antagonist activity which have been found to be general throughout related series. Other structure-activity relationships concerning both antagonist and analgesic properties, which appear to be more specific for this type of compound, were also discovered.

In the following summary of the known structure-activity data, discussion will concern only compounds in which the pentacylic skeleton of the morphine molecule has not been modified. Comparisons of the activities of nalorphine analogues with those of morphinans, benzomorphans, and ethenotetrahydrothebaines can be found in several recent reviews (1, 5, 18).

The first report of a morphine antagonist was that of Pohl in 1915 (23) who studied N-allylnorcodeine, which had been synthesized by von Braun (29). In 1941 Hart and McCawley (21) reported that N-allylnormorphine was a more potent antagonist than N-allylnorcodeine, but it subsequently appeared that the compound they studied was probably O,N-diallylnormorphine (11). Pure N-allylnormorphine was first synthesized in 1942 by Weijlard and Erickson (31) in the Merck Laboratories. Its activity in animals as a morphine antagonist was demonstrated by Hart (11) and by Unna (27), and it was also shown to inhibit the effects of other narcotic analgesics (13). Its effectiveness in man was demonstrated by Eckenhoff (8), and Wikler (32) showed that it would precipitate immediate withdrawal symptoms in humans physically dependent on morphine. Isbell (14) found that nalorphine produced neither physical nor psychic dependence after prolonged administration to postaddicts, although subsequent studies have shown that a mild physical dependence unlike that of morphine can be produced (20). It was introduced into medical use in 1952.

Two years later, in studies designed to discover whether combinations of nalorphine and morphine could produce satisfactory analgesia with reduced respiratory depression, Lasagna and Beecher (17) found that nalorphine was a potent analgesic. Keats and Telford (15) demonstrated that it was equipotent with morphine in the clinic. This was the first example of a potent analgesic without dependence liability. However, there was a sufficiently high incidence of psychotomimetic effects to preclude its use for pain relief.

During this period a large number of nalorphine analogues had been studied as morphine antagonists in the tests for analgesia then available (10, 34). However, these tests did not show any significant analgesic action for nalorphine or other antagonist analogues. As research continued toward strong analgesics with added antagonist action which should prevent development of dependence, test methods were developed to show the analgesic effect of this type of compound. However, chemical interest had moved to totally synthetic compounds, with the result that most of the structural analogues of nalorphine have never been studied in the newer tests. Knowledge of their activities is limited largely to antagonist potencies.

SYNTHESIS

The only structural change in the morphine molecule which has been found to produce antagonist action is replacement of the N-methyl group by certain other alkyl or cycloalkyl groups. The first synthesis of nalorphine is shown in Fig. 1 and represents the method used by Clark et al. (6) for the synthesis of 70 nalorphine analogues and by Green et al. (10) for the synthesis of another 16. This is basically the method originally used by von Braun to prepare N-allylnorcodeine (29) and another series of analogues including the N-cyclopropylmethyl- and cyclobutylmethyl-norcodeines (30). Subsequent discovery of the tendency of cycloalkylmethyl halides to re-arrange, and the properties reported for the products cast doubt on their identity (1, 24). In 1964 Gates and Montzka (9) prepared a series of N-cyclopropylmethyl analogues of strong analgesics, among them the mor-phine analogue. They reasoned that the chemical similarity between the allyl and cyclopropylmethyl groups might indicate that they would also have similar effects on biological activity. The Gates synthesis is shown in Fig. 2; it has become the generally used method for preparing N-cyclo-alkylmethyl derivatives.

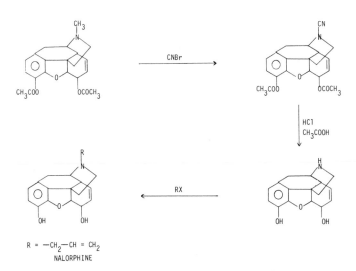

FIG. 1. Synthesis of nalorphine [Weijlard and Erickson (31)].

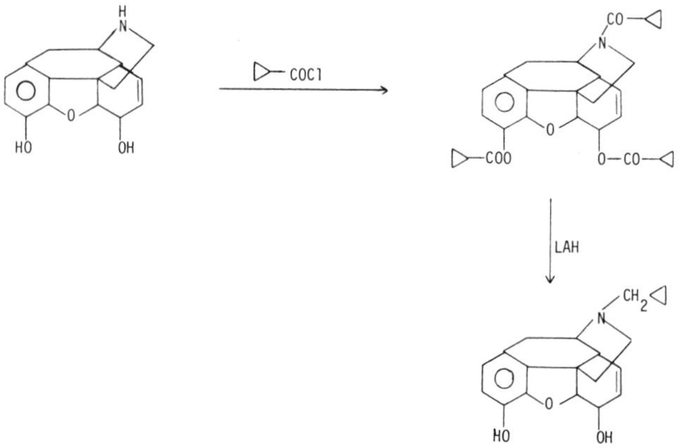

FIG. 2. Synthesis of N-cyclopropylmethylnormorphine [Gates and Montzka (9)].

STRUCTURE-ACTIVITY RELATIONSHIPS

In Fig. 3 are shown those N-analogues of morphine which have detectable narcotic antagonist activity, and in Fig. 4 those which showed no antagonism. Most of the data are those of Winter et al. (34) as noted. They used the tail-flick method in rats and tested repeatedly over a period of time so that the total analgesic effect was measured. Antagonist potencies relative to nalorphine were determined by comparing dose-response[1] curves for antagonism of a standard dose of morphine. Green et al. (10) studied some of the same compounds using both heat and pressure methods in rats. Antagonist ED_{50}'s were determined for reduction of the elevation in pain threshold caused by a standard dose of morphine. The value for the cyclopropylmethyl analogue represents antagonism of the effect of meperidine in another modification of the tail-flick test (9). In general there was good agreement between the results of Winter and Green, and the instances in which Winter's values were higher may represent a longer duration of action of the compound.

Available data indicate similar effects of these substituents on the antagonist action of other morphine analogues, but with some exceptions. N-Propyl analogues in the codeine series are generally less potent than the allyl analogues. N-Isobutylnorcodeine analogues were totally inactive,

---

[1] It has been reported that 7,8-dihydro-5',6'-dimethylcyclohex-5'-eno[1',2':8:14]morphinone is an antagonist 1/10 as potent as nalorphine, but this involves addition of a sixth ring to the morphine structure (18).

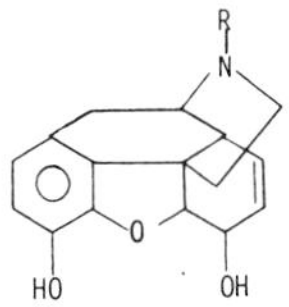

R		
—CH_2—CH = CH_2	1	
—CH_2CH_2—CH_3	0.7-1	a,b
—CH_2—C(—CH_3) = CH_2	1+	a
—CH_2—◁	3*	c
—CH_2—CH = CH—CH_3	0.1	a,b
—CH_2—CH(—CH_3)—CH_3	0.1	a

R		
—CH_2CH_3	<0.1	a
—$CH_2CH_2CH_2CH_3$	<0.1	a,b
—$CH_2CH_2CH_2CH_2OH$	<0.1	a
—CH_2C(=O)—CH_3	<0.1	a
—CH_2—C≡CH	<0.1	b

FIG. 3. Relative antagonist potencies of N-substituted normorphines [(*a*) Winter et al. (34); (*b*) Green et al. (10); (*c*) Gates et al. (9)].

whereas N-isobutyldihydronormorphine was 60% as potent as its allyl congeners. Other examples have confirmed that N-cyclopropylmethyl analogues are the most potent antagonists (2, 3, 7, 9), but N-cyclopropyl-methyl-5-methyldihydromorphine is a potent analgesic without antagonist properties (25, 28).

These data indicate severe structural limitations on the substituents which confer antagonist potency on morphine congeners. A straight chain of at least three carbons is required and is also optimal. Extending the length to four reduces potency, and to five or more, restores morphine-like activity. Branching at the second carbon is allowable and may be advantageous. A double bond is not a requirement, but may increase potency. Substitution with polar atoms decreases activity.

Modification of other parts of the molecule affects antagonist potency as shown by the examples in Fig. 5. The most striking effect is that of the 14-hydroxyl group (IX, naloxone). This effect is consistent throughout the series, as is discussed by Dr. Blumberg in the following chapter. There is a definite indication that a free phenolic function is needed for maximum potency. A 7,8-double bond appears to enhance activity and a 6-hydroxyl group decreases it. These same relationships are emphasized by the N-

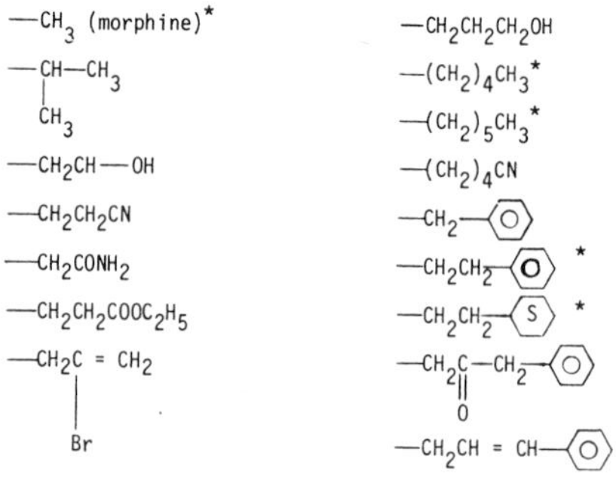

—CH3 (morphine)*
—CH—CH3
CH3
—CH2CH—OH
—CH2CH2CN
—CH2CONH2
—CH2CH2COOC2H5
—CH2C = CH2
Br
—CH2CH2CH2OH
—(CH2)4CH3*
—(CH2)5CH3*
—(CH2)4CN
—CH2—
—CH2CH2— *
—CH2CH2— S *
—CH2C—CH2—
O
—CH2CH = CH—

*Strong analgesic

FIG. 4. N-Substituted normorphine analogues without antagonist activity [Winter et al. (34)].

CH2CH = CH2
N
I
HO
O
OH
(Nalorphine) 1
II
CH3COO
OCOCH3
0.5
III
CH3COO
0.3
IV
H
1.3
V
CH3COO
OCOCH3
0.1
VI
OH
0.7
VII
2.2
VIII
1.8
IX
HO
13d

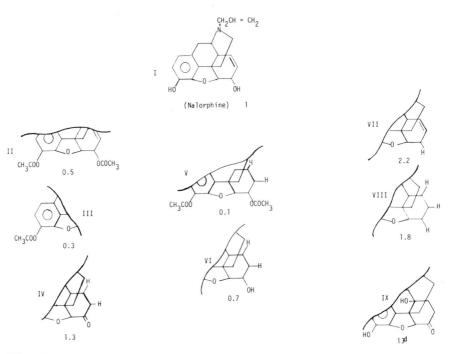

FIG. 5. Relative antagonist potencies of nalorphine analogues [Winter et al. (34); (*d*) Blumberg et al. (4)].

allylcodeine analogues shown in Fig. 6. The potency of N-allylnorcodeine reported by Green was much lower than Winter's value. However, Green did not study the other compounds shown, so comparisons are made using the higher values. The potency of the 14-hydroxy analogue XVIII was determined by Minakami et al. (22), who used Green's test method but measured total analgesia as did Winter.

The fact that nalorphine was a more potent antagonist than N-allyl-norcodeine raised the question of correlation of antagonist potencies of N-allyl analogues with analgesic potencies of the parent N-methyl compounds. Winter (34) concluded that there was no quantitative correlation. Archer and Harris (1) compared a series of 11 pairs of compounds and concluded there was a definite association between the two activities. Subsequently, it was reported that N-allyl or N-cyclopropylmethyl analogues of certain extremely potent ethenothebaine analgesics were devoid of antagonist activity. It must be assumed that in some cases at least, the structural features associated with analgesic and antagonist potency differ.

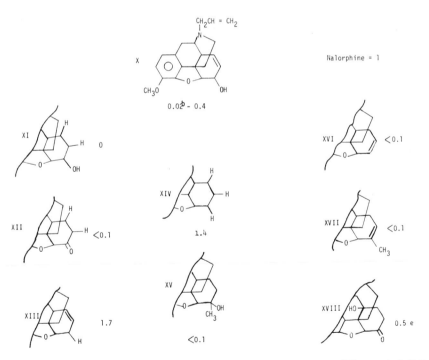

FIG. 6. Relative antagonist potencies of N-allylnorcodeine analogues [Winter et al. (34); (*b*) Green et al. (10); (*e*) Minakami et al. (22)].

Martin (19) has discussed the evidence that different modes of binding to receptors or different sites may be involved.

ANALGESIC STUDIES

At the time that the clinical analgesic effect of nalorphine was discovered, neither it nor any of its analogues had shown a significant analgesic effect in any animal test (26). In order to investigate the relationship between analgesic and antagonist potencies, Keats and Telford (26) evaluated a series of narcotic antagonists in the clinic, including the nalorphine analogues shown in Table 1. These were selected because of slightly different profiles in animal tests (N-methallylnormorphine had a much steeper dose-response curve than nalorphine) (34). The results confirmed the predicted antagonist activity, and also showed some separation between antagonist and psychotomimetic effects. The hoped for separation of analgesic and unwanted side effects was not seen.

It is of interest to compare these results with studies of Kosterlitz and Watt (16) (Table 2). Their test, which is based on opposite modifications of the effect of electrical stimulation of guinea pig ileum by narcotic agonists and antagonists, has established that compounds in either category actually have both actions. The overall pharmacological activity is dependent on which action predominates. The relative activities shown are calculated from the parameters given by Kosterlitz. The "effective antagonist activities" were designated by him, with 2.0 being considered the dividing line between pharmacological agonists and antagonists. The low agonist activity of the N-methallyl analogue correlates well with its lack of analgesia in Keat's study, and also explains its high pharmacological antagonist action. Values for naloxone are given for reference, since it is considered to be a "pure" antagonist without analgesic activity.

During the last 15 years few studies of nalorphine analogues have been reported (exclusive of 14-hydroxy analogues). It was established by Winter and Flataker (33), using a modification of the Randall Sellito test which demonstrated equal analgesic effects for morphine and nalorphine at low doses, that N-cyclopropylnormorphine was an analgesic, three to four times as potent as morphine.

Sargent and May (25) have reported that N-cyclopropylmethylnordesomorphine is an antagonist that is twice as potent as nalorphine with analgesic activity approximately one quarter that of morphine in the mouse hot-plate test and without physical dependence capacity in the monkey — a remarkable combination for a morphine analogue.

It is evident that structure-activity relationships among nalorphine

TABLE 1. *Clinical studies of nalorphine analogues*

Analogues	Activity in rats[a]		Clinical Activity[b]			
	Analgesic	Antagonist	Dose in man mg/70 kg	Analgesia	Antagonism of respiratory depression	Psychoto-mimetic effect
Nalorphine	weak	potent	10	++	++	++
N-Propylnormorphine	none	potent	20	±	+++	+
N-Methallylnormorphine	none	potent	20	±+	++	0
N-Allyldihydronorcodeinone	weak	weak	50	+	++	+
Morphine	potent	none	10	++	0	0

[a] Winter et al. (34).
[b] Telford et al. (26).

29

TABLE 2. *Actions of nalorphine analogues on guinea pig ileum*

Analogue	Agonist activity	Antagonist activity	Effective antagonist activity
Morphine	1	0.05	0.8
Nalorphine	2.8	1	5.4
N-Methallylnormorphine	0.1	0.09	14.7
Naloxone	<0.0006	3.8	>56,000

Kosterlitz and Watt (16).

analogues are far too complex to be understood on the basis of available data. Some predictions can be made by reasoning from the much more extensive knowledge about related series, but these cannot be expected to explain the unique properties of epoxymorphinans.

REFERENCES

1. Archer, S., and Harris, L.: Narcotic antagonists. Prog. Drug. Res. *8*:262–322, 1965.
2. Bartels-Keith, J.: Northebaine and N-allylnorthebaine. J. Chem. Soc. (London) C Org. Chem. 617–620, 1966.
3. Bartels-Keith, J. R., and Hills, D. W.: Derivatives of nororipavine and 8,14-dihydronororipavine. J. Chem. Soc. (London) C Org. Chem. 434–438, 1966.
4. Blumberg, H., Dayton, H., and George, M.: Combinations of the analgesic oxymorphine with the narcotic antagonist N-allyloxymorphone. Fed. Proc. *21*:327, 1962.
5. Casey, A. F.: Analgesics and their antagonists: Recent developments. Prog. Med. Chem. *7*:229–284, 1970.
6. Clark, R., Pessolano, A., Weijlard, J., and Pfister, K.: N-Substituted epoxymorphinans. J. Amer. Chem. Soc. *75*:4963–4969, 1958.
7. Deneau, G. A., Villarreal, J., and Seevers, M. H.: Evaluation of new compounds for morphine-like physical dependence. Addendum 2, Minutes of Twenty-eighth Meeting, Committee on Problems of Drug Dependence, 1966.
8. Eckenhoff, J. E., Elder, J. D., and King, B. D.: The effect of N-allylnormorphine in treatment of opiate overdose. Am. J. Med. Sci. *222*:115, 1951.
9. Gates, M., and Montzka, T.: Some potent morphine antagonists possessing high analgesic activity. J. Med. Chem. *7*:127–131, 1964.
10. Green, A. F., Ruffell, G. K., and Walton, E.: Morphine derivatives with antianalgesic action. J. Pharmacol. *6*:390–397, 1954.
11. Hart, E. R., and McCawley, E. L.: Pharmacology of N-allylnormorphine as compared with morphine. J. Pharmacol. Exp. Ther. *82*:339–348, 1944.
12. Hart, E. R.: N-Allylnorcodeine and N-allylnormorphine. J. Pharmacol. Exp. Ther. *73*:19, 1941.
13. Huggins, R. A., Glass, W. G., and Bryan, A. R.: Protective action of N-allylnormorphine against the respiratory depression produced by some compounds related to morphine. Proc. Soc. Exp. Biol. Med. *75*:540–541, 1950.
14. Isbell, H.: Attempted addiction to nalorphine. Fed. Proc. *15*:442, 1956.
15. Keats, A. S., and Telford, J.: Nalorphine, a potent analgesic in man. J. Pharmacol. Exp. Ther. *117*:190–196, 1956.
16. Kosterlitz, H. W., and Watt, A. J.: Kinetic parameters of narcotic agonists and antagonists. Brit. J. Pharmacol. *33*:276–277, 1968.

17. Lasagna, L., and Beecher, H. K.: Analgesic effectiveness of nalorphine and nalorphine combinations in man. J. Pharmacol. Exp. Ther. *112*:356–363, 1954.
18. Lewis, J. W., Bentley, K. W., and Cowan, A.: Narcotic analgesics and antagonists. Ann. Rev. Pharmacol. *11*:241–270, 1971.
19. Martin, W. R.: Opioid antagonists. Pharmacol. Rev. *19*:463–521, 1967.
20. Martin, W. R., and Gorodetsky, C. W.: Demonstration of tolerance to and dependence on nalorphine. J. Pharmacol. Exp. Ther. *150*:437, 1965.
21. McCawley, E. L., Hart, E. R., and Marsh, D. F.: Preparation of N-allylnormorphine. J. Amer. Chem. Soc. *63*:314, 1941.
22. Minakami, H., Tagaki, H., Kobayashi, S., Deguchi, T., Kumakura, S., Iwai, I., and Seki, I.: Morphine antagonistic actions of N-propargyl-14-hydroxydihydronormorphinone and related compounds. Life Sci. *10*:503–507, 1962.
23. Pohl, J.: N-Allylnorcodeine. Z. Exp. Path. Ther. *17*:370, 1915.
24. Roberts, J. D., and Mazur, R. H.: Interconversion reactions of cyclobutyl, cyclopropyl-carbinyl and allylcarbinyl derivatives. J. Amer. Chem. Soc. *73*:2509–2513, 1951.
25. Sargent, L. J., and May, E. L.: Agonist-antagonists derived from desomorphine and metopon. J. Med. Chem. *13*:1061–1063, 1970.
26. Telford, J., Papadopoulos, C. N., and Keats, A. S.: Morphine antagonists as analgesics. J. Pharmacol. Exp. Ther. *133*:116, 1961.
27. Unna, K.: Antagonistic effect of N-allylnormorphine upon morphine. J. Pharmacol. Exp. Ther. *79*:27–31, 1943.
28. Villarreal, J., and Seevers, M. H.: Evaluation of new compounds for morphine-like physical dependence. Addendum 6. Minutes of the Thirty-third Annual Meeting. Committee on Problems of Drug Dependence, 1971.
29. von Braun, J.: Untersuchungen über Morphium-Alkaloide. Ber. Dtsh. Chem. Ges. *49*:977–989, 1916.
30. von Braun, J., Kuhn, M., and Siddiqui, S.: Ungesattige Reste in chemischer und pharmakologischer Beziehung. Ber. dtsh. Chem. Ges. *59*:1081–1090, 1926.
31. Weijlard, J., and Erickson, A. E.: N-Allylnormorphine. J. Amer. Chem. Soc. *64*:869–870, 1942.
32. Wikler, A. R., Carter, L., Fraser, H. F., and Isbell, H.: Precipitation of "abstinence syndromes" by single doses of N-allylnormorphine in addicts. Fed. Proc., *11*:402, 1952.
33. Winter, C. A., and Flataker, L.: Reaction thresholds to pressure in edemetous hindpaws of rats and responses to analgesic drugs. J. Pharmacol. Exp. Ther. *150*:165, 1965.
34. Winter, C. A., Orahovats, P. A., and Lehman, E. G.: Analgesic activity and morphine antagonism of compounds related to nalorphine. Arch. Interm. Pharmacodyn. Ther. *110*:186–202, 1957.

Narcotic Antagonists, edited by M. C. Braude, L. S. Harris, E. L.
May, J. P. Smith, and J. E. Villarreal. *Advances in Biochemical
Psychopharmacology, Vol. 8.* Raven Press, New York © 1974.

Naloxone, Naltrexone, and Related Noroxymorphones

Harold Blumberg and Hyman B. Dayton

Endo Laboratories, Garden City, New York 11530

Oxymorphone, or 7,8-dihydro-14-hydroxymorphinone, is a potent narcotic analgesic, that is approximately 10 times as active as morphine
sulfate. Noroxymorphone is a weak narcotic analgesic, approximately one-
third as active as morphine when injected subcutaneously into mice and
rats. N-Substituted noroxymorphone derivatives have been compared subcutaneously for analgesic activity by the phenylquinone test in mice and
rats, and for narcotic antagonist activity by prevention of the oxymorphone
Straub tail in mice, by counteraction of narcosis in rats, and by counteraction of respiratory rate depression in rabbits. N-Allylnoroxymorphone,
or naloxone, has little or no analgesic activity, but is a potent narcotic antagonist, approximately 10 to 30 times as active as nalorphine. The N-3,3-
dimethylallyl derivative is about one-third as active as morphine as an analgesic, and about one-half as active as nalorphine as an antagonist. The N-
propynyl derivative has little or no analgesic activity, but is about as active
as nalorphine as an antagonist. The N-cyclobutylmethyl derivative is
slightly better than morphine as an analgesic, and is two to five times as
active as nalorphine as an antagonist. N-Cyclopropylmethylnoroxymor-
phone, or naltrexone or EN-1639, has limited analgesic activity, being
inactive in the mouse and showing some activity with a low ceiling effect in
the rat. However, it is a potent narcotic antagonist, approximately 30 to 40
times as active as nalorphine and two to three times as active as naloxone.
When administered orally for narcotic blockade in rats, naltrexone HCl is
about eight times as active and about three times as long acting as naloxone
HCl on a milligram dose basis.

In 1956 we were working with oxymorphone (7,8-dihydro-14-hydroxy-
morphinone), a narcotic analgesic approximately 10 times as potent as
morphine sulfate. Inasmuch as the N-methyl narcotic analgesic itself was
much more active than morphine, we were interested in the possibility
that the N-allyl derivative might be correspondingly a much more active
narcotic antagonist than N-allylnormorphine, or nalorphine, and also might
be free of some of the undesirable side effects of the latter, such as respiratory depression and psychotomimetic reactions.

N-Allylnoroxymorphone or naloxone (Fig. 1) was synthesized by M. J.

33

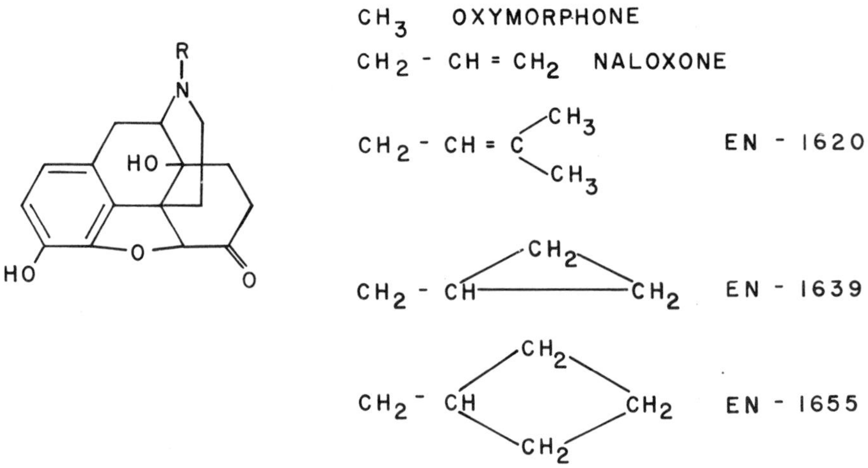

CH₃   OXYMORPHONE

$CH_2 - CH = CH_2$ NALOXONE

$$CH_2 - CH = C \Big\langle {}^{CH_3}_{CH_3} \qquad EN - 1620$$

$$CH_2 - CH \underset{\displaystyle CH_2}{\overbrace{\hspace{2cm}}} CH_2 \qquad EN - 1639$$

$$CH_2 - CH \underset{\displaystyle CH_2}{\overset{\displaystyle CH_2}{\diamondsuit}} CH_2 \qquad EN - 1655$$

FIG. 1. Naloxone and related noroxymorphones.

Lewenstein and J. Fishman in 1960. In the spring of 1961 it was reported by Blumberg, Dayton, George, and Rapaport (3) that naloxone was indeed a potent narcotic antagonist in animals, at least 10 times as active as nalorphine. Later that year Lunn, Foldes, Moore, and Brown (19) reported that naloxone was likewise a potent and well-tolerated narcotic antagonist in man, and Foldes and associates initiated an extensive series of clinical studies on naloxone (13, 14).

In view of the high narcotic antagonist potency and good tolerance found in naloxone when the N-allyl substitution was made, it seemed desirable to investigate other N-substitutions in the noroxymorphone series. With the chemical collaboration of Z. Matossian, and later of I. J. Pachter, we started a program in 1962 on the synthesis and testing of various N-substituted derivatives formed from noroxymorphone and the respective alkyl and cycloalkyl bromides. Archer, Harris, and co-workers (1) and Harris and Pierson (15) had just reported on their interesting series of benzomorphan compounds, notably pentazocine and cyclazocine; therefore similar N-substitutions were among the first tried in the noroxymorphone series (7), as shown in Fig. 1. The N-3,3-dimethylallyl derivative, or EN-1620, was synthesized by Matossian and Pachter in 1963. The N-cyclopropylmethyl derivative (EN-1639 naltrexone) and the N-cyclobutylmethyl derivative, EN-1655, were synthesized by Matossian and evaluated by us in 1963.

Some of the pharmacological properties of these compounds have been briefly described (6). The present report deals with additional studies on structure-activity relationship with respect to analgesic and narcotic antagonist activity.

METHODS

The animals used were CF#1–S (Carworth Farms) male albino mice weighing 20 to 25 g, CFN (Carworth Farms) male albino rats weighing 100 to 160 g, and New Zealand White female rabbits (Perfection Breeders) weighing 2.5 to 4.0 kg. The drugs used were morphine sulfate (Merck), nalorphine hydrochloride (Merck), naloxone hydrochloride (Endo), and oxymorphone hydrochloride (Endo). The other compounds employed were synthesized at Endo Laboratories; all were water-soluble.

Analgesia was determined in mice and rats by the phenylquinone test of Siegmund, Cadmus, and Lu (23), as modified by Blumberg et al. (8), using a 30-min observation period. In addition, the compounds were tested by the mouse, hot-plate method of Eddy and Leimbach (11), and by the same method adapted for rats.

Narcotic antagonism was determined in mice, rats, and rabbits. In mice the test used was prevention of the Straub-tail reaction that is produced by the injection of oxymorphone HCl at 2 mg/kg s.c. The test drugs were injected subcutaneously 15 min before the oxymorphone challenge, and the mice were observed for 30 min after the oxymorphone injection. The Straub-tail reaction was scored as follows: 0 — tail not raised from cage floor; 1 — tail raised only to horizontal; 2 — tail raised close to 45°; 3 — tail raised vertically to nearly 90°. Each mouse was scored for the maximum reaction during each 5-min observation period, and the total score for the six periods was recorded. If the total score was reduced to 50% or less of the average score (usually 16 to 18) of the saline-injected control group, narcotic antagonism was considered positive for that mouse. Three or more dosage levels, with 10 mice per level, were used for each compound. The ED_{50} (95% confidence limits) was calculated as the dose of the drug which produced a 50% or more decrease in Straub-tail score in 50% of the animals, using the method of Litchfield and Wilcoxon (18).

Narcotic antagonism was determined subcutaneously in rats by counter-action of the oxymorphone-induced loss-of-righting reflex, as previously described (8). Some results were calculated as the $ED_{50} \pm SE$, by the method of Miller and Tainter (21). In rabbits narcotic antagonism was estimated simply by counteraction of the oxymorphone-induced depression of the respiratory rate. Rabbits in restrainers were quieted for 30 min for a control period and then were injected with oxymorphone HCl at 2 mg/kg i.v., which regularly reduced the respiratory rate to 75/min or less within 30 min. The antagonist was then injected intravenously, and respiratory rate was counted by visual observation after 1, 2, and 5 min, and at 5-min intervals thereafter for a total of 30 min. Three or more dose levels, with 10 rabbits per level, were used for each drug. The ED_{50} (95% C.L.) was calculated as the dose which produced a peak 100% counteraction of the respiratory rate depression, based on each rabbit's control rate, in 50% of the rabbits during the 30-min observation period. Usually the peak effect occurred within 10 min.

RESULTS

Analgesia

The analgesic activities of the noroxymorphones, as compared with morphine sulfate and oxymorphone hydrochloride on the mouse and rat phenylquinone writhing tests, are presented in Table 1. Noroxymorphone itself is a weak narcotic, as indicated by the production of the Straub-tail reaction in mice and narcosis in rats at moderately high subcutaneous doses. As an analgesic it was slightly weaker than morphine in the mouse and approximately one-third as active as morphine in the rat on the phenylquinone tests; it was approximately one-fifth as active as morphine on the mouse and rat hot-plate tests.

The N-substituted noroxymorphones all appeared to be nonnarcotic as indicated by the absence of both the Straub-tail effect in mice and narcosis in rats. Also, they showed no significant analgesic activity on the hot-plate test with the CF#1-S mice and the CFN rats that were routinely used. Naloxone, a practically "pure" narcotic antagonist in mammals at therapeutic dosages (2), showed essentially no analgesic activity on the phenylquinone tests. The N-cyclopropylmethyl derivative, naltrexone, was inactive in the mouse; in the rat it showed limited activity with a low ceiling for its maximum analgesic effect, suggesting weak agonist action. The N-propynyl derivative was also inactive in the mouse. The N-dimethylallyl derivative was approximately one-third as active as morphine in the mouse and rat. The most active analgesic was the N-cyclobutylmethyl derivative, which was nearly twice as potent as morphine in the mouse and close to four times in the rat.

Naloxone counteracted the phenylquinone-test analgesia shown by these N-substituted noroxymorphones, just as it counteracts the phenylquinone-test analgesic activity of cyclazocine, pentazocine, and other narcotic antagonist analgesics (5). Although the limited analgesia shown by nal-

TABLE 1. *Noroxymorphones–phenylquinone writhing test analgesia, s.c.*

Compound	Mouse		Rat	
	ED$_{50}$ (95% C.L.) (mg/kg)	Potency	ED$_{50}$ (95% C.L.) (mg/kg)	Potency
Morphine sulfate	.80 (.64–.97)	1.0	.26 (.18–.38)	1.0
Oxymorphone HCl	.046 (.027–.078)	17	.020 (.013–.030)	13
Noroxymorphone HCl	1.0 (.73–1.38)	.80	.71 (.47–1.07)	.37
N-Allyl NOM[a] HCl (naloxone)	>100	<.008	>100	<.003
N-Cyclopropylmethyl NOM HCl	>100	<.008	.14 (.064–.31)	1.9[b]
N-Propynyl NOM HCl	>100	<.008		
N-Dimethylallyl NOM HCl	2.0 (1.1–3.6)	.40	.74 (.57–.96)	.35
N-Cyclobutylmethyl NOM HCl	.39 (.19–.82)	2.0	.06 (.038–.096)	4.3

[a] Noroxymorphone
[b] Low ceiling effect

trexone in the rat could also be counteracted by naloxone, the weakness of the agonist component in naltrexone was demonstrated by the fact that naltrexone itself could in turn counteract the phenylquinone-test analgesia of cyclazocine and other narcotic antagonist analgesics (2).

Narcotic Antagonist Activity

A. *Counteraction of Oxymorphone Straub-Tail in Mice*

The N-substituted noroxymorphones were evaluated subcutaneously for narcotic antagonist activity by prevention of the oxymorphone-induced Straub tail in mice. The results are shown in Table 2, in comparison with nalorphine hydrochloride. The weakest antagonist was the N-dimethylallyl derivative, which had a relative potency of only 0.26 as compared to nalorphine as 1.0. The N-propynyl derivative was nearly equal to nalorphine, with a potency of 0.70; this is in agreement with the evaluation made by Minakami et al. (22) on the basis of different types of tests. The N-cyclobutylmethyl derivative was moderately active, with a potency of 2.5. Naloxone had a potency of 10 on this test. The N-cyclopropylmethyl derivative, naltrexone, was approximately three times as active as naloxone, with a potency of 31.

TABLE 2. *Noroxymorphones: Narcotic antagonist activity. Counteraction of oxymorphone Straub tail in mouse, s.c.*

Compound	ED_{50} (95% C.L.) (mg/kg)		Potency
Nalorphine HCl	1.45	(.95–2.15)	1.0
Naloxone HCl	.14	(.09–.23)	10
N-dimethylallyl NOM[a] HCl	5.6	(4.2–7.5)	.26
N-propynyl NOM HCl	2.1	(1.3–3.3)	.70
N-cyclobutylmethyl NOM HCl	.57	(.36–.92)	2.5
N-cyclopropylmethyl NOM HCl	.047	(.031–.071)	31

[a] Noroxymorphone

B. *Counteraction of Oxymorphone Narcosis in Rats*

When tested for narcotic activity subcutaneously by counteraction of oxymorphone-induced narcosis or loss-of-righting reflex in rats, the N-substituted noroxymorphones gave the results presented in Table 3. Again the N-dimethylallyl derivative was the weakest, with a relative potency of 0.64; the N-cyclobutylmethyl derivative was moderately active, 4.8;

TABLE 3. *Noroxymorphones: Narcotic antagonist activity. Counter-action of oxymorphone narcosis in rat, s.c.*

Compound	ED_{50} (95% C.L.) (mg/kg)	Potency
Nalorphine HCl	.90 (.58–1.39)	1.0
Naloxone HCl	.051 (.030–.080)	18
N-dimethylallyl NOM[a] HCl	1.4 (.74–2.7)	.64
N-cyclobutylmethyl NOM HCl	.19 (.12–.30)	4.8
N-cyclopropylmethyl NOM HCl	.023 (.014–.037)	39

[a] Noroxymorphone

naloxone was 18; and naltrexone was 39, or approximately twice as active as naloxone.

C. *Counteraction of Oxymorphone Respiratory-Rate Depression in Rabbits*

Three of the N-substituted noroxymorphones have also been compared with nalorphine intravenously for counteraction of oxymorphone-induced depression of respiratory rate in rabbits. As demonstrated in Table 4, the N-dimethylallyl derivative was again the weakest, with a relative potency of 0.25; naloxone was 19; and naltrexone was 42, again nearly twice as active as naloxone. Although the determination of respiratory rate alone would miss the effect of any significant differences in respiratory amplitude, in practice this simple method appears to yield comparative results in a third species, the rabbit, which are consistent with the results obtained in mice and rats by other methods. As a matter of fact, these results with naloxone and nalorphine agree rather well with a previous comparison in which naloxone was found to be approximately 15 times as active as nalorphine in counteracting oxymorphone- and morphine-induced respiratory depression in rabbits as determined by minute volume measurement (4).

TABLE 4. *Noroxymorphones: Narcotic antagonist activity. Counter-action of oxymorphone respiratory rate depression in rabbits, i.v.*

Compound	ED_{50} (95% C.L.) (mg/kg)	Potency
Nalorphine HCl	.85 (.65–1.08)	1.0
Naloxone HCl	.045 (.032–.063)	19
N-dimethylallyl NOM[a] HCl	3.4 (2.3–4.9)	.25
N-cyclopropylmethyl NOM HCl	.020 (.013–.030)	42

[a] Noroxymorphone

Other Narcotic Antagonist Studies

Kosterlitz and Watt (17) have compared these N-substituted noroxymorphones for agonist and narcotic antagonist activity by means of the coaxially stimulated isolated guinea pig ileum. By this method there was moderately good agreement with the previously discussed live animal studies. With reference to nalorphine as 1.0, the narcotic antagonist potencies were approximately: N-dimethylallyl 0.1, N-cyclobutylmethyl 1.5, naloxone 4.0, and naltrexone 12.0. On the other hand, the agonist activities were approximately the following, with respect to morphine as 1.0: N-cyclobutylmethyl 1.0 and N-dimethylallyl 0.2. Naltrexone showed only very slight agonist activity, and naloxone had virtually none.

Some narcotic antagonist activities have also been reported in monkeys, as determined by precipitation of abstinence after subcutaneous injection into the morphine-dependent animals. Deneau et al. (10) found that the N-dimethylallyl derivative was approximately 0.1 as active as nalorphine, and Deneau and Seevers (9) rated naloxone as nearly seven times as active. Villarreal and Seevers (24) reported that naltrexone was six to 13 times as potent as nalorphine, which should make it slightly more active than naloxone; they also found that naltrexone was longer acting than naloxone. The comparative potencies in monkeys appear to be in approximate agreement with the rodent data, although tending to be slightly lower in comparison with nalorphine.

Some narcotic antagonist data are also available for man. In surgical patients, Foldes and associates (13) estimated naloxone to be 30 times as potent as nalorphine when the antagonists were given intravenously to counteract narcotic respiratory and circulatory depression. In morphine-dependent addicts, Jasinski et al. (16) found naloxone to be five to eight times as potent as nalorphine subcutaneously in precipitating abstinence, and Martin, Jasinski, and Mansky (20) found naltrexone (EN-1639) to be twice as active as naloxone, which should make it close to 13 times as potent as nalorphine. Naltrexone was also longer acting than naloxone.

Oral Narcotic Antagonist Activity: Comparison of Naloxone and Naltrexone for Narcotic Blockade

Early experiments in rats showed that naloxone was an effective narcotic antagonist by oral administration, but the dosages required were much higher than by injection. Fink et al. (12) have demonstrated that comparatively large oral doses of naloxone hydrochloride can block the effects of heroin injection in man. However, due to the relatively short duration of action of naloxone and its high degree of inactivation after oral administration, Zaks et al. (25) found that a single dose of as much as 3,000 mg of naloxone hydrochloride was necessary to produce 24-hr narcotic blockade. In view of the special interest shown in oral naltrexone hydrochloride by Dr. W. R. Martin at the Addiction Research Center for producing narcotic blockade in post-addicts, the results of a comparison of oral naloxone and oral naltrexone in rats will be described.

Oral narcotic antagonist activity was determined by prevention of oxymorphone-induced, loss-of-righting reflex in the rats. The preventive method was the same as the previously described (8) subcutaneous curative method except that the antagonists were administered by stomach tube 30 min before the subcutaneous injection of 1 mg/kg of oxymorphone hydrochloride instead of 30 min after. If a rat did not lose its righting reflex within 20 min, it was considered to show narcotic antagonism.

The results are shown in Table 5. Although, after subcutaneous injection naltrexone hydrochloride is only approximately twice as active as naloxone hydrochloride in counteracting oxymorphone-induced loss-of-righting reflex, it appears to be nearly eight times as active as naloxone hydrochloride in the oral prevention or blocking of this narcotic effect.

The duration of oral narcotic antagonist action was determined in rats by holding the dosage constant at the approximate 80% equi-antagonist protective levels, i.e., naloxone hydrochloride 16 mg/kg and naltrexone 2 mg/kg, and varying the time by giving the oxymorphone challenge subcutaneously at 30, 60, 120, 180, and 240 min after the oral administration of the antagonists. As illustrated in Fig. 2, the times required for a 50% decrease in narcotic antagonist activity (considering the 30-min determination as the initial point) were approximately 58 min for naloxone hydrochloride and approximately 169 min for naltrexone hydrochloride. Therefore, it appears that the narcotic-blocking action of oral naltrexone hydrochloride in rats was about three times as long as that of an equiantagonist dose of oral naloxone hydrochloride, even though the naltrexone hydrochloride dose was only one-eighth that of naloxone hydrochloride.

TABLE 5. *Oral narcotic antagonist activity in rats determined by prevention of oxymorphone loss-of-righting reflex*

Antagonist	$ED_{50} \pm SE$ (mg/kg)	Activity
Naloxone HCl	8.0 ± 2.7	1
Naltrexone HCl	0.98 ± 0.18	8

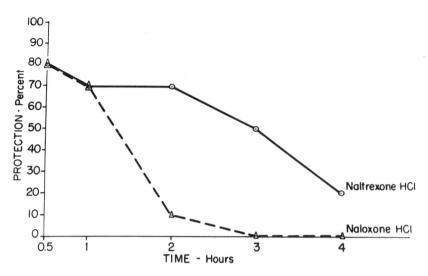

FIG. 2. Naloxone HCl and naltrexone HCl: duration of narcotic blockade orally in rats, as measured by protection against oxymorphone HCl loss-of-righting reflex. Drug dosages: naloxone HCl 16 mg/kg p.o., naltrexone HCl 2 mg/kg p.o., and oxymorphone HCl 1 mg/kg s.c.

If naltrexone hydrochloride is about eight times as active and about three times as long acting as naloxone hydrochloride orally in rats, it would appear to be nearly 24 times as effective as naloxone hydrochloride on a mg basis for narcotic blockade. Martin et al. (20) have estimated that a 50- to 100-mg oral dose of naltrexone hydrochloride would probably provide 24-hr narcotic blockade in man, whereas Zaks et al. (25) found that approximately 3,000 mg of oral naloxone hydrochloride would probably be required for the same duration of blockade. These facts suggest that, in man, naltrexone hydrochloride might be 30 to 60 times as effective as naloxone hydrochloride on a mg basis, or conversely, that oral narcotic blockade might be attained with naltrexone hydrochloride at $1/30$ to $1/60$ of the dose required with naloxone hydrochloride.

REFERENCES

1. Archer, S., Albertson, N. F., Harris, L. S., Pierson, A. K., Bird, J. G., Keats, A. S., Telford, J., and Papadopoulos, C. N.: Narcotic antagonists as analgesics. Science *137*:541–543, 1962.
2. Blumberg, H., and Dayton, H. B.: Naloxone and related compounds. *In:* Agonist and Antagonist Actions of Narcotic Analgesic Drugs, edited by H. W. Kosterlitz, H. O. J. Collier, and J. E. Villarreal, pp. 110–119. University Park Press, Baltimore, 1973.
3. Blumberg, H., Dayton, H. B., George, M., and Rapaport, D. N.: N-allylnoroxymorphone: A potent narcotic antagonist. Fed. Proc. *20*:311, 1961.

4. Blumberg, H., Dayton, H. B., and Wolf, P. S.: Narcotic antagonist activity of naloxone. Fed. Proc. *24*:676, 1965.
5. Blumberg, H., Dayton, H. B., and Wolf, P. S.: Counteraction of narcotic antagonist analgesics by the narcotic antagonist naloxone. Proc. Soc. Exp. Biol. Med. *123*: 755–758, 1966.
6. Blumberg, H., Dayton, H. B., and Wolf, P. S.: Analgesic and narcotic antagonist properties of noroxymorphone derivatives. Toxicol. Appl. Pharmacol. *10*:406, 1967.
7. Blumberg, H., Pachter, I. J., and Matossian, Z.: 14-Hydroxydihydronormorphinone derivatives. U.S. Pat. No. 3,332,950, July 25, 1967.
8. Blumberg, H., Wolf, P. S., and Dayton, H. B.: Use of writhing test for evaluating analgesic activity of narcotic antagonists. Proc. Soc. Exp. Biol. Med. *118*:763–766, 1965.
9. Deneau, G. A. and Seevers, M. H.: Evaluation of morphine-like physical dependence in the rhesus monkey (Macaca mulatta). Bulletin, Drug Addiction and Narcotics, Addendum 1, 24, 1963.
10. Deneau, G. A., Villarreal, J. E., and Seevers, M. H.: Evaluation of new compounds for morphine-like physical dependence in the rhesus monkey. Bulletin, Problems of Drug Dependence, Addendum 2, 4, 1966.
11. Eddy, N. B., and Leimbach, D.: Synthetic analgesics II. dithienylbutenyl- and dithienylbutylamines. J. Pharmacol. Exp. Ther. *107*:385–393, 1953.
12. Fink, M., Zaks, A., Sharoff, R., Mora, A., Bruner, A., Levit, S., and Freedman, A. M.: Naloxone in heroin dependence. Clin. Pharmacol. Ther. *9*:568–577, 1968.
13. Foldes, F. F., Duncalf, D., and Kuwabara, S.: The respiratory, circulatory, and narcotic antagonistic effects of nalorphine, levallorphan, and naloxone in anaesthetized subjects. Can. Anaesth. Soc. J. *16*:151–161, 1969.
14. Foldes, F. F., Lunn, J. N., Moore, J., and Brown, I. M.: N-allylnoroxymorphone: A new potent narcotic antagonist. Amer. J. Med. Sci. *245*:23–30, 1963.
15. Harris, L. S., and Pierson, A. K.: Some narcotic antagonists in the benzomorphan series. J. Pharmacol. Exp. Ther. *143*:141–148, 1964.
16. Jasinski, D. R., Martin, W. R., and Haertzen, C. A.: The human pharmacology and abuse potential of N-allylnoroxymorphone (naloxone). J. Pharmacol. Exp. Ther. *157*:420–426, 1967.
17. Kosterlitz, H. W., and Watt, A. J.: Kinetic parameters of narcotic agonists and antagonists. Reported to the *Committee on Problems of Drug Dependence*, 30th meeting, 1968.
18. Litchfield, J. T., and Wilcoxon, F.: A simplified method of evaluating dose-effect experiments. J. Pharmacol. Exp. Ther. *96*:99–113, 1949.
19. Lunn, J. N., Foldes, F. F., Moore, J., and Brown, I. M.: The influence of N-allyloxymorphone on the respiratory effects of oxymorphone in anaesthetized man. Pharmacologist *3*:66, 1961.
20. Martin, W. R., Jasinski, D. R., and Mansky, P. A.: Characteristics of the blocking effects of EN-1639A (N-cyclopropylmethyl-7,8-dihydro-14-hydroxynormorphinone HCl). Reported to the *Committee on Problems of Drug Dependence*, 33rd meeting, 1971.
21. Miller, L. C., and Tainter, M. L.: Estimation of the ED_{50} and its error by means of logarithmic-probit graph paper. Proc. Soc. Exp. Biol. Med. *57*:261–264, 1944.
22. Minakami, H., Takagi, H., Kobayashi, S., Deguchi, T., Kumakura, S., Iwai, I., and Seki, I.: Morphine antagonistic actions of N-propargyl-14-hydroxydihydronormorphinone hydrochloride and related compounds. Life Sci. *1*:503–507, 1962.
23. Siegmund, E., Cadmus, R., and Lu, G.: A method for evaluating both nonnarcotic and narcotic analgesics. Proc. Soc. Exp. Biol. Med. *95*:729–731, 1957.
24. Villarreal, J. E., and Seevers, M. H.: Evaluation of new compounds for morphine-like physical dependence in the rhesus monkey. Bulletin, Committee Problems of Drug Dependence, Addendum 1, 2, 1970.
25. Zaks, A., Jones, T., Fink, M., and Freedman, A. M.: Naloxone treatment of opiate dependence. J. Am. Med. Assoc. *215*:2108–2110, 1971.

Narcotic Antagonists, edited by M. C. Braude, L. S. Harris, E. L. May, J. P. Smith, and J. E. Villarreal. *Advances in Biochemical Psychopharmacology, Vol. 8.* Raven Press, New York © 1974.

Levallorphan and Related Compounds

W. Leimgruber, E. Mohacsi, H. Baruth, and L. O. Randall

Hoffmann-La Roche Inc., Nutley, New Jersey 07110

The need for new narcotic antagonists which are free of undesirable side effects prompted the search for novel morphinans structurally related to levallorphan. The discovery that the rate of acid-catalyzed cyclizations of 1-benzyl-substituted N-methyloctahydroisoquinolines (Grewe approach) can be greatly enhanced by replacement of the N-methyl by an N-formyl group led to a new, efficient, and versatile synthesis of morphinans. By this approach, a considerable number of new morphinans were prepared, in racemic and enantiomeric forms, which are oxygenated in the 1, 2, 3, or 4 position and whose substituents on nitrogen include the allyl, dimethyl-allyl, and cyclopropylmethyl groups.

Among these compounds, (+)-2-hydroxy-N-cyclopropylmethylmor-phinan hydrochloride was selected for extensive pharmacological evaluation because of its unexpected morphine antagonist properties. Since this morphinan, whose structure is unique in terms of absolute configuration for an antagonist, did not suppress abstinence symptoms in morphine-dependent monkeys, chronic toxicity studies have been initiated in view of possible clinical trials in man.

INTRODUCTION

Levallorphan is well established as a clinically effective antidote for opiates which produce severe respiratory depression (6). This drug, which belongs to the morphinan class of compounds, is unique because it is made by total synthesis (10) rather than by structural modification of a natural product. Recently, two metabolites of levallorphan have been isolated from rat urine and identified (3, 12, 13). Although levallorphan has many of the pharmacological properties of the morphine-like analgesics, its clinical use as an analgesic and/or an antitussive agent is precluded because of the disturbing mental effects that are produced. This drug is also far from ideal as an antagonist. Since there exists a pressing need for new narcotic antagonists that are free of undesirable side effects, we initiated a search for novel morphinans structurally related to levallorphan.

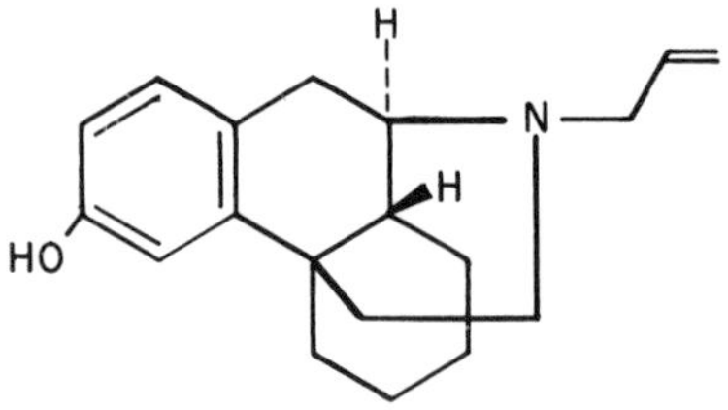

Levallorphan

CHEMISTRY

Our recent discovery (18) that the rate of acid catalyzed cyclizations of 1-benzyl-substituted N-methyloctahydroisoquinolines [Grewe approach (7)] can be greatly enhanced by replacement of the N-methyl by an N-formyl group has led to a new, efficient, and versatile synthesis of morphinans[1] whose principle is outlined in Fig. 1.

In this figure, 1-methoxybenzyl-substituted N-formyloctahydroisoquinolines (I) are cyclized under mild conditions to N-formylmorphinians of structure II. We found, for example, that 1-(p-methoxybenzyl)-N-formyl-1, 2,3,4,5,6,7,8-octahydroisoquinoline, upon heating at 70°C for 20 hr in phosphoric acid (which contains a small amount of sulfuric acid), affords 3-methoxy-N-formylmorphinan in more than 90% yield. This cyclization proceeds at a rate which is 400 times that of the corresponding N-methyl compound. The remaining transformation of N-formylmorphinans (II) to N-alkylmorphinans of the general structure III can be easily achieved by conventional methods.

By this synthetic approach, we prepared a considerable number of new morphinans (III), in racemic and enantiomeric forms, which are oxygenated in the 1, 2, 3, or 4 position and whose substituents on nitrogen include the allyl, dimethylallyl, and cyclopropylmethyl groups.

The pharmacological evaluation of these compounds in terms of morphine antagonist activity has thus far been restricted to the 2- and 3-oxygenated morphinans summarized in Table 1.

METHODS

The lack of response to narcotic antagonists in the usual animal tests for analgesia stimulated a search for tests that can detect analgesics of this

---

[1] Based on these findings, we have also developed a new synthesis of benzomorphans which utilizes the same principle (17).

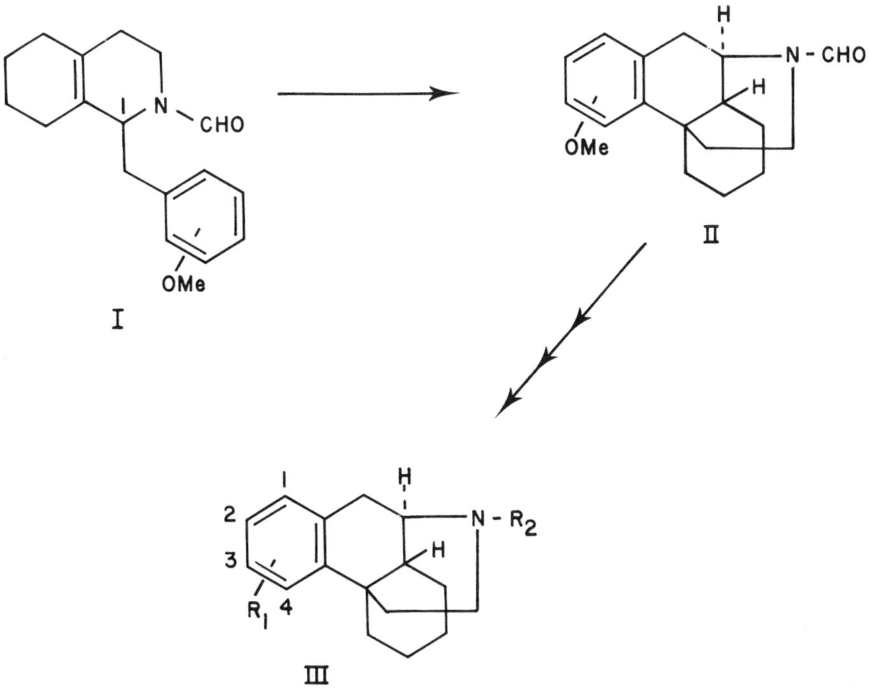

R_1 = -OH, -OMe, -OAC

R_2 = -H, -Me, $-CH_2-CH=CH_2$, $-CH_2-CH=CMe_2$, $-CH_2-$◁

FIG. 1. Synthesis of morphinans.

class. Several investigators (4, 14, 16) have reported that the phenylquinone writhing test of Siegmund, Cadmus, and Lu (15) may be an effective tool for evaluating the analgesic activity of narcotic antagonists. Blumberg (4) reported a correlation between the ED_{50} values in the prevention of writhing in mice and rats and the analgesic properties of narcotic antagonists in man. In a modification of the writhing test involving the numerical sum of writhing episodes in response to phenylquinone irritation, analgesic activity was found in a series of 2- and 3-oxygenated morphinans (Table 1). The ED_{50} was calculated according to the method of Litchfield and Wilcoxin (11).

An assay procedure based upon an adaptation of the tail-flick method (1, 2, 8) was used for determining the narcotic antagonist effects of these morphinans against the analgesic response to 10 mg/kg of morphine in mice. Narcotic antagonists were administered subcutaneously 10 min prior to morphine. Pain thresholds were measured 30 min after morphine ad-

TABLE 1. *Morphinans: antagonist and analgesic activity*

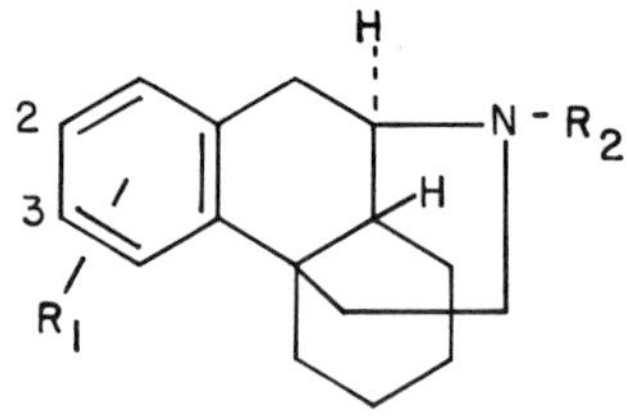

Compound	R_1	R_2	OI*	Antagonist activity mice (tail-flick) AD_{50} (mg/kg s.c.)	Analgesic activity mice (writhing ED_{50} (mg/kg s.c.)
1[a](10)	HO-(3)	—CH₂—CH=CH₂	(−)	0.39	0.29
2[b](10)	HO-(3)	—CH₂—CH=CH₂	(+)	inactive (>32)[f]	55.0
3[b]	HO-(3)	—CH₂—CH=C(CH₃)₂	(−)	inactive (>32)	0.30
4[c](5)	HO-(3)	—CH₂—◁	(−)	0.25	0.036
5[c]	HO-(3)	—CH₂—◁	(+)	inactive (>32)	34.0
6[d]	AcO-(3)	—CH₂—◁	(+)	inactive (>32)	22.0
7[c]	HO-(2)	—CH₂—CH=CH₂	(−)	24.5	20.0
8[c]	HO-(2)	—CH₂—CH=CH₂	(+)	inactive (>32)	30.0
9[c]	HO-(2)	—CH₂—CH=C(CH₃)₂	(−)	inactive (>32)	33.0
10[c]	HO-(2)	—CH₂—CH=C(CH₃)₂	(+)	inactive (>32)	33.0
11[c]	HO-(2)	—CH₂—◁	(−)	9	1.12
12[c]	HO-(2)	—CH₂—◁	(+)	7	13
13[d]	AcO-(2)	—CH₂—◁	(−)	inactive (>32)	1.95
14[d]	AcO-(2)	—CH₂—◁	(+)	inactive (>32)	48.0
Morphine[e]				—	0.41
Nalorphine[b]				0.52	0.40

[a] Tartrate, [b] hydrobromide, [c] hydrochloride, [d] oxalate, [e] sulfate, [f] *i.e.*, not active at doses up to 32 mg/kg s.c.
* Optical isomerism.

ministration. Morphine, when given alone, typically produces a 75% increase in reaction time 30 min after treatment. The percent antagonism of morphine analgesia was calculated according to the formula of Harris and Pierson (9).

DISCUSSION

In comparison to morphine, the 3-substituted levorotatory morphinans **1** (levallorphan), **3** and **4** (cyclorphan) are strong analgesics. Compounds **1** and **4** are strong morphine antagonists in the range of nalorphine, whereas **3** is not an antagonist at the doses tested. The dextrorotatory compounds **5** and **6** are weak analgesics and lack morphine antagonist activity. Compound **2**, the dextrorotatory antipode of levallorphan, is inactive in the morphine-antagonism test.

The 2-substituted levorotatory morphinans **11** and **13** are strong analgesics although **7** and **9** are weak analgesics. Both **7** and **11** are moderately active as morphine antagonists whereas **9** and **13** are inactive. The 2-substituted dextrorotatory compounds **8**, **12**, and **14** are weak analgesics. In conformity with the results on 3-substituted morphinans, compounds **8**, **10**, and **14** are inactive as morphine antagonists. Surprisingly, compound **12** [(+)-2-hydroxy-N-cyclopropylmethylmorphinan] like nalorphine exhibits significant antagonist activity as well as analgesic activity.

12

CONCLUSION

Among the compounds discussed, (+)-2-hydroxy-N-cyclopropylmethyl-morphinan hydrochloride was selected for extensive pharmacological evaluation because of its unexpected morphine antagonist properties. Since this morphinan, whose structure is unique in terms of absolute configuration for an antagonist, did not suppress abstinence symptoms in morphine-dependent monkeys, chronic toxicity studies have been initiated in view of possible clinical trials in man.

ACKNOWLEDGMENTS

We wish to thank Mr. L. Berger for his assistance in the preparation of this manuscript.

REFERENCES

1. D'Amour, F. E., and Smith, D. L.: A method for determining loss of pain sensation. J. Pharmacol. Exp. Ther. *72*:74–79, 1941.
2. Bass, W. B., and Vander Brook, M. J.: A note on an improved method of analgetic evaluation. J. Am. Pharm. Assoc. (Sci. Ed.) *41*:569–570, 1952.
3. Blount, J. F., Mannering, G. J., Mohacsi, E., and Vane, F.: Isolation, X-ray analysis and synthesis of a metabolite of (−)-3-hydroxy-N-allylmorphinan (levallorphan). J. Med. Chem. *16*:352–355, 1973.
4. Blumberg, H., Wolf, P. S., and Dayton, H. B.: Use of writing test for evaluating analgesic activity of narcotic antagonists. Proc. Soc. Exp. Biol. Med. *118*:763–766, 1965.
5. Gates, M., and Montzka, T. A.: Some potent morphine antagonists possessing high analgesic activity. J. Med. Chem. *7*:127–131, 1964.
6. Goodman, L. S., and Gilman, A.: The Pharmacological Basis of Therapeutics, pp. 252 and 268. The Macmillan Co., New York, New York, 1970.
7. Grewe, R., and Mondon, A.: Synthesen in der Phenanthren-Reihe, VI. Mitteil: Synthese des Morphinans. Chem. Ber. B*81*:279–286, 1948.
8. Gross, F.: Eine einfache Methode zur quantitativen Analgesie-prufung. Helv. Physiol. Acta. *5*:C31–33, 1947.
9. Harris, L. S., and Pierson, A. K.: Some narcotic antagonists in the benzomorphan series. J. Pharmacol. Exp. Ther. *143*:141–148, 1964.
10. Hellerbach, J., Grussner, A., and Schnider, O.: (−)-3-Hydroxy-N-allylmorphinan und Verwandte Verbindungen. Helv. Chim. Acta. *39*:429–440, 1956.
11. Litchfield, J. T., and Wilcoxon, F.: A simplified method of evaluating dose-effect experiments. J. Pharmacol. Exp. Ther. *96*:99–113, 1949.
12. Mannering, G. J., and Schanker, L. S.: Metabolic fate of levo-3-hydroxy-N-allylmorphinan (levallorphan). J. Pharmacol. Exp. Ther. *124*:296–304, 1958.
13. Mohacsi, E., Blount, J. F., and Mannering, G. J.: (−)-N-Allyl-3,6-dihydroxymorphinan, a new metabolite of levallorphan. In: Abstracts of the 13th National Medicinal Chemistry Symposium, p. 17, Iowa City, Iowa, June, 1972.
14. Pearl, J., and Harris, L. S.: Inhibition of writhing by narcotic antagonists. J. Pharmacol. Exp. Ther. *154*:319–323, 1966.
15. Siegmund, E., Cadmus, R., and Lu, G.: A method of evaluating both nonnarcotic and narcotic analgesics. Proc. Soc. Exp. Biol. Med. *95*:729–731, 1957.
16. Taber, R. I., Greenhouse, D. D., and Irwin, S.: Inhibition of phenylquinone-induced writhing by narcotic antagonists. Nature *204*:189–190, 1964.
17. U.S. Patent No. 3,553,223, January 5, 1971: Acid catalyzed cyclization of tetrahydropyridines containing an electron withdrawing group on the nitrogen.
18. U.S. Patent No. 3,634,429, January 11, 1972: Morphinan derivatives and preparation thereof.

Narcotic Antagonists, edited by M. C. Braude, L. S. Harris, E. L. May, J. P. Smith, and J. E. Villarreal. *Advances in Biochemical Psychopharmacology, Vol. 8.* Raven Press, New York © 1974.

Cyclorphan and Related Compounds

Marshall Gates

University of Rochester, Rochester, New York 14627

Three methods for the preparation of isocyclorphan are described and discussed briefly. A modification of the Grewe cyclization is the best and appears to be modifiable for larger scale preparation. A possible mechanism for the formation of *trans*-isomorphinans in the Grewe cyclization is discussed. A possible new stereospecific synthesis of isomorphinans is discussed briefly.

That the cyclopropylmethyl group, when substituted for the N-methyl group of codeine, confers narcotic antagonistic properties on the substance so produced was discovered many years ago (3), but this observation lay fallow until the early sixties when the work of Archer (2) and his co-workers, and Gates and Montzka (5) demonstrated the generality of this earlier observation. The most potent antagonists now known bear this distinguishing substituent.

Among the substances prepared and studied in the early sixties were cyclorphan (I), which has the natural morphine configuration at C_{14}, and its C_{14} epimer isocyclorphan (II).

Both of these substances are potent antagonists. Cyclorphan is, in addition, a potent agonist resembling cyclazocine in its pharmacological properties. Isocyclorphan in contrast, at least on the basis of small animal tests (10), has little or no agonistic activity[1] and is therefore of interest as an an-

---

[1] The results obtained by Winter using the inflamed paw technique (10) suggested that isocyclorphan was inactive as an agonist. More recent results with the phenylquinone writhing test indicate that the agonist activity of isocyclorphan (AD_{50} 6.5 mg/kg) is about 1/300 that of cyclorphan (AD_{50} 0.02 mg/kg) and about 1/200 that of cyclazocine (AD_{50} 0.03 mg/kg).

tagonist prophylactic against readdiction in post-addicts. This chapter deals largely with the various synthetic methods which have been employed to produce the *trans*-morphinan ring system of isocyclorphan and with the synthesis of certain related substances.

Isocyclorphan, or at least the *trans*-morphinan ring system from which it can be obtained, has been prepared by three methods: total synthesis by the method of Gates and Webb (6); partial synthesis from thebaine; and synthesis by a modification of the Grewe method.

The first of these methods proceeds as follows:

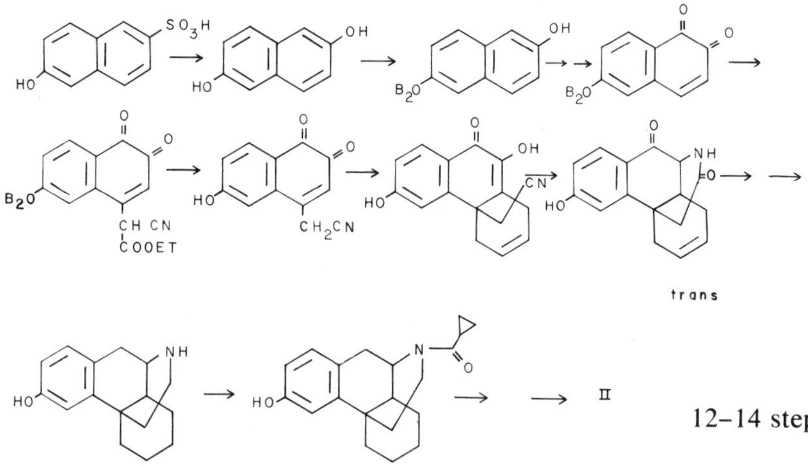

trans

12–14 steps

The preparation of isocyclorphan from the naturally occurring alkaloid thebaine has been carried out as follows (5):

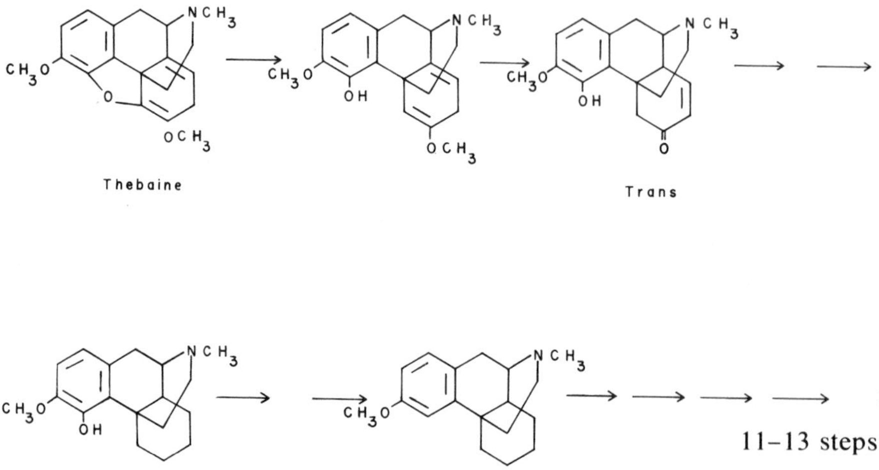

11–13 steps

An alternative synthesis from thebaine, all steps of which have not yet been carried through, is the following:

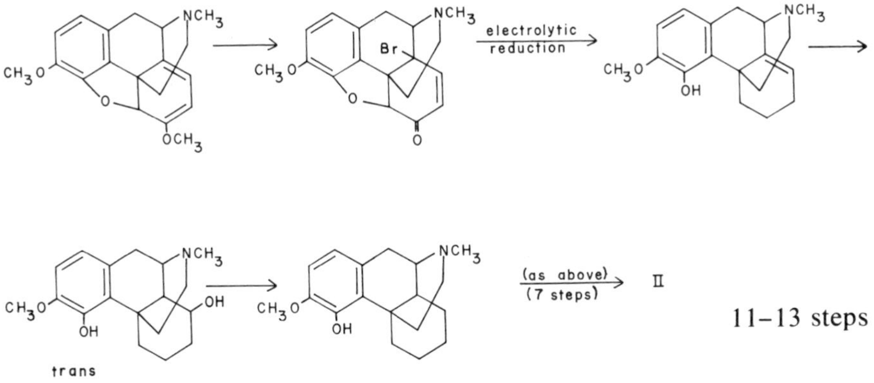

electrolytic reduction

(as above)
(7 steps) → II

11–13 steps

trans

Those skilled in organic synthesis will recognize that all of the above methods are long, tedious, and inefficient.

The original Grewe synthesis of morphinans (7,9) which involved the acid catalyzed cyclization of 1-benzyloctahydroisoquinolines, normally yields mostly morphinans (*cis*) rather than isomorphinans (*trans*), but Fry and May showed that by using aluminum halides as cyclization catalysts substantial amounts of *trans*-benzomorphans were produced during the cyclization of benzyltetrahydropyridines (1). We have found that a similar use of aluminum bromides in the morphinan cyclization yields substantial quantities of isomorphinans. Thus the synthesis of isocyclorphan by this method proceeds as follows:

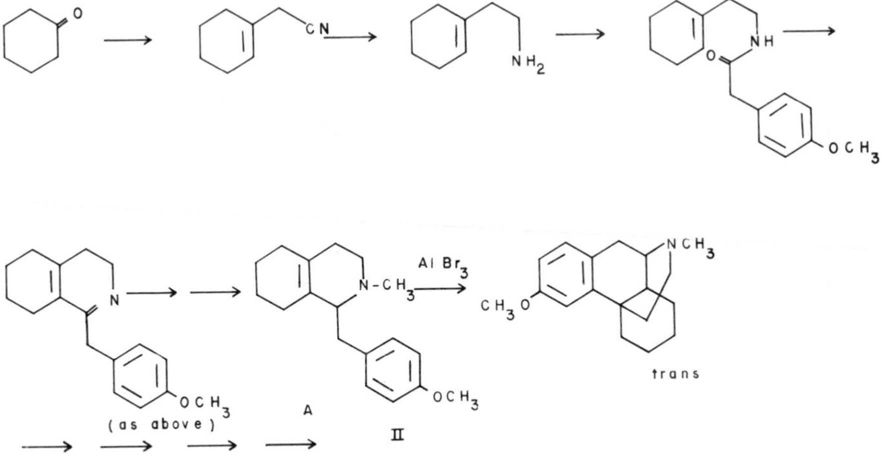

AlBr₃

trans

(as above)
A
II

This synthesis is scarcely less lengthy than those outlined earlier, but fortunately the intermediate A, in optically active form, is a commercial product, and its availability through the courtesy of Hoffmann-LaRoche greatly reduced the effort required for us to prepare moderate quantities of II. Furthermore, there is every reason to believe that should it become necessary to obtain isocyclorphan in quantity, further modification of this synthesis will greatly improve its efficiency. Such modifications might comprise the use of cyclopropylmethyl or better yet cyclopropylcarbonyl rather than methyl as substituents on the nitrogen of A.

At present, owing to the production of only limited amounts of isocyclorphans in this cyclization, it is necessary to separate the *cis* and *trans* forms. This can be done efficiently by making use of the great differences in the rates of quaternization of 3-methoxy-N-methylmorphinan (III) and isomorphinan (IV), the former of which reacts 270 times as rapidly with methyl iodide as the latter. A similar, but less marked difference in rates of quaternization of N-methylbenzomorphans was noted earlier by May and his coworkers (4) who correctly ascribed the difference to conformational effects.

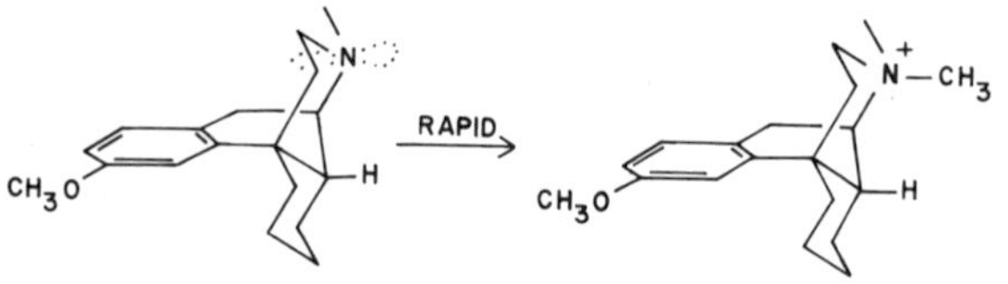

III

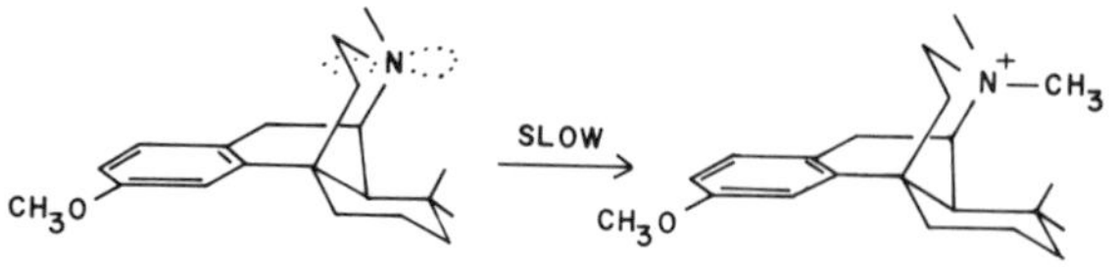

IV

Conditions have been found under which III is essentially completely converted to its highly polar quaternary salt and IV is scarcely attacked.

We are also investigating the preparation of the intermediate V, analogous to A above, which should cyclize stereospecifically to II:

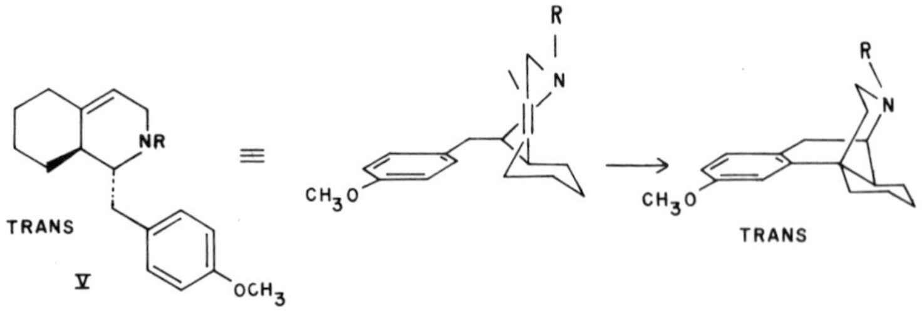

V

A word or two of speculation as to the mechanistic course of this cyclization seems in order. Why does the use of the powerful Lewis acid aluminum
bromide produce a higher *trans-cis* ratio in the cyclization product than the
use of strong protic acids? We believe the answer is to be found in the structures of the corresponding intermediates in these electrophilic aromatic
substitutions:

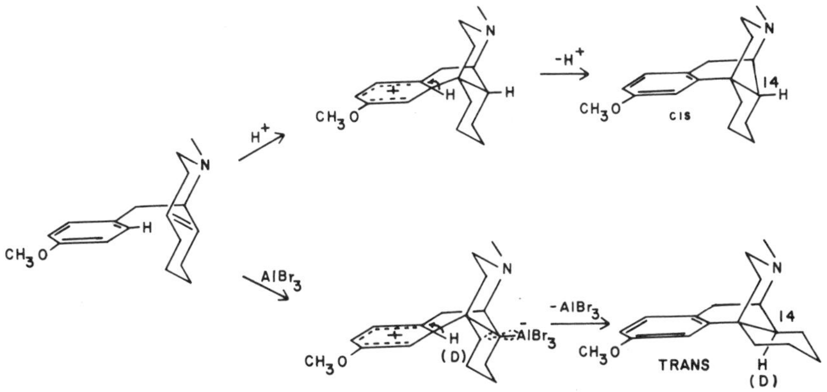

In cyclization initiated by proton addition to the double bond of the starting benzyloctahydroisoquinoline, the intermediate loses a proton from the
aromatic ring to form the *cis* product, whereas in cyclizations initiated by
aluminum bromide, the intermediate must also lose aluminum bromide. We
think it does so by intramolecular *electrophilic* substitution at C_{14} with in-
version of this center.[2] If this is so, starting material containing deuterium
in the positions *ortho* to the benzylic carbon should yield *trans* product with
deuterium at C_{14}. This hypothesis is currently being tested experimentally.

Another synthetic route to isomorphinans which we are investigating is
the following:

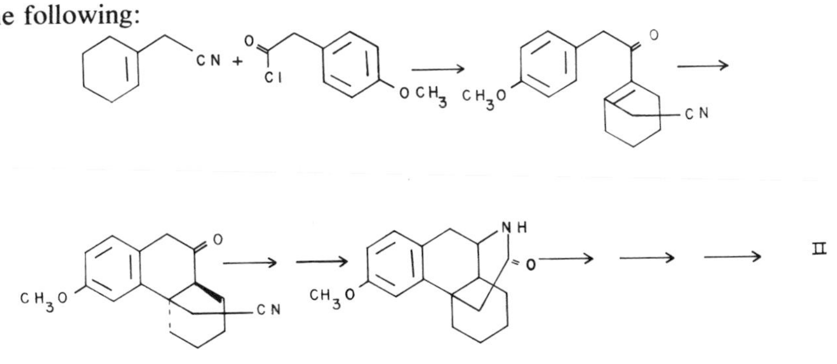

___

[2] This explanation was first suggested to us by Mr. Dennis Werber, then of these laboratories.

The rationale behind this synthetic scheme is that the ketone VI is epimerizable at C_{14} and is more stable as the *trans* modification. Cyclization by a sequence involving a Ritter reaction should then lead to the *trans* lactam VII. Although the first reaction in this sequence has been reported not to occur (8), we have found conditions under which it goes in good yield. So far we have not been able to carry out the second cyclization.

A second phase of our work in this area involves the preparation of substances with new substituents on and near the nitrogen atom. The substances now used for the prophylactic treatment of post-addicts to prevent readdiction have been for the most part by-products of research directed toward other goals, usually the preparation of new analgesics, and only recently has the preparation of narcotic antagonists specifically for this prophylactic treatment been undertaken.

We are preparing a series of compounds in both the cyclorphan and isocyclorphan series with new small-ring substituents on nitrogen and with cyclopropyl group and olefinic functions near the nitrogen atom. None of these substances has yet been tested for physiological activity.

REFERENCES

1. Ager, J. H., Fullerton, S. E., Fry, E. M., and May, E. L.: Structures related to morphine XXVI. Cyclization experiments with 2-benzyl-1,3,4-trialkyl-1,2,5,6-tetrahydropyridines. Improved yields of β-5,9-dialkyl-6,7-benzomorphans. J. Org. Chem. 28:2470–2472, 1963.
2. Archer, S., Albertson, N. F., Harris, L. S., Pierson, A. K., and Bird, J. G.: Pentazocine. Strong analgesics and analgesic antagonists in the benzomorphan series. J. Med. Chem. 7:123–127, 1964.
3. von Braun, J., Kuhn, M., and Siddiqui, S.: Ungesättigte Reste in chemischer and pharmakologischer Beziehung (V). Ber. 59:1081–1090, 1926.
4. Fullerton, S. E., May, E. L., and Becker, E. D.: Structures related to morphine XXIII. Stereochemistry of 5,9-dialkyl-6,7-bensomorphans. J. Org. Chem. 27:2144–2147, 1962.
5. Gates, M., and Montzka, T. A.: Some potent morphine antagonists possessing high analgesic activity. J. Med. Chem. 7:127–131, 1964.
6. Gates, M., and Webb, W. G.: The synthesis and resolution of 3-hydroxy-N-methylisomorphinan. J. Am. Chem. Soc. 80:1186–1194, 1958.
7. Grewe, R., and Mondon, A.: Synthesen in der Phenanthren-Reihe, VI: Synthese des morphinans. Ber. 81:279–286, 1948.
8. Henecka, H.: Neue synthesen in der morphinanreihe. Ann. Chem. 583:110–128, 1953.
9. Schnider, O., and Grussner, A.: Synthese von oxy-morphinanen. Helv. Chim. Acta. 32:821–828, 1949.
10. Winter, C. A., and Flataker, L.: Reaction thresholds to pressure in edematous hindpaws of rats and responses to analgesic drugs. J. Pharmacol. and Exptl. Ther. 150:165–171, 1965.

Narcotic Antagonists, edited by M. C. Braude, L. S. Harris, E. L. May, J. P. Smith, and J. E. Villarreal. *Advances in Biochemical Psychopharmacology, Vol. 8.* Raven Press, New York © 1974.

Synthetic 14-Hydroxymorphinan Narcotic Antagonists

Irwin J. Pachter

Bristol Laboratories, Syracuse, New York

As part of an extensive program at Bristol Laboratories devoted to the combat of narcotic abuse and addiction, we sought to prepare a narcotic antagonist which was fully synthetic, made from readily available starting materials, as potent parenterally as naloxone, as long-acting and orally active as cyclazocine, and free from undesirable side effects at therapeutic doses. Our efforts led to the synthesis of BC-2605 (structure I) which, on the basis of animal experiments, has the properties desired. Chemically, BC-2605 is D,L-N-cycloprophylmethyl-3,14-dihydroxymorphinan. It bears some structural similarities to other potent antagonists such as naloxone (II) and cyclazocine (III). A notable feature of BC-2605 is the 14-hydroxy group which is present in naloxone but not in any of the synthetic narcotic antagonists prepared up to this time.

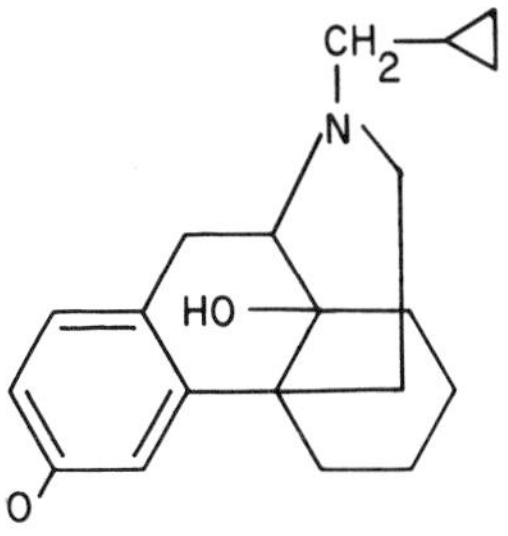

I 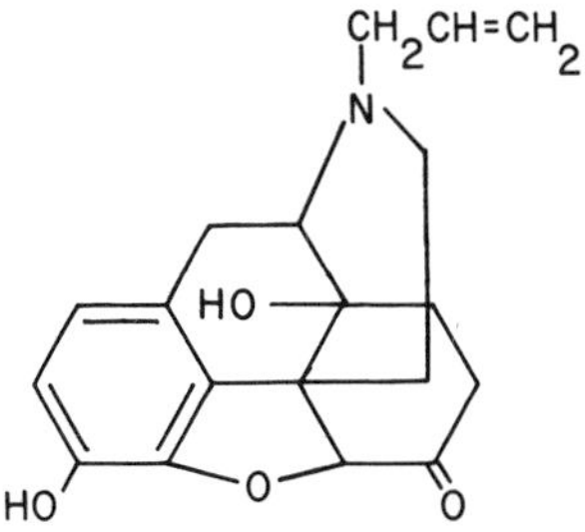   II 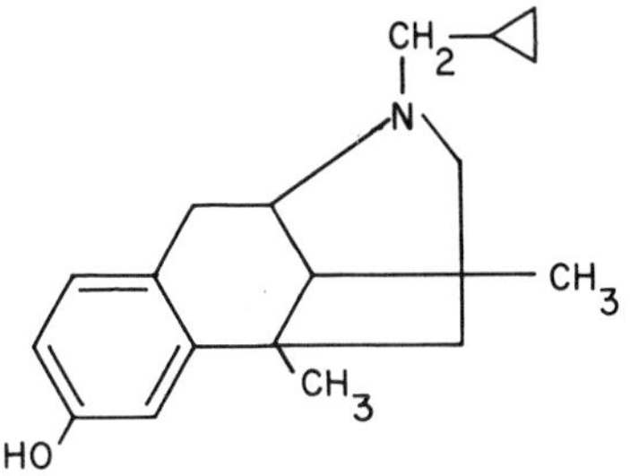   III

Resolution showed that all of the antagonist action resided in the levo isomer and, accordingly, clinical trials were initiated with L-BC 2605. Other analogues in the 14-hydroxymorphinan series proved to be potent analgetics and antitussives. The active compounds and their biological activity will be described.

In mid 1970 Bristol Laboratories began an extensive program devoted to the combat of narcotic abuse and addiction. As part of this program we sought narcotic antagonists which possessed more optimal combinations of potency, long action, and freedom from side effects than those currently available.

57

Four of the cleanest antagonists thus far evaluated in man are shown in Fig. 1. A feature common to these compounds is the 14-hydroxy group. This group appears to enhance potency and decrease disorienting side effects. Its presence, therefore, is an asset.

The four compounds are relatively short-acting in comparison to similar substances which lack the oxygen bridge. While the oxygen bridge is not a primary site of metabolism, it seems to promote metabolic deactivation at the 3-position. Its presence appears to be a liability and it should be eliminated.

In Fig. 2 are the structures of two morphinans synthesized by Professor Marshall Gates of the University of Rochester. One of these, cyclorphan, was evaluated in man. It was found to be an active analgetic but produced serious dysphoria. As an antagonist it was two to four times as potent as

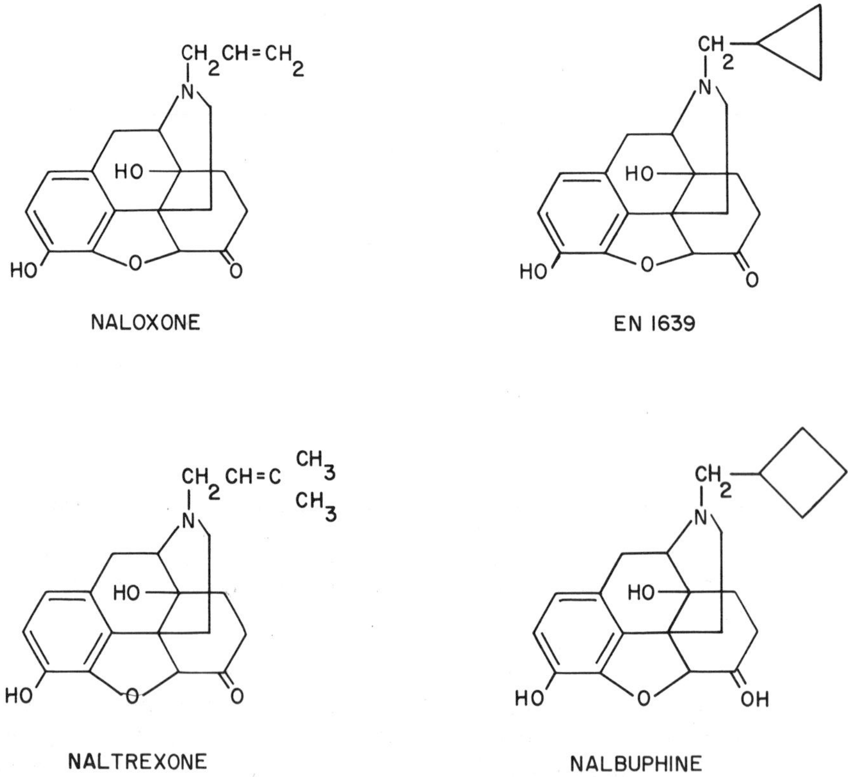

FIG. 1. Structures of four synthetic narcotic antagonists Common feature is 14-hydroxy group.

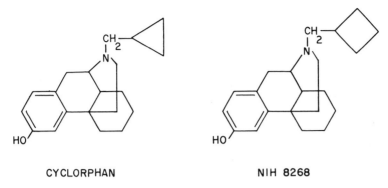

CYCLORPHAN   NIH 8268

FIG. 2. Structures of two morphinans synthesized at University of Rochester.

nalorphine; as an agonist, it was 11 times more potent than morphine. The other compound, NIH 8268, was not an antagonist at all. Instead it was found to be 40 times as potent as morphine in suppressing abstinence in monkeys.

It was interesting to determine the effect on pharmacology of the introduction of the 14-hydroxy group into these compounds. The synthesis of the products of Fig. 3 was accordingly undertaken. These substances lack the oxygen bridge and were expected to be very long-acting.

Their synthesis was achieved by the chemists of Bristol Laboratories of Canada. Time does not permit a description of the chemical reactions. (These were described by Dr. Ivo Monkovic at the Thirteenth National Medicinal Chemistry Symposium of the American Chemical Society at Iowa City, Iowa, on June 19, 1972.)

In Table 1 are some analgetic and narcotic antagonist data on the new

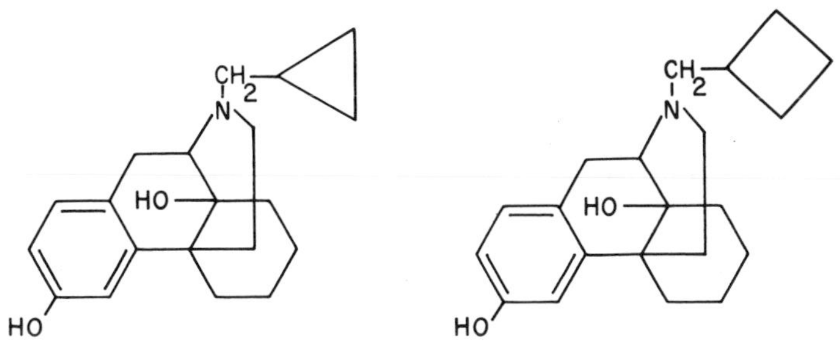

Levo-BC 2605   Levo-BC 2627

FIG. 3. Structures of two morphinans lacking oxygen bridge.

TABLE 1. *Analgetic and narcotic antagonist activity in the mouse and the rat*

Compound	ED_{50} (mg/kg, s.c.)	
	Analgetic activity (mouse writhing test)	Antagonist activity (morphine Antag.—R.T.F.)
L-BC-2605	12.8	0.012
L-BC-2627	0.051	0.43
Cyclazocine	0.047	0.040
Pentazocine	4.9	12.2
Naloxone	>80	0.010

compounds. L-BC 2605 was somewhere between naloxone and cyclazocine in narcotic antagonist potency. Its agonist effects were weak; its duration of action was very long. Bristol undertook Phase I evaluation in man and found the compound to have only about one-tenth the side effect liability of cyclazocine. Parenteral doses of 1 to 3 mg/day were well tolerated for a week.

I will present some of the data on L-BC 2605 derived from human studies at Lexington by Dr. Jasinski (*personal communication*). At Lexington, L-BC 2605 was found to have about one-eighth the side effect potential of cyclazocine and to be very long acting. Doses of 0.25 to 0.4 mg per patient precipitated withdrawal in morphine-addicted individuals. The effects lasted for over 24 hr and were not reversed by an injection of 60 mg of morphine. By contrast, the effects of a 0.4 mg dose of naloxone would have disappeared in approximately 3 hr. This illustrates a very important point: potency determinations without due consideration to duration of action are of little significance. Oral studies with L-BC 2605 are planned for the future. If comparisons can be made with cyclazocine, oral doses of 2.5 to 5.0 mg of L-BC 2605 should be enough to block the action of 25 mg of morphine or heroin for a day.

TABLE 2. *Antitussive activity in the guinea pig*

Compound	ED_{50} (mg/kg)	
	Subcutaneous (2 hr)	Oral (2 hr)
L-BC 2627	0.34	2.55
Pentazocine	43.70	—
Codeine	42.75	31.98
Morphine	3.80	10.00
Dextromethorphan	41.50	33.60

TABLE 3. *Subcutaneous antitussive activity in the dog*

	Average % inhibition	
Dose (mg/kg)	1 hr	2 hr
L-BC 2627		
0.10	100	82
0.02	73	70
0.005	39	19
Codeine		
4.0	98	95
2.0	72	33
1.0	4	10

The second compound shown in Fig. 3, L-BC 2627, was found to be a weak antagonist but a powerful analgetic, comparable to cyclazocine in potency and many times more active than pentazocine. More unusual than its analgetic action is its extraordinary antitussive effect; narcotic antagonists have not previously been reported to be antitussive. Assays involving electrical stimulation of wires implanted in tracheal tissue of guinea pigs and dogs have shown that L-BC 2627 is approximately 100 times more potent than codeine and dextromethorphan when administered subcutaneously (Tables 2 and 3). L-BC 2627 is also very potent orally (Table 2), although oral potency of narcotic antagonists in man is usually underestimated when based on animal data. Oral cyclazocine, for example, is far more potent in man than would have been predicted from potency estimates based on activity in rodents.

One of the stated objectives of the Government has been to find syn-

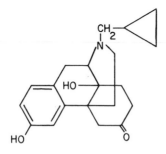

FIG. 4. Structure of the L-6-oxo analogue of BC 2605.

thetic replacements for opium and its derivatives. Compounds such as L-BC 2627 may go a long way toward meeting this objective since they are potential replacements for codeine, the major opium derivative of commercial use.

Among the morphinans, another compound stands out. This is the L-6-oxo analogue of BC 2605 shown in Fig. 4. It was first synthesized at the Shionogi Company in Japan. Lacking the oxygen bridge, this close relative of EN 1639 is very long acting and more potent than L-BC 2605, cyclazocine, or naloxone. It deserves to be developed for study in man.

Narcotic Antagonists, edited by M. C. Braude, L. S. Harris, E. L.
May, J. P. Smith, and J. E. Villarreal. *Advances in Biochemical
Psychopharmacology, Vol. 8.* Raven Press, New York © 1974.

Cyclazocine and Congeners

Noel F. Albertson

Sterling-Winthrop Research Institute, Rensselaer, New York 12144

The synthesis of cyclazocine, known chemically as 2RS,6RS, 11RS-3-
cyclopropylmethyl-1,2,3,4,5,6-hexahydro-*cis*-6,11-dimethyl-2,6-methano-
3-benzazocin-8-ol, was reported by Archer and co-workers in 1964. To
date, modification of 10 of the 11 ring positions in cyclazocine has been
achieved. In this chapter, some of the methods that have been reported in
the chemical and patent literature and employed in the author's laboratory
to modify the nonaromatic positions are described. The effect of structural
changes on antagonist activity is presented. In general, substitution at
positions one or four causes considerable decrease in activity whereas alkyl
substitution at positions five, six, or eleven has a lesser effect. Analgesic
and antagonist activity may be modified independently.

INTRODUCTION

The synthesis of cyclazocine, *1,* was reported by Archer and co-workers
in 1964 (6). Nor base *2* (18) was acylated and reduced or alkylated to
give 2RS,6RS,11RS-3-cyclopropylmethyl-1,2,3,4,5,6-hexahydro-*cis*-6,11-
dimethyl-2,6-methano-3-benzazocin-8-ol, *1,* (5).

Modification of 10 of the 11 ring positions in cyclazocine has been
achieved. In this chapter some of the methods of modifying the nonaromatic
portions of the molecule and their effects on narcotic antagonist activity
are described. Not all of these methods have been applied to the synthesis
of benzomorphans bearing antagonist side chains.

METHODS

Because of the versatility of the original synthesis, as well as the fact that
some newer methods are merely modifications of it, May's method of synthesis is outlined below.

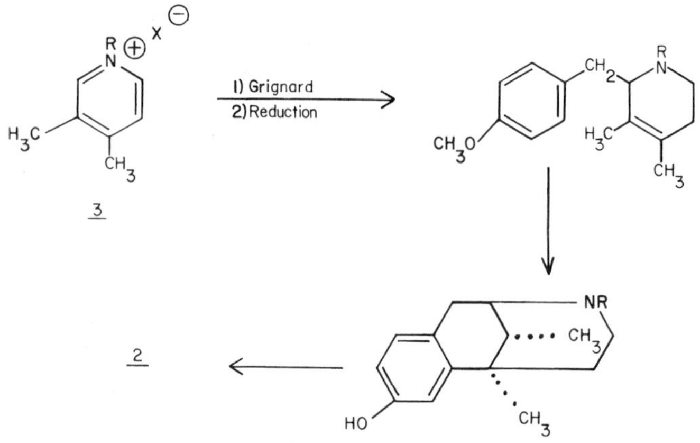

3,4-Lutidine methiodide (*3*, R = CH$_3$) is treated with the anisyl Grignard to give a dihydropyridine which is reduced to the tetrahydropyridine *4* (R = CH$_3$). Cyclization with HBr leads to *5* (R = CH$_3$) (21, 38, 39, 41).

The von Braun cyanogen bromide method was used for N-demethylation (18, 38, 40). The phenolic group was protected by acetylation. Hydrolysis of the N-cyano-O-acetyl intermediate gave nor base *2*.

Introduction of substituents into position one has recently been reported by Ziering and co-workers (70). They oxidized the methyl ether of *5* (R = CH$_3$) with chromium trioxide to introduce a ketone group giving 2SR,6RS,11RS-3,4,5,6-tetrahydro-8-methoxy-*cis*-3,6,11-trimethyl-2,6-methano-3-benzazocin-1(2H)-one, *6*, a compound that had been prepared some years ago in our laboratory.

Reaction of ketone *6* with phenyllithium afforded the phenyl carbinol. The 1RS,2SR,6RS,11RS configuration is in agreement with our independent work. The benzylic oxygen was removed catalytically to give a compound having a reported antagonist ED$_{50}$ of 1.1 mg/kg, s.c. Cleavage of the ether group decreased the antagonist activity of the resulting 1,2,3,4,5,6-hexahydro-3,6,11-trimethyl-1-phenyl-2,6-methano-3-benzazocin-8-ol to an ED$_{50}$ of 2.5. This result is the opposite of that observed when an antagonist side chain is present. The Ziering group did not report on any structures that would be expected to be potent antagonists; they limited themselves to N-methyl compounds.

Treatment of ketone *6* with methyllithium, dehydration to the *exo* methylene compound and reduction to the 1-methyl derivative gave a compound with a reported antagonist ED$_{50}$ of 6.25 mg/kg, s.c. (70). The intermediate compounds were inactive. Cleavage of the ether group increased the antagonist value to 0.6 mg/kg, s.c. This compound is surprisingly active as an antagonist for an N-methyl benzomorphan.

In our initial work leading to substitution at position one, the methyl ether of nor base *2* was oxidized with chromium trioxide to give the 2SR, 6RS, 11RS-3,4,5,6-tetrahydro-8-methoxy-*cis*-6,11-dimethyl-2,6-methano-3-benzazocin-1(2H)-one, *7*, in yields of 80 to 90% or better (45). Hydrolysis afforded 2SR,6RS,11RS-3,4,5,6-tetrahydro-8-hydroxy-*cis*-6,11-dimethyl-2,6-methano-3-benzazocin-1(2H)-one, *8*. Either nor base was readily alkylated. The ketone group could then be modified. Some biological test results are summarized in Table 1.

Chemical syntheses have provided some 1-substituted 2,6-methano-3-benzazocines which have not been used to make antagonists. For example, the following have been reported: 1,2,5,6-tetrahydro-5-cyano-2-hydroxy-1, 1-dimethyl-2,6-methano-3-benzazocin-4(3H)-one (58); 2,3,5,6-tetrahydro-

TABLE 1. *Change in* R_1

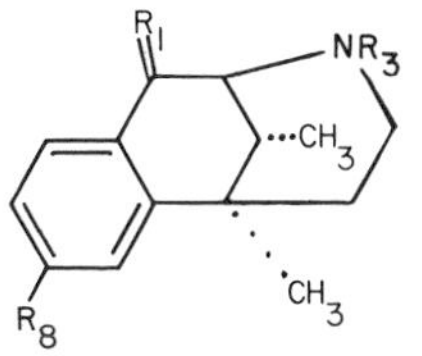

		Antagonist AD$_{50}$ s.c.		
R_3	R_8	$R_1 = H_2$	$R_1 = O$	$R_1 = $ eq OH, H
H	OH	11	1.15	
"	MeO		>80	
CH$_3$	OH	>10	29	
n—C$_3$H$_7$	"	0.019	1.8	
CH$_2$CH=CH$_2$	MeO		ca. 40	37
"	OH	0.047	1.6	0.98
CH$_2$—△	H	0.66	NDR	
"	MeO	0.146	48	
"	OH	0.019	2.0	11 flat
"	OAc	0.012	3.0	
CH$_2$CH=CMe$_2$	OH	3.9	>80	
CH$_2$—△ (trans) cis 6-Et-11-Me	"	0.014	2.8	
CH$_2$—△ trans 6-Et-11-Me	OH	0.024	NDR	
CH$_2$—△ 6-Et-des-11-Me	OH	0.014	4.2	
CH$_2$—△	OH	0.21	14	

3-methyl-6R-2,6-methano-3-benzazocin-1,4-dione where R is methyl (48) or phenyl (61); 3,4,5,6-tetrahydro-3,6-dimethyl-2,6-methano-3-benzazocin-1(2H)-one (44); 3,4,5,6-tetrahydro-6-cyano-3-methyl-2,6-methano-3-benzazocin-1(2H)-one (33) and the corresponding 6-phenyl compound (49); 3,4,5,6-tetrahydro-3-methyl-2,6-methano-3-benzazocin-1 (2H)-one (29); and 3,4,5,6-tetrahydro-3-methyl-2,6-methano-3-benzazocin-1(2H)-one oxime and 1-acetamido-1,2,3,4,5,6-tetrahydro-3-methyl-2,6-methano-3-benzazocine (59).

No antagonists modified at position two have been reported although a nor base bearing a 2-OH group has been described (58).

The simplest position to modify is position three if the nor base is available. The von Braun method for converting the N-methyl benzomorphan to the nor base has already been mentioned. Diethyl azodicarboxylate proved superior to cyanogen bromide in the case of a nonquaternary benzomorphan (29), and alkyl chloroformates have been used in some cases by the Geigy group (10). The resulting urethane group is not always easy to remove.

The N-methyl compound may be refluxed with an acid chloride to give an amide and methyl chloride. For example, refluxing the acetoxy derivative of 1,2,3,4,5,6-hexahydro-*cis*-3,6,11-trimethyl-2,6-methano-3-benzazocin-8-ol with cyclopropylcarbonyl chloride in toluene gives the 3-cyclopropylcarbonyl derivative. Reduction with diisobutylaluminum hydride gives cyclazocine (46).

An alternative approach to the nor base was investigated in this laboratory some time ago. This consisted of replacing the methyl iodide in the May synthesis with benzyl chloride so that R in formulas *3, 4,* and *5* became $CH_2C_6H_5$. This permitted the removal of R by catalytic hydrogenation (4). The overall yield of nor base by this method is now more than twice that of the original May procedure. This same procedure was recently published by Kametani and co-workers (28).

One variation based on the N-benzyl benzomorphan involves quaternization with an alkyl halide such as cyclopropylmethyl chloride. Treatment of the quaternary with sodium thiophenoxide preferentially cleaves the benzyl group to leave the cyclopropylmethyl on the nitrogen. Cyclazocine has been made in this manner (31). In a related scheme, R in *3, 4,* and *5* is 1-naphthylethyl. This group is removed after quaternization by heat or base (52).

In another modification, compound *4* ($R{=}CH_2C_6H_5$) was hydrogenated to the nor base and then formylated. Reduction of the basicity of the nitrogen enabled the cyclization step to be performed under milder conditions than with the N-alkyl intermediate (35). The ratio of β to α isomer increased by this procedure; i.e., more *trans* dimethyl product is obtained than with the N-benzyl (67).

The use of anisyl chloride in place of benzyl chloride for the preparation of *3* has been reported (36).

The desired N-alkyl side chain may be introduced at the first step if it will survive the remaining operations. This method was introduced by Ager and May (2) who used it to prepare the first antagonist in the benzomorphan area, namely, 5 (R=CH$_2$CH$_2$CH$_3$). The activity of this compound as an antagonist was pointed out by Archer (6). The use of allyl, crotyl, or dimethylallyl halides to quaternize 3,4-lutidine to give *3* (R=alkenyl) which is converted to *4* and *5* with phosphoric acid has been reported (8, 9, *cf.* 23). The yields are not given for the hydroxy benzomorphans, and the method is not useful for the synthesis of pentazocine in spite of the patent claims.

The cyclopropylmethyl and *cis*-3-chloroallyl side chains proved to be the most potent. Compounds with an allylic side chain which is part of a five- (3) or six- (14) membered ring, either *exo* or *endo*, are relatively weak as antagonists. Data for various 3-substituted 2,6-methano-3-benzazocines appear in Table 2.

The simplest synthesis of 4-substituted 2,6-methano-3-benzazocines makes use of the May synthesis in which the desired 4-substituent appears in the 6-position of the starting pyridine. Parfitt and Walters (50) prepared 2RS, 4SR, 6RS-3-cyclopropylmethyl-1,2,3,4,5,6-hexahydro-4,6-dimethyl-2, 6-methano-3-benzazocines by this procedure. They reported that this compound did not suppress the abstinence syndrome of morphine-dependent monkeys. In our laboratory it was found that introduction of a 4-methyl group into cyclazocine (by a different synthetic route) reduced antagonist activity more than 4,000-fold. A larger group at position four caused a lesser, but still substantial, decrease in activity (67). Toxicity was increased.

Robinson and Anderson (54) report the synthesis of 3-cyclopropyl-methyl-4-ethyl-1,2,3,4,5,6-hexahydro-6-methyl-2,6-methano-3-benzazocin-8-ol and 1,2,3,4,5,6-hexahydro-4,6-dimethyl-3-methylenecyclopropyl-methyl-2,6-methano-3-benzazocin-8-ol, but give no antagonist data beyond the statement that "benzomorphan derivatives of this invention in general have been found to show little or no antagonist activity." Some of these compounds were prepared by a Steven's rearrangement, a method first used by Fry and May in benzomorphan work (19).

A patent (53) by the same inventors covering 4,6,11-trialkyl substitution of the 2,6-methano-3-benzazocin-8-ol nucleus also claims little or no antagonist activity in agreement with our results.

4-Dehydro-2,6-methano-3-benzazocines have been synthesized (37).

TABLE 2. *Changes in R_3 of 2,6-methano-3-benzazocin-8-ol*

No.	R_3	AD_{50}
	$R_1 = H_2$; $R_6 = R_{11} = $ cis-CH_3	
1	H	11
2	CH_3	>10
3	n—C_3H_7	0.019
4	$CH_2CH{=}CH_2$	0.047
5	$CH_2C{\equiv}CH$	0.078
6	$CH_2CH{=}CHCl$ (*cis*)	0.018
7	" (*trans*)	0.039
8	$CH_2CH{=}CCl_2$	5.1
9	$CH_2C(Cl){=}CH_2$	4.2
10	$CH_2CH(CH_3){=}CH_2$	0.094
11	$CH_2CH{=}CMe_2$	3.9
12	$CH_2C(CH_3){=}CMe_2$	0.62
13	c—C_5H_9	0.150
14	CH_2CN	17
15	CH_2—c—C_3H_5	0.019
16	CH_2—c—C_4H_7	0.37
17	CH_2—c—C_5H_9	0.28
18	CH_2—c—C_6H_{11}	14.5
19	—c—C_5H_9	0.150
20	2-cyclopenten-1-yl	2.7
21	1-cyclopentenylmethyl	0.17 flat
22	D-*trans*-2-methylcyclopropylmethyl	0.15
23	L-*trans*-2-methylcyclopropylmethyl	0.026
24	CH_2CH_2—c—C_3H_5	0.092
25	$CH_2CH_2COCH_3$	1.7
26	CH_2C—CH_3 (with O O epoxide: CH_2——CH_2)	0.07
27	$CH_2CH{=}C(CH_3)Cl(Z)$	0.48
28	$CH_2CH{=}C(CH_3)Cl(E)$	1.4
29	$CH_2C(CH_3){=}C(CH_3)Br$	Inact.
	$R_1 = O$; $R_6 = R_{11} = $ cis-CH_3	
30	H	1.15
31	$CH_2CH{=}CH_2$	1.6
32	CH_2—c—C_3H_5	2.0
33	$CH_2CH_2CH_3$	1.8
34	$CH_2CH{=}CMe_2$	>80
35	CH_3	29
	$R_1 = O$; $R_6 = $ Et; $R = CH_3$ (*cis*)	
36	CH_2—c—C_3H_5	NDR

Substitution at position five has been accomplished by Fry (17).[1] Sodium borohydride reduction of a 4-alkyl or 3,4-dialkylpyridine quaternary salt in the presence of cyanide ions gives a tetrahydropyridine bearing a 6-cyano group. This group is readily replaced by a Grignard reagent. Upon cyclization, the 3-substituent of the pyridine ring becomes the 5-substituent in the 2,6-methano-3-benzazocine ring. The original work described the preparation of 1,2,3,4,5,6-hexahydro-3,5,6-trimethyl-2,6-methano-3-benzazocine. No antagonist side chains were prepared.

Parfitt and Walters (50) prepared 3-cyclopropylmethyl-1,2,3,4,5,6-hexahydro-5,6-dimethyl-2,6-methano-3-benzazocine, but no antagonist data were given. Actually, this compound had already been prepared in our laboratory; data for this and some related compounds appear in Table 3.

TABLE 3. *Changes in* R_4

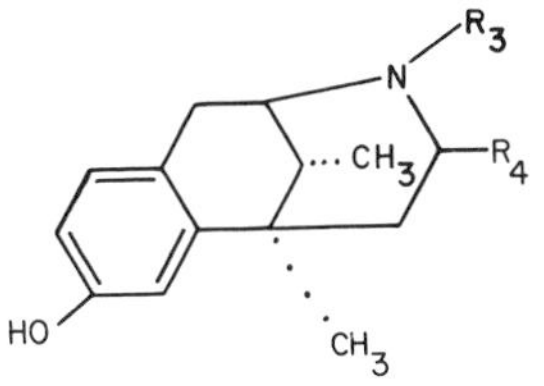

R_3	R_4	Antag. AD_{50} s.c.
CH_3	H	>10
	CH_3	>80
$CH_2-c-C_3H_5$	H	0.019
	CH_3	>80

A recent paper by Thyagarajan and May (65) provides a new route to the intermediates needed for 5-substitution. Treatment of *9* with butyl lithium

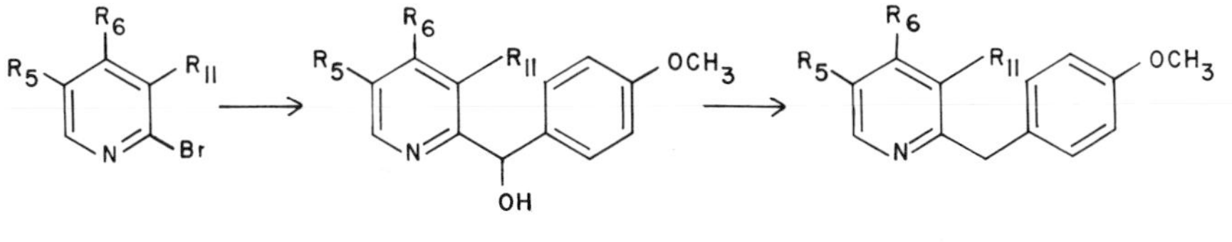

9   *10*   *11*

---

[1] Dr. B. F. Tullar supplied the author with nor bases of 5,6-dialkyl-2,6-methano-3-benzazocin-8-ols before the work of Fry appeared. However, this approach was laborious, and the Fry method has since been used in our laboratory.

followed by anisaldehyde gives *10*. This is reduced to *11*, quaternized, reduced with $NaBH_4$, and cyclized. R_5, R_6, and R_{11} of pyridine *9* become substituents in positions 5, 6, and 11 in the tricyclic methanobenzazocine.

Perry and Albertson had prepared *10* ($R_5 = H$; $R_6 = R_{11} = CH_3$) in very poor yield by the Emmert reaction between 3,4-lutidine, aluminum amalgam, and anisaldehyde, and also by oxidation of the analogous *11* (51).

A potential route to 5-substituted compounds is suggested by the synthesis of 1,2,5,6-tetrahydro-5-cyano-2-hydroxy-1,1-dimethyl-2,6-methano-3-benzazocin-4(3H)-one (58). However, the 1,1-dialkyl groups would be necessary for this approach. It is doubtful that any antagonists made in this area would be very potent.

One may note that 3-alkyl-1,2,3,4,5,6-hexahydro-2,6-methano-3-benzazocin-8-ols unsubstituted in the 11-position are light sensitive and very readily undergo photochemical oxidation to give colored products. Substitution of either the axial or equatorial hydrogen by alkyl or hydroxyl prevents this.

Variations in the 6-position of the 2,6-methano-3-benzazocine ring requires a variation in the 4-position of the starting pyridine if the May synthesis is employed. Introduction of simple alkyl groups into pyridine is readily accomplished by treating the appropriate pyridine with an acid anhydride and zinc. Thus, propionic anhydride introduces an n-propyl group, for example (7, 68, 69). Alkylation of 4-methylpyridine with $NaNH_2$ and an alkyl halide has also been used (13).

Another May synthesis of benzomorphans permits considerable variation in the substitution of positions 6 and 11 (42, 47, 56). However, the method is lengthy and suffers from low overall yields.

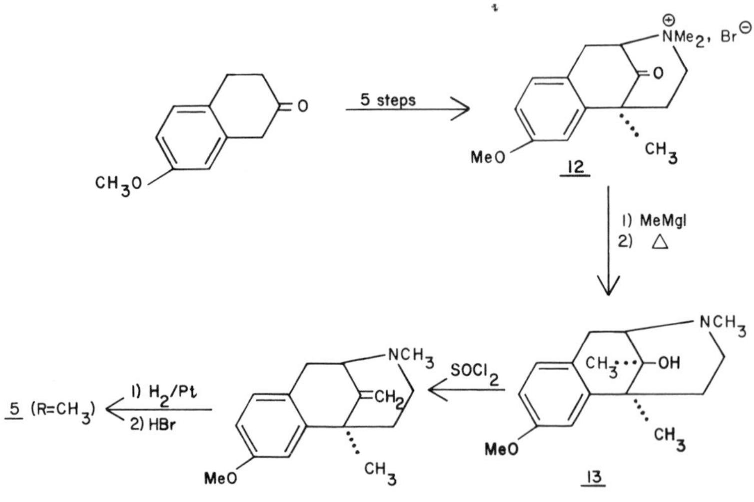

Stereochemical control of the addition to the ketone group of *12* is possible (32, 42, 43, 55).

Substitution of methyl ethyl ketone for cyclohexanone in the very elegant morphinane synthesis of Schnider and Hellerbach (57) should lead to a benzomorphan. The author tried this approach in 1959 but abandoned it after the first few steps. Henecka and Schubert were more persistent workers — by working with mixtures for several steps they succeeded in synthesizing *15* as a pair of epimers purified by chromatography (24).

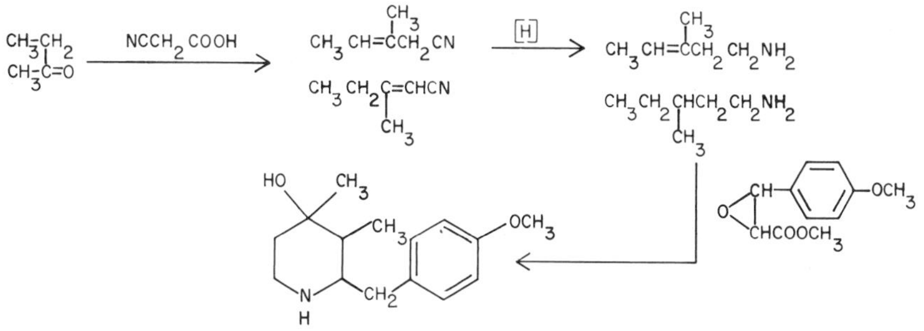

Cyclization afforded a benzomorphan. The same synthetic route has recently been reported by a Japanese group (27). This route has been applied to other ketones at S-WRI. One synthesis was successful and one failed because the double bond could not be kept in the right position.

Perhaps the greatest variations in position six are cited in a German patent issued to F. B. Block and F. H. Clarke (11), but yields are not given. However, Dr. Clarke will be detailing his own work in this area with particular reference to the 6-phenyl series.

An interesting variation in position six in 2,6-methano-3-benzazocines unsubstituted in position eleven started with 2-(*p*-methoxybenzyl)-1-methyl-4-piperidone, *16*, obtainable from the commercially available 4-methoxypyridine N-oxide in 18% overall yield by a procedure worked out at the NIH (60, 61). Takeda and May have cyclized *16* to obtain 1,2,3,4,5,6-hexahydro-3-methyl-2,6-methano-3-benzazocine-6,8-diol. This was inactive as an analgesic at 100 mg/kg, s.c. (63). The analogue in which the 6-OH was replaced by a 6-methyl had an ED_{50} of 3.0 mg/kg, s.c.

The previously mentioned 3,4,5,6-tetrahydro-6-cyano-3-methyl-2,6-methano-3-benzazocin-1(2H)-one (33) has been used to prepare 1-oxygenated-6-acyl-1,2,3,4,5,6-hexahydro-2,6-methano-3-benzazocines for use as analgesics (12).

Variations in the 11-position depend generally upon modifications in synthesis already described. At present there is one important difference between substitution at the 11-position and the 1, 4, or 5-position; in the former case it is possible to synthesize both axial and equatorial isomers, whereas in 1, 4, or 5-substitution only one isomer has been isolated in useful amounts.

Cyclization of tetrahydropyridine *4* gives mixtures of the α or *cis* and β or *trans* isomers of *5*. The relative amounts depend upon the nature of R and upon the cyclization conditions. A study of the latter parameter was made at the NIH (1). The use of aluminum bromide in carbon disulfide often leads to *trans* isomers where the use of HBr gives predominantly the *cis* isomer (25, 26). In our laboratory we noted that R = $CH_2C_6H_5$ gives less *trans* isomer than R = CH_3, whereas R = CHO gives more *trans*.

Jacobson and May (25) found that the alkyl groups on the pyridine ring also influence isomer ratio. No *trans* isomer could be detected upon cyclization of 2-benzyl-3,4-diethyl-1-methyl-1,2,5,6-tetrahydropyridine with hydrobromic acid even though the 3,4-dimethyl intermediate leads to a mixture of *cis* and *trans*.

The absolute configuration of the 11-substituent in the 6,11-dimethyl series was determined by rate of quaternization with methyl iodide and by nuclear magnetic resonance studies (20). The published spectral data are most helpful in assigning configurations to new compounds.

The usual synthesis of benzomorphan *5* starting from pyridinium quaternary *3* leads predominantly to the *cis* isomer. Fry has found that if the product of the Grignard reaction is isolated as a perchlorate salt it may be converted to either a *cis* or *trans* 2-benzyl-1,3,4-trimethyl-2,3-dihydropyridinium salt. Cyclization then leads to stereo-specific benzomorphan syntheses (17). This method has been used in the 6,11-diethyl series (25).

The β-tetralone synthesis referred to earlier (*cf.* 12), although suffering from low overall yields, has been used for stereospecific synthesis (15, 16, 32, 42, 43, 55, 56).

Diborane has been added to the desmethoxy analogue of *14* and the product oxidized with H_2O_2 to give 11-hydroxymethyl compound (34). Tanabe Seiyaku Co., Ltd. has a patent application covering this and related compounds (64).

Both the axial and equatorial 11-acetamido-1,2,3,4,5,6-hexahydro-3,6-dimethyl-2,6-methano-3-benzazocines have been prepared (59). The

17

requisite 11-keto compound was prepared from *17* by halogenation, hydrolysis, and treatment with base (62).

The chemistry of the 11,11-dialkyl-2,6-methano-3-benzazocines will be reviewed by Dr. Paul Janssen.

DISCUSSION

Biological data are summarized in the accompanying tables for some of the compounds prepared at Sterling-Winthrop Research Institute. Antagonist data were obtained by the tail-flick procedure (22) in Mrs. Pierson's laboratory.

Table 1 indicates that introduction of a keto or equatorial hydroxyl group into position one invariably reduces antagonist activity when an antagonist side chain is present. Comparison of the first two compounds shows that such a change increased the activity of the nor base. It is interesting to note that 3-cyclopropylmethyl-6-ethyl-3,4,5,6-tetrahydro-8-hydroxy-11-methyl-2,6-methano-3-benzazocin-1(2H)-one, showing no dose response as an antagonist, has an agonist ED_{50} of 0.044 mg/kg, s.c., in the acetylcholine writhing test compared to a value of 0.15 for cyclazocine.

TABLE 4. *Changes in* R_5

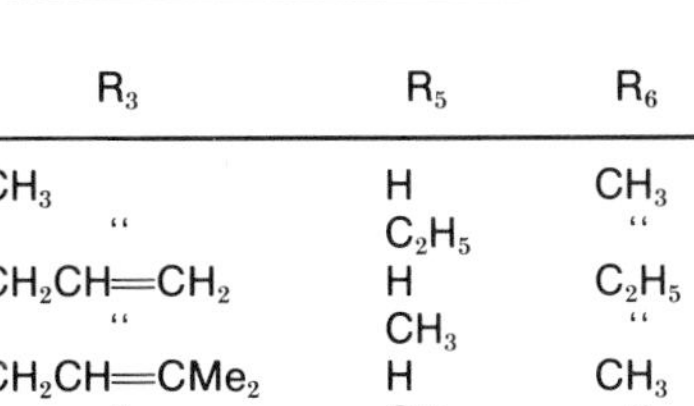

R_8	R_3	R_5	R_6	Antag. AD_{50} s.c.
$R_8 = OH$	CH_3	H	CH_3	18
	"	C_2H_5	"	9.0
	$CH_2CH{=}CH_2$	H	C_2H_5	0.032
	"	CH_3	"	0.037
	$CH_2CH{=}CMe_2$	H	CH_3	1.05
	"	CH_3	"	2.8
$R_8 = H$	$CH_2CH{=}CH_2$	H	CH_3	0.11
	"	CH_3	"	5.2
	$CH_2{-}c{-}C_3H_5$	H	"	0.026
	"	CH_3	"	0.52

Table 2 shows that maximum activity is obtained with a cyclopropyl-methyl or *cis*-3-chloroallyl side chain on nitrogen. Other three carbon side chains, including the 2-propanone cyclic ethylene ketal, *28,* are almost as active. The substitution of a terminal chlorine on the allyl group (*6* and *7*) increases activity, but a single chlorine in the 2-position (*9*) or two chlorines in the terminal position (*8*) greatly reduce activity. A 2-methyl group is less harmful (*10*). Enlarging the cyclopropane ring decreased activity (*15* to *18*).

TABLE 5. *Changes in* R_6

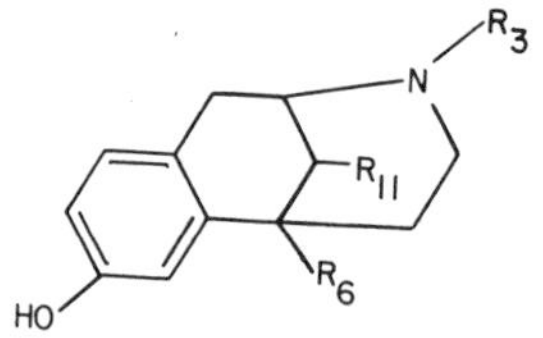

R_{11}	R_3	R_6	Antag. AD_{50} s.c.
H	CH_2—△	H	0.036
	"	CH_3	0.026
	"	C_2H_5	0.021
	"	n—C_3H_7	0.027
	$CH_2CH=CH_2$	CH_3	0.110
	"	C_2H_5	0.032
	"	n—C_3H_7	0.014
CH_3	"	CH_3	0.047
	"	C_2H_5	0.049
	"	n—C_3H_7	0.011
	$CH_2CH=CHCl(cis)$	CH_3	0.018
	"	n—C_3H_7	0.017
	$CH_2CH=CCl_2$	CH_3	5.1
	"	C_2H_5	>20
	$CH_2C\equiv CH$	CH_3	0.078
	"	C_2H_5	0.071
	CH_2—c—C_3H_5	CH_3	0.019
	"	C_2H_5	0.024
	"	n—C_3H_7	0.009
	CH_2—c—C_4H_7	CH_3	0.37
	"	C_2H_5	0.45
	$CH_2CH_2COCH_3$	CH_3	1.7
	"	C_2H_5	26 i.p.
	$CH_2CH=Me_2$	CH_3	3.9
	"	C_2H_5	10.9

The very limited data of Table 3 suggests that a substituent in the 4-position is undesirable.

Table 4 suggests that introduction of a small alkyl group at the 5-position has a relatively minor effect on antagonist activity in the 8-hydroxy series. In the desoxy series, activity is decreased at least 20-fold by a 5-methyl group.

Introduction of a small alkyl group into position six or eleven has little effect on antagonist activity as noted in Tables 5 and 6. The first compound in Table 6 shows that a quaternary carbon is not needed for activity.

The 6,11-*trans* isomers generally show greater activity than the *cis* isomers as agonists (Table 7). There is relatively little difference between the *cis* and *trans* isomers as antagonists. The active isomer of cyclazocine has the 2R,6R,11R configuration (30).

TABLE 6. *Change in* R_{11}

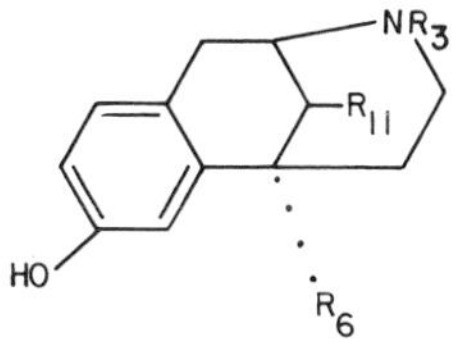

cis− *trans*	R_6	R_{11}	R_3	Antag. AD_{50} s.c.
−	H	H	CH_2—c—C_3H_5	0.036
−	CH_3	"	"	0.026
c	"	CH_3	"	0.019
c	"	C_2H_5	"	0.005
−	"	H	$CH_2CH=CH_2$	0.110
c	"	CH_3	"	0.047
−	C_2H_5	H	"	0.032
c	"	CH_3	"	0.049
−	CH_3	H	$CH_2C(CH_3)=CH_2$	0.55
c	"	CH_3	"	0.094
−	"	H	2-cyclopentenylmethyl	>20
c	"	CH_3	"	0.17 flat
−	"	H	$CH_2CH=CMe_2$	1.1
c	"	CH_3	"	3.9
Same with R_1 = carbonyl				
−	C_2H_5	H	CH_2—c—C_3H_5	14
c	"	CH_3	"	NDR
t	"	"	"	4.2
c	"	C_2H_5	"	>80

TABLE 7. *6,11*-cis *versus* *6,11*-trans $(R_6 = R_{11} = CH_3; R_8 = OH)$

	Antag. AD_{50} s.c.	
R_3	*cis*	*trans*
$CH_2CH_2CH_3$	0.019	0.056
$CH_2CH=CH_3$	0.047	0.019
$CH_2-c-C_3H_5$	0.019	0.014
$CH_2-c-C_4H_7$	0.37	0.060
$CH_2-c-C_5H_9$	0.28	0.92
1-Cyclopentenylmethyl	0.17 flat	1.6
$CH_2CH=CHCl(cis)$	0.18	0.047
$CH_2C(CH_3) = CH_2$	0.094	1.1
$CH_2CH = CMe_2$	3.9	3.3
$Ch_2-C-C_3H_5{}^a$	0.024	0.014

$^a R_6 = C_2H_5$

CONCLUSIONS

In general, substitution at positions one or four causes considerable decrease in antagonist activity whereas the introduction of alkyl substituents at positions five, six, or eleven has a lesser effect. Differences in antagonist activity between *cis* and *trans* 6,11-dialkyl-2,6-methano-3-benzazocin-8-ols are very minor. Agonist and antagonist activity may be modified independently. A quaternary carbon is not necessary for potent antagonist activity.

ACKNOWLEDGMENTS

The work in the benzomorphan area was undertaken at Dr. Archer's suggestion and he directed much of this work. Mrs. Pierson supplied biological data, and Dr. Tullar and his group made available many intermediates. We had helpful discussions with Dr. L. Harris during his tenure at S-WRI. Laboratory assistance was provided by F. C. McKay, W. F. Michne, E. D. Parady, R. L. Perry, R. L. Salsbury, and M. P. Wentland. To each we are grateful.

REFERENCES

1. Ager, J. H., Fullerton, S. E., Fry, E. M., and May, E. L.: Structures related to morphine. XXVI. Cyclization experiments with 2-benzyl-1,3,4-trialkyl-1,2,5,6-tetrahydropyri-

dines. Improved yields of β-5,9-dialkyl-6,7-benzomorphans. J. Org. Chem. *28*:2470–2472, 1963.

2. Ager, J. H., and May, E. L.: Structures related to morphine. XIII. 2-Alkyl-2'-hydroxy-5,9-dimethyl-6,7-benzomorphans and a more direct synthesis of the 2-phenethyl compound (NIH 7519). J. Org. Chem. *25*:984–986, 1960.

3. Albertson, N. F., and Archer, S.: U.S. Pat. 3,632,591 (to Sterling Drug Inc.).

4. Albertson, N. F., and Wetterau, W. F.: The synthesis of pentazocine. J. Med. Chem. *13*:302–303, 1970. Belg. Pat. 719, 408; Can. Pat. 855,699 (to Sterling Drug Inc.)

5. Archer, S.: U.S. Pat. 3,372,165 (to Sterling Drug Inc.).

6. Archer, S., Albertson, N. F., Harris, L. S., Pierson, A. K., and Bird, J. G.: Pentazocine. Strong analgesics and analgesic antagonists in the benzomorphan series. J. Med. Chem. *7*:123–127, 1964.

7. Arens, J. F. and Wibaut, J. P.: Eine neue Methode zur Einfuhrung von Alkylgruppen in die 4-Stelle im Pyridinmolekul 50 Mitteilung uber der Derivate von Pyridin und Chinolin. Rec. Trav. Chim. *61*:59–68, 1942.

8. Atami, T.: Jap. Pat. 27748/71 and 27751/71 (to Sumitomo).

9. Atsumi, T., Kobayashi, Y., Takebayashi, Y., and Yamamoto, H.: Brit. Pat. 1,263,372; Ger. Pat. 1,927,724; U.S. Pat. 3,631,051 (to Sumitomo).

10. Australian Pat. 285,463; Brit. Pat. 1,092,394; Can. Pat. 795,345 (to Geigy Chemical Corp.).

11. Block, F. B., and Clarke, F. H.: Can. Pat. 797,849; cf. U.S. Pat. 3,480,638 (to Geigy Chemical Corp.).

12. Block, F. B., and Schroder, A. H.: U.S. Pat. 3,687,957 (to Geigy Chemical Corp.).

13. Brown, H. C., and Murphy, W.: A convenient synthesis of monoalkylpyridines; a new prototropic reaction of 3-picoline. J. Am. Chem. Soc. *73*:3308–3312, 1951.

14. B.S.M. 7523M; Neth. Applic. 6716638 (to Boehringer Sohn.).

15. Chignell, C., Ager, J. H., and May, E. L.: Structures related to morphine XXVIII. Alternative synthesis of α- and β-2,9-dimethyl-2'-hydroxy-5-propyl-6,7-benzomorphan. J. Med. Chem. *8*:235–238, 1964.

16. Chignell, C., and May, E. L.: Structures related to morphine. XXIX. Further experiments on the stereo-controlled reduction of 9-methylene-6,7-benzomorphans. J. Med. Chem. *8*:385–386, 1964.

17. Fry, E. M.: Stereospecific tautomerism in a 1,2-dihydropyridine. A β-benzomorphan synthesis. J. Org. Chem. *28*:1869–1874, 1963. 6-Cyano-1,2,5,6-tetrahydropyridines in the preparation of 1,2-dihydropyridines. Tautomerism of the dienes. Ibid. *29*:1647–1650, 1964.

18. Fry, E. M., and May, E. L.: Mannich derivatives of analgesic agents. J. Org. Chem. *24*:116–117, 1959.

19. Fry, E. M., and May, E. L.: The Stevens rearrangement in the benzomorphan synthesis. J. Org. Chem. *26*:2592–2594, 1961.

20. Fullerton, S. E., May, E. L. and Becker, E. D.: Structures related to morphine. XXIII. Stereochemistry of 5,9-dialkyl-6,7-benzomorphans. J. Org. Chem. *27*:2144–2147, 1962.

21. Gordon, M., and Lafferty, J.: U.S. Pat. 2,959,594 (to Smith, Kline and French).

22. Harris, L. S., and Pierson, A. K.; Some narcotic antagonists in the benzomorphan series. J. Pharmacol. Exp. Ther. *143*:141–148, 1964.

23. Hellerbach, J., Grussner, A., and Schnider, O.: Hydroxy-morphinane. (—)-3-Hydroxy-N-allyl-morphinan und verwandte Verbindungen. Helv. Chim. Acta *39*:429–440, 1956.

24. Henecka, H., and Schubert, H.: Brit. Pat. 1,078,286. For the cyclization step see French Pat. 1,484,542 or Can. Pat. 841,616 (all to Farb. Bayer AK.).

25. Jacobson, A. E. and May, E. L.: Structures related to morphine. XXVII. α- and β-5,9-diethyl-2-methyl-6,7-benzomorphans. J. Med. Chem. *7*:409–412, 1964.

26. Joshi, B., and May, E. L.: Structures related to morphine. XXXII. α- and β-2,9-dimethyl-5-propyl-6,7-benzomorphan from 3-methyl-4-propylpyridine. J. Med. Chem. *8*:696–697, 1965.

27. Kametani, T., Kigasawa, K., Hayasaka, M. Wakisaka, K., Satoh, F., Aoyama, T., and

Ishimaru, H.: Syntheses of benzomorphans and related compounds. Part III. An alternative synthesis of 3-substituted -1,2,3,4,5,6-hexahydro-8-hydroxy-2,6-methano-6,11-dimethyl-3-benzazocine. J. Heterocyclic Chem. 8:769–771, 1971.

28. Kametani, T., Kigasawa, K., Hiiragi, M., Hayasaka, T., Wagatsuma, N., and Wakisaka, K.: Syntheses of benzomorphan and related compounds. Part I. Synthesis of N-substituted -1,2,3,4,5,6-hexahydro-8-hydroxy-2,6-methano-6,11-dimethyl-3-benzazocine. J. Heterocyclic Chem. 6:43–48, 1969.

29. Kanematsu, K., Takeda, M., Jacobson, A. and May, E. L.: Synthesis of 6,7-benzomorphan and related nonquaternary carbon structures with marked analgetic activity. J. Med. Chem. 12:405–408, 1969.

30. Karle, I. L., Gilardi, R. D., Fratini, A. V., and Karle, J.: Crystal Structures of Dl-cyclazocine and L-cyclazocine, HBr. H₂O and the absolute configuration of L-cyclazocine. HBr. H₂O (2-cyclopropylmethyl-2'-hydroxy-5,9-dimethyl-6,7-benzomorphan). Acta Crystallogr., Sect. B, 25:1469–1479, 1969.

31. Kigasawa, K., Hiiragi, M., Wagatsuma, N., and Kusama, O.,: U.S. Pat. 3,644,373; French Pat. 2,025,561; Brit. Pat. 1,246,192 (to Grelan Pharmaceutical Co.).

32. Kugita, J., and May, E. L.: Structures related to morphine. XVI. Stereochemical chemical control of addition of hydrogen to 9-oxobenzomorphans. J. Org. Chem. 26:1954–1957, 1961.

33. Kugita, H., Saito, S., and May, E. L.: Structures related to morphine. XXII. A Benzomorphan congener of meperidine. J. Med. Chem. 5:357–361, 1962.

34. Kugita, J., and Takeda, M.: Synthesis of morphin-like structures. I. 9-Hydroxy-methyl-2,5-dimethyl-6,7-benzomorphan. Chem. Pharm. Bull. Japan 11:986–989, 1963. II. 2'-Methoxy-9-hydroxymethyl-2,5-dimethyl-6,7-benzomorphan. Ibid., 12:1163–1166, 1964.

35. Leimgruber, W., and Mohacsi, E.: Belg. Pat. 726,427; Can. Pat. 874,969; Brit. Pat. 1,198,750; Swiss Pat. 513,863 (to Hoffman-LaRoche).

36. Leimgruber, W., and Ziering, A.: U.S. Pat. 3,546,239 (to Hoffmann-LaRoche).

37. Lewis, J. W.: Brit. Pat. 1,224,918 (to Reckitt and Coleman Prods.).

38. May, E. L.: U.S. Pat. 3,138,603 (to U.S.A.).

39. May, E. L., and Ager, J. H.: Structures related to morphine. XI. Analogs and a diastereoisomer of 2'-hydroxy-2,5,9-trimethyl-6,7-benzomorphan. J. Org. Chem. 24:1432–1435, 1959.

40. May, E. L., and Eddy, N.: A new potent synthetic analgesic. J. Org. Chem. 24:294–295, 1959.

41. May, E. L., and Fry, E. M. Structures related to morphine. VIII. Further synthesis in the benzomorphan series. J. Org. Chem. 22:1366–1369, 1957.

42. May, E. L., and Kugita, J.: Structures related to morphine. XV. Stereochemical control of methyl-metallo additions to 9-oxobenzomorphans. J. Org. Chem. 26:188–193, 1961.

43. May, E. L., Kugita, H., and Ager, J. H.: Structures related to morphine. XVII. Further stereochemical studies with 9-oxobenzomorphans. J. Org. Chem. 26:1621–1624, 1961.

44. May, E. L., and Murphy, J. G.: Structures related to morphine. III. Synthesis of an analog of N-methylmorphinan. J. Org. Chem. 20:257–263, 1955.

45. Michne, W. F., and Albertson, N. F.: Analgetic 1-oxidized-2,6-methano-3-benzazocines. J. Med. Chem. 15:1278–1281, 1972. Belg. Pat. 768,084 (to Sterling Drug Inc.).

46. Moriyama, H., Yamamoto, J., Nagata, J., and Tamaki, T.: U.S. Pat. 3,634,433 (to Sumitomo Chem. Co., Ltd.).

47. Murphy, J. G., Ager, J. H., and May, E. L.: Structures related to morphine. XIV. 2'-Hydroxy-5-methyl-2-phenethyl-6,7-benzomorphan, the 9-demethyl analog of NIH 7519 (Phenazocine) from 3,4-dihydroxy-7-methoxy-2(1H) naphthalenone. J. Org. Chem. 25:1386–1388, 1960.

48. Nelson, W. L., and Nelson, K. F.: Cyclic lactams. II. 1,7-Dimethyl-2,3-benzo-7-azabicyclo[4.3.0]nonane-4,8-dione and 3,6-dimethyl-1,2,3,4,5,6-hexahydro-2,6-methano-3-benzazocine-1,4-dione from 4-methyl-1-tetralone-4-acetic acid. J. Org. Chem. 36:607–609, 1971.

49. Netherlands Pat. Applic. 6606056 (to Geigy Chem. Corp.).
50. Parfitt, R., and Walters, S.: Synthesis and analgetic activity of 3- and 4-methyl-6,7-benzo-morphans. J. Med. Chem. *14*:565–568, 1971.
51. Perry, R. L., and Albertson, N. F. Unpublished observations.
52. Petersen, J., and Ross-Petersen, K.: Ger. Pat. Applic. 2,057,115; Neth. Pat. Applic. 7016907 (to Aktieselkabet Grindstedvaerket).
53. Robinson, F., and Anderson, P.: Brit. Pat. 1,261,481 (to Merck and Co.).
54. Robinson, F., and Anderson, P.: Brit. Pat. 1.261,693 (to Merck and Co.).
55. Saito, S., and May, E. L.: Structures related to morphine. XVIII. Stereocontrol of addition of hydrogen and methyl-metallo reagents to 5-ethyl-2-methyl-9-oxo-6,7-benzomorphan. J. Org. Chem. *26*:4536–4540, 1961.
56. Saito, S., and May, E. L.: Structures related to morphine. XXI. An alternative synthesis of diastereoisomeric 2'-hydroxy-2,5,9-trimethyl-6,7-benzomorphan. J. Org. Chem. *27*:1087–1089, 1962.
57. Schnider, O., and Hellerbach, K.: Synthese von Morphinanen. Helv. Chim. Acta *33*:1437–1448, 1950.
58. Shelver, W., and Rao, N. G.: The synthesis of potential analgesics. Diss. Abstr. *28*, 2364B–2365B, 1967.
59. Shiotami, S., and Mitsuhashi, K.: Structure-activity relation of analgesics. XII. Syntheses of acetamidoazabenzobicyclo[3.3.1]nonanes. Yakugaku Zasshi *92*:97–100, 1972.
60. Takeda, M., Jacobson, A. E., Kanematsu, K., and May, E. L.: 4-Methoxy-1-methyl-pyridinium iodide. Grignard products and transformations thereof. J. Org. Chem. *34*:4154–4157, 1969.
61. Takeda, M., Jacobson, A. E., and May, E. L.: 4-Methoxy-1-methylpyridinium iodide. Stevens rearrangement of borohydride reduction product. J. Org. Chem. *34*:4158–4160, 1969.
62. Takeda, M., and Kugita, H.: Jap. Pat. 7121026 (to Tanabe Seiyaku Co. Ltd.).
63. Takeda, M., and May, E. L.: Acyl derivatives of 5-hydroxy-6,7-benzomorphans. Prodine congeners. J. Med. Chem. *13*:1223–1224, 1970.
64. Tanabe Seiyako Co. Ltd.: Jap. Pat. Applic. 217/65. Derwent Japanese Patents Report Vol. 4, Nos. 1 and 2. Published 2/16/65.
65. Thyagarajan, G., and May, E. L.: Improved synthesis of 2-benzyl-1,2,5,6-tetrahydro-pyridines. Precursors of analgetic 6,7-benzomorphans. J. Heterocyclic Chem. *8*:465–468, 1971.
66. Walker, G. N., and Alkalay, D.: New benzomorphan ring closure in the synthesis of 5-phenylbenzomorphans. J. Org. Chem. *31*:1905–1911, 1966.
67. Wentland, M. P., and Albertson, N. F.: Unpublished observations.
68. Wibaut, J. P., and Arens, J. F.: Die Bereitung von 4-Athylpyridin aus Pyridin, Essig-saureanhydrid, Essigsaure und Zinkstaub; Uber die hierbei verlaufenden chemischer Reactionen und gebildeten Zwischenprodukte. Rec. Trav. Chim. *60*:119–137, 1941.
69. Wibaut, J. P., and Vromen, S.: Preparation of 3-methyl-4-alkylpyridines from 3-methyl pyridine. Rec. Trav. Chim. *67*:545–550, 1948.
70. Ziering, A., Malatestinic, N., Williams, T., and Brossi, A.: 3'-Methyl, 8-methyl- and 8-phenyl derivatives of 5,9-dimethyl-6,7-benzomorphans. J. Med. Chem. *13*:9–13, 1970.

Narcotic Antagonists, edited by M. C. Braude, L. S. Harris, E. L.
May, J. P. Smith, and J. E. Villarreal. Advances in Biochemical
Psychopharmacology, Vol. 8. Raven Press, New York © 1974.

Antagonists in the 5-Phenyl-Benzomorphan Series

F. H. Clarke, R. T. Hill, J. K. Saelens, and N. Yokoyama

Research Department, Pharmaceutical Division, CIBA-GEIGY Corporation, Summit,
New Jersey 07901, and Ardsley, New York 10502

The clinical pharmacology of the orally effective, potent analgesic GPA
1657 (l-β-2'-hydroxy-2,9-dimethyl-5-phenyl-6,7-benzomorphan) is described as well as its antagonist properties in animals. The structure of GPA
1657 in relation to other potent analgesics is discussed. The pharmacology
of a number of classical antagonist derivatives related to GPA 1657 is described. Of these, GPA 2163, the 2-propargyl analogue, is a pure antagonist
that is less potent than nalorphine. The 2-dimethylallyl analogue, GPA
2443, was evaluated in man and found to be inactive orally as an analgesic
and very weak intramuscularly. The corresponding 2-cyclobutylmethyl
analogue, GPA 3154, was more potent than GPA 2443 in animals but displayed symptoms of intolerance at relatively low doses in man. The 2-cyclo-
butylmethyl analogue of the 9-desmethyl series, GPA 4622, showed a
potential for physical dependence capacity in a chronic study in the monkey. In conclusion, the search continues for a potent analgesic free of abuse
potential. In the meantime, perhaps a potent oral analgesic will be found
with advantages over morphine.

INTRODUCTION

When our studies began in 1962, antagonists of morphine and similar
narcotics were confined to congeners of potent analgesics in the morphine,
morphinan, and benzomorphan series in which the usual N-methyl group
was replaced by one of a small family of substituents (1). Among these, the
cyclopropylmethyl, cyclobutylmethyl, and allyl type substituents were most
prominent (1). By tests in use at that time, these antagonists were generally
not detected as analgesics in mice and rats. It was very unusual then to
find that a potent analgesic in mice, the levorotatory isomer of a 5-phenyl-
2,9-dimethyl benzomorphan (31) (GPA 1657) precipitated withdrawal
symptoms in monkeys treated chronically with morphine (28).

RESULTS AND DISCUSSION

In man, GPA 1657 has been demonstrated to be a potent analgesic both
orally and parenterally. A 10-mg oral dose of GPA 1657 has a greater anal-

81

gesic activity for a longer period of time than 60 to 90 mg of codeine (23, 24), and 2.5 mg of oral GPA 1657 is equivalent to 50 mg of oral pentazocine (4). Parenterally, GPA 1657 has a potency twice that of morphine (12). Certain side effects associated with morphine analgesia are observed, such as respiratory depression, dizziness, and nausea, but their incidence does not exceed that seen with morphine at comparable analgesic doses (7). The analgesia produced by GPA 1657 is reported to be pleasant (25), indicating a euphoriant effect comparable to morphine at therapeutically useful doses. GPA 1657 is apparently resistant to the development of tolerance since a global, uncontrolled study demonstrated that pain could be alleviated in chronically ill patients without increasing dosage over periods as long as 90 days (13). No indication of addiction or withdrawal symptoms has been reported in efficacy studies on over 1,100 patients. One might conclude that in normal clinical use physical dependence to GPA 1657 would rarely be encountered. Nevertheless, in an extensive study on two volunteer former addicts with daily oral doses of GPA 1657 as large as 720 mg, Jasinski, Martin, and Hoeldtke (10) of the Mental Health Addiction Research Center reported "that GPA 1657 has a significant potential to produce dependence of the morphine type in man." Even in their studies, however, GPA 1657 provided only partial suppression of morphine abstinence, and they were unable to exceed single parenteral doses of 20 mg (10).

GPA 1657 is a 5-phenyl-benzomorphan derivative (Fig. 1), and the finding that it is a potent analgesic adds one more link to a growing chain of evidence concerning the structural requirements for analgesia. Thus, although Beckett (3) had originally placed meperidine in the mold of morphine and suggested that the phenyl group was axial to the piperidine ring, May and Murphy (17) showed that a phenyl-morphan (with an equatorial phenyl group) had analgesic properties only slightly less than meperidine.

Slowly, however, evidence was accumulated to suggest that there are no definitive conformational requirements of the phenyl group for analgesic action (19). Finally, an X-ray study has shown that the phenyl group of meperidine has an equatorial configuration as in phenyl-morphans (26). In some respects then, the 5-phenyl-benzomorphans combine features of both meperidine and morphine, and we hoped to find congeners with new and interesting properties. This was certainly the case with GPA 1657.

It will not be necessary to review the synthetic route to the 5-phenyl-benzomorphans (31), since it followed the well-established path discovered by Grewe (6) for the morphinans that was applied many times by May in the 5-alkyl-benzomorphan series (6). It is interesting to observe that the 9-methyl substituent of GPA 1657 is in the axial or β-orientation relative to the piperidine ring (31). It is also of interest that GPA 1657 is the levoro-

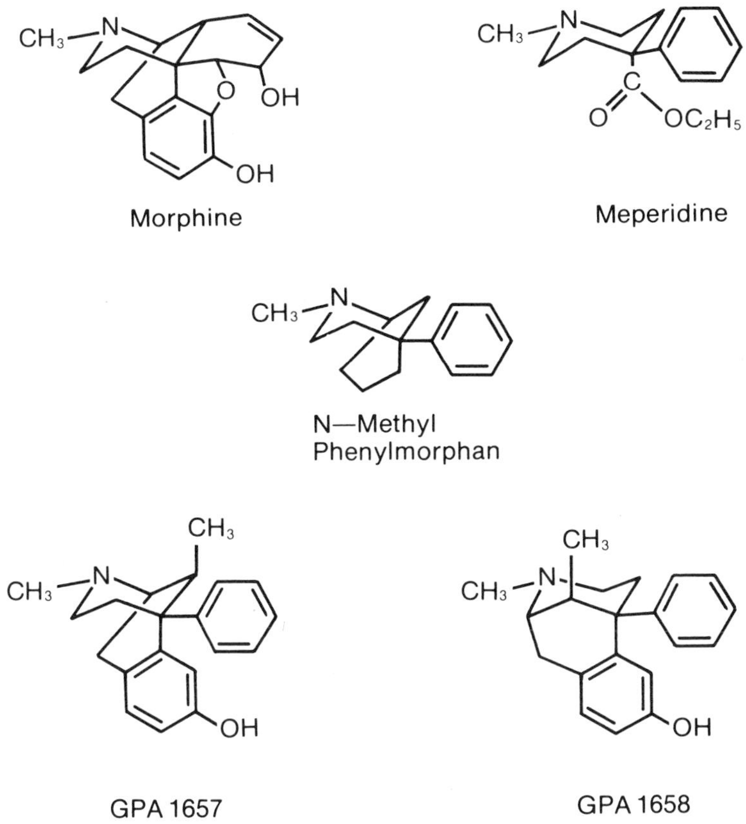

FIG. 1. Conformations of GPA 1657 and other potent analgesics.

tatory isomer and that it has been shown with an X-ray study to have the same absolute configuration as morphine (31). In itself this is no surprise for the l-isomers of the 5,9-dialkyl-benzomorphans also have the same absolute configuration as morphine (22). However, the pharmacology of GPA 1657 and its optical isomer (Table 1) are of special interest (9). GPA 1657, its racemate (GPA 1579), and even the d-isomer (GPA 1658) are all analgesics but GPA 1657 is the most active (31). In the morphinan and benzomorphan series one usually finds that d-isomers are very weak or inactive as analgesics (6).

With regard to physical dependence capacity, it was first found that the racemate GPA 1579 caused only a slight suppression of morphine withdrawal symptoms in the monkey (28). However, we were surprised to find not only that GPA 1658 was an analgesic but that it possessed a high level

TABLE 1. *Analgesic isomers of the 5-phenyl-benzomorphan series*[a]

Effect and test	Racemate (GPA 1579)	l-Isomer (GPA 1657)	d-Isomer (GPA 1658)	Morphine
Analgesia				
Hot plate ED_{50}	0.5 sc	0.2 sc	3.4 sc	1.2 sc
Tail-flick	5 sc	2 sc	20 sc	4 sc
Max. effect dose	10 po	10 po	40 po	16 po
PQW[b] ED_{50}		0.5 sc	4.2 sc	1 sc
		6.0 po		8.9 po
Antagonism				
Morphine analgesia Tail-flick	none	partial	none	
Physical dependence capacity Single dose result (monkey)	slight suppression	no support weak antagonist	almost complete suppression	

[a] Numbers are doses in mg/kg administered subcutaneously (sc), intraperitoneally (ip), or orally (po).
[b] Phenylquinone writhing test.

of physical dependence capacity and caused complete suppression of morphine withdrawal symptoms in the monkey at 5 mg/kg (28).

Perhaps one should not be surprised when a d-isomer of the benzomorphan series behaves like morphine. A close look at skeletal models of GPA 1657 and GPA 1658 reveals that they are remarkably similar and that the main difference in shape is a small rotation of the axial benzene ring. This is not the case with the morphinans which are highly asymmetric molecules.

Nevertheless, GPA 1657 is even more unusual. It not only failed to suppress morphine withdrawal symptoms in the monkey, it actually precipitated abstinence symptoms in the morphine-dependent monkey and behaved like a mild, nalorphine-like morphine antagonist (18, 28). Morphine antagonism could even be demonstrated in the mouse using the tail-flick test for analgesia (9). Although the antagonist properties of GPA 1657 were not overtly observed in man (10), the important analgesic properties were soon evident, as discussed above.

In an attempt to produce drugs with the nalorphine or naloxone type of antagonism, we directed our attention toward classical antagonist derivatives. The properties of some of these are summarized in Table 2. Here we see the usual substituents: propargyl, allyl, dimethylallyl, cyclopropylmethyl and cyclobutylmethyl. Both optical isomers of 9-β-methyl compounds were prepared as well as a number of 9-desmethyl compounds. Among the

TABLE 2. *Antagonists of the 5-phenyl-benzomorphan series*[a]

9-β-Methyl Cpds.	l-Isomer		d-Isomer	
	Joint effect	Analgesia	Joint effect	Analgesia
N—CH$_2$C≡CH	A/20/sc	None/sc TF		
N—CH$_2$CH=CH$_2$	A/40/sc	None/sc TF	P/320/sc	slight/ac TF
N—CH$_2$CH=CMe$_2$	A/40/sc	40/sc TF	P/160/sc	45/sc PQW
N—CH$_2$◁	A/20/sc	slight/sc TF	P/80/sc	80/sc TF 100/sc PQW
N—CH$_2$◇	A/25/sc	12/sc TF 180/po TF 25/sc PQW 125/po PQW		None/sc PQW

9-Desmethyl Cpds.	Racemate		Isomer
	Joint effect	Analgesia	Analgesia
N—CH$_2$C≡CH	A/20/sc	None/sc TF	
N—CH$_2$CH=CH$_2$	A/200/po	None/sc PQW None/po PQW	
N—CH$_2$CH=CMe$_2$	P/40/sc	15/sc PQW	
N—CH$_2$◁	A/10/sc	80/sc TF 18/sc PQW 33/po PQW	(d) 45/sc PQW
N—CH$_2$◇		6.2/sc PQW 120/po PQW	(l) 2.8/sc PQW 40/po PQW

[a] Numbers are doses in mg/kg administered subcutaneously (sc) or orally (po). Joint effect is the activity (antagonist or potentiator) in the tail-flick test when administered with morphine. Tests for analgesia are tail-flick (TF) or phenylquinone writhing (PQW) tests.

9-β-methyl compounds, the l-isomers are all morphine antagonists and the d-isomers potentiated morphine analgesia. We would expect the d-isomers to cause physical dependence. As analgesics, most of the antagonists were weak, as expected, in animals. However, for two compounds with dimethyl-allyl and cyclobutylmethyl substituents, respectively, analgesia could be demonstrated in the mouse, particularly with the phenylquinone writhing test. Of the 9-desmethyl compounds, the most interesting was the cyclo-butylmethyl derivative, the l-isomer which showed potent analgesia in mice.

Four of the antagonists were studied in considerable depth, and their structures are illustrated in Fig. 2. GPA 2163, the N-propargyl analogue of GPA 1657, was found by Kosterlitz and Watt (15) to be a pure antagonist in the guinea pig ileum. Indeed, our own studies could detect no analgesia

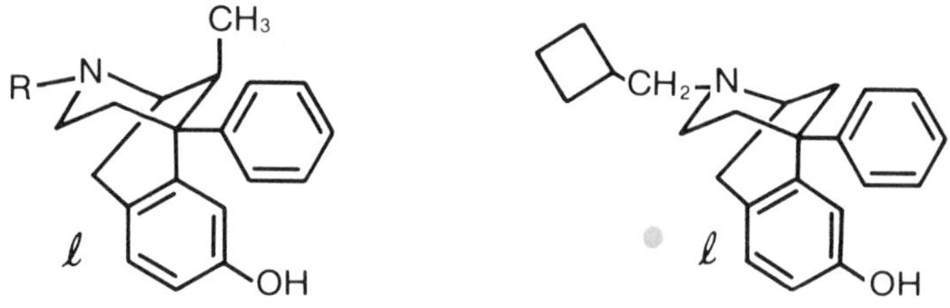

GPA 1657 R = CH₃
GPA 2163 R = CH₂ - C ≡ CH
GPA 2443 R = CH₂CH = C (CH₃)₂
GPA 3154 R = CH₂—◇

GPA 4622

FIG. 2. 5-Phenyl-benzomorphan antagonists.

parenterally in the mouse using the tail-flick or phenylquinone writhing tests. There was evidence of some delayed analgesia, orally, which suggested metabolism to an active metabolite. The compound caused a precipitation of abstinence in partially withdrawn monkeys which lasted for 15 hr, whereas a comparably effective dose of nalorphine lasted only 2 to 3 hr. GPA 2163 showed no evidence of physical dependence in the mouse jumping test (21). However, as an antagonist, GPA 2163 is only 10 to 50% as potent as nalorphine (29); for this reason, it was not studied in man for its potential in the prevention of narcotic abuse.

Our primary interest in the synthesis of these antagonists was to find an analgesic which does not cause physical dependence. GPA 2443, with a dimethylallyl substituent on the 5-phenyl-benzomorphan nucleus was quite naturally compared to pentazocine in its pharmacological evaluation. In the mouse tail-flick test, GPA 2443 was approximately equipotent to or slightly more potent than pentazocine by the intraperitoneal, subcutaneous, and oral routes of administration. As a morphine antagonist, GPA 2443 was slightly more potent than pentazocine but less potent than nalorphine in the tail-flick test. It did not substitute for morphine in the non-withdrawn monkey, and in withdrawn monkeys signs of morphine withdrawal were exacerbated at a dose of 2 mg/kg (5).

After 3-month toxicity studies in the rat and monkey, GPA 2443 was evaluated in man. No significant analgesic effect was observed following oral doses (11) ranging from 5 to 400 mg; intramuscular doses from 30 to 100 mg showed an estimated, relative potency of only one-fourteenth that of morphine (8). In human studies it was found that plasma levels were lower and urinary excretion of GPA 2443 was less than expected from comparable studies on pentazocine reported in the literature. A half-life of 60 to 90 min was observed following intravenous injection in monkeys. Although definitive studies were not performed, it was concluded that a rapid metabolism could have accounted for the lack of analgesia of GPA 2443 in man (16).

Kosterlitz and Watt (15) observed that N-cyclobutylmethyl derivatives of 14-hydroxydihydromorphinone are more potent agonists than their cyclopropylmethyl analogues. This is the case in the 5-phenyl-benzomorphan series as well, and the next two compounds studied possess a cyclobutylmethyl substituent. The analogue with a 9-β-methyl substituent, GPA 3154, was an analgesic in mice and rats both orally and parenterally. The analgesic effect was weak, however, so that based on experience with known analgesics it was predicted that oral doses of 75 to 150 mg would be required for adequate analgesia in man. GPA 3154 was a more potent antagonist than pentazocine in the mouse, and exaggerated morphine abstinence was observed in the monkey (27). There was no evidence of withdrawal following nalorphine challenge after 60 to 90 days of chronic administration to the monkey (5). After appropriate sub-chronic toxicity studies, GPA 3154 was evaluated for oral tolerance in man. Unfortunately, although doses of 1 to 15 mg produced no signs or symptoms of intolerance, moderate, drug-related CNS effects were observed at 25 and 35 mg (30). Since it was anticipated that much higher doses would be required for clinical analgesia, this compound was not studied further.

GPA 4622 is also a cyclobutylmethyl derivative, but in this case the 9-methyl substituent is missing from the 5-phenyl-benzomorphan nucleus. This compound was a moderately potent analgesic in mice and rats; it was completely negative in the mouse jumping test for physical dependence (21). However, in a chronic study in the monkey, withdrawal symptoms were observed 60 days after challenge with nalorphine and also after abrupt withdrawal of GPA 4622 (20). This is rather a severe test for morphine physical dependence, but since the adverse effect was found in the monkey it was decided not to proceed to studies in man.

CONCLUSIONS

The studies outlined above illustrate some of the problems encountered in a classical approach to the preparation of morphine antagonists in the 5-phenyl-benzomorphan series. These difficulties are probably typical of those experienced by other laboratories engaged in the search for a deep analgesic that is free of abuse potential. Many of the medical aspects of this search were discussed at the 1972 Cornell University symposium on analgesics. During this meeting, Dr. William Beaver (2) pointed out that an orally effective potent analgesic free of tolerance development is needed in medicine today. Perhaps such a drug with advantages over morphine will emerge as fallout while the search continues for the final objective.

ACKNOWLEDGMENTS

The authors wish to thank Drs. K. Brunings and G. Lukas of this Department and Drs. E. DeMaar, D. Tedeschi, and M. Weiner formerly with CIBA-GEIGY Corporation for participation in the work we have described. We also wish to express appreciation to the late Dr. N. B. Eddy and to Dr. E. L. May, Chief of Medicinal Chemistry of the National Institutes of Health for helpful advice. For the physical dependence studies in man, we thank Dr. W. R. Martin and Dr. D. R. Jasinski of the NIMH Addiction Research Center in Lexington, Kentucky. We also thank Drs. M. Seevers and J. Villarreal of the University of Michigan and Drs. F. Coulston, D. Serrone, and I. Rosenblum of the Albany Medical College for studies of physical dependence in monkeys.

REFERENCES

1. Archer, S., and Harris, L. S.: Narcotic antagonists. *In:* Jucker, E. Progress in Drug Research, Birkhauser-Verlag, Basel. *8*:261–320, 1965.
2. Beaver, W. T.: Sloan Kettering Institute for Cancer Research, N.Y., N.Y.
3. Beckett, A. H.: Stereochemical factors in biological activity, analgesics, *In:* Jucker, E.: Progress in Drug Research, Birkhauser-Verlag, Basel. *1*:519–529, 1959.
4. Chilton, N. W.: Temple University School of Dentistry, personal communication.
5. Coulston, F., and Serrone, D.: Institute of Experimental Pathology and Toxicology, Albany Medical College, personal communication.
6. Eddy, N. B., and May, E. L.: Synthetic analgesics, Part II B., 6,7-Benzomorphans, pp. 115–137, Pergamon Press, N.Y., 1966.
7. Forrest, W. H., Jr.: personal communication. See also Minutes 30th Meeting of Committee on Problems of Drug Dependence, NAS-NRC, 1968, Appendix 29, 5531–5551.
8. Forrest, W. H., Jr.: Veterans Administration Hospital, Palo Alto, California, personal communication.
9. Hill, R. T., and Lukas, G.: Some pharmacological and toxicology properties of GPA 1657, a new hexahydro-2,6-methano-3-benzazocine. Minutes, 29th Meeting of Committee on Problems of Drug Dependence, NAS-NRC, 1967, Appendix 14, 4946–4955.
10. Jasinski, D. R., Martin, W. R., and Hoeldtke, R.: Studies of the dependence-producing properties of GPA 1657, Profadol, and Propiram in man, Clin. Pharmacol. Therap. *12*:613–649, 1971.
11. Kantor, T. G., Hopper, M., Cohen, G., and Streem, A.: personal communication. See also Minutes, 33rd Meeting of Committee on Problems of Drug Dependence, NAS-NRC, 1971, 225–238.
12. Keats, A. S., and Telford, J.: personal communication. See also Minutes 30th Meeting of Committee on Problems of Drug Dependence, NAS-NRC, 1968, Appendix 28, 5514–5530.

13. Korman, S.: Kingsbrook Jewish Medical Center, Brooklyn, N.Y., personal communication.

14. Kosterlitz, H. W., and Watt, A. J.: personal communication. See also Minutes 30th Meeting of Committee on Problems of Drug Dependence, NAS-NRC, 1968, Appendix 10, 5342–5349.

15. Kosterlitz, H. W., and Watt, A. J.: personal communication. See also Minutes 31st Meeting of Committee on Problems of Drug Dependence, NAS-NRC, 1969, 5819–5826.

16. Lukas, G., and Redalieu, E.: Research Department, Pharmaceuticals Division, CIBA-GEIGY Corporation, personal communication.

17. May, E. L., and Murphy, J. G.: Structures related to morphine. II. An isomer of N-methylmorphinan. J. Org. Chem. *19*:618–622, 1954.

18. Similar observations have been observed with other benzomorphan derivatives; see May, E. L., and Takeda, M.: Optical isomers of miscellaneous strong analgetics. J. Med. Chem. *13*:805–807, 1970.

19. Portoghese, P. S., Mikhail, A. A., and Kopferberg, H. J.: Sterrochemical studies on medicinal agents. VI. Bicyclic bases. Synthesis and pharmacology of epimeric bridged analogs of meperidine, 2-methyl-5-phenyl-5-carbethoxy-2-azabicyclo[2,2,1]heptane. J. Med. Chem. *11*:219–225, 1968.

20. Rosenblum, I.: Institute of Experimental Pathology and Toxicology, Albany Medical College, personal communication.

21. Saelens, J. K., Granat, F. R., and Sawyer, W. K.: The mouse jumping test – A simple screening method to estimate the physical dependence capacity of analgesics. Arch. Int. Pharmacodyn. Ther. *190*:213–218, 1971.

22. Sawa, Y. K., and Irisawa, J.: Elimination of the 4-hydroxyl group of the alkaloids related to morphine. VII. Synthesis of the active 2′-hydroxy-2-methyl-5,9-diethyl-6,7-benzomorphan derivatives. *Tetrahedron 21*:1129, 1965.

23. Sevelius, H., McCoy, J., Merrill, J. A., and Colemore, J. P.: personal communication. See also Minutes 30th Meeting of Committee on Problems of Drug Dependence, NAS-NRC, 1968, Appendix 24, 5469–5475.

24. Sunshine, A., Laska, E., Kantor, T. G., Sharkey, I., and Hopper, M.: personal communication. See also Minutes 30th Meeting of Committee on Problems of Drug Dependence, NAS-NRC, 1968, Appendix 30, 5552–5558.

25. Sunshine, A.: personal communication. See also Minutes 29th Meeting of Committee on Problems of Drug Dependence, NAS-NRC, 1967, Appendix 15, 4956.

26. Van Koningsveld, H.: The crystal and molecular structure of pethidine hydrobromide. Rec. Trav. Chim. *89*:375–378, 1970.

27. Villarreal, J. E.: Department of Pharmacology, University of Michigan. Ann Arbor, personal communication.

28. Villarreal, J. E., and Seevers, M. H.: personal communication. See also Minutes, 29th Meeting of Committee on Problems of Drug Dependence, NAS-NRC, 1967, Addendum 1, 12.

29. Villarreal, J. E., and Seevers, M. H.: personal communication. See also Minutes, 30th Meeting of Committee on Problems of Drug Dependence, NAS-NRC, 1968, Addendum 2, 5.

30. Wingfield, W. L.: Virginia State Prison, Richmond, personal communication.

31. Yokoyama, N., Block, F. B., and Clarke, F. H.: 1,2,3,4,5,6-Hexahydro-6-phenyl-2,6-methano-3-benzazocines. II. J. Med. Chem. *13*:488–492, 1970.

Narcotic Antagonists, edited by M. C. Braude, L. S. Harris, E. L. May, J. P. Smith, and J. E. Villarreal. *Advances in Biochemical Psychopharmacology, Vol. 8.* Raven Press, New York © 1974.

Structure-Activity Relationships in Narcotic Antagonists with N-Furylmethyl Substituents

Herbert Merz, Adolf Langbein, Klaus Stockhaus, Gerhard Walther, and Helmut Wick

C. H. Boehringer Sohn, Ingelheim, Germany

N-Furylmethyl derivatives of the 2'-hydroxy-6,7-benzomorphan series have been synthesized and evaluated for antagonistic, analgesic, and toxic properties in mice. Depending on the nature of the N-furyl-methyl group, pure antagonists, agonists-antagonists, or strong analgesics can be obtained. The most active compounds are almost as potent as naloxone as antagonists or equipotent to morphine as analgesics. Monkey experiments have shown that representatives of the pure antagonist, the agonist-antagonist, and even the strong analgesic type are devoid of physical dependence capacity. In order to study scope and limitations of structural features of narcotic antagonists, the N-furylmethyl substituent as well as the benzomorphan moiety have been modified systematically. Furthermore, N-furylmethyl analogues of other strong analgesics have been prepared. The effects of such structural variations on selected pharmacological parameters are summarized and structure-activity relationships are discussed. Representatives of the new compounds may be useful as anti-heroin agents or nonaddicting strong analgesics.

INTRODUCTION

The use of such substituents as propyl, allyl, propargyl, cyclopropyl-methyl, and related groups has been well established in the design of narcotic antagonists (20, 2, 11, 12, 19, 9). In spite of major endeavors in this fascinating field, especially during the last two decades, no essentially new N-substituents effecting opioid antagonist (19) activity have been described.

Consequently, we have been searching for unusual groups capable of conferring antagonistic properties to the molecules of strong analgesics. In the course of this work N-furfuryl derivatives of the 2'-hydroxy-6,7-benzomorphan series have been synthesized; they proved to be potent antagonists in mice. Proceeding from these findings, the scope and limitations of this novel structural feature of narcotic antagonists have been studied: The N-furylmethyl group as well as the benzomorphan moiety have been modified (21). Furthermore, N-furylmethyl analogues of other strong analgesics have been prepared.

We now wish to summarize the effects of such structural variations on selected pharmacological parameters and to discuss structure-activity relationships in narcotic antagonists with N-furylmethyl substituents.

METHODS

Chemical Structure and Syntheses

The chemical structures of the new N-furylmethyl compounds are generalized in Fig. 1. M represents the moiety of a strong analgesic which is structurally related to morphine, and R^1 represents the furan nucleus that may be substituted for H, Me, or Et.

Syntheses may be accomplished on various routes. The following methods, both starting from the corresponding nor-compounds, are most convenient and provide the reaction products in good to excellent yields (Fig. 2). According to method (A), the nor-compound concerned is alkylated with the appropriate chloromethyl-furan thus directly yielding the N-furylmethyl derivative. Using method (B), the nor-compound is acylated with the appropriate furoyl chloride to the corresponding furamide intermediate, which, on reduction, yields the wanted N-furylmethyl compound. Further details have been published in the patent literature (6–8) or will be published in the near future.

Pharmacological Methods

The new substances and appropriate standards were tested for analgesia, morphine antagonism, and toxicity in mice. Promising representatives were

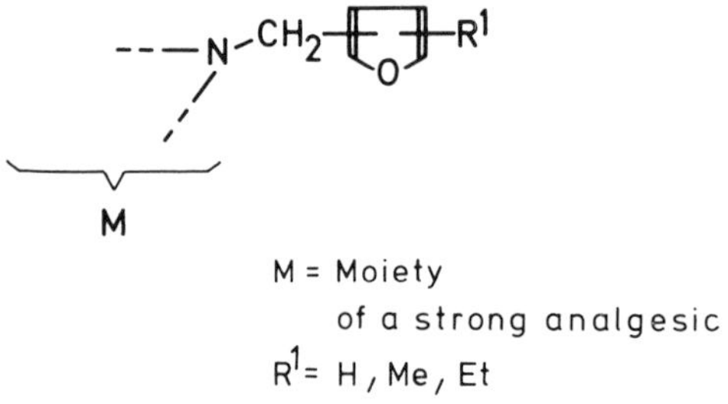

$$---\!-\!N\!-\!CH_2\!-\!\!\left[\!\!\begin{array}{c}\\O\end{array}\!\!\right]\!\!-\!R^1$$

M

M = Moiety
    of a strong analgesic
R^1 = H , Me , Et

FIG. 1. N-Furylmethyl analogues of strong analgesics.

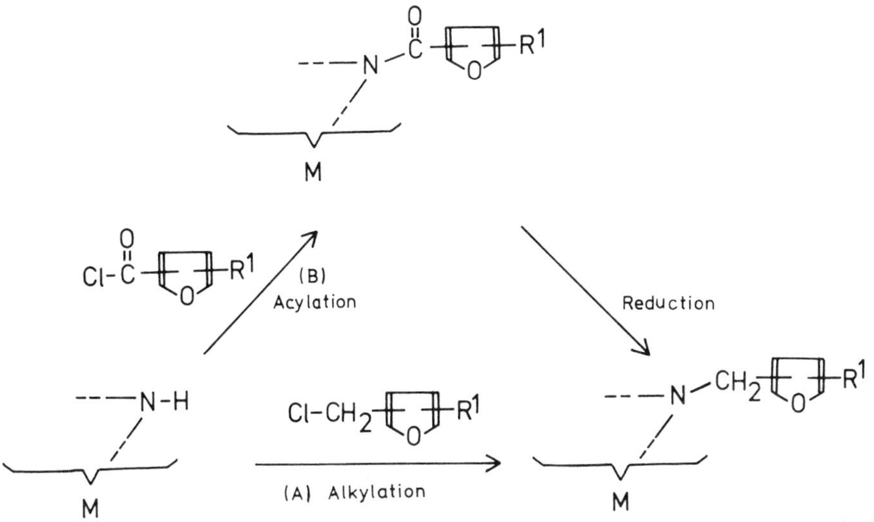

FIG. 2. Syntheses of N-furylmethyl compounds.

also evaluated for physical dependence capacity and morphine antagonism in monkeys. The following techniques were employed:

(a) *Analgesia (Mice)*

NMRI-mice (both sexes, 16 to 20 g, 10 animals per dose) were used. The test compounds were administered s.c. as aqueous solutions of their methanesulfonic or hydrochloric acid salts. Analgesic activity (ED-values, mg/kg s.c.) was estimated using the following methods: tail-clip method according to Haffner (16); hot-plate method according to Woolfe and MacDonald (25); and writing test according to Blumberg, Wolf, and Dayton (4).

(b) *Morphine Antagonism (Mice)*

Antagonistic activity was estimated using Haffner's tail-clip method: after injection of morphine hydrochloride (15 mg/kg s.c., corresponding to its ED_{80}) and the test dose of the antagonist, the analgesic activity was determined. On the basis of the results obtained from various suitable dose ratios the AD_{50} (50% suppression of the original morphine analgesia) was calculated.

(c) *Toxicity (Mice)*

NMRI-mice (both sexes, 16 to 20 g, 10 animals per dose) were used. The test compounds were administered as aqueous solutions of their methane-sulfonic or hydrochloric acid salts. After an observation period of 14 days the LD_{50}-values were calculated according to Litchfield and Wilcoxon (18).

(d) *Morphine Antagonism (Monkeys)*

Antagonistic properties in nonwithdrawn morphine-dependent rhesus monkeys were evaluated by Villarreal and Seevers (23), Ann Arbor, Michigan, according to a procedure published earlier (10).

(e) *Physical Dependence Capacity (Monkeys)*

Physical dependence capacity in withdrawn morphine-dependent rhesus monkeys was estimated by Villarreal and Seevers (23) according to a procedure published earlier (10).

RESULTS

More than 1,500 compounds of the general formula (Fig. 1) have been synthesized and numerous pharmacological data have been obtained. This chapter is intended as a summary rather than a complete publication of details. Consequently, only selected data, in particular those throwing light upon structure-activity correlations, are listed in the following tables. A blank in the columns for analgesic or antagonistic activity means that those effects were not observed up to toxic doses.

DISCUSSION

Results and structure-activity relationships in the novel N-furylmethyl compounds (Fig. 1) will be discussed under the following headings: variation of the N-furylmethyl substituent, and modification of the moiety M.

Variation of the N-Furylmethyl Substituent

In order to demonstrate the effects of the N-substituent the α-5,9-di-methyl-2'-hydroxy-6,7-benzomorphan molecule is used as a suitable moiety, M.

In Table 1 the effects of the most common furylmethyl residue, the

TABLE 1. *N-substituted α-5,9-dimethyl-2'-hydroxy-6,7-benzomorphans*

Compound number	1	2	3	4
N-Substituent -R	$-CH_2-CH=CH_2$	$-CH_2-$(furyl, O)	$-CH_2-$(thienyl, S)	$-CH_2-$(phenyl)
Salt HX =	HCl	CH_3SO_3H	HCl	HCl
Analgesia Writhing, Mice, ED_{50}, mg/kg, s.c.	—	18	—	—
Antagonism Suppression of Analgesia, Mice, AD_{50}, mg/kg, s.c.	0.5	1.0	10	>10

furfuryl group, are compared to those of other related known or new N-substituents. The N-furfuryl derivative *2* is a strong antagonist equipotent to nalorphine and at least half as potent as its "classical" N-allyl counterpart *1* (5, 15, 1). The closely related N-thenyl analogue *3*, on the other hand, is only $1/10$ as potent and the N-benzyl analogue *4* (14) is even weaker. This marked decline in antagonistic potency seems to reflect the corresponding decrease in allyl character of the substituents due to an increasing delocalization of the double bonds of their aromatic rings. Thus the trend observed in antagonistic activities supports our primary idea that the furfuryl group with its inherent allyl character is a useful residue in the design of narcotic antagonists. We also observed those differentiated antagonistic potencies in other 2'-hydroxy-6,7-benzomorphans, 3-hydroxy-morphinans, and in related series of strong analgesics. As a rule, the N-thenyl derivatives are $1/10$ as potent as the N-furfuryl analogues, whereas the N-benzyl analogues are even weaker or inactive.

Lengthening of the methylene bridge between the benzomorphan nitrogen and the furan ring of the N-furfuryl derivative *2* (Table 1) to an ethylene chain results in the N-[2-(2-furyl)ethyl] homologue described in the literature (13). Whereas the former is a nalorphine-like antagonist with little analgesic activity, the latter is a morphine-like analgesic which proved to be almost 30 times as effective as morphine in the mouse writing test.

Modification of the N-furylmethyl group by isomerization or by substitution of the furan nucleus causes considerable change in the pharmacological properties: either compounds with modified-action profiles or inactive substances may be obtained. The most interesting prototypes of the α-5,9-dimethyl-2-furylmethyl-2'-hydroxy-6,7-benzomorphan series are shown in Table 2. Depending on the nature of the N-furylmethyl substituent, the compound is either a potent pure antagonist (compound 5), an agonist-antagonist (compounds 2 and 6), or a strong analgesic agonist (compound 7). Since these four substances have been studied extensively in our laboratories and in others, the code numbers of C. H. Boehringer Sohn (Mr), of the National Institutes of Health (NIH), and the University of Michigan (UM) are listed in Table 2. Detailed pharmacological data of these prototypes and appropriate standards are presented in Table 3:

Mr 1256-MS, devoid of analgesic activity, represents the pure antagonist type. In mice it is as potent as nalorphine whereas in monkeys it is half as active as the standard.

Mr 1029-MS and *Mr 1268-MS* are both agonists-antagonists but opposite as far as their relative activities are concerned. In Mr 1029-MS the antagonistic properties comparable to those of its isomer Mr 1256-MS dominate over a weak analgesic activity, which can only be detected in the sensitive writhing test. In Mr 1268-MS, on the other hand, strong analgesic properties comparable to those of pentazocine dominate over a weak questionable antagonistic activity which can be demonstrated in mice but not in monkeys.

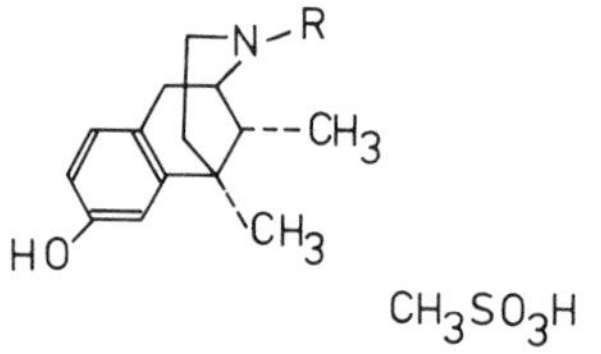

TABLE 2. *Action profiles of α-5,9-dimethyl-2-furylmethyl-2'-hydroxy-6,7-benzomorphans*

Compound number	5	2	6	7
N-Substituent –R	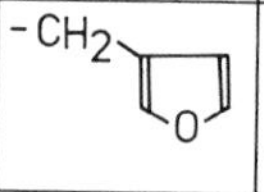 $-CH_2$ (furyl)	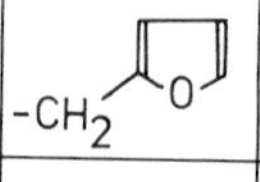 $-CH_2$ (furyl)	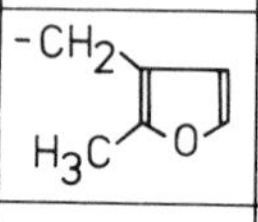 $-CH_2$, H_3C (furyl)	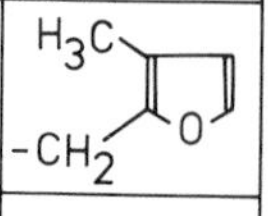 H_3C, $-CH_2$ (furyl)
Code numbers	Mr1256-MS NIH 8738 UM 912	Mr 1029-MS NIH 8740 UM 914	Mr 1268-MS NIH 8735 UM 909	Mr 1353-MS NIH 8737 UM 911
Antagonism	+ + +	+ + +	+	none
Analgesia	none	+	+ +	+ + +
Action profile	Antagonist	Antagonist-(Agonist)	Agonist (Antagonist)	Agonist

TABLE 3. *Pharmacological data of*
α-5,9-dimethyl-2-furylmethyl-2'-hydroxy-6,7-benzomorphans

Substance	Analgesia (Mice)			Antagonism		PDC (Monkeys)	Straub Tail (Mice)	Toxicity (Mice)
				(Mice)	(Monkeys)	Physical Dependence Capacity		
	Tail Clip ED_{50}	Hot Plate ED_{100}	Writhing ED_{50}	Suppression of Analgesia AD_{50}	Precipitation of Abstinence Nalorphine=1			LD_{50}
	mg/kg, s.c.			mg/kg, s.c.				mg/kg, s.c.
Mr 1256-MS	—	—	—	1.0	1/2	none	—	180
Mr 1029-MS	—	—	18	1.0	1/2	none	—	292
Mr 1268-MS	—	3.2	1.8	20	—	none	±	156
Mr 1353-MS	12	1.6	0.6	—	—	none	—	305
Morphine-hydrochloride	11	1.2	0.5	—	—	high	+	500
Pentazocine-hydrochloride	—	7.0	1.4	8.0	1/40	none	±	220
Nalorphine-hydrochloride	—	(+)	0.5	1.0	1	none	—	560

Mr 1353-MS, finally, seems to be devoid of antagonistic properties. This compound is rather a strong analgesic almost as potent as morphine but different from morphine as to side effects. Thus, in spite of its high analgesic activity even in the tail-clip test, no Straub tail phenomenon was observed in mice. Since the Straub activity in relation to toxicity (Straub index $LD_{50}:ED_{50}$) is reported (22) to be predictive for the addiction liability of morphine-like analgesic compounds, Mr 1353-MS should be a nonaddicting strong analgesic. This notion is strongly supported in monkey experiments carried out by Villarreal and Seevers (23). Each of the four prototypes shown in Table 3, including the strong analgesic Mr 1353-MS, was estimated to possess no physical dependence capacity in withdrawn monkeys. The absence of morphine-like side effects in Mr 1353-MS suggests very weak antagonistic efficacy not traceable in the tests presently available.

Further chemical work concerning variations of the N-furylmethyl group is in progress in our laboratories.

Modification of the Moiety M

The correlation of distinct action profiles with the nature of the N-furyl-methyl substituent involved is not limited to the α-5,9-dimethyl-2'-hydroxy-6,7-benzomorphan molecule but seems to be a principle of much broader scope. The very same correlation is evident in related structures such as other 2'-hydroxy-6,7-benzomorphans and 3-hydroxy-morphinans.

Results of Optical Resolution

As expected from well-documented findings in the benzomorphan series (11), optical resolution of the four racemic prototypes discussed above results in *levo* antipodes with enhanced activities and almost inactive *dextro* counterparts (Table 4). The action profiles, however, are not affected. Supposing that the (+)-forms are inert, the (−)-forms should be twice as potent as the corresponding racemic compounds, an assumption which proved right with the exception of the pure antagonist compound Mr 1256-MS. In this

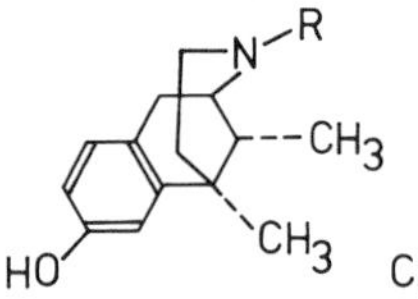

TABLE 4. *Optically active* α-5,9-*dimethyl*-2-*furylmethyl*-2'-*hydroxy*-6,7-*benzomorphans*

Compound		Analgesia	Antagonism	Toxicity
Number		Writhing Mice ED$_{50}$	Suppression of Analgesia	LD$_{50}$
-R	Isomer	mg/kg, s.c.	AD$_{50}$, mg/kg, s.c.	mg/kg, s.c.
5 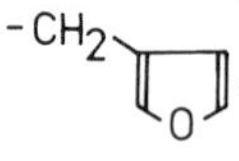	(±)	—	1.0	180
-CH$_2$	(−)	—	0.1	110
	(+)	—	30	223
2 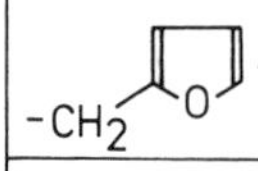	(±)	18	1.0	292
	(−)	—	0.5	182
-CH$_2$	(+)	30	30	253
6 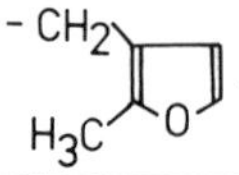	(±)	1.8	20	156
-CH$_2$	(−)	0.7	—	108
H$_3$C	(+)	—	—	177
7 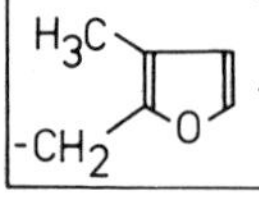	(±)	0.6	—	305
H$_3$C	(−)	0.35	—	182
-CH$_2$	(+)	—	10	375

case optical resolution yields a *levo* antipode 10 times as potent as its racemic mother compound. This effect may be explained by an inhibitory interaction of the two antipodes.

Effects of O-Substituents

The effects of O-substitution summarized in Table 5 were anticipated from
known findings in the benzomorphan series (11). The analgesic or antagonistic effects of the four prototypes either remain unchanged or increase due
to acetylation of the phenolic hydroxy group. On the contrary, methylation
of the phenolic hydroxy group markedly decreases both the analgesic and
the antagonistic activities. The action profile remains unchanged.

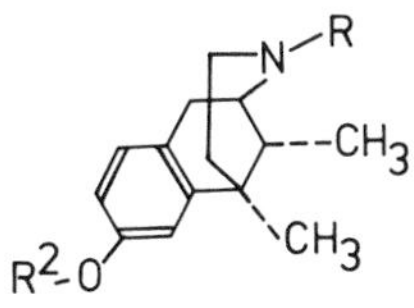

TABLE 5. *O-substituted*
α-5,9-dimethyl-2-furylmethyl-
2'-hydroxy-6,7-benzomorphans

Compound			Analgesia	Antagonism
			Writhing, Mice	Suppression of
-R	Number	-R^2	ED_{50}	Analgesia, Mice
			mg/kg, s.c.	AD_{50}, mg/kg, s.c.
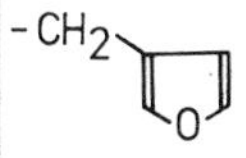 -CH₂ (furan)	5	H	—	1.0
	8	CH_3	—	10
	9	$COCH_3$	—	0.3
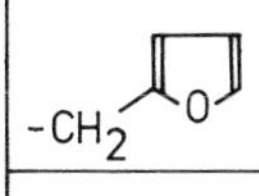 -CH₂ (furan)	2	H	18	1.0
	10	CH_3	—	—
	11	$COCH_3$	12	0.5
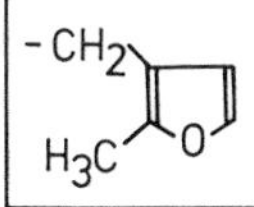 -CH₂ H_3C (furan)	6	H	1.8	20
	12	CH_3	7.0	—
	13	$COCH_3$	0.9	—
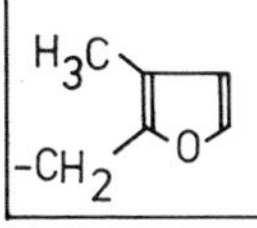 H_3C -CH₂ (furan)	7	H	0.6	—
	14	CH_3	8.6	—
	15	$COCH_3$	0.1	—

Influence of 5- and 9-Alkyl Substituents

Lengthening or shortening of the alkyl chains in the 5 and 9 positions of the benzomorphan system modifies the analgesic or antagonistic efficacy but does not influence the action profiles of the four prototypes.

In the 5-monoalkyl series (Table 6) maximum analgesic activity is observed in the 5-ethyl compounds *22*, *26*, and *30*, and the compounds with longer or shorter 5-alkyl chains are less effective. The antagonistic activity, on the other hand, is less affected by the length of the 5-alkyl group. It is interesting that compounds *16* and *20* with a nonquaternary carbon in position 5 (R^3 = H) are strong antagonists with potencies comparable to those of their quaternary homologues.

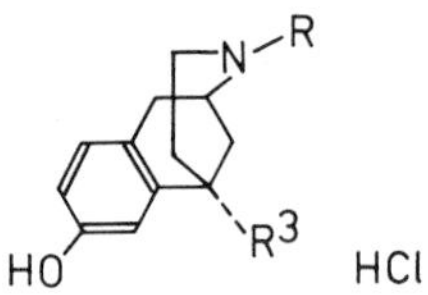

TABLE 6. *5-Alkyl-2-furylmethyl-2'-hydroxy-6,7-benzomorphans*

Compound -R	Number	-R^3	Analgesia Writhing, Mice ED_{50} mg/kg, s.c.	Antagonism Suppression of Analgesia, Mice AD_{50}, mg/kg, s.c.
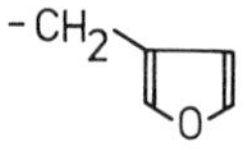 -CH₂ (furyl)	16	H	—	0.5
	17	Me	—	1.0
	18	Et	—	1.0
	19	Pr	—	0.5
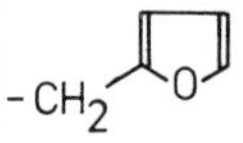 -CH₂ (furyl)	20	H	—	3.0
	21	Me	26	6.0
	22	Et	3.8	3.0
	23	Pr	11	3.0
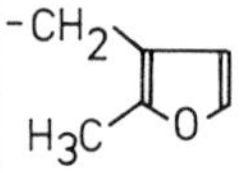 -CH₂ (H₃C furyl)	24	H	—	
	25	Me	—	—
	26	Et	1.0	—
	27	Pr	4.0	—
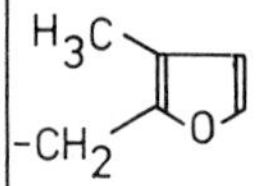 H₃C (furyl) -CH₂	28	H	11	
	29	Me	0.5	—
	30	Et	0.6	—
	31	Pr	2.0	—

In the 5,9-dialkyl series (Table 7) maximum analgesic activity is displayed in the compounds possessing alkyl groups with a total length of three carbon atoms. The same is reported on benzomorphans with other N-substituents (11). The antagonistic activity, however, is less sensitive to changes in the alkyl substituents in the 5- and 9-positions.

Effect of the Steric Orientation of the 9-Alkyl Group

The effect of the steric orientation of the 9-alkyl group is demonstrated in Table 8. Only in the pure antagonist type is no difference in potency of the α-compound and its β-diastereoisomer observed. In all other cases the β-compounds are less potent as antagonists and analgesics than their

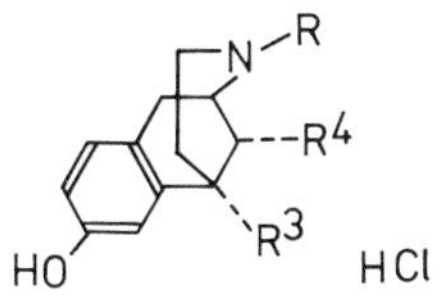

TABLE 7. *5,9-Dialkyl-2-furylmethyl-2'-hydroxy-6 7-benzomorphans*

Compound -R	Number	-R³	-R⁴	Analgesia Writhing, Mice ED₅₀ mg/kg, s.c.	Antagonism Suppression of Analgesia, Mice AD₅₀, mg/kg, s.c.
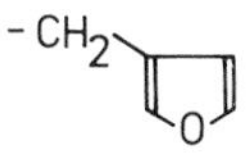 -CH₂ (furyl)	5	Me	Me	—	1.0
	32	Me	Et	—	0.5
	33	Et	Me	—	0.5
	34	Et	Et	—	0.3
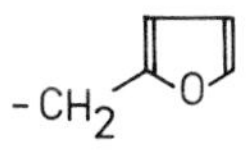 -CH₂ (furyl)	2	Me	Me	18	1.0
	35	Me	Et	8.6	0.5
	36	Et	Me	1.1	2.0
	37	Et	Et	4.0	2.0
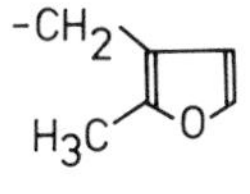 -CH₂ (H₃C-furyl)	6	Me	Me	1.8	20
	38	Me	Et	1.7	2.0
	39	Et	Me	1.0	—
	40	Et	Et	1.0	—
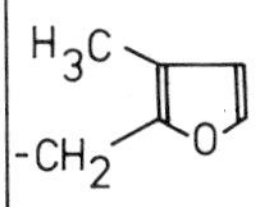 H₃C (furyl) -CH₂	7	Me	Me	0.6	—
	41	Me	Et	0.5	—
	42	Et	Me	0.4	—
	43	Et	Et	1.2	—

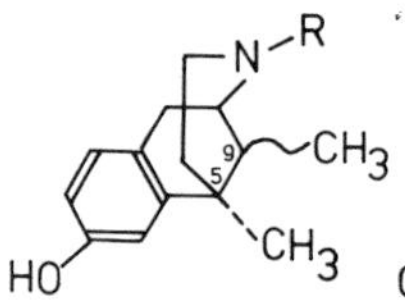

TABLE 8. *Diastereoisomeric 5,9-dimethyl-2-furylmethyl- 2'-hydroxy-6,7-benzomorphans*

CH_3SO_3H

Compound - R	Number	Isomer	Analgesia Writhing Mice ED_{50} mg/kg, s.c.	Antagonism Suppression of Analgesia, Mice AD_{50}, mg/kg s.c.	Toxicity LD_{50} mg/kg s.c.
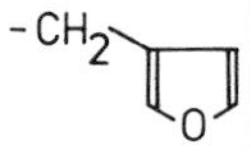 $-CH_2$ (furyl)	5	α	—	1.0	180
	44	β	—	1.0	285
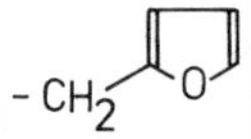 $-CH_2$ (furyl)	2	α	18	1.0	292
	45	β	—	3.0	380
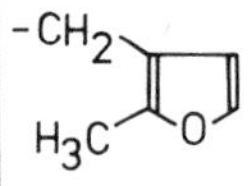 $-CH_2$, H_3C (furyl)	6	α	1.8	20	156
	46	β	11	—	680
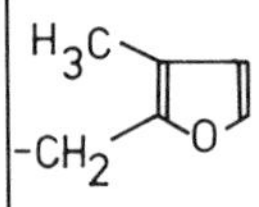 H_3C, $-CH_2$ (furyl)	7	α	0.6	—	305
	47	β	3.2	—	740

α-counterparts. Again the action profile is retained. The β-compounds possess the lower toxicities throughout. Very similar observations concerning known benzomorphan antagonists are described in the literature (9).

N-Furylmethyl Derivatives of the Morphinan Series

The close relationship between the benzomorphan and morphinan structures suggested the synthesis of N-furylmethyl-3-hydroxymorphinans. As shown in Table 9, the approved variants of the furylmethyl group provide morphinans with action profiles similar to those of the corresponding benzomorphans discussed above. In monkey experiments carried out by Villarreal and Seevers (23) the N-furfuryl derivatives 49 had no physical dependence

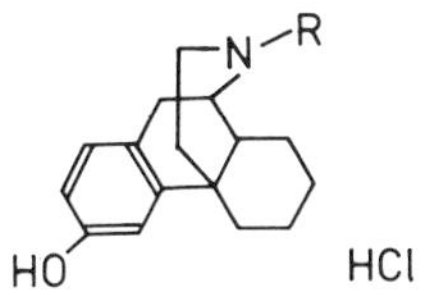

TABLE 9. *N-Furylmethyl-3-hydroxy-morphinans*

Compound - R	Number	Isomer	Analgesia Writhing, Mice ED_{50} mg/kg, s.c.	Antagonism Suppression of Analgesia, Mice AD_{50}, mg/kg, s.c.
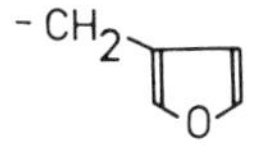 - CH₂ (furyl)	48	(±)	—	0.8
		(−)	—	0.3
		(+)	—	—
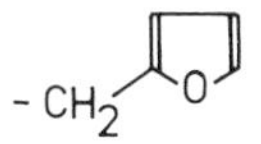 - CH₂ (furyl)	49	(±)	—	0.8
		(−)	—	0.5
		(+)	—	8.0
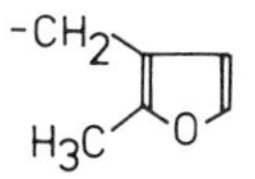 -CH₂ (methylfuryl) H₃C	50	(±)	1.0	—
		(−)	0.3	—
		(+)	—	—
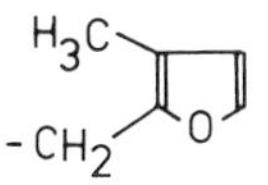 H₃C -CH₂ (methylfuryl)	51	(±)	0.5	—
		(−)	0.2	—
		(+)	—	—

capacity, and the racemic compound and the *levo* isomer were antagonists $^{1}/_{30}$ and $^{1}/_{4}$ as potent as nalorphine. It is interesting to note that antagonistic activity is observed not only in the (−)-3-hydroxy-morphinans with an appropriate N-furylmethyl substituent, but also in their racemic counterparts, whereas the antagonistic effects of N-allyl-3-hydroxy-morphinan are reported (3) to be confined to the (−)-isomer (levallorphan).

N-Furylmethyl Analogues of Other Strong Analgesics

In N-furylmethyl analogues of other strong analgesics such as morphine and its congeners the relationship between the nature of the N-furylmethyl substituent and the action profile is less distinct. With growing complexity of the molecule, the influence of the N-substituent seems to cease and the structure of the moiety M seems to become more important. Since our studies concerning those compounds are not yet completed, a detailed discussion is impossible. Nevertheless, Table 10 gives an idea of the extended scope of this novel structural feature of narcotic antagonists. Known N-allyl antagonists (compounds *a*), derived from L-metazocine, levorphanol, desomorphine, morphine, oxymorphone, and 6,14-endo-etheno-tetrahydro-nororipavine, are compared to their N-(3-furylmethyl) analogues (compounds *b*). As expected from the nature of the N-furylmethyl group involved, all the compounds are pure antagonists. The N-(3-furylmethyl)-benzomorphan *5b* and the closely related compounds *48b* and *52b* surpass

TABLE 10.

N-Furylmethyl analogues of strong analgesics

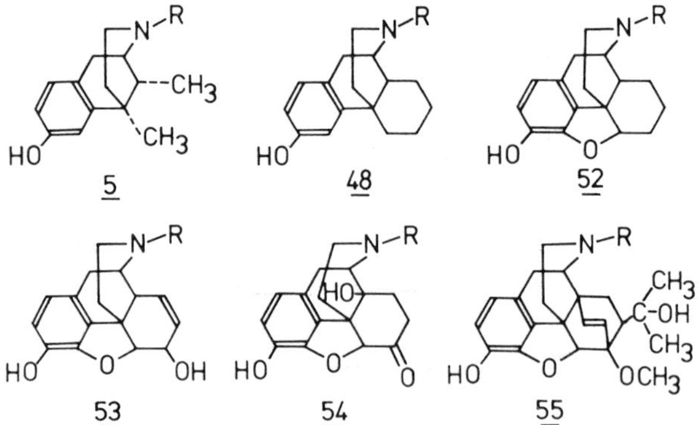

(-) - Compounds; Hydrochlorides

Compound − R		Antagonism Suppression of Analgesia, Mice: AD$_{50}$, mg/kg, s.c.						
a -CH$_2$-CH=CH$_2$	Number	5a	48a	52a	53a	54a	55a
	AD$_{50}$	0.5	0.3	0.3	1.0	0.05	0.3
b - CH$_2$	Number	5b	48b	52b	53b	54b	55b
	AD$_{50}$	0.1	0.3	0.2	2.0	0.2	3.0

their N-allyl analogues *5a* and *48a* (levallorphan) and *52a* in potency. On the contrary, in the more complex molecules the N-(3-furylmethyl) derivatives *53b*, *54b*, and *55b* are less effective as antagonists than their N-allyl counterparts *53a* (nalorphine), *54a* (naloxone), and *55a*.

So far the N-furylmethyl analogues of meperidine have failed to display any antagonistic activity. Since we were able, however, to demonstrate antagonistic properties in certain bemidones (17), we synthesized N-furylmethyl-norbemidones and related compounds. Some of them showed questionable antagonistic activity. Consequently, two compounds of this series, N-furfuryl- and N-(5-methyl-furfuryl)-4-(m-hydroxyphenyl)-4-methoxycarbonyl-piperidine, were studied in monkeys (23). These substances were estimated to possess low or intermediate-high physical dependence capacity. Similar results had been obtained with the corresponding N-allyl derivative (24).

CONCLUSIONS

The idea that the furylmethyl group might be an N-substituent useful in the design of narcotic antagonists due to its inherent allyl character has proved to be successful. N-Furylmethyl analogues of analgesics structurally related to morphine are novel compounds with antagonistic and/or analgesic properties. In the 2'-hydroxy-6,7-benzomorphan and the 3-hydroxy-morphinan series the action profile is first of all governed by the nature of the N-furylmethyl substituent. Pure antagonists comparable to naloxone, agonists-antagonists with differentiated effects, or analgesics as potent as morphine but devoid of physical dependence capacity can be obtained. With the growing complexity of the molecule, the influence of the N-furylmethyl group seems to become less pronounced. Studies of those compounds are in progress and demonstrate the extended scope of the novel structural element of narcotic antagonists. Like the N-allyl group, however, the N-furylmethyl substituents fail to confer antagonistic properties to meperidine, bemidone, and their congeners.

The studies of N-furylmethyl analogues of strong analgesics and related compounds are being continued in our laboratories. Furthermore, experiments concerning a potential correlation of the differentiated pharmacological properties with physicochemical parameters are being done. Finally, selected representatives of the new N-furylmethyl compounds are being investigated as to their subacute and chronic toxicities. Appropriate substances may be useful as anti-heroin agents or as nonaddicting strong analgesics.

REFERENCES

1. Archer, S., Albertson, N. F., Pierson, A. K., Bird, J. G., Keats, A. S., Telford, J., and Papadopoulos, C. N.: Narcotic antagonists as analgesics. Science 137:541–543, 1962.
2. Archer, S., and Harris, L. S.: Narcotic antagonists. In: Progress in Drug Research 8:261–320. Edited by E. Jucker. Birkhäuser Verlag, Basel, 1965.
3. Benson, W. M., O'Gara, E., and Van Winkle, S.: Respiratory and analgesic antagonism of dromoran by 3-hydroxy-N-allyl-morphinan. J. Pharmacol. Exp. Ther. 106:373, 1962.
4. Blumberg, H., Wolf, P. S., and Dayton, H. B.: Use of writhing test for evaluating analgesic activity of narcotic antagonists. Proc. Soc. Exp. Biol. Med. 118:763–766, 1965.
5. Boehringer Sohn, C. H.: 2'-Hydroxy-5,9-dimethyl-6,7-benzomorphane. Deutsche Patentschrift 1420015; Oct. 16, 1959.
6. Boehringer Sohn, C. H.: 2-Furylmethyl-α-5,9-dialkyl-6,7-benzomorphane, deren Säureadditionssalze sowie Verfahren zu deren Herstellung. Deutsche Offenlegungsschrift 2105735.2; Feb. 8, 1971.
7. Boehringer Sohn, C. H.: N-Furylmethyl-morphinane, deren Säureadditionssalze sowie Verfahren zu deren Herstellung. Deutsche Offenlegungsschrift 2107989.0; Feb. 19, 1971.
8. Boehringer Sohn, C. H.: N-Furylmethyl-5-alkyl-6,7-benzomorphane, deren Säureadditionssalze sowie Verfahren zu deren Herstellung. Deutsche Offenlegungsschrift 2108954.3; Feb. 25, 1971.
9. Casy, A. F.: Analgesics and their antagonists: Recent developments. In: Progress in Medicinal Chemistry 7:229–284. Edited by G. P. Ellis and G. B. West. Butterworths, London, 1970.
10. Deneau, G. A., and Seevers, M. H.: Evaluation of new compounds for morphine-like physical dependence in the rhesus monkey. Addendum to the report of the Committee on Drug Addiction and Narcotics. 27th annual meeting, Houston, Texas, 1963.
11. Eddy, N. B., and May, E. L.: 6,7-Benzomorphans. In: Synthetic Analgesics Part IIB. Edited by J. Rolfe. Pergamon Press, London, 1965.
12. Fraser, H. F., and Harris, J. S.: Analgesics and their antagonists. Ann. Rev. Pharmacol. 7:277–300, 1967.
13. Gordon, M., and Lafferty, J. J.: Aralkylbenzomorphan derivatives. U.S. Pat. 2,924,603; Feb. 9, 1960. To Smith Kline & French Laboratories. Ref. in Chem. Abstr. 54, P 1855b, 1960.
14. Gordon, M., and Lafferty, J. J.: Isobenzomorphan derivatives. U.S. Pat. 2, 959,954; Nov. 8, 1960. To Smith Kline & French Laboratories. Ref. in Chem. Abstr. 55, P 9433i, 1961.
15. Gordon, M., Lafferty, J. J., and Tedeschi, D. H.: A new potent analgetic antagonist. Nature, 92:1089, 1961.
16. Haffner, F.: Experimentelle Prüfung schmerzstillender Mittel. Dtsch. Med. Wochenschrift 55:731–733, 1929.
17. Langbein, A., Merz, H., Stockhaus, K., and Wick, H.: Narcotic antagonists of the 4-phenylpiperidine series. Report of the First International Conference on Narcotic Antagonists. Nov. 26–29, 1972, Airlie House, Warrenton, Virginia.
18. Litchfield, J. T., Jr., and Wilcoxon, F.: A simplified method of evaluation of dose-effect experiments. J. Pharmacol. Exp. Ther. 96:99–113, 1949.
19. Martin, W. R.: Opioid antagonists. Pharmacol. Rev. 9:463–521, 1967.
20. May, E. L., and Sargent, L. J.: Morphine and its modifications. In: Medicinal Chemistry 5: Analgetics. Edited by G. deStevens. Academic Press, New York and London, 1965.
21. Merz, H., Langbein, A., Stockhaus, K., and Wick, H.: Novel opioid antagonists of the 2'-hydroxy-6,7-benzomorphan series. Unpublished communication to the Committee on Problems of Drug Dependence. 34th annual meeting, Ann Arbor, Michigan.
22. Shemano, J., and Wendel, H.: A rapid screening test for potential addiction liability of new analgesic agents. Toxicol. Appl. Pharmacol. 6:334–339, 1964.

23. Villarreal, J. E., and Seevers, M. H.: Addendum to the report of the 34th annual meeting of the Committee on Problems of Drug Dependence, Ann Arbor, Michigan, 1972.
24. Villarreal, J. E., and Seevers, M. H.: Addendum to the Report of the 31st annual meeting of the Committee on Problems of Drug Dependence, Palo Alto, California, 1969.
25. Woolfe, G., and MacDonald, A. D.: The evaluation of the analgesic action of pethidine hydrochloride (Demerol). J. Pharmacol. Exp. Ther. *80*:300–307, 1944.

Narcotic Antagonists, edited by M. C. Braude, L. S. Harris, E. L.
May, J. P. Smith, and J. E. Villarreal. *Advances in Biochemical
Psychopharmacology, Vol. 8.* Raven Press, New York © 1974.

Potent Long-Acting Antagonists of the
9,9-Dialkylbenzomorphan Series

Paul A. J. Janssen

Janssen Pharmaceutica, Research Laboratoria, Beerse, Belgium

A collaborative research effort between the chemical research department of ACF Chemiefarma N. V. (Amsterdam, The Netherlands) and the
pharmacological research department of Janssen Pharmaceutica N. V.
(Beerse, Belgium) resulted in the discovery of an extensive series of 9,9-
dialkylbenzomorphan-derivatives (I) (Fig. 1). In this chapter I will briefly
outline the most important results of our work.

Starting with alkyl 2,2-dimethyl-3-oxo-4-phenylbutyrates (II), the corresponding 3-aminobutyrates (III) were prepared in three steps via a Schiff
base and reduction. The N-methylated propionic ester derivatives (IV)
yielded the 2-benzyl-1,3,3-trimethyl-4-piperidones (V) via a Dieckmann
cyclization. These could be converted into the 4-substituted 2-benzyl-1,3,3-
trimethyl-4-piperidinols (VI), which served as the direct precursors of a
series of 5-substituted 2,9,9-trimethyl-6,7-benzomorphans (VII). Exchange
of the N-methyl group for a variety of substituents was achieved by conventional methods leading to the nor-compounds (VIII) and a large series
of racemic benzomorphans of type IX. Several optical enantiomers were
also prepared and obtained in pure form.

All compounds were pharmacologically tested in aqueous solution for
morphine-like and nalorphine-like activity in rats, by subcutaneous route,
using the previously described tail-withdrawal test, the fentanyl-antagonism
test, and the acetic-acid-writhing test.

The relationship between structure and activity in this series of 9,9-
dialkylbenzomorphans of general structure I can be described as follows:

1. All pharmacological activity of the racemates is due to the *levo*-
rotatory isomer, the *dextro*-isomers being virtually inactive and the *levo*-
isomer being about twice as active as the *racemic* mixture.

2. The most active compounds are derived from 9,9-dimethylbenzo-
morphan (VII), other 9,9-dialkylbenzomorphans being less active.

3. As compared with the known 9-methyl-6,7-benzomorphan derivatives
such as phenazocine, cyclazocine, and pentazocine, the new 9,9-dimethyl-

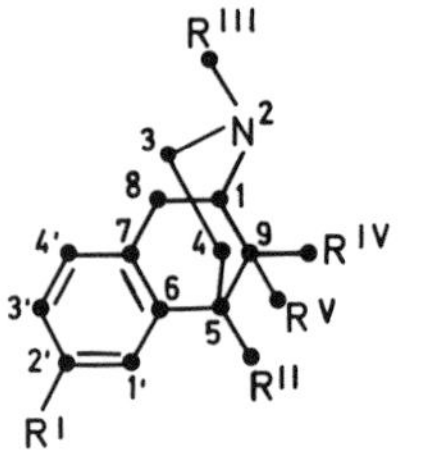
R^III
N^2
3
8
1
4'
7
4
9
R^IV
3'
6
R^V
5
2'
1'
R^II
R^I

I

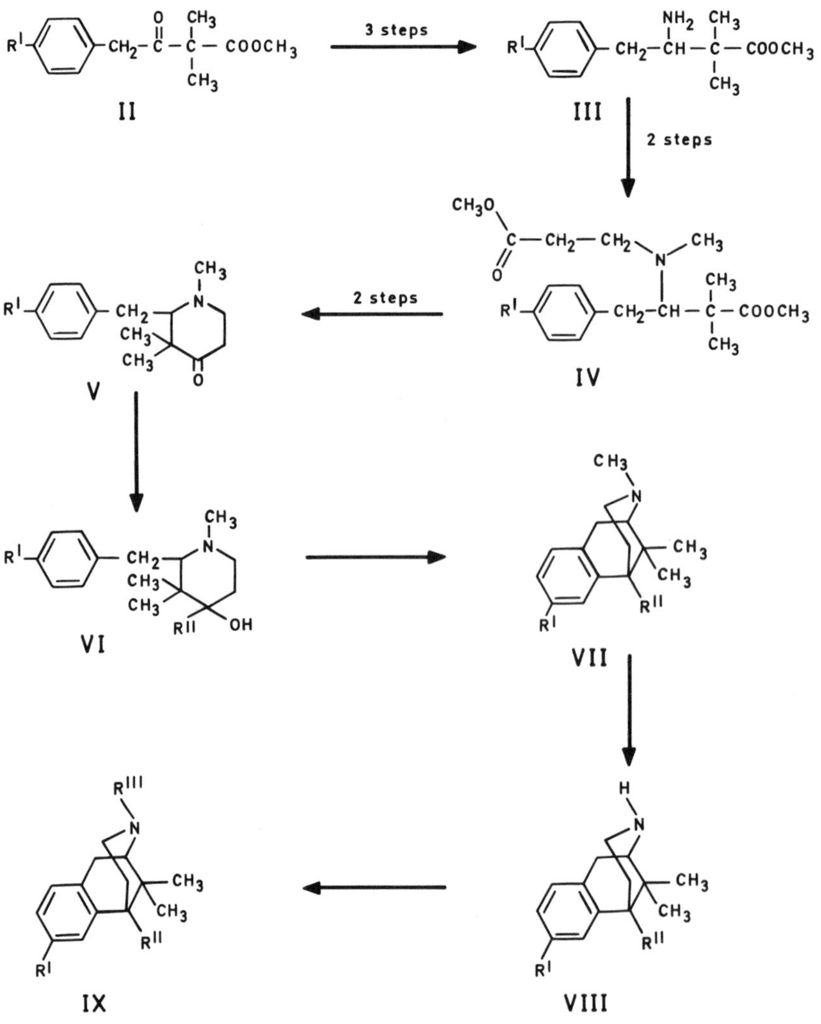
II
3 steps
III
2 steps
IV
2 steps
V
VI
VII
VIII
IX

analogues are found to possess very similar pharmacological profiles. They are, however, as a rule, several times more potent and particularly *much longer acting.*

4. High morphine-like or nalorphine-like potency is associated (a) with a phenolic OH-substituent in position 2′ of the aromatic ring or a classical derivative thereof, such as methoxy or acetoxy and (b) with a lower alkyl substituent, preferably methyl or ethyl, in position 5 (I).

5. As in the known 9-methyl-6,7-benzomorphan-series, potent morphinomimetic activity is associated with substituents such as CH_3 or $CH_2CH_2C_6H_5$ on the basic nitrogen, whereas substituents such as N-allyl, N-cyclopropylmethyl, N-ethyl, N-*n*-propyl, N-propargyl, or N-cyclobutylmethyl give rise to potent nalorphine-like antagonistic activity.

To summarize, it was found that the introduction of a second methyl group in 9-monomethyl-6,7-benzomorphan-derivatives leads to pharmacologically, similarly acting 9,9-dimethyl-6,7-benzomorphans that are both more potent and longer acting.

Narcotic Antagonists, edited by M. C. Braude, L. S. Harris, E. L. May, J. P. Smith, and J. E. Villarreal. *Advances in Biochemical Psychopharmacology, Vol. 8.* Raven Press, New York © 1974.

Antagonists in the Homobenzomorphan Series

Mikio Takeda, Mikihiko Konda, Hirozumi Inoue, Seiichi Saito, Hiroshi Kugita, and Seiichi Nurimoto*

Organic Chemistry Research Laboratory, Tanabe Seiyaku, Co. Ltd., Toda, Saitama, Japan

The marked analgesic activities of 2'-hydroxy-2,6,10-trimethyl-7,8-homobenzomorphans (VIa,b) have suggested further studies on the N-substituted derivatives in this series as possible analgesics and/or narcotic antagonists. BrCN treatment of 2'-methoxy-2,6,10α-trimethyl-7,8-homobenzomorphan (XI), followed by LiAlH₄ reduction, afforded the N-nor compound (XIII). A similar treatment of the 10β-methyl isomer (XIV), on the other hand, exclusively yielded the ring fission product (XV). The N-benzyl-hexahydro-benzo[f]-quinoline derivative (XXV) was converted to the 10-oxo-N-benzylhomobenzomorphan (XXVI) by an application of a novel rearrangement of heterocyclic enamines via bromination as reported previously. XXVI was ultimately converted to the N-nor compounds (XIII) and (XVII) by a series of similar reactions described previously for the N-methyl derivative. Various N-substituted homobenzomorphans (XXIX) and (XXX) were synthesized from (XIII) and (XVII) respectively and tested for analgesic and antagonistic activities. The 6,10-*trans*-dimethyl-N-cyclopropylmethyl derivative (XXXc) exhibits marked antagonist activity comparable to nalorphine with no appreciable agonist property. Generally, this "pure" antagonist property is observed in all 6,10-*trans*-dimethyl series. The homologue (XXIXb) of pentazocine is devoid of antagonist activity.

Seven-membered homologues of some piperidine derivatives are known to have analgesic activity (5). Although the benzomorphan derivatives have been extensively explored as analgesics and/or narcotic antagonists, no reports have appeared on their homologues.[1]

We have, therefore, initiated the study on seven-membered homologues of benzomorphan derivatives. Our first approach (14) to the homobenzomorphan derivatives followed the conventional method of benzomorphan synthesis from β-tetralone (9). Thus, 2'-methoxy-2,6-dimethyl-10-oxo-

---

* Tanabe Seiyaku, Osaka, Japan.

[1] Very recently, the synthesis of the two C-homobenzomorphan derivatives was reported by Shiotani et al. (11).

7,8-homobenzomorphan[2] (IIIa) was prepared by cyclization of the bromo ketone (I) followed by pyrolysis. Since the elimination product (IV) was concurrently formed in both steps, IIIa was obtained in rather low yield[3] (Fig. 1). Through the 10-methylene derivative (V), IIIa was ultimately converted to 2'-hydroxy-2,6,10-trimethyl-homobenzomorphans (VIa,b). More recently, an improved synthesis of IIIa, a key intermediate in the above synthesis, was achieved by a novel rearrangement of the heterocyclic enamine (IXa) via bromination (13) (Fig. 2).

The N-carbethoxy compound (VIIIa) gave the hexahydro-benzo[f]-quinoline derivative (IXa) on alkaline hydrolysis. Bromination of IXa, followed by treatment with aqueous ammonium hydroxide, yielded 81% 10-oxo homobenzomorphan (IIIa). Similarly, the dihydrobenz[e]indoline derivative (IXb) yielded the 9-oxo benzomorphan (IIIb).

The marked analgesic activities (14) of 2'-hydroxy-2,6,10-trimethyl-homobenzomorphans (VIa,b) have suggested further study on the N-substituted derivatives in this series as possible analgesics and/or narcotic antagonists.

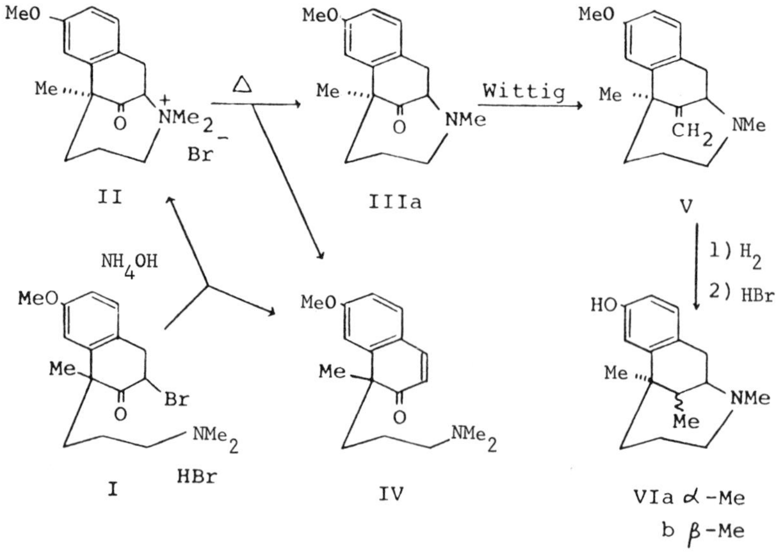

---

[2] *Chemical Abstracts* name: 3,7-dimethyl-9-methoxy-12-oxo- 1,2,4,5,6,7-hexahydro-2,7-methano-3H-3-benzazonine. The term "homobenzomorphan" has been given to this series of derivatives with numbering analogous to that of benzomorphan (14).

[3] A similar observation has been reported in the benzomorphan series (9).

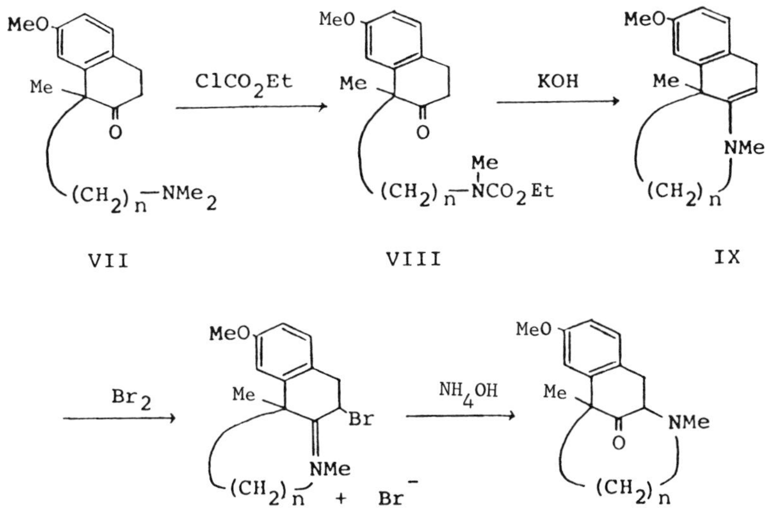

VII   VIII   IX

X   III

a. n=3   b. n=2

Cyanogen bromide treatment of 2'-methoxy-2,6,10α-trimethyl-homo-benzomorphan (XI) in CHCl$_3$ gave a good yield of the N-cyano derivative (XII), which was reduced with LiAlH$_4$ to the N-nor compound (XIII). A similar treatment of the 10β-methyl derivative (XIV), on the other hand, exclusively afforded the ring fission product (XV) with a recovery of XIV hydrobromide. Structural assignment for the anomalous product (XV) was made largely from nuclear magnetic resonance (nmr) spectra (δ 5.75 1H broad triplet, olefinic proton; 1.80 3H broad singlet, C=C—CH$_3$). Treatment of XIV with ethyl chloroformate (1) also resulted in the formation of XVI (Fig. 3). Different behavior of the two isomers (XI) and (XIV) in their reactions with cyanogen bromide prompted us to examine a similar reaction on the isomeric pair of benzomorphans (XVIIIa,b). The 9α-methyl derivative (XVIIIa) gave the expected (8) N-cyano derivative (XIXa) in a quantitative yield, whereas the 9β-methyl isomer (XVIIIb) yielded XIXb and again the ring fission product (XX) in 3:1 ratio, respectively. The presence of the double bond in a benzene conjugated position in this instance was established by nmr and ultraviolet spectra. Although no satisfactory explanation on these anomalous results can be offered at present, the pro-

XI XII XIII

XVII XIV XV X=CN

XVI X=CO$_2$Et

XX

nounced tendency of the more hindered N-methyl derivatives[4] (XIV) and (XVIIIb) to undergo ring cleavage is noteworthy. When treated with diethyl azodicarboxylate (6), XIV afforded a very small amount of the N-nor compound (XVII).

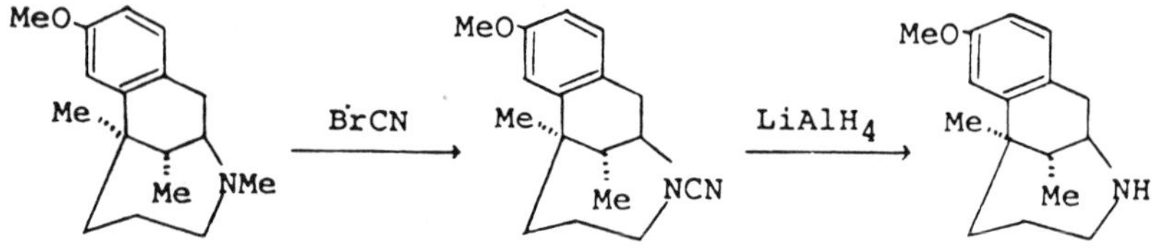

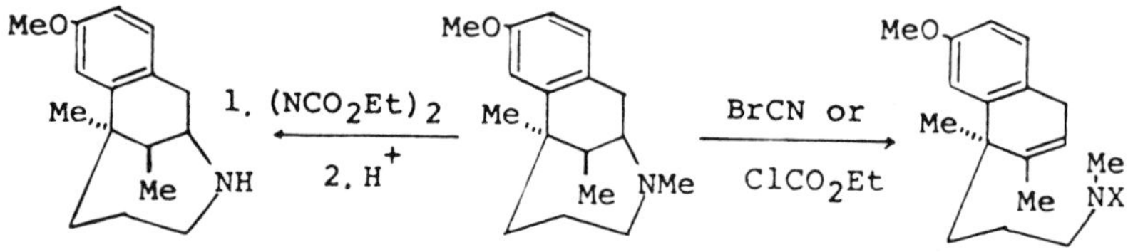

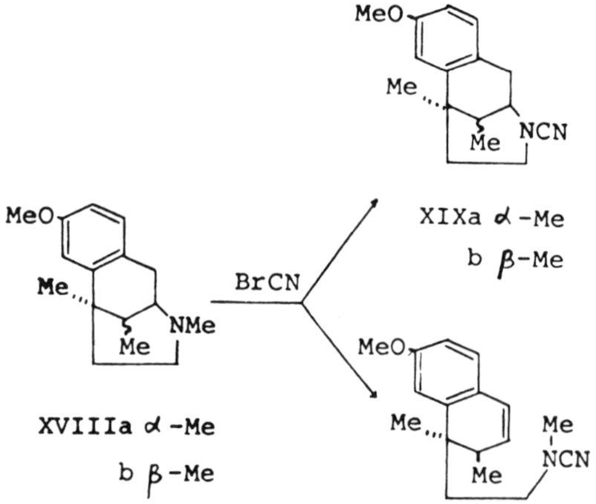

[4] β-Alkyl substituents in the benzomorphan and its homologue, equatorially oriented for the hydroaromatic ring, are close enough to the nitrogen to cause steric hindrance.

Conventional methods of N-demethylation thus proved refractory for
XIV and we took an alternative route to XVII via the N-benzyl enamine
(XXV). Through the cyano ketone (XXII), XXV was synthesized from
3,4-dihydro-7-methoxy-1-methyl-2(1H)-naphthalenone   (XXI)   by   the
method outlined in Fig. 4. The reactions were all relatively straightforward

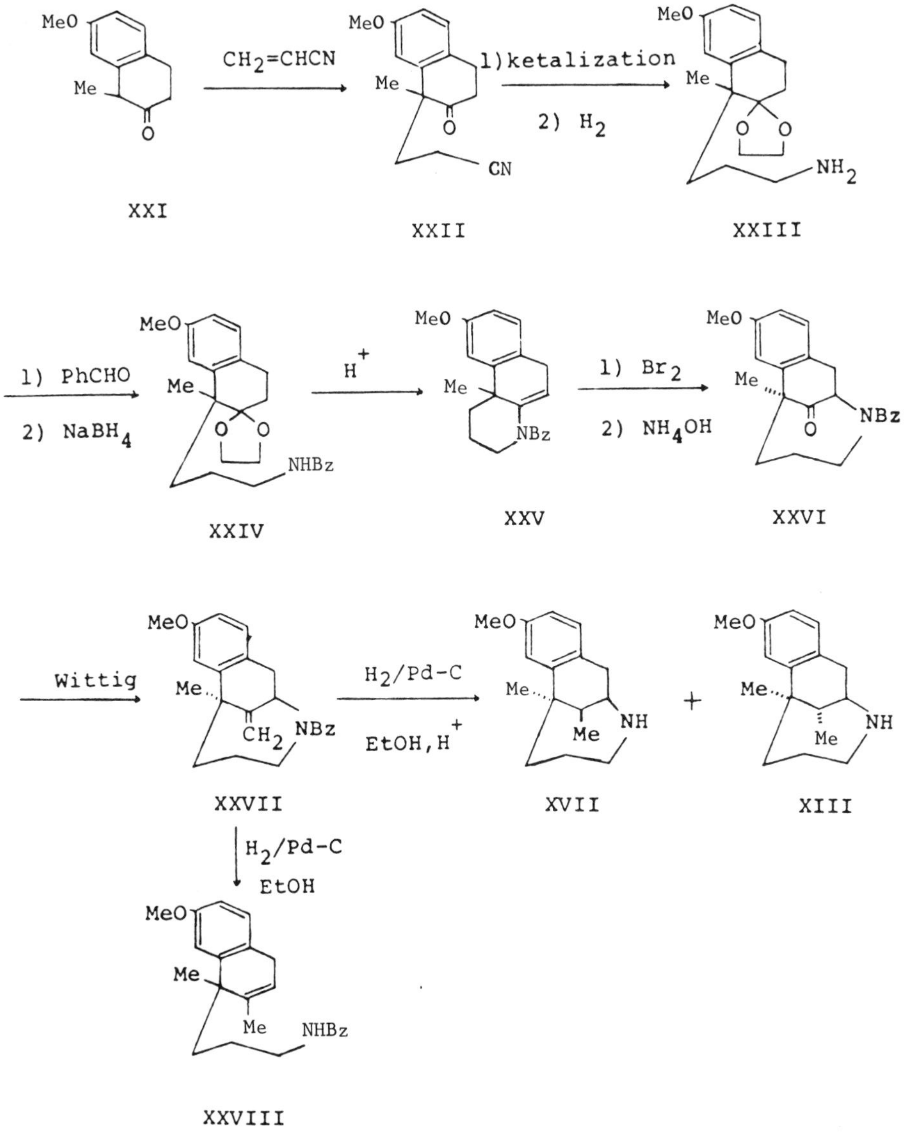

and good yields were obtained. The rearrangement of XXV to the 10-oxo derivative (XXVI) proceeded in 40% yield. The low yield might be due to the weak basicity of XXV (pK$_a$ 7.00) compared with that of the N-methyl relative (IXa, pK$_a$ 9.65). XXVI with methylenetriphenylphosphorane gave the 10-methylene compound (XXVII) in 77% yield. Hydrogenation (Pd-C in EtOH-aq. HCl) of XXVII effected both hydrogenolysis of the N-benzyl group and saturation of the methylene group and gave the 10β-methyl (XVII) and the 10α-methyl isomer (XIII) in yield of 64.3% and 21.4%, respectively. In nmr spectra, the 10-methyl signal of the α-isomer (XIII) appeared at higher field (0.34 ppm) than that of the β-isomer (XVII) in agreement with the reported observation in the benzomorphan series (4). N-Methylation of XVII and XIII to XIV and XI respectively proved their identity. In an effort to obtain XIII predominantly, XXVII was hydrogenated in EtOH alone.[5] The major product in this instance, however, was found to be the ring fission product (XXVIII).[6] Susceptibility to cleavage of C$_1$—N bond has been thus observed throughout the series of homobenzomorphan derivatives.

Finally, various N-substituted derivatives (XXIX) and (XXX) were prepared from the N-nor compounds (XIII) and (XVII) respectively by usual methods and tested for analgesic and antagonist activities.

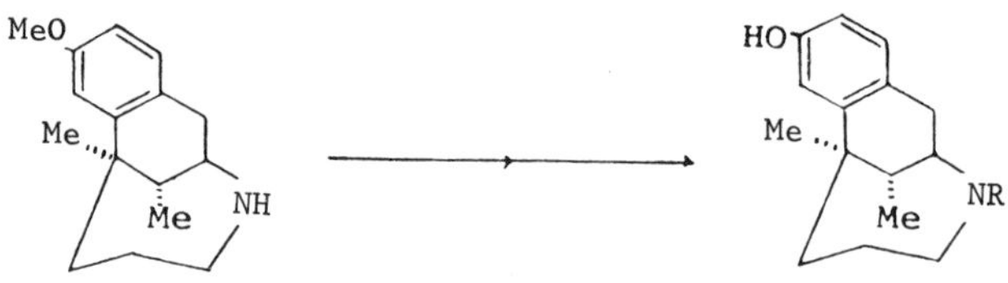

XIII

XXIX

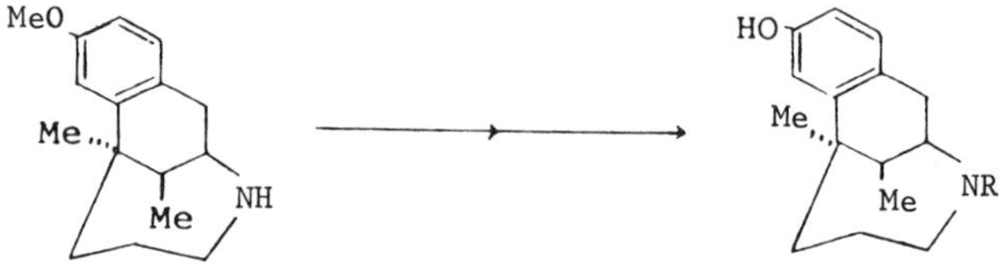

XVII

XXX

---

[5] Stereoselective formation of the α-methyl derivatives has been reported in the benzomorphan series (10).

[6] An analogous finding has been reported for the N-methyl derivative (V) (14).

PHARMACOLOGY

Table 1 gives a pharmacologic summary of the representative N-substituted homobenzomorphans. The two N-cyclopropylmethyl derivatives (XXIXc) and (XXXc) exhibit the marked antagonist activities comparable to levallorphan. The *cis* isomer (XXIXc), the homologue of cyclazocine, is about three times as potent as the *trans* isomer (XXXc) in this property. However, (XXIXc) is also agonist (analgesic) and quite toxic. The *trans* counterpart (XXXc), on the other hand, demonstrates no appreciable agonist activity. The *cis* N-dimethylallyl derivative (XXIXb), the homologue of pentazocine, is found to be devoid of antagonist activity and a weaker analgesic than pentazocine, and the *trans* isomer (XXXb) and the *trans* N-allyl compound (XXXa) are weak and moderate antagonists

TABLE 1. *Analgesic and antagonist activities of homobenzomorphans*

R: a, —CH$_2$CH=CH$_2$ b, —CH$_2$CH=CMe$_2$ c, —CH$_2$—◁

Compound[a]	LD$_{50}$	ED$_{50}$	AD$_{50}$
	(mouse, mg/kg, s.c.)		
XXIXb	183.7	ca 20	>30
XXIXc	55.1	3.9	0.021
XXXa	113.5	>22.5	0.32
XXXb	89.7	>22.5	3.8
XXXc	104.0	>22.5	0.069
Nalorphine	670.0	4.5	0.078
Pentazocine	190.1	4.5	6.0
Levallorphan		>22.5	0.040

Analgesic activity determined by AcOH writhing method (7). When tested by the hot-plate method (3), no analgesic activities were observed up to 22.5 mg/kg for these compounds.

Antagonist activity versus morphine analgesia (10 mg/kg), determined by Haffner's method (12).

[a] Administered as HCl salts in H$_2$O.

respectively with no analgesic activities. Thus, the *trans*-6,10-dimethyl-homobenzomorphans (XXXa,b,c) are all devoid of agonist property with weak to strong antagonist activity and seem to fall under the category of "pure" antagonist. This property, on the other hand, is not apparent in the *cis* counterparts (XXIXb,c). This is a most striking result in structure-activity relationship. Regarding the effect of modifying the substituent on nitrogen, the order of antagonist activity is N-cyclopropylmethyl > N-allyl > N- dimethylallyl. This parallels the experience in the 5,9-dimethyl benzomorphan series (2). In the rhesus monkey[7] the antagonist activity of XXXc is approximately $1/_3$ that of nalorphine but of longer duration. Its peak effect is sustained about three times longer than nalorphine. Thus, the compound (XXXc) is a possible candidate for clinical trial as "pure" antagonist.

CONCLUSION

Replacement of the N-methyl group by N-allyl and related groups in the homobenzomorphan analgesics resulted in appearance of antagonist activities. 2'-Hydroxy-2-cyclopropylmethyl-6,10β-dimethyl-7,8-homobenzomorphan (XXXc) exhibits the marked antagonist activity comparable to nalorphine with no appreciable agonist property.

ACKNOWLEDGMENTS

The authors express their gratitude to Dr. Everette L. May, National Institutes of Health, for his aid and useful discussions in this series of work. Thanks are also due to Mr. M. Yamazaki, Director of Organic Chemistry Research Laboratory, Dr. N. Sugimoto and Dr. S. Sugasawa, Professor Emeritus of Tokyo University, for their interest and encouragement.

REFERENCES

1. Abdel-Monem, M. M., and Portoghese, P. S.: N-Demethylation of morphine and structually related compounds with chloroformate esters. J. Med. Chem. *15*:208–210, 1972.
2. Archer, S., and Harris, L. S.: Narcotic antagonist. Prog. Drug Res. *8*:261–320, 1965.
3. Eddy, N. B., and Leimbach, D.: Synthetic analgesics II. Dithienylbutenyl- and dithienylbutylamines. J. Pharmacol. Exp. Ther. *107*:385–393, 1953.
4. Fullerton, S. E., May, E. L., and Becker, E. D.: Structures related to morphine. XXIII. Stereochemistry of 5,9-dialkyl-6,7-benzomorphans. J. Org. Chem. *27*:2144–2147, 1962.
5. Hardy, Jr., R. A., and Howell, M. G.: Synthetic analgetics with morphine-like action. *In:*

---

[7] We are indebted to Dr. J. E. Villarreal, Department of Pharmacology, University of Michigan, for this observation (*personal communication,* also ref 15).

Analgetics, edited by G. de Stevens, pp. 206–211. Academic Press, New York and London, 1965.

6. Kanematsu, K., Takeda, M., Jacobson, A. E., and May, E. L.: Synthesis of 6,7-benzomorphan and related nonquaternary carbon structures with marked analgetic activity. J. Med. Chem. *12*:405–408, 1969.

7. Koster, R., Anderson, M., and de Beer, E. J.: Acetic acid for analgesic screening. Fed. Proc. *18*:412, 1959.

8. May, E. L., and Eddy, N. B.: Structures related to morphine. XII. (±)-2'-Hydroxy-5,9-dimethyl-2-phenethyl-6,7-benzomorphan (NIH 7519) and its optical forms. J. Org. Chem. *24*:1435–1437, 1959.

9. Murphy, J. G., Ager, J. H., and May, E. L.: Structures related to morphine. XIV. 2'-Hydroxy-5-methyl-2-phenethyl-6,7-benzomorphan, the 9-demethyl analog of NIH 7519 (phenazocine) from 3,4-dihydro-7-methoxy-2(1H)-naphthalenone. J. Org. Chem. *25*:1386–1388, 1960.

10. Saito, S., and May, E. L.: Structures related to morphine. XXI. An alternative synthesis of diastereoisomeric 2'-hydroxy-2,5,9-trimethyl-6,7-benzomorphans. J. Org. Chem. *27*:1087–1089, 1962.

11. Shiotani, S., Kometani, T., and Mitsuhashi, K.: Studies on structure-activity relationship of analgetics. XIII. Syntheses of homobenzomorphans and related compounds. (1). Chem. Pharm. Bull. *20*:277–283, 1972.

12. Takagi, H., Inukai, T., and Nakama, M.: A modification of Haffner's method for testing analgesics. Jap. J. Pharmacol. *16*:287–294, 1966.

13. Takeda, M., Inoue, H., Konda, M., Saito, S., and Kugita, H.: An improved synthesis of a 9-oxo-6,7-benzomorphan and its homolog. A novel rearrangement of heterocyclic enamines via bromination. J. Org. Chem. *37*:2677–2679, 1972.

14. Takeda, M., and Kugita, H.: Homologs of benzomorphan derivatives. I. J. Med. Chem. *13*:630–634, 1970.

15. Villarreal, J. E., and Seevers, M. H.: Evaluation of new compounds for morphine-like physical dependence in the rhesus monkey. Addendum 6, Minutes of the 33rd Meeting of the Committee on Problems of Drug Dependence, National Research Counsil, National Academy of Sciences, 1971.

Narcotic Antagonists, edited by M. C. Braude, L. S. Harris, E. L. May, J. P. Smith, and J. E. Villarreal. *Advances in Biochemical Psychopharmacology, Vol. 8.* Raven Press, New York © 1974.

Ring C-Bridged Derivatives of Thebaine and Oripavine

John W. Lewis

Reckitt and Colman, Research Laboratories, Pharmaceutical Division, Hull, England

Diels-Alder adducts of thebaine have been the source of a series of analgesics in which the opportunity for structural variation at peripheral sites has led to a wide range of agonist-antagonist profiles. The series of oripavine tertiary alcohols prepared from the thebaine-methyl vinyl ketone adduct in particular has yielded analgesics of extremely high potency. N-Alkenyl, N-propyl, and especially N-cyclopropylmethyl analogues of these narcotics are, in many cases, potent antagonists of morphine. Diprenorphine is a relatively "pure" antagonist whereas buprenorphine has powerful agonist actions combined with easily demonstrable antagonist characteristics. Diprenorphine antagonizes the analgesic actions of buprenorphine; the two compounds differ only in the tertiary alcohol function. The actions of the two antagonists in animals are characterized by relatively long durations of action, by lack of behavioral effects, and by low dependence liability. From preliminary studies in man, buprenorphine appears to be an effective analgesic lacking dysphoric effects.

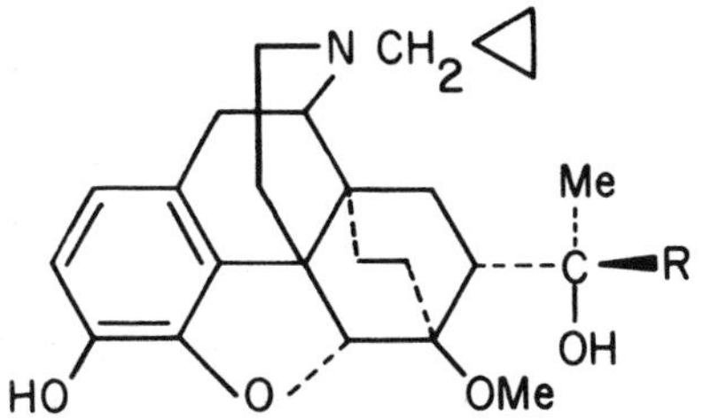

Diprenorphine R = Me

Buprenorphine R = tBu

INTRODUCTION

The search for analgesics superior to morphine has largely concerned derivatives of the alkaloid itself and simpler synthetic compounds having some of the characteristics of the morphine structure. The widely explored series of ring C-bridged derivatives of thebaine and oripavine developed by Bentley and his co-workers reverse this trend in that they are more complex than morphine (for a recent full review of the chemistry of these series see reference 2). In these series the opportunity for structural varia-

123

tions at peripheral sites has led to compounds of very widely differing analgesic profiles and potencies.

CHEMISTRY

The series are derived from Diels-Alder adducts of thebaine, **1**, especially those, **2**, with alkyl vinyl ketones (R^1 = alkyl) and alkyl acrylates (R^1 = O-alkyl) (4). The Diels-Alder reaction is under electronic control and, in these cases, gives only C-7-substituted 6,14-*endo*ethenotetrahydro-thebaines with no trace of the C-8 substituted compounds even with a large-scale operation (for numbering of the carbon atoms in the bridged ring derivatives see Fig 1). The reactions result almost entirely in the production of 7α-compounds, **2** (Fig. 2).

The adducts, **2**, react readily with Grignard reagents to give alcohols, **3** (8). The most extensively studied series is that of the tertiary alcohols derived from the ketone, **2** (R^1 = Me). The normal Grignard reaction, which in most cases is accompanied by competing reduction of the ketone and by rearrangement, gives tertiary alcohols of structure **3** with uniform stereochemistry as a result of the formation of a six-membered, cyclic intermediate which demands a highly stereospecific attack on the carbonyl group from above the plane of the C-7 to C-19 bond. The secondary alcohol by-product of the Grignard reaction has the *S*-configuration, **3** (R^1 = Me, R^2 = H). The diastereoisomeric alcohol, **3** (R^1 = H, R^2 = Me), is produced by Meerwein-Ponndorf reduction of the ketone, **2** (R^1 = Me) (8).

The thebaine derivatives of structure **3** can be demethylated to give the corresponding phenols, derivatives of oripavine (5). Because rearrangement readily occurs under acid conditions, demethylation can only be achieved by alkali, in particular by potassium hydroxide in diethylene glycol at approximately 210°C. A number of the thebaines of structure **3** are very potent analgesics; the corresponding oripavines are even more active, in some cases several thousand times greater than morphine.

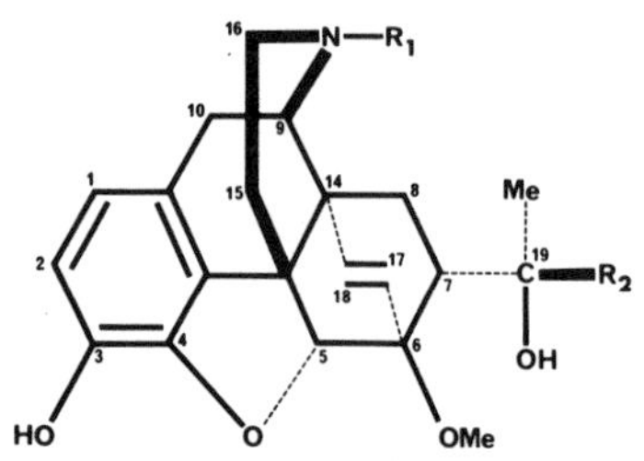

FIG. 1. Structure of the 6,14-*endo*-ethenotetrahydrooripavine tertiary alcohols.

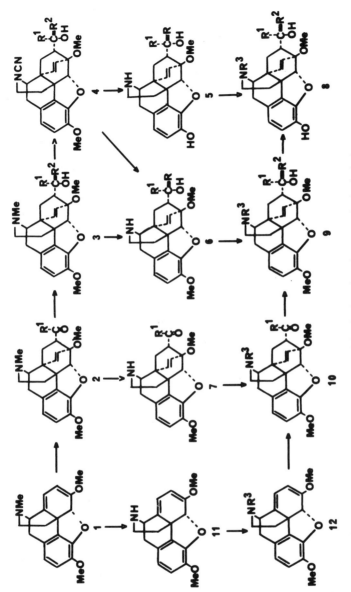

FIG. 2. Synthesis of N-substituted derivatives of the 6,14-*endo*-ethenotetrahydrothebaine and the oripavine series.

125

In the search for new morphine antagonists and partial agonists the alcohols, **3**, were converted to the corresponding nor-oripavines, **5**, and nor-thebaines, **6**, via the N-cyanonorthebaines, **4** (5). The latter, prepared from tertiary bases, **3**, by reaction with cyanogen bromide, are converted to the secondary bases with caustic alkalis in diethylene glycol at temperatures of 180°C and above. At 180°C the products are largely the nor-thebaines, **6**; at higher temperature (210°C) the nor-oripavines **5** are predominantly formed.

The bases of structure **3** can also be converted to the secondary bases, **6**, via their adducts with ethyl azodicarboxylate. The adducts are converted to the secondary bases by mild treatment with acids (5). The ketones and esters of structure **2**, which are readily rearranged under alkaline conditions (6), are smoothly converted to secondary bases, **7**, by the azodicarboxylate method.

The secondary bases, **5**, **6**, and **7**, have been directly alkylated to new tertiary bases, **8**, **9**, and **10**, in which the group R^3 is alkyl up to C_5, allyl, 2-methylallyl, 3,3-dimethylallyl, and propargyl (5). The N-cyclopropyl-methyl (CPM) derivatives in the series, **8** and **9**, are accessible from the secondary bases by acylation with cyclopropylcarbonyl chloride followed by reduction with lithium aluminium hydride (5).

The N-CPM ketones and esters of structure **10** were prepared by Diels-Alder reactions from N-cyclopropylmethylnorthebaine, **12** (R^3 = CPM) (27), which was obtained from thebaine by azodicarboxylate N-demethylation to **11** followed by the previously mentioned procedure of acylation and lithium aluminium hydride reduction (3). The N-substituted tertiary alcohols, **9**, can also be prepared from the ketones and esters, **10**, by reaction with Grignard reagents, and O-demethylation of the thebaine derivatives, **9**, gives the corresponding oripavines **8**.

An alternative route to the N-CPM ketones of structure **10** involves direct acylation and reduction of the dimethyl acetals of the nor-ketones, **7**. O-Demethylation of the ketone acetals can be achieved with caustic alkali to afford a route to the N-CPM oripavine ketones (18).

For the preparation of N-substituted tertiary alcohols of the analogous 6,14-ethano series, the modification of the above procedures is illustrated in Fig. 3 for the preparation of the interesting N-CPM derivatives diprenorphine, **18** (R = Me), and buprenorphine, **18** (R = tBu) (cf 5). The 6,14-etheno group is hydrogenated (with 10% palladium on carbon) as the ketone, **2** (R^1 = Me), since the tertiary alcohol group hinders access to the double bond. The ethano-ketone, **13**, is treated with the appropriate Grignard reagent to give the tertiary alcohols, **14**. N-Demethylation with cyanogen bromide followed by treatment at 210°C in diethylene glycol with caustic

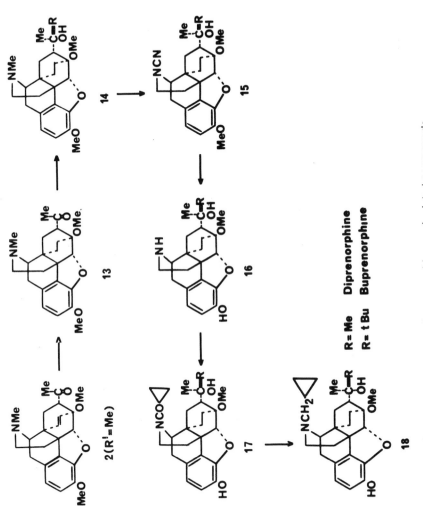

FIG. 3. Synthesis of diprenorphine, buprenorphine, and related compounds.

127

potash gives the nor-oripavine derivatives, **16**, which are converted to the N-CPM derivatives, **18**, by lithium aluminium hydride reduction.

The stability of the oripavines, **18**, in aqueous solution is governed by acid catalyzed rearrangement (9) below pH 3 and oxidative-phenol-coupling reactions above pH 6. The optimum pH is about 4; diprenorphine and buprenorphine give stable formulations at this pH.

The chemistry of the bridged thebaine derivatives is very extensive and morphine antagonists have been found in a number of series not specifically discussed in this review. They have not, in general, proved as interesting as the tertiary alcohols. The reader is referred to the original literature for details on chemistry and structure-activity relationships. Series lacking any C-7 substituent (25) or having at C-7α, an alkyl group (7) or a hetero-cyclic group (17), have members which are antagonists and partial agonists as do the series of 7-ketones (25) and 7,7- (24) and 7,8-disubstituted com-pounds (26). The series of N-substituted tertiary alcohols, **8** and **9**, have been subject to removal of the C-3 oxygen function (23) and introduction of a C-16 alkyl group (22) with interesting results.

TESTING METHODS

Earlier evaluation of the N-alkenyl and N-cyclopropylmethyl members of the tertiary alcohol series used the conventional rat tail-pressure (10) and phenylquinone-writhing (10) tests for agonist activity, and antagonism of the analgesic action of morphine was assessed by the rat tail-pressure test (10). It was believed that agonist activity in the tail-pressure test as well as in the hot-plate and tail-flick tests reflected unacceptably high levels of physical dependence in man. That this need not be the case was revealed when cyclazocine was examined; in the tail-pressure test it showed signifi-cant activity as an analgesic but also antagonized the action of morphine. In contrast, no member of the bridged thebaine or oripavine series showed unequivocally both agonist and antagonist actions in this test.

Use of the tail-flick test in both rats and mice with hot water as the nociceptive stimulus (19) allowed a more detailed evaluation of the agonist-antagonist profiles of representative samples of the series of N-substituted tertiary alcohols, **8**, **9**, and **18**, to be made. By varying the temperature of the water, graded intensities of stimulus became available and an assessment of the intrinsic activity of partial agonists could be made. It was also found that this test is much more sensitive to narcotic antagonists than the tail-pressure test and that compounds of the oripavine series which showed only agonism in the latter test were shown to be morphine antagonists in the tail-flick tests.

Both morphine antagonism and physical dependence liability have been evaluated in mice and primates (19). The ability to precipitate abstinence effects in the morphine-dependent animals reflects morphine antagonist character when direct dependence studies are carried out on naive animals.

STRUCTURE-ACTIVITY RELATIONSHIPS

Replacement of N-methyl groups of narcotic analgesics by allyl and related alkenyl groups and by cyclopropylmethyl groups often leads to compounds that are able to antagonize the effects of the narcotics. Most narcotic antagonists also show analgesic effects to a greater or lesser extent, i.e., they have varying levels of intrinsic activity. Thus in studying the relationship between structure and activity in a series of narcotic antagonists, intrinsic activity has to be accorded at least as great importance as potency.

For the series of tertiary carbinols of structures **8** and **9**, the effects on activity in the tail-pressure test of varying R^1, R^2, and R^3 are shown in Tables 1–4 for the N-allyl and N-CPM derivatives to illustrate relationships which have been established by studying a wide range of nitrogen substi-

TABLE 1. *Activities of bases of structure 9 (R^3 = ally)*
in the rat tail-pressure test

R^2 / R^1	Me	Et	n Pr
Me	110^a	$>100^{b,a}$	$>100^{b,a}$
Et	15^a	44^a	
n Pr	2.7^a		
n Bu	1.05^a		

^{a} ED_{50} mg/kg, i.p. or s.c.
^{b} AD_{50} mg/kg, i.p. or s.c.

TABLE 2. *Activities of bases of structure 9 (R^3 = CPM) in the rat*
tail-pressure test

R^2 / R^1	Me	Et	n Pr	n Bu
Me	1.45^b	2.5^b	$>100^{b,a}$	9.0^a
Et	10^b	70^b		
n Pr	0.3^a	3.0^a		
n Bu	0.95^a			

^{a} ED_{50} mg/kg, i.p. or s.c.
^{b} AD_{50} mg/kg, i.p. or s.c.

TABLE 3. Activities of bases of structure 8 (R^3 = allyl) in the rat tail-pressure test

R^2 \ R^1	Me	Et
Me	0.21^b	0.42^b
Et	4.2^b	0.48^b
n Pr	0.033^a	

^{a} ED_{50} mg/kg, i.p. or s.c.
^{b} AD_{50} mg/kg, i.p. or s.c.

TABLE 4. Activities of the bases of structure 8 (R^3 = CPM) in the rat tail-pressure test

R^2 \ R^1	Me	Et	n Pr	n Bu
Me	0.013^b	0.06^b	0.52^b	0.35^a
Et	0.02^b	0.26^b		
n Pr	0.002^a			
n Bu	0.026^a			

^{a} ED_{50} mg/kg, i.p. or s.c.
^{b} AD_{50} mg/kg, i.p. or s.c.

tuents. In general, the groups giving rise to the highest proportion of narcotic antagonists are n-propyl, allyl, and cyclopropylmethyl. The oripavines, **8** (Tables 3 and 4), have greater morphine antagonist character than the corresponding thebaines, **9** (Tables 1 and 2), i.e., lower intrinsic activity. This is very clearly shown for the N-allyl compounds where demethylation of the weakly analgesic thebaines (Table 1) gives rise to oripavines which are strong morphine antagonists (Table 3). In contrast to the drop in intrinsic activity there is always a large increase in potency in going from the thebaine to the corresponding oripavine.

The size of the alkyl groups in the tertiary alcohol function and the configuration of C-19 have a profound effect on intrinsic activity. The latter rises as R^2 increases in size. This is illustrated by the sharp contrast in both N-allyl and N-CPM series of oripavines when R^1 = methyl (Tables 3 and 4) between the bases where R^2 = ethyl and R^2 = n-propyl. The ethyl carbinols are powerful antagonists in the tail-pressure test but the propyl carbinols, which are derivatives of etorphine, **8** ($R^1 = R^3$ = Me, R^2 = Pr), are extremely powerful analgesics and show no antagonism of morphine in the same test. N-Cyclopropylmethylnoretorphine is an analgesic 1,000 times more potent than morphine whereas its diasteroisomer (19S series) is a morphine antagonist of nalorphine's potency. However, the etorphine derivative is a morphine antagonist in the tail-flick test ($0.3 \times$ nalorphine) and this kind of activity is generally shown by the oripavines of structure **8** ($R^3 = $ CPM), which show only analgesia in the tail-pressure test. As in the N-methyl series, potency increases as R^2 becomes larger, reaching a maximum in the propyl-butyl range.

The N-CPM bases have greater agonist character as the size of R^1 increases in structures **8** and **9**. In the series where $R^2 = $ methyl the change from morphine antagonism to agonism in the tail-pressure test comes when R^1 changes from propyl to butyl. The transition is less marked than the corresponding one for R^2, because potency decreases with increasing R^1 especially between $R^1 = $ ethyl and $R^1 = $ propyl, whereas the reverse is true for R^2 for this size of group.

Alletorphine, **8** ($R^1 = $ Me, $R^2 = $ Pr, $R^3 = $ allyl), is 50 to 100 times more potent than morphine as an analgesic in rats but shows very much lower depression of respiration at an equianalgesic dose (11); however, this separation of effects apparently does not hold for mice (16). In single-dose studies in withdrawn, morphine-dependent monkeys alletorphine showed some signs of suppression but others of exacerbation of the withdrawal effects indicating a partial agonist character (29). The narcotic antagonist component was not of a sufficiently high order to prevent primary dependence being established in naive monkeys (19). In man alletorphine was shown to be an effective analgesic in postoperative and cancer patients but in the latter group it produced a high incidence of dysphoric effects (14).

The increase of intrinsic activity observed as R^1 or R^2 changes from methyl to butyl in the N-CPM bases of structures **8** and **9** is similarly shown in the series of N-CPM ketones and esters of structure **10**. This is illustrated in Tables 5 and 6 for the rat-tail pressure test. In the ketone series the crossover from morphine antagonism to analgesia occurs between the propyl and butyl ketones. The increase of agonism in the early part of the series is reflected in the activities in the antiwrithing test for the ketones which are morphine antagonists in the tail-pressure test.

Our more recent work has involved 6,14-ethano derivatives particularly the alcohols of the oripavine series having N-CPM substituents. The primary alcohol and the diatereoisomeric methyl secondary alcohols are powerful antagonists of very low intrinsic activity (Table 7). Diprenorphine [M-5050] has a very similar profile; its length of action as an antagonist is intermediate between that of naloxone and cyclazocine (21). It is virtually inactive in the mouse antiwrithing and rat antibradykinin tests (10) but shows some activity in the hot-plate (28) and rat antiwrithing (15) tests. It

TABLE 5. *Activities of ketones of structure 10 ($R^3 = CPM$)*

R^1 in structure 10	Rat-tail pressure		Mouse antiwrithing $ED_{50}{}^a$
	$ED_{50}{}^a$	$AD_{50}{}^a$	
Me	IA	1.2	70
Et	IA	2.1	7.8
n Pr	IA	20	1.3
n Bu	0.64	IA	
n Pent	0.85	IA	

^{a} mg/kg, i.p. or s.c.
IA = inactive

TABLE 6. *Activities of esters of structure 10 ($R^3 = CPM$) in the rat tail-pressure test*

R^1 in structure 10	$ED_{50}{}^a$	$AD_{50}{}^a$
OMe	IA	9.5
OEt	IA	8.9
On Pr	100	IA
On Bu	5.4	IA
On Pent	2.6	IA

^{a} mg/kg, i.p. or s.c.
IA = inactive

is marketed (as Revivon®) in the U.K. for the reversal of immobilization in animals brought about by etorphine (Immobilon®).

In contrast to the lower members of the alcohol series, the propyl and butyl tertiary alcohols are not antagonists in the tail-pressure test but are powerful analgesics in this test. In the tail-flick test in mice all the bases of structure **18** so far examined antagonize the analgesic actions of morphine (Table 8). The interesting combination of agonism and antagonism in the tail-flick test shown by the partial agonists of structure **18** is highlighted by the nature of their dose-response curves. They show a maximum response at usually less than complete analgesia, and higher doses produce lower effect. This is illustrated in Fig. 4 for buprenorphine **18** (R = tBu); a similar although less striking effect was demonstrated for cyclazocine. Only the report by Blane and Dugdall (13) that in the antibradykinin test in rats, high doses of pentazocine in the presence of morphine had no analgesic effect, parallels the present observation which may be an example of "auto-

TABLE 7. Activities of ethano-oripavine tertiary alcohols

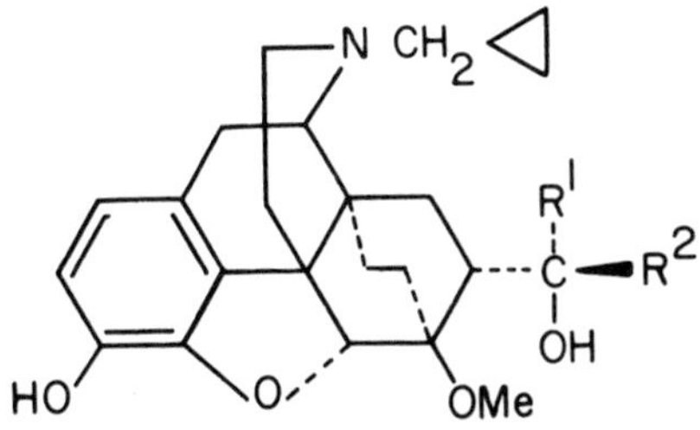

R^1	R^2	Rat tail-pressure $ED_{50}{}^a$	Antiwrithing $ED_{50}{}^a$
H	H	0.025	>100
H	Me	0.011	>100
Me	H	0.02	>100
Me	Me	0.008	>100
Me	Et	0.002	0.094

^{a} mg/kg, s.c. or i.p.

TABLE 8. Activities of ethano-oripavines of structure 18

R	Rat tail-pressure $ED_{50}{}^a$	A Mouse antiwrithing $ED_{50}{}^a$	B Mouse tail-flick $AD_{50}{}^a$	$\dfrac{B}{A}$
Me	>100	>100	0.003	$<3 \times 10^{-5}$
Et	>100	0.094	0.014	0.15
n Pr	0.008	0.003	5.6	1867
i Pr	0.015	0.045	0.023	0.51
n Bu	0.041	0.012	1.7	142
i Bu	0.133	0.068	0.163	2.4
s Bu	0.004	0.006	0.95	15.8
t Bu	0.024	0.033	0.220	6.7
Nalorphine	>100	2.1	0.95	0.45
Morphine	1.8	0.64	>100	>156

^{a} mg/kg, i.p. or s.c.

inhibition" as defined by Ariens, van Rossum, and Simonis (1). A compound acting on two receptors produces an agonist response at one receptor but as its concentration increases it interacts with a second receptor leading to noncompetitive antagonism of its own agonist effect at the first receptor.

In Table 8 for the series of bases of structure **18** the ratio of the ED_{50}'s in the mouse tail-flick, morphine-antagonism test and the mouse antiwrithing test is shown as a measure of intrinsic activity. There are very large in-

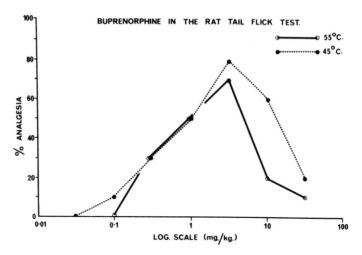

FIG. 4. Dose-response curve for buprenorphine in the rat tail-flick test.

creases in intrinsic activity as R in structure **18** changes from methyl to ethyl and from ethyl to n-propyl. The difference between the methyl and n-propyl derivatives is such that the analgesic action of the latter in the tail-pressure test is antagonized by the former with an ED_{50} value of 0.27 mg/kg, i.p.

In passing from the n-propyl to n-butyl there is a fall in intrinsic activity and the branched propyl and butyl derivatives all have activities at this level or lower. The ratio for the isopropyl carbinol is similar to that for the ethyl analogue; it is, therefore, surprising that in the rat tail-pressure test the former is a very potent agonist and the latter a very potent antagonist (Table 7).

Buprenorphine has been selected for clinical evaluation as a result of its interesting animal pharmacology (20) and encouraging results from healthy human volunteers. It is a partial agonist with powerful agonist effects in the conventional rodent tests balanced by strong morphine antagonist actions. In addition to antagonizing the analgesic actions of morphine in the tail-flick test, the latter actions are shown in reversal of morphine-induced mydriasis in mice, by precipitation of abstinence effects in morphine-dependent monkeys, and by the production of the jumping syndrome in morphine-pelleted mice (20). Buprenorphine does not produce physical dependence on chronic administration to monkeys and mice (19). It acts more than twice as long as morphine in the tail-pressure test.

In clinical pharmacology studies (12) no signs of dysphoria with doses of buprenorphine up to 2 μg/kg, i.v. or i.m., and 40 μg/kg, p.o., were observed. Significant blockade of experimental thermal pain was shown at these doses. The side effects were nausea, sedation, miosis, and constipation.

REFERENCES

1. Ariens, E. J., van Rossum, J. M., and Simonis, A. M.: Affinity, intrinsic activity, and drug interactions. Pharmacol. Rev. 9:225–228, 1957.
2. Bentley, K. W.: The morphine alkaloids. *In:* The Alkaloids, Vol. 13, edited by R. F. Manske, pp. 75–120. Academic Press, New York, 1971.
3. Bentley, K. W., Bower, J. D., and Lewis, J. W.: Novel analgesics and molecular rearrangements in the morphine-thebaine group XVI. Some derivatives of 6,14-*endo*-etheno-7,8-dihydromorphine. J. Chem. Soc. C.:2569–2572, 1969.
4. Bentley, K. W., and Hardy, D. G.: Novel analgesics and molecular rearrangements in the morphine-thebaine group I. Ketones derived from 6,14-*endo*-ethenotetrahydrothebaine. J. Amer. Chem. Soc. 89:3267–3273, 1967.
5. Bentley, K. W., and Hardy, D. G.: Novel analgesics and molecular rearrangements in the morphine-thebaine group III. Alcohols of the 6,14-*endo*-ethenotetrahydrooripavine series and derived analogs of n-allylnormorphine and -norcodeine. J. Amer. Chem. Soc. 89:3281–3292, 1967.
6. Bentley, K. W., Hardy, D. G., Crocker, H. P., Haddlesey, D. I., and Mayor, P. A.: Novel analgesics and molecular rearrangements in the morphine-thebaine Group VI. Base-catalysed rearrangements in the 6,14-*endo*-ethenotetrahydrothebaine series. J. Amer. Chem. Soc. 89:3312–3321, 1967.
7. Bentley, K. W., Hardy, D. G., Lewis, J. W., Readhead, M. J., and Rushworth, W. I.: Novel analgesics and molecular rearrangements in the morphine-thebaine group VIII. 7-Alkyl-6,14-*endo*-ethenotetrahydrothebaine and related compounds. J. Chem. Soc. C.:826–830, 1969.
8. Bentley, K. W., Hardy, D. G., and Meek, B.: Novel analgesics and molecular rearrangements in the morphine-thebaine group II. Alcohols derived from 6,14-*endo*-etheno- and 6,14-*endo*-ethanotetrahydrothebaine. J. Amer. Chem. Soc. 89:3273–3280, 1967.
9. Bentley, K. W., Hardy, D. G., and Meek, B.: Novel analgesics and molecular rearrangements in the morphine-thebaine group IV. Acid-catalysed rearrangements of alcohols of the 6,14-*endo*-ethenotetrahydrothebaine series. J. Amer. Chem. Soc. 89:3293–3303, 1967.
10. Blane, G. F.: Blockade of bradykinin-induced nociception in the rat as a test for analgesic drugs with particular reference to morphine antagonists. J. Pharm. Pharmacol. 19:367–373, 1967.
11. Blane, G. F., Boura, A. L. A., Leach, E. C., Gray, W. D., and Osterberg, A. C.: Dissociation of analgesic and respiratory depressant properties in N-substituted analogues of etorphine. J. Pharm. Pharmacol. 20:796–798, 1968.
12. Blane, G. F., and Campbell, D.: *Unpublished work.*
13. Blane, G. F., and Dugdall, D.: Interactions of narcotic antagonists and antagonist analgesics. J. Pharm. Pharmacol. 20:547–552, 1968.
14. Blane, G. F., Robbie, D. S., and Swerdlow, M.: *Unpublished work.*
15. Blumberg, H.: *Private communication.*
16. Bousfield, J. D., and Rees, J. M. H.: The analgesic and respiratory depressant activities of N-allylnoretorphine and morphine in the mouse. J. Pharm. Pharmacol. 21:630–632, 1969.
17. Brown, J. J., and Hardy, R. A., Jr.: 7-Heterocyclic dodides and morphides. Brit. Pat. 1243 838.
18. Brown, J. J., Hardy, R. A., Jr., and Nora, C. T.: Substituted *endo*-ethenocodides and morphides. Brit. Pat. 1223 444.

19. Cowan, A.: Evaluation of the physical dependence capacities of oripavine-thebaine partial agonists in patas monkeys. This volume.
20. Cowan, A., Harry, E. J. R., Lewis, J. W., and McFarlane, I. R.: *Unpublished work.*
21. Cowan, A., Lewis, J. W., and McFarlane, I. R.: *Unpublished work.*
22. Lewis, J. W., Mayor, P. A., and Haddlesey, D. I.: Novel analgetics and molecular rearrangements in the morphine-thebaine group, 30. J. Med. Chem. 16, 1973 (Jan. '73.)
23. Lewis, J. W., and Readhead, M. J.: Novel analgetics and molecular rearrangements in the morphine-thebaine group XVIII 3-deoxy-6,14-*endo*-etheno-6,7,8,14-tetrahydrooripavines. J. Med. Chem. *13*:525–527, 1970.
24. Lewis, J. W., and Readhead, M. J.: Novel analgesics and molecular rearrangements in the morphine-thebaine group XXI. Alcohols derived from 7-methyl-*epi*-nepenthone. J. Chem. Soc. C.:2296–2298, 1971.
25. Lewis, J. W., Readhead, M. J., and Smith, A. C. B.: Novel analgetics and molecular rearrangements in the morphine-thebaine group, 28. J. Med. Chem. 16, 1973 (Jan '73).
26. Lewis, J. W., and Rushworth, W. I.: Novel analgesics and molecular rearrangements in the morphine-thebaine group XVII. Compounds related to the thebaine-maleic anhydride adduct. J. Chem. Soc. C.:560–564, 1970.
27. Lewis, J. W., and Taylor, J. B.: *Unpublished work.*
28. May, E. L.: *Private communication.*
29. Villarreal, J. E.: *Private communication.*

Narcotic Antagonists, edited by M. C. Braude, L. S. Harris, E. L. May, J. P. Smith, and J. E. Villarreal. *Advances in Biochemical Psychopharmacology, Vol. 8.* Raven Press, New York © 1974.

Bridged Amino Tetralins

Meier E. Freed, John R. Potoski, Elisabeth H. Freed, Melvyn I. Gluckman, and Jerry L. Malis

Wyeth Laboratories Inc., Radnor, Pennsylvania 19087

A series of new bridged 2-amino tetralins demonstrate qualitatively similar patterns of analgesic and narcotic antagonist activity in animals. In the rat tail-flick test, where morphine intramuscularly has an ED_{50} of approximately 1.7 mg/kg, nine members of the bridged amino tetralin series have intramuscular ED_{50}'s ranging from 0.1 to 95.0 mg/kg. All of these compounds also possess the ability to reverse the depressant properties of a high dose of morphine in rats. Their ED_{50}'s for this effect range from 3.0 to about 200 mg/kg. With one exception the analgesic effect of all the amino tetralins is greater than the antagonistic effect. In monkey leg-shock titration studies, all compounds tested were analgesic by the intramuscular route. The minimal analgesic dose varied from 0.25 to 2.5 mg/kg. In general, order of potency in the monkey was correlated with order of potency in the rat. The optimal size of the bridge was five carbon atoms. Ethyl substitution on the bridge-head carbon conferred more analgesic potency than a methyl substitution. A hydroxy substitution on the aromatic ring conferred greater analgesic potency than a methoxy substitution.

INTRODUCTION

A continuing search for non-narcotic analgesics revealed the activity of a number of members of a series of bridged amino tetralins with the general structure:

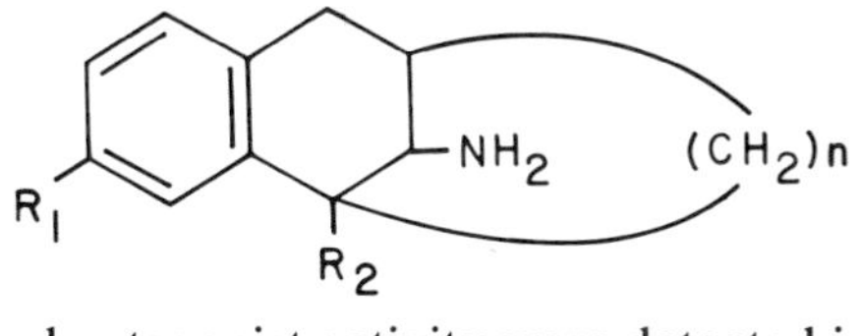

Both analgesic and antagonist activity were detected in rats and monkeys. There is a tendency for the more potent antagonists to be the more potent analgesics. Analgesic potency in the rat ranged from 20 times to $1/50$ that of morphine. Antagonist potency ranged from about $1/2$ to $1/100$ that of nalorphine.

137

METHODS

Rat Tail Flick

Analgesia was measured by a modification of the D'Amour and Smith (2) method. Rats, 10 per group, were tested for their reaction time, three times at 10-min intervals. Drugs were administered by the various routes indicated under Results, and the animals tested at 20-min intervals for 2 hr. Analgesia was considered to be present in those animals, showing reaction times equal to or greater than one and one-half times the average of the three pre-drug tests on two or more consecutive measures.

Monkey Leg Shock

Chaired rhesus monkeys were trained to lever press to regulate the intensity of an electric shock delivered through aluminum foil boots. This is a modification (4) of the method of Weiss and Laties (7). The shock automatically increased every 2 sec through 32 steps of increasing current. Each lever press reduced the succeeding shock by one step. After a stable baseline (threshold) was reached, drugs were administered and changes in threshold determined over varying periods of time up to 4 hr.

The effects of antagonists were determined by administering them during the plateau of analgesic effect and determining change in threshold.

Antagonism of Morphine (Rats)

One-half hour after the subcutaneous administration of morphine, 50 mg/kg, rats were examined for loss of righting reflex (1). Drugs were then administered intramuscularly and animals examined every 20 min for return of righting reflex. The experiment was terminated at 2 hr after drug or before if morphine controls demonstrated return of righting reflex.

Antagonism of Morphine (Mice)—Jump Test

A modification of the method of Saelens et al. (6) was used. Groups of 10 mice (CR-1, 18 to 22 g) were given morphine sulfate, 100 mg base/kg, intraperitoneally at 9:00 A.M., 12:15 P.M., and 3:30 P.M. on each of two successive days. On the third day, animals received morphine again at 9:00 A.M. and 12:15 P.M. At 2:00 P.M. antagonists were given intraperitoneally, and jumping was measured for 5 min. Appropriate controls for nalorphine and naloxone were run.

RESULTS

The first compound of this series (III [Wy-14,910], Table 1) to be tested at the University of Michigan in both withdrawn and nonwithdrawn morphine-dependent monkeys caused exacerbation of abstinence in the former and a dose-related precipitation of abstinence in the latter (5). As a prototype of the series, this compound was compared with morphine and a number of narcotic antagonists to determine its profile of activity.

Dose-response curves for analgesic effect, using the rat tail-flick method, are compared for Wy-14910, morphine, nalorphine, and pentazocine in Fig. 1. By the intramuscular route, Wy-14910 is about six times more potent than morphine which in turn is three to six times more potent than nalorphine and pentazocine. With pentazocine it was never possible to increase the number of animals demonstrating analgesia to much above 60%. Table 1 presents the rat analgesic ED_{50}'s of the four compounds of Fig. 1, and presents some data on their acute toxicity by various routes of administration. Wy-14910 by the intraperitoneal or oral route of administration had a potency approximately equal to that of morphine. By the intramuscular route, Wy-14910 was about six times as potent as morphine. Both nalorphine and pentazocine demonstrated analgesic activity in this test but were considerably less potent than either Wy-14910 or morphine. No analgesic activity was observed with oral pentazocine up to a dose of 50 mg/kg. No convulsions or deaths were noted with the highest doses of Wy-14910 administered by any route. Wy-14910 proved to have an acute safety ratio greater than morphine.

Figure 2 shows the effects of cyclazocine, pentazocine, and Wy-14910 in the monkey analgesia test. After intramuscular administration, the maximal effect of Wy-14910 and cyclazocine is reached in about 15 min.

TABLE 1. *Analgesia and safety in rats*

Compound	ED_{50}, (mg/kg)			Potency × morphine			Safety ratio (LD_{50}/ED_{50})		
	i.p.	i.m.	p.o.	i.p.	i.m.	p.o.	i.p.	i.m.	p.o.
Wy-14910	3.1	0.26	10	1.3	6.5	1.1	>128	>380	>80
Morphine	4.0	1.7	11	1	1	1	>50	100	60
Nalorphine	25	6.3	—	0.16	0.27	—	—	—	—
Pentazocine	11	7.2	*	0.36	0.24	—	>16	>22	—

* No measurable analgesia up to 50 mg/kg p.o.

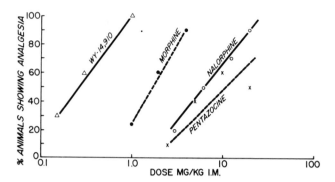

FIG. 1. Analgesic effect as measured by the D'Amour and Smith (2) tail-flick method. Each point represents data from groups of 10 animals and is the percentage of animals demonstrating analgesia according to the criteria given in Methods.

The onset of the maximal effect of pentazocine is about double, approximately 30 min. Intramuscular doses of the above compounds and morphine required to produce a 100% increase in threshold were determined and found to be: cyclazocine, 1.5 mg/kg; pentazocine, 8.0 mg/kg; Wy-14910, 1.2 mg/kg; and morphine, 2.0 mg/kg.

Narcotic antagonists reverse the acute analgesic effect of morphine

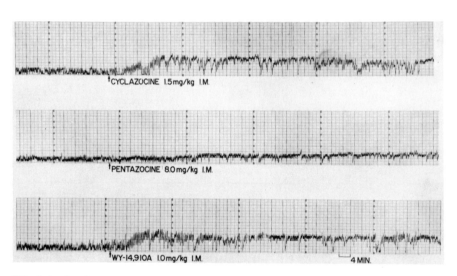

FIG. 2. Analgesia as measured by the monkey leg-shock titration procedure as described in Methods. Compounds were administered intramuscularly at the arrows. The distance between the numbered horizontal lines represents approximately four shock steps (about 0.15 mA/step).

in monkeys (3). Naloxone (1 mg/kg, i.m.) completely reversed the analgesic effect of morphine, Wy-14910, pentazocine, and cyclazocine. Nalorphine (2 mg/kg, i.m.), on the other hand, had no effect on the analgesic effect of cyclazocine whereas it completely reversed the effects of morphine. At the 2 mg/kg dose shown, nalorphine produced only a partial block of the analgesic effects of Wy-14910 and pentazocine. In other studies, doses up to 8 mg/kg also produced only a partial block. Figure 3 demonstrates some of these effects. The analgesic effect of cyclazocine was clearly un-affected by nalorphine and completely reversed by naloxone. The partial reversal by nalorphine, of the analgesic effect of pentazocine and Wy-14910 is seen as a cycling phenomenon.

Antagonist activity was determined in two ways. In rats, the acute effects of morphine were reversed by the various compounds with ED_{50}'s as follows: naloxone, 0.2 mg/kg; cyclazocine, 0.4 mg/kg; nalorphine, 1.0 mg/kg; Wy-14910, 48 mg/kg; and pentazocine, 160 mg/kg. In the mouse jump test, naloxone and nalorphine produced jumping in all animals at doses of 1.7 and 17 mg/kg, respectively. On the other hand, Wy-14910 produced no jumping in any of the morphinized mice at a dose of 20 mg/kg; doses of 63 and 200 mg/kg were toxic. Seven of nine mice convulsed and six of nine mice died in the former group whereas all animals convulsed and died in the latter group. This toxicity was only slightly less in non-mor-phinized mice. At the high dose, eight of 10 animals convulsed and again all died. At the 63 mg/kg dose, two of 10 convulsed and died.

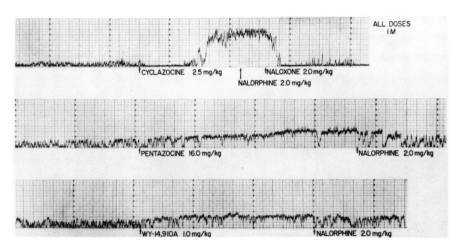

FIG. 3. Reversal of the agonist effect of cyclazocine, pentazocine, and Wy-14910 by naloxone or nalorphine in the monkey leg-shock titration method.

TABLE 2. Comparison of the analgesic and antagonist activity of members of the bridged amino tetralin series

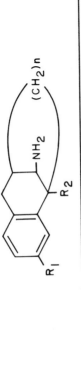

Compound[a]	R_1	R_2	n	Rat			Monkey		
				Morphine Antagonism ED_{50} (mg/kg, i.m.)	Analgesia ED_{50} (mg/kg, i.m.)	Antagonism Analgesia	Minimal Analgesic dose (mg/kg, i.m.)	Maximum dose tried (mg/kg, i.m.)	Analgesia antagonism by nalorphine
I	OH	Me	5	6.5	0.45	14.0	1.5	10	No
I (L)	OH	Me	5	3.0	0.09	33.0	0.25	8	No
I (D)	OH	Me	5	88.0	95.0	0.9	–	–	–
II	OMe	Me	5	–	4.5 (i.p.)	–	<5.0	20	Yes (T)[b]
III	OH	Et	4	48.0	0.25	200	1.0	20	Yes (P)[b]
III (L)	OH	Et	4	8.5	0.1	85	2.0	8	No
III (D)	OH	Et	4	100.0	2.0	50	–	–	–
IV	OMe	Et	4	140.0	12.0	12.0	2.5	20	No
V	OMe	Me	4	200.0	25.0	8	–	–	–
VI	OH	Me	4	37.5	2.0	19	2.5	12	No

[a] All compounds are racemates with the exceptions of those followed by (L) or (D) which designate levo- and dextrorotatory optical isomers, respectively.

[b] T and P refer to total and partial antagonism by nalorphine.

Table 2 presents a comparison of some of the more interesting analogues. The following structure-activity relationships are suggested from the data. The levorotatory isomer is more potent than the dextrorotatory isomer [compare I (l) and III (l) with I (d) and III (d)].

In one example, I versus VI, the five-bridged compound is more potent than the four-bridged compound. Although not listed, the three-bridged compounds were less active than the four-bridged analogues. A hydroxy group at R_1 confers greater potency than a methoxy group at this position (compare I vs. II and III vs. IV). Those compounds which are the most potent antagonists (in the acute morphine test) are also potent analgesics. The reverse is not necessarily true, e.g., III. The more potent analgesics in rats were also potent analgesics in the monkey. Of the compounds tested, with only two (II and III) was the analgesic effect in monkeys reversed by nalorphine, the latter being only partially reversed.

DISCUSSION

The above series of bridged amino tetralins possess both analgesic and antagonist activity as measured in rats and monkeys. III was reported to be about $\frac{1}{5}$ as potent as nalorphine as an antagonist in the morphine-dependent monkey (5). In rats, III was about $\frac{1}{50}$ as active as nalorphine in antagonizing the acute depressant effects of morphine, and it was essentially inactive in the mouse jump test where both nalorphine and naloxone were very active. In this specific case then, there would appear to be little correlation between the mouse jump test and the other tests used to measure antagonist activity. Further, the morphine-dependent monkey is a more sensitive test than the acute rat test for assaying antagonists. This is borne out further by recent information (5) that I and IV are also antagonists in the non-withdrawn morphine-dependent monkey, at minimal subcutaneous doses of 0.5 and 2 mg/kg, respectively.

In our studies, the analgesic effect of III in monkeys was partially reversed by nalorphine and completely reversed by naloxone. As indicated above, III was stated to be an antagonist in morphine-dependent monkeys. Since the activity of "agonist/antagonist" type analgesics can be reversed by some antagonists, this is not a good measure of "morphine-like" character of an analgesic.

CONCLUSIONS

A new series of bridged amino tetralins has been demonstrated to have both agonist and antagonist properties. Structure-activity relationships indicate that potent antagonist activity is associated with potent agonist activity whereas the reverse is not necessarily true. One member of the series (III) which was an antagonist in tests using morphine-dependent monkeys and acutely morphinized rats was inactive in the mouse jump test, suggesting that the latter test may be inadequate for screening for antagonist activity. In monkeys the analgesic activity of this compound was reversed by naloxone and partially reversed by nalorphine, suggesting that such reversal is not in itself a measure of morphine-like character of an analgesic, since the compound was shown to be an antagonist in morphine-dependent monkeys.

REFERENCES

1. Blumberg, H.: personal communication.
2. D'Amour, F. E., and Smith, D. L.: A method for determining loss of pain sensation. J. Pharmacol. Exp. Ther. *72*:74–79, 1941.
3. Malis, J. L.: Analgesic testing in primates. *In:* Symposium on Agonist and Antagonist Action of Narcotic Analgesic Drugs. Aberdeen, Scotland, July, 1971.
4. Malis, J., and Gluckman, M. I.: Assaying narcotic antagonist drugs for analgesic activity in rhesus monkeys. This volume.
5. May, E. L.: personal communication.
6. Saelans, J. K., Granat, F. R., and Sawyer, W. R.: The mouse jumping test—A simple method to estimate the physical dependence capacity of analgesics. Arch. Int. Pharmacodyn. *190*:213–218, 1971.
7. Weiss, B., and Laties, V. G.: Analgesic effects in monkeys of morphine, nalorphine, and a benzomorphan narcotic antagonist. J. Pharmacol. Exp. Ther. *143*:169–173, 1964.

Narcotic Antagonists, edited by M. C. Braude, L. S. Harris, E. L. May, J. P. Smith, and J. E. Villarreal. *Advances in Biochemical Psychopharmacology, Vol. 8*. Raven Press, New York © 1974.

Arylpyrrolidines as Narcotic Antagonists

D. A. McCarthy

Department of Pharmacology, Research and Development Division, Parke, Davis & Company, Ann Arbor, Michigan 48106

During the past 20 years the arylpyrrolidines have been the subject of an extensive search for potent analgesics with minimal dependence liability. Predictive animal testing in rodents allowed the identification of several compounds having sufficient antinociceptive activity to warrant work-up for human clinical trials. Among these, prodilidine (1,2-dimethyl-3-phenyl-3-propionoxypyrrolidine), profadol [*m*-(1-methyl-3-propyl-3-pyrrolidinyl) phenol], and the D and L isomers of profadol have received the most attention. The mixed agonist-antagonist actions of profadol have been defined, at least in part. For example, morphine antagonist actions have been demonstrated in morphine-dependent monkeys. Agonist actions leading to a mild-to-moderate physical dependence have also been reported to occur in monkeys chronically maintained on profadol. This dependence may be unmasked by either abrupt withdrawal or by challenge with morphine antagonists. The studies leading to the selection of profadol from among a large number of related arylpyrrolidines sought to achieve a favorable dissociation of antinociceptive action from such morphine-like actions as are responsible for the production of euphoria and physical dependence. Since antinociception was the primary consideration upon which the systematic preparation and testing of compounds was based, it is not surprising that these studies have not led to discovery of highly selective opiate-opioid antagonists among the arylpyrrolidines. Studies seeking to discover a selective analgesic were never intended to identify highly selective morphine antagonists. However, these studies now provide a basis for developing a strategy for the exploration of the pyrrolidine ring as a framework for compounds having a high degree of selectivity as morphine antagonists. Two compounds, *m*-[1-(cyclopropylmethyl)-3-methyl-3-pyrrolidinyl]phenol (*m*CMPP) and *m*-(1-allyl-3-methyl-3-pyrrolidinyl)phenol (*m*AMPP) will be used as examples and discussed in comparison with profadol.

At the beginning of this section, Dr. Harris called attention to the major molecular modifications of the morphine molecule that have been found to be compatible with the retention of morphine-like pharmacologic activity as well as selective (specific) opiate antagonistic actions. Following this theme various authors have elaborated on the structure-activity relationships occurring as various portions of the nonphenyl ring system are stripped away from the parent molecule. This "molecular striptease" has progressively extended to a point at which the morphine molecule may well have been reduced to the bare essentials necessary for a morphine-like action. I hope to show that this "stripping" has not extended to a point where further observation ceases to cause excitement.

My comments about this chemical class will be mainly historical and speculative for several reasons: (a) interest in the arylpyrrolidines as a potential source of analgesic drugs is not new and has been reviewed (1), (b) the chemistry and structure-activity relationship studies have been published in detail elsewhere, (c) the recognition that the arylpyrrolidine nucleus may serve as a framework for synthesis and selection of highly selective opiate-opioid antagonists is relatively new and as yet almost entirely unexplored, (d) observations made by myself or under my direction have only very recently been made, are scanty, and at best are incompletely documented.

Historically, chemical and pharmacological work was directed entirely toward examining the speculation that analgesics could be found among the arylpyrrolidines, and that because they differ as much as they do from morphine structure, they might lack those properties responsible for the production of tolerance and physical dependance.

This goal appeared achievable in view of the knowledge, then relatively new, that nalorphine possessed considerable analgesic activity as well as the ability to antagonize the acute effects of narcotic analgesics and to precipitate the abstinence syndrome in dependent subjects. Most of the synthetic work was carried out in the Hounslow, England, laboratories of Parke-Davis by Drs. Bowman, Davoll, Cavalla, and Lockhart, supported by their assistants. A large number of new compounds were prepared, including more than 60 arylpyrrolidines. The pharmacologic evaluation, at first directed almost entirely toward obtaining presumptive evidence for analgesic activity, was initially carried out in our Detroit and Ann Arbor laboratories by Winder and his associates and later also by Collier in Hounslow. Nine basic research publications describe the chemistry, the antinociceptive and structure-activity relationships resulting from these studies (1–7, 10, 11). In addition, numerous other investigations regarding the pharmacology and clinical utility of profadol have been published. At the same time, other groups were also examining the arylpyrrolidines as potential analgesics. Early in the study, prodilidine was separately and independently discovered by the Parke-Davis group and by scientists working in the Mead-Johnson Research Laboratories. Prodilidine enjoyed only limited clinical trials. Interest in it diminished rapidly, especially in our own laboratories with the discovery of profadol, a more potent analgesic which later proved to have an especially interesting spectrum of pharmacologic activity (12). The structures of prodilidine, profadol, and two other arylpyrrolidines as well as two reference compounds are shown in Fig. 1.

When profadol was first discovered early in 1960, it was not immediately recognized that the compound had antagonistic properties. It has a fairly respectable antinociceptive potency, and Winder et al. had reported it to be 2.5 to 4 times as potent as codeine or meperidine in the tail-pressure squeak test for antinociceptive activity (12). This antinociceptive activity in rats was antagonized by nalorphine (12), yet studies carried out at the addiction laboratory of the University of Michigan showed that profadol would not alleviate the morphine-abstinence syndrome in morphine-dependent monkeys. Its opiate antagonist properties were not detected at first. It should be recalled that the first objective of the laboratory search was discovery of drugs high in antinociceptive potency. Hence, all structure-activity relationship studies continued to direct synthesis to this end. Later, when the morphine-antagonistic properties were established by Deneau, Villarreal, and Seevers at the addiction laboratory of the University of Michigan, the research strategy shifted to a search among the arylpyrrolidines for compounds having both high potency in tests for antinociception and in tests for morphine antagonism. The search for morphine antagonism was justified on the assumption that this property would minimize dependence liability. It later proved disappointing when this assumption was tempered by the discovery that mixed agonist-antagonists can possess the capacity to produce a low level of physical dependence. This discovery placed another demand upon the search for an even greater selectivity of analgesic action. The demand for selectivity is now so great that we have abandoned, at least for the present, the search for an "ideal analgesic" among the arylpyrrolidines.

Today priorities seem to be changing, and we appear to be swept up by those who support the assumption that a serious sociologic, moral, and legal problem can somehow be treated pharmacologically. I personally have serious reservations about the validity of this premise. However, with respect to the arylpyrrolidines it seems important to frame a new question: "Does our present knowledge provide a sufficient basis for extending the investigation of pyrrolidines as a framework for the preparation of specific morphine antagonists?" Examination of such published data (5–7) as are available, limited data yet to be published (1,2), and some recently obtained observations lead one to believe that the answer to the question is a *qualified yes.* *"Qualified"* because of (a) the nature of the therapeutic objective, (b) the present existence of highly potent drugs in this category, and (c) the

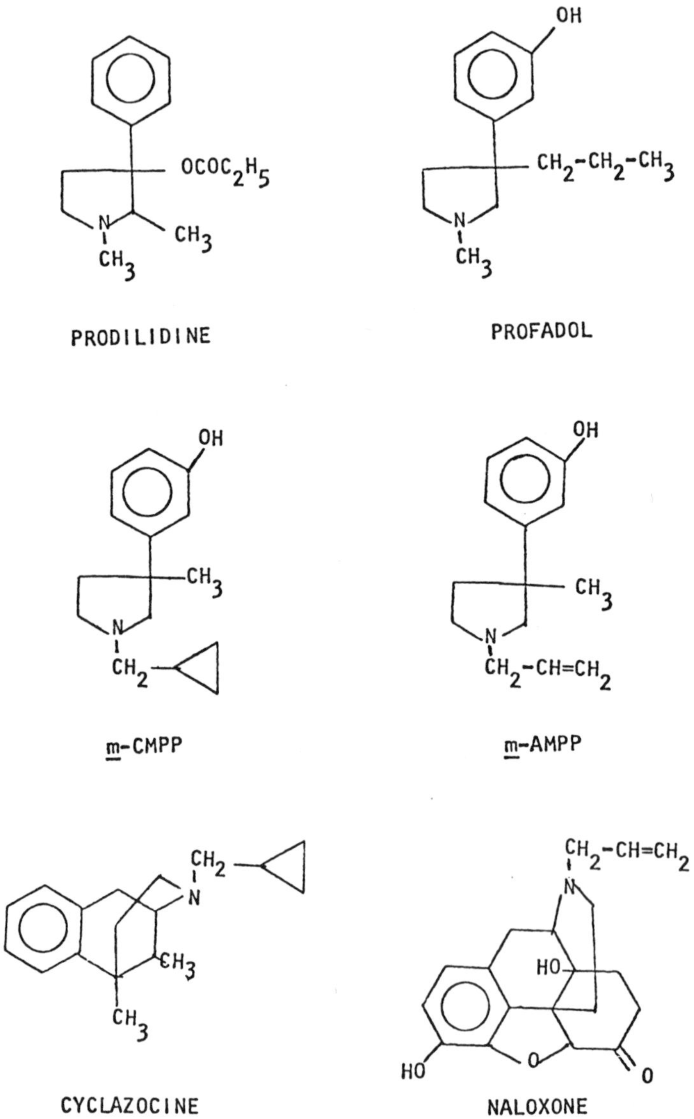

FIG. 1. Structures of prodilidine, profadol, and two other arylpyrrolidines as well as two reference compounds, cyclazocine and naloxone.

astronomical costs associated with new drug development. *"Yes,"* because past experience with in-depth structure-activity relationship studies on several other chemical series have shown that nearly all levels of dissociation of agonistic and antagonistic properties are achievable when an appropriate strategy is applied to solve the problem.

Arguing by analogy also supports the "yes" answer. Chemical series such as the morphine derivatives, oripavines, morphinans, and benzomorphans, when subjected to an appropriate research strategy have yielded or are yielding a full spectrum of activities ranging from highly selective agonists to highly selective antagonists. Why not the arylpyrrolidines? One has only to have the acumen to detect these qualitative shifts and to examine activity in a way appropriate to detect them. Such a strategy could now be applied.

Past experience also favors the possibility that molecular manipulation and a battery of effective presumptive tests can rapidly direct synthesis toward achieving the kind of pharmacologic properties we seek. Whereas a sizeable number of the more recently synthesized arylpyrrolidines were examined for activity as antagonists, this was not the case during roughly the first decade of the study. Also since the study was directed toward discovery of a potent analgesic, compounds not showing this property were not examined for antagonist actions. More importantly, modifications of chemical structure which would lead to reduction or loss of antinociceptive activity, regardless of the consequence such modifications might have had on opiate antagonism, were never pursued.

In support of this position let us examine data taken from a manuscript by Bowman et al. (1,2) and two papers by Collier et al. (8,9). I have extracted data presented in Table 1 as an example of the remarkable shifts in selectivity of action which are achieved with relatively modest configurational alterations among only one series of profadol analogues. Results obtained from evaluation of other antagonists and using the same methods are included for comparison. Several conclusions can be drawn from the data presented in this table:

TABLE 1. *Modification of narcotic agonist: antagonist ratio with structural modification of profadol structure*

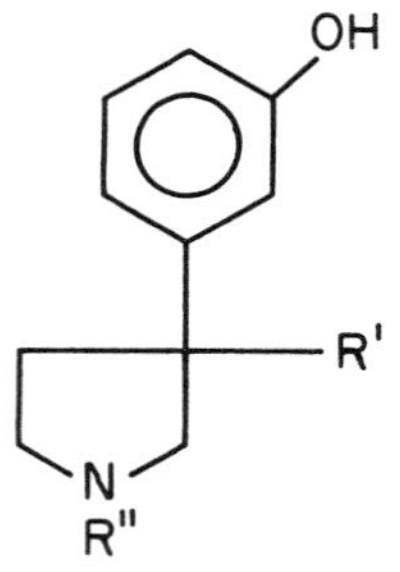

Compound designation	R''→ $-CH_2-CH=CH_2$ R'→				R''→ cyclopropyl-methyl R'→		
	R'	I.S.[a]	MAD$_{50}$[b] mg/kg, s.c.	Potency relative to naloxone	I.S.[a]	MAD$_{50}$[b] mg/kg, s.c.	Potency relative to naloxone
m-CMPP	$-CH_3$	3.12	1.7	0.006	22.22	0.9	0.011
m-AMPP	$-CH_2CH_3$	0.92	1.3	0.008	0.41	1.4	0.007
	$-CH_2-CH_2-CH_3$	0.78	3.7	0.003	0.07	4.3	0.002
	$-CH(CH_3)CH_3$	1.00	2.5	0.004	0.25	3.0	0.003
	$-CH_2-CH(CH_3)CH_3$	0.23	1.5	0.007	0.06	1.7	0.006
	$-CH_2-C(CH_3)_2CH_3$	0.29	1.6	0.006	0.06	3.3	0.003

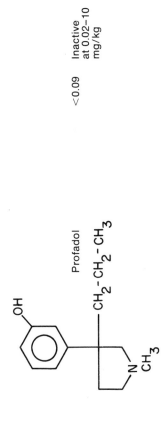

Profadol   <0.09   Inactive at 0.02–10 mg/kg   <0.001

Standards	I.S.[a]	MAD_{50}[b] mg/kg, s.c.	Potency relative to naloxone
Naloxone	6,370	0.01	1.0
Nalorphine	33.3	0.54	0.19
Cyclazocine	1.33	0.06	0.17
Levallorphan	71.7	0.06	0.17

[a] I.S. = index of specificity.
ED_{50} for agonist active (antiwrithing test in mice)/MAD_{50} for antagonist activity (antagonism of morphine antinociception in mice)
[b] MAD_{50} = median effective dose as a suppressant of morphine antinociception.
Data taken from Collier and associates[1,2,8,9]

151

(1) Within this very limited series of chemical variations on the profadol structure, selectivity for antagonistic action (by the criteria employed by Collier) ranges over 300-fold.

(2) Relative to the reference standards, at least one of the compounds when tested in mice was found to be approximately 17 times more selective than cyclazocine, but only about two-thirds as selective as nalorphine.

(3) Although there appears to have been an adequate separation of agonist and antagonist action in the compound *m*-CMPP and, especially, *m*-AMPP, it should be noted that the antagonist potency of these arylpyrrolidines remains considerably lower than the reference standards with which the compound was compared.

Data recently obtained in our laboratories by Miss J. Wax are shown in Table 2. The data reported were obtained from a test in which the nociceptive-threshold-elevating effect of morphine was antagonized by the test substances. Whereas these studies led to somewhat different absolute values, potencies relative to naloxone were found to be very comparable.

Certainly the decision that a given compound is selectively antagonistic to morphine would have to have supporting data beyond the antagonism of

TABLE 2. *Antimorphine activity in rat tail-pinch test*[a]

Drug	ED_{50}[b] (mg/kg)	Potency relative to naloxone
Naloxone	0.025 $(0.019–0.035)_{95\%}$	1
Nalorphine	0.33 (0.25–0.44)	0.076
Levallorphan	0.15 (0.12–0.18)	0.17
dl-Profadol	>3.00	<0.008
Cyclazocine	0.15 (0.12–0.21)	0.17
m-CMPP	2.6 (1.7–4.8)	0.010
m-AMPP	5.6 (3.6–11)	0.004

[a] A dose of morphine, previously established as the ED_{95} for elevating the NCT of rats beyond 200% of the level required to cause squeaking in vehicle-treated rats, was used. All treatments were given subcutaneously. Vehicle volume for drug administration was 1.0cc/100g and doses and potencies are expressed in terms of the active base content of the test drugs. Overall randomization of treatments was employed. Thirty min after treatment, NCT's were determined with the observer "blind" to the individual animal's treatment. The relationship between the proportion of the animals with NCT's less than or equal 200% the average NCT for vehicle-treated animals and the dosage of the test substance on a log scale were subjected to standard probit analysis.

[b] ED_{50}'s were obtained in independent regression experiments except cyclazocine. This was computed from the combined slope of a valid comparative bioassay of cyclazocine and naloxone.

morphine antinociception. In our laboratory we are prepared to examine the ability of a drug to precipitate an abstinence syndrome in monkeys physically dependent upon morphine. Monkeys restrained using the Michigan arm and harness system are maintained in a dependent state by the continuous intravenous infusion of morphine at the rate of 0.5 mg/kg (as free base) per hour. Three hours before challenge with the test drug, the morphine injection is terminated. The test substance is then given i.m., and the monkeys are observed remotely using closed-circuit television. Their movements within the cage are monitored using an acoustic motion detection system. At present we have attempted to establish only the minimum i.m. dose of the test substance that will precipitate unequivocal abstinence signs plus increased recordable movements within the cage that exceed saline controls by a factor of at least two. Since the degree of physical dependence developed in monkeys on continuous infusion of morphine is a function of time exposed to that drug, and since different monkeys have different patterns of motor behavior during withdrawal, more than one monkey is treated with each dose of the test substance using a randomized block cross-over design. In addition naloxone and nalorphine are used as reference standards. Comparisons between treatments are made within the same animal about the same time in his dependence history. We are now partly through a comparison of compounds *m*-CMPP and *m*-AMPP with standards. As shown in Table 3, using this test, we find the compounds to be respectively approximately 0.03 and 0.01 as potent as naloxone. This test confirms morphine antagonism in a primate species as it relates to the phenomenon of physical dependence. Although there are obvious differ-

TABLE 3. *Preliminary estimates of morphine-antagonist potency as determined by unmasking morphine dependence in* M. mulatta

Drug	No. of monkeys	Estimated minimum dose[a] mg/kg, i.m.	Potency relative to naloxone
Naloxone	3	.010	1
Nalorphine	1	.050	0.2
dl-Profadol	2	<4	>0.003
d-Profadol	1	<4	>0.003
l-Profadol	1	≤8	>0.001
m-CMPP	3	0.4	0.03
m-AMPP	1	1	0.01

[a] Minimum i.m. dose required to produce unequivocal abstinence signs as determined by observation and by increased in-cage movements recorded by an ultrasonic motion detection system.

ences in quantitative estimates of potency, the agreement between two different laboratories and three separate test objects seems to be sound enough to support the claim that these two compounds do indeed possess morphine-antagonistic activity.

Certain arylpyrrolidines have been identified among a series containing compounds with both prominent mixed opiate-opioid antagonist and agonist properties. In these compounds, the antagonist properties dominate the agonist (antinociceptive). This suggests that some members of other series of arylpyrrolidines, that were previously synthesized and tested for their antinociceptive activity and found weak in this regard, should now be resynthesized and reexamined to establish a basis for structure-activity relationship studies. The ultimate objective would be a highly selective narcotic antagonist with properties amenable to formulation in a depot or repository form.

It seems probable that small alkyl and/or alkylene substitutions at 2, 3, and/or 4 on the pyrrolidine nucleus coupled with an alkyl or cyclopropyl-methyl substituent on the pyrrolidine nitrogen would upgrade the potency and the selectivity of this series of compounds. Only synthesis and testing to this end will provide the desired answers.

REFERENCES

1. Bowman, R. E., Collier, H. O. J., Hattersley, P. J., Lockhart, I. M., Peters, D. J., Schneider, C., Webb, N. E., and Wright, M.: *m*-[3-Alkyl-1-(cyclopropylmethyl)-3-pyrrolidinyl]phenols: A group of antinociceptive agents that antagonise morphine. J. Chem. Soc. submitted for publication.
2. Bowman, R. E., Collier, H. O. J., Lockhart, I. M., Schneider, C., Webb, N. E., and Wright, M.: *m*-(3-Alkyl-1-allyl-3-pyrrolidinyl)phenols: A group of antinociceptive agents that antagonise morphine. J. Chem. Soc. submitted for publication.
3. Cavalla, J. F., Davoll, J., Dean, M. J., Franklin, C. S., Temple, D. M., Wax, J., and Winder, C. V.: Analgetics based on the pyrrolidine ring. J. Med. Pharm. Chem. 4:1–19, 1961.
4. Cavalla, J. F., Selway, R. A., Wax, J., Scotti, L., and Winder, C. V.: Analgetics based on the pyrrolidine ring. II. J. Med. Pharm. Chem. 5:441–451, 1962.
5. Cavalla, J. F., Jones, R., Welford, M., Wax, J., and Winder, C. V.: Analgetics based on the pyrrolidine ring. III. J. Med. Chem. 7:412–415, 1964.
6. Cavalla, J. F., Bishop, D. C., Selway, R. A., Webb, N. E., Winder, C. V., and Welford, M.: Analgetics based on the pyrrolidine ring. IV. J. Med. Chem. 8:316–326, 1965.
7. Cavalla, J. F., Lockhart, I. M., Webb, N. E., Winder, C. V., Welford, M., and Wong, A.: Analgetics based on the pyrrolidine ring. V. J. Med. Chem. 13:794, 1970.
8. Collier, H. O. J., Dinneen, L. C., Johnson, C. A., and Schneider, C.: The abdominal constriction response and its suppression by analgesic drugs in the mouse. Brit. J. Pharmacol. 32:295–310, 1968.
9. Collier, H. O. J., and Schneider, C.: Profiles of activity in rodents of some narcotic and narcotic antagonist drugs. Nature 244:610, 1969.
10. Lockhart, I. M., Webb, N. E., Wright, M., Winder, C. V., and Varner, P.: Analgetics based on the pyrrolidine ring. VI. J. Med. Chem. 15:930–934, 1972.

11. Lockhart, I. M., Webb, N. E., Wright, M., Winder, C. V., and Hare, M. A.: Analgetics based on the pyrrolidine ring. VII. J. Med. Chem. *15*:687–690, 1972.
12. Winder, C. V., Welford, M., Wax, J., and Kaump, D. H.: Pharmacologic and toxicologic studies of *m*-(1-methyl-3-propyl-3-pyrrolidinyl)phenol (Cl-572), an analgetic and antitussive agent. J. Pharmacol. Exp. Ther. *154*:161–175, 1966.

Narcotic Antagonists, edited by M. C. Braude, L. S. Harris, E. L. May, J. P. Smith, and J. E. Villarreal. *Advances in Biochemical Psychopharmacology, Vol. 8.* Raven Press, New York © 1974.

Narcotic Antagonists of the 4-Phenylpiperidine Series

Adolf Langbein, Herbert Merz, Klaus Stockhaus, and Helmut Wick

C. H. Boehringer Sohn, D-6507 Ingelheim, Germany

The structure-activity relationships in the field of narcotic antagonists have been considered anew. According to conclusions drawn by some investigators, narcotic antagonists are not to be obtained in the 4-phenylpiperidine series. This view is derived from structural principles present in the morphine, morphinan, and benzomorphan molecules but not in the 4-phenylpiperidines. In opposition to this generally accepted opinion, distinct narcotic antagonists of the 4-phenylpiperidine type have been found. Based on the results of our investigations, the following structural features promote morphine-antagonist properties to 4-phenylpiperidine derivatives: (1) A free phenolic hydroxyl group in the *m*-position of the aromatic nucleus is an important element for activity; (2) An ester function, preferably the methoxycarbonyl group, is necessary for optimal antagonist action; (3) N-substituents with cyclic or noncyclic, allyl-like structures are appropriate for antimorphine properties. The allyl group itself is not suitable for antagonism.

INTRODUCTION

It is well documented in the literature that certain N-substituents such as allyl, cyclopropylmethyl, and related groups confer narcotic antagonist properties to morphine-like compounds (2,6,13,14). According to a generally accepted hypothesis, however, antagonistic activity should be confined to structures closely related to morphine (1,2). In particular a rigid molecule containing at least three rings which cannot have a planar structure and/or a phenethylamine fragment are claimed to be essential. Consequently, narcotic antagonists of the meperidine series should not exist.

In the course of our syntheses in the 4-phenylpiperidine series, however, we did find compounds with definite antagonistic properties in mice. In pursuit of these surprising findings we have extended our work in order to trace the structural features involved in antagonistic activity of 4-phenylpiperidines. We now wish to report on syntheses of 4-phenylpiperidine antagonists, to summarize selected pharmacological data, and to discuss structure-activity relationships.

157

CHEMICAL STRUCTURE AND SYNTHESIS OF NEW 4-PHENYLPIPERIDINES

In this chapter the chemical structure and the synthetic route of new 4-phenylpiperidines are described. As demonstrated in Fig. 1, the new N-alkyl derivatives (II) were prepared by alkylation of known 4-phenyl-

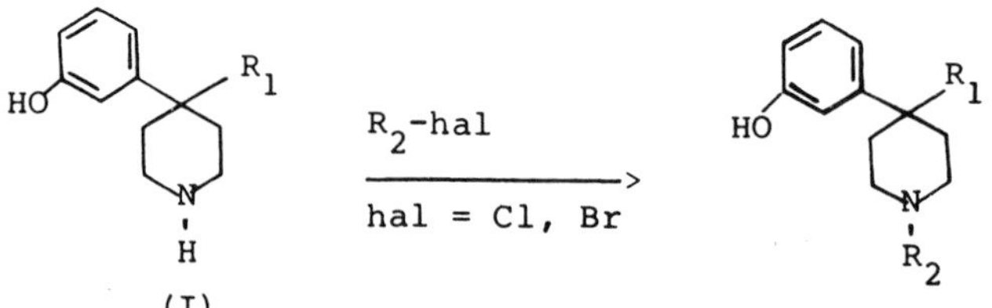
R1
HO
N
H
R2-hal
hal = Cl, Br
R1
HO
N
R2

(I) (II)

Bemidone series:

R_1= COO-alkyl; alkyl= CH_3, C_2H_5

Ketobemidone series:

R_1= CO-alkyl; alkyl= CH_3, C_2H_5

Known allyl-like N-substituents:

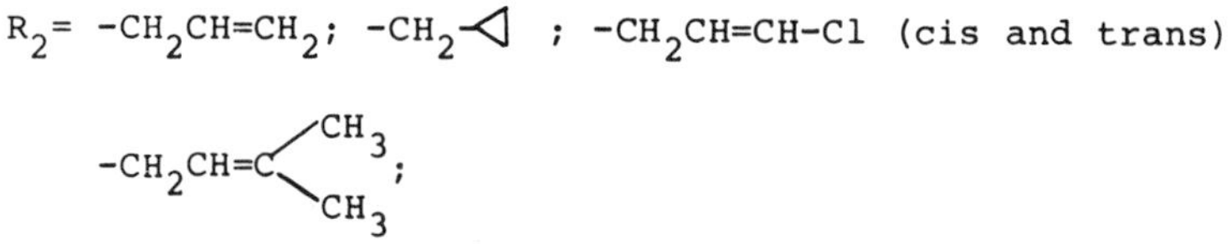
R2= -CH2CH=CH2; -CH2- ; -CH2CH=CH-Cl (cis and trans)
-CH2CH=C
CH3
CH3
;

New cyclic allyl-like N-substituents:

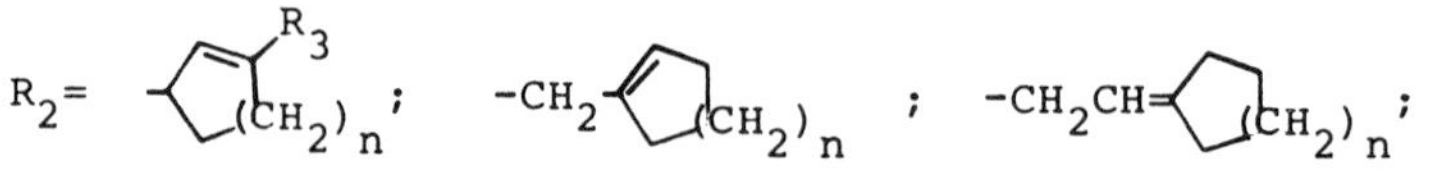
R3
R2=
(CH2)n ;
-CH2
(CH2)n ;
-CH2CH=
(CH2)n ;

n= 1-4; R_3= H, Cl

New furylmethyl N-substituents:

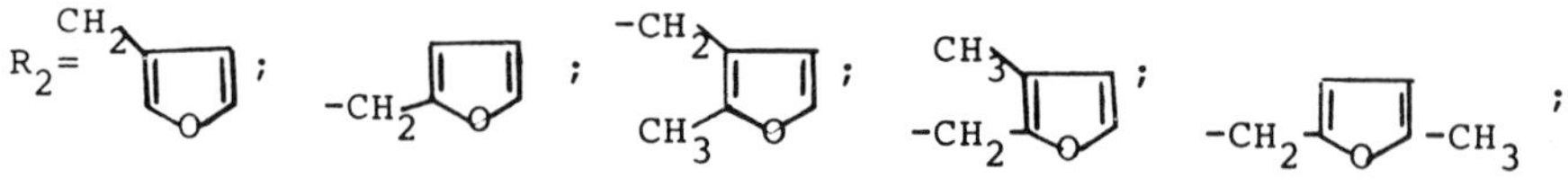
CH2
R2= ;
-CH2 ;
-CH2
CH3 ;
CH3
-CH2 ;
-CH2 -CH3 ;

FIG. 1. Synthesis and structure of new 4-phenylpiperidines.

piperidines (I) with chlorides or bromides of different structures. The tertiary bases resulted in very good yields. Purification was accomplished by crystallization of the free bases or the acid addition salts. The cycloalkenyl, cycloalkenylmethyl, and cycloalkylidenethyl halides like the furylmethyl halides can be obtained by known methods. Experimental details are reported in the patent literature or will be published in the near future (4,5,11,16,17).

PHARMACOLOGICAL METHODS

The new 4-phenylpiperidines were tested for analgesia and morphine antagonism in mice. Promising compounds were evaluated for morphine antagonism and physical dependence capacity in monkeys. The following techniques were used:

Analgesia (Mice)

NMRI-mice (both sexes, 16 to 20 g, 10 animals per dose) were used. The test compounds were administered s.c. as solutions of their methanesulfonic or hydrochloric acid salts in water. Analgesic activity (ED-values, mg/kg s.c.) was estimated using the following methods: (a) tail-clip method according to Haffner (12), (b) hot-plate method described by Woolfe and MacDonald (26), and (c) writing test as reported by Blumberg, Wolf, and Dayton (3).

Morphine Antagonism (Mice)

Antagonistic activity versus morphine analgesia was estimated using Haffner's tail-clip method. After successive injections of morphine hydrochloride (15 mg/kg s.c., corresponding to its ED_{80}) and the test dose of the antagonist, the analgesic activity was determined. Using the results obtained with various suitable dose ratios, an AD_{50} (50% suppression of the original morphine analgesia) was calculated. The antagonistic AD_{50} of the corresponding compound was compared with the AD_{50} of nalorphine. These relative values are recorded in Tables 1 and 2.

Morphine Antagonism (Monkeys)

The evaluation for antagonistic properties in nonwithdrawn, morphine-dependent rhesus monkeys was carried out by Deneau, Seevers, and Villarreal, in Ann Arbor, Michigan (9, 10, 21–24).

TABLE 1: New 4-phenylpiperidines and their pharmacological properties

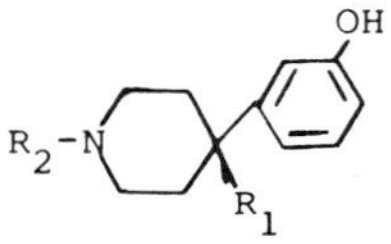

Code number CHBS	UM	NIH	R_1	R_2	ANALGESIA Straub tail Mouse	Tail-clip ED$_{50}$ mg/kg,s.c.	Hot-plate ED$_{100}$ mg/kg,s.c.	Writing ED$_{50}$ mg/kg,s.c.	ANTAGONISM Mouse a)	Monkey b)	PDC Monkey c)
Mr 77-MS	756	8452	COOCH$_3$	-CH$_2$CH=CH$_2$	+	30-50	-	35	none	-	high
Mr 471-MS	767	8453	COOCH$_3$	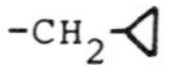 -CH$_2$-△	-	-	-	12	1/30 N	1/100 N	none
Mr 473-MS	560	8170	COOCH$_3$	-CH$_2$-CH=CH-Cl	-	-	-	13,5	-	1/200 N	none
Mr 417-MS	558	8168	COOCH$_3$	-CH$_2$-CH=CH-Cl	-	-	9,5	9	1/20 N	1/50 N	none
Mr 432-MS			COOCH$_3$	-CH$_2$CH=C(CH$_3$)CH$_3$	-	-	-	35	+	-	
Mr 623-MS	659	8285	COOCH$_3$	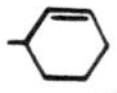 -CH$_2$-(cyclohexenyl)	-	-	4,5	29	-	1/80 N	none
Mr 635-MS	658	8284	COOCH$_3$	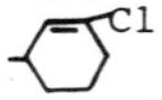 -CH$_2$-(Cl-cyclohexyl)	-	-	-	17	1/20 N	1/200N	none
Mr 669-MS	698	8384	COOCH$_3$	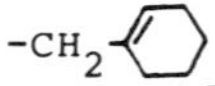 -CH$_2$-(cyclohexenyl)	-	-	-	-	-	mild	+
Mr 600-MS	660	8286	COOCH$_3$	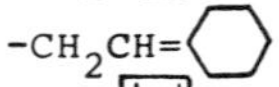 -CH$_2$CH=(cyclohexyl)	-	-	20	40	1/3 N	1/3 N	none
Mr 85-CL	855	8637	COOCH$_3$	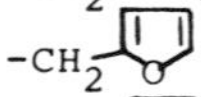 -CH$_2$-(furyl)	+	-	2	1,8	-	-	low
Mr 1196-MS	856	8638	COOCH$_3$	-CH$_2$-(furyl)-CH$_3$	+	-	5	0,6	-	-	high

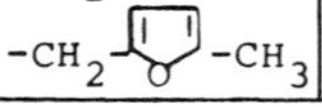

a Suppression of morphine analgesia in mice. nalorphine (N) = 1 (see Pharmacological Methods)
b Precipitation of abstinence in nonwithdrawn monkeys performed by Deneau, Seevers, and Villarreal
c Physical dependence capacity in withdrawn monkeys

TABLE 2: Pharmacological results of new bemidone and ketobemidone derivatives

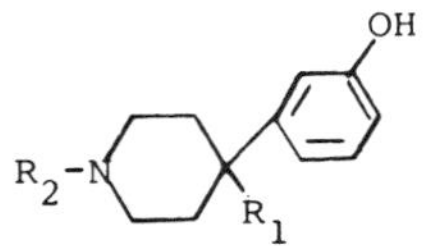

Code number					ANALGESIA				ANTAGONISM		PDC
CHBS	UM	NIH	R₁	R₂	Mouse				Mouse	Monkey	Monkey
			R_1	R_2	Straub tail	Tail-clip ED$_{50}$	Hot-plate ED$_{100}$	Writing ED$_{50}$	a)	b)	c)
						mg/kg,s.c.	mg/kg,s.c.	mg/kg,s.c.			
Mr 61-CL			COOC$_2$H$_5$	-CH$_2$CH=CH$_2$	±	-	-	5,6	±		none
Mr 424-MS	559	8169	COOC$_2$H$_5$	-CH$_2$CH=C<CH$_3$/CH$_3$	-	-	-	35	1/30 N	1/100 N	none
Mr 513-CL	621	8237	COOC$_2$H$_5$	-CH$_2$-△	-	-	-	-	+	1/100 N	none
Mr 418-MS	648	8261	COOC$_2$H$_5$	-CH$_2$-CH=CH-Cl	-	-	53	17,5	+	+	none
Mr 2-CL			COC$_2$H$_5$	-CH$_2$CH=CH$_2$	+	31	10	1,2	-	-	
Mr 12-MS	619	8235	COC$_2$H$_5$	-CH$_2$CH=C<CH$_3$/CH$_3$	+	-	20	50	-	+	none
Mr 415-MS	620	8236	COC$_2$H$_5$	-CH$_2$-CH=CH-Cl	+	15	1,6	1,5	-	-	high
Mr 16-CL			COC$_2$H$_5$	-CH$_2$-△	(+)	-	4	1,1	-		

[a] Suppression of morphine analgesia in mice, nalorphine (N) = 1 (see Pharmacological Methods)
[b] Precipitation of abstinence in nonwithdrawn monkeys (9, 10, 21–24)
[c] Physical dependence capacity in withdrawn monkeys

161

Physical Dependence Capacity (Monkeys)

Physical dependence capacity in withdrawn, morphine-dependent, rhesus monkeys was estimated by Deneau, Seevers, and Villarreal in Ann Arbor, Michigan (9, 10, 21–24).

RESULTS

The new 4-phenylpiperidines are depicted together with their properties in Tables 1 and 2. As outlined in the discussion, the methyl ester analogues are well distinguished from the bemidone and ketobemidone congeners, consequently, they are recorded in a separate table (Table 1). The pharmacological results of a selected number of bemidone and ketobemidone derivatives are shown in Table 2. Because some compounds were tested not only in our, but also in other, laboratories, different code numbers are recorded in the tables (C. H. Boehringer Sohn: CHBS-Mr numbers; University of Michigan: UM; National Institutes of Health: NIH).

DISCUSSION

Appropriate substitution on the nitrogen atom of the 4-(*m*-hydroxy-phenyl)-piperidine molecule results in compounds with analgesic and antagonistic activity. The methyl ester analogue of bemidone proved to be the most suitable 4-phenylpiperidine in the design of antagonists. The nature of the N-substituent profoundly influences analgesia and narcotic antagonist activity. Compounds with certain well-established N-substituents of allyl-like structure are active antagonists. The most effective of these is the *trans* 3-chloroallyl derivative *Mr 417*. In mice and monkeys it surpasses the *cis* isomer *Mr 473* and the cyclopropylmethyl analogue *Mr 471*. These distinct antagonists were estimated to have no physical dependence capacity in withdrawn monkeys. In nonwithdrawn animals they precipitated abstinence. Additionally, they display analgesic activity in mice without morphine-like side effects. The N-dimethylallyl derivative *Mr 432* has low antagonistic activity although the analgesic effect is still maintained. Interesting enough, the allyl analogue *Mr 77* has no antagonist properties. On the contrary, this compound is effective in the Haffner tail-clip test and induces the Straub-tail phenomenon (20). Since the Straub activity and the effectiveness in the Haffner test are usually related to morphine-like side effects (19), then the allyl derivative should be an analgesic with addiction liability. This assumption is supported by the results of the monkey experiments; *Mr 77* was able to substitute for morphine in dependent monkeys.

Replacement of the N-methyl residue by cyclic substituents with allyl-like structures provides compounds with sustained antagonistic activity. Four selected representatives with six-member rings in the N-residue are recorded in Table 1. These drugs are inactive in the Haffner test and failed to show the Straub phenomenon. *Mr 635* and *Mr 600* are antagonists both in mice and monkeys whereas Mr *623* displays antagonistic activity only in monkeys. The most potent substance is approximately $^1/_3$ as active in mice and monkeys as nalorphine, the most effective antagonist of the 4-phenylpiperidine series.

Substitution of the nitrogen atom of 4-phenylpiperidines with furylmethyl groups fails to produce antagonists. These drugs display Straub-tail activity and do not suppress morphine analgesia in mice. Monkey experiments demonstrated a morphine-like profile of action.

The bemidone molecule is not as suitable to obtain narcotic antagonism as the methyl ester analogue. The cyclopropylmethyl derivative *Mr 513* and the equipotent dimethylallyl analogue *Mr 424* exert very weak antagonistic action in mice and monkeys. The corresponding allyl compound *Mr 61* displays analgesia with questionable antagonism.

The derivatives of ketobemidone exhibit no antagonistic activity at all. They proved to be morphine-like analgesics with positive Straub phenomenon and physical dependence capacity in monkeys. They behave like meperidine congeners.

CONCLUSIONS

In the design of narcotic antagonists the structure-activity relationships have to be considered anew. As we have demonstrated, it is possible to obtain narcotic antagonists in the 4-phenylpiperidine series. It is common knowledge that morphine (III), levorphanol (IV), and metazocine (V) are suitable molecules to furnish compounds with anti-morphine action. These drugs are featured by free phenolic groups in the same relative position of the aromatic nucleus. The failure of antagonism in the allyl counterpart of meperidine (VI) (6, 7, 8, 25) is due primarily to the lack of the hydroxy substituent as already suggested (15). The absence of this group in penta-zocine (VII) and in the allyl analogue SKF 10, 047 (VIII) produces the same effect (Fig. 2) (18).

Obviously not only the *m*-hydroxy group but also other structural elements are responsible for optimal antagonist action. An ester function, preferably the methoxycarbonyl group, promotes a nalorphine-like activity.

Last but not least, the nature of the N-substituent profoundly influences the properties of the corresponding compounds. In the 4-phenylpiperidine

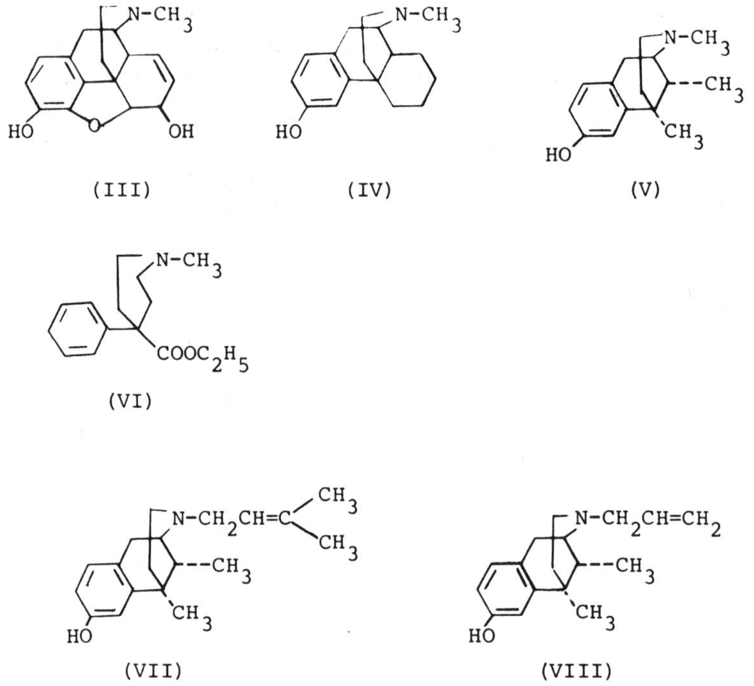

(III)   (IV)   (V)

(VI)

(VII)   (VIII)

FIG. 2. Structures of known analgesics and narcotic antagonists.

series, substituents with cyclic or noncyclic, allyl-like structures are appropriate for morphine antagonistic activity whereas the allyl residue is not.

REFERENCES

1. Archer, S., Albertson, N. F., Harris, L. S., Pierson, A. K., and Bird, J. G.: Pentazocine. Strong analgesics and analgesic antagonists in the benzomorphan series. J. Med. Chem. 7: 123–131, 1964.
2. Archer, S., and Harris, L. S.: Narcotic antagonists. In: Progress in Drug Research, edited by E. Jucker. 8:261–320, Birkhäuser Verlag, Basel, 1965.
3. Blumberg, H., Wolf, P. S., and Dayton, H. B.: Use of writhing test for evaluating analgesic activity of narcotic antagonists. Proc. Soc. Exp. Biol. Med. 118:763–766, 1965.
4. Boehringer Sohn, C. H.: Ger. pat. 1, 288, 605 (appln. July 21, 1964).
5. Boehringer Sohn, C. H.: Ger. Offenlegungsschrift 2, 109, 155 (appln. Feb. 26, 1971).
6. Casy, A. F.: Analgesics and their antagonists: Recent developments. In: Progress in Medicinal Chemistry, edited by G. P. Ellis and G. B. West. 7:229–284, Butterworths, London, 1970.
7. Casy, A. F., Simmonds, A. B., and Staniforth, D.: 1-Allyl and 1-(3,3-dimethylallyl) analogues of pethidine and its reversed ester. J. Pharm. Pharmacol. 20:768–774, 1968.
8. Costa, P. J., and Bonnycastle, D. D.: The effect of levallorphan tartrate, nalorphine HCl and WIN 7681 (1-allyl-4-phenyl-4-carbethoxypiperidine) on respiratory depression

and analgesia induced by some active analgesics. J. Pharmacol. Exp. Therap. *113*:310–318, 1955.

9. Deneau, G. A., and Seevers, M. H.: Evaluation of new compounds for morphine-like physical dependence in the rhesus monkey. Published in the addendum of the report of the committee on drug addiction and narcotics, 27th annual meeting, Houston, Texas, 1965.

10. Deneau, G. A., Villarreal, J. E., and Seevers, M. H.: Evaluation of new compounds for morphine-like physical dependence in the rhesus monkey. Published in the addendum of the report of the committee on problems of drug dependence, 28th annual meeting, New York, New York, 1966.

11. Freter, K., Merz, H., Schroeder, H.-D., and Zeile, K.:US-pat. 3, 627, 772 (appln. Nov. 13, 1969).

12. Haffner, F.: Experimentelle Prüfung schmerzstillender Mittel, Dtsch. Med. Wochenschrift. *55*:731–733, 1929.

13. Martin, W. R.: Opioid antagonists. Pharmacol. Rev. *19*:463–521, 1967.

14. May, E. L., and Sargent, L. J.: Morphine and its modifications. *In*: Analgesics, edited by G. de Stevens, *5*:171–172, Academic Press, New York, 1965.

15. May, E. L.: Agonists and antagonist actions of narcotic analgesic drugs. Chemistry. Synthetic compounds. Paper presented at the symposium on agonist and antagonist action of narcotic analgesics, Aberdeen, 1971. Personal communication.

16. Merz, H., Schroeder, H.-D., Langbein, A., and Zeile, K.: US-pat. 3, 462, 427 (appln. June 8, 1966).

17. Merz, H., Schroeder, H.-D., Langbein, A., and Zeile, K.: US-pat. 3, 438, 990 (appln. June 29, 1966).

18. Merz, H., Langbein, A., Stockhaus, K., and Wick, H.: Unpublished results.

19. Shemano, J., and Wendel, H.: A rapid screening test for potential addiction liability of new analgesic agents. Toxicol. Appl. Pharmacol. *6*:334–339, 1964.

20. Straub, W.: Eine empfindliche biologische Reaktion auf Morphin. Dtsch. Med. Wochenschrift. *37*:1462, 1911.

21. Villarreal, J. E., and Seevers, M. H.: Evaluation of new compounds for morphine-like physical dependence in the rhesus monkey. Published in the addendum of the report of the committee on problems of drug dependence, 29th annual meeting, Lexington, Kentucky, 1967.

22. Villarreal, J. E., and Seevers, M. H.: Evaluation of new compounds for morphine-like physical dependence in the rhesus monkey. Published in the addendum of the report of the committee on problems of drug dependence, 30th annual meeting, Indianapolis, Indiana, 1968.

23. Villarreal, J. E., and Seevers, M. H.: Evaluation of new compounds for morphine-like physical dependence in the rhesus monkey. Published in the addendum of the report of the committee on problems of drug dependence, 31st annual meeting, Palo Alto, California, 1969.

24. Villarreal, J. E., and Seevers, M. H.: Evaluation of new compounds for morphine-like physical dependence in the rhesus monkey. To be published in the addendum of the report of the committee on problems of drug dependence, 34th annual meeting, Ann Arbor, Michigan, 1972.

25. Winter, C. A., Orahovats, P. D., and Lehman, E. G.: Analgesic activity and morphine antagonism of compounds related to nalorphine. Arch. Int. Pharmacodyn. Thér. *110*: 186–202, 1957.

26. Woolfe, G., and MacDonald, A. D.: The evaluation of the analgesic action of pethidine hydrochloride (Demerol). J. Pharmacol. Exp. Ther. *80*:300–307, 1944.

Narcotic Antagonists, edited by M. C. Braude, L. S. Harris, E. L.
May, J. P. Smith, and J. E. Villarreal. *Advances in Biochemical
Psychopharmacology, Vol. 8.* Raven Press, New York © 1974.

Narcotic Antagonist Activity of Substituted 1,2,4,5-Tetrahydro-3H,3-Benzazepines

John E. Giering, Thomas A. Davidson, B. Vithal Shetty, and Aldo P. Truant

Pennwalt Corporation, Rochester, New York 14623

The bicyclic-ring system of the 1,2,4,5-tetrahydro-3H,3-benzazepines
can be viewed as a simplification of the tricyclic benzomorphans with removal of the methylene-bridge carbon and contraction of the eight-membered azocine ring by one carbon. This provides a rationale for synthesis
of a series of benzazepines and evaluation of analgesic and narcotic antagonist activities. The benzazepine-ring system was synthesized either by
cyclization of the intermediate *o*-phenylenediacetonitriles or by Friedel-
Crafts cyclization of the appropriate N-methanesulfonyl-N-phenethyl-
glycine to the 3H,3-benzazepin-1-one followed by reduction and demesyla-
tion. Oxymorphone mydriasis, morphine-induced analgesia, respiratory
depression, enhancement of locomotor activity, and physical dependence
in animals were used to assess narcotic antagonist characteristics. Analgesia was evaluated by phenylbenzoquinone writhing. Compounds with
hydroxy or methoxy groups in the 7 position and with hydrogen, methyl,
ethyl, propyl, or cyclopropylmethyl groups as substituents on the nitrogen
were weak or inactive as antagonists and analgesics. The 7-hydroxy-benza-
zepines with dimethylallyl or allyl substituents on the nitrogen had the
greatest antagonist action which was less than that of naloxone and equivalent to, or less than, nalorphine, depending upon the test method and route
of administration. Duration of antagonism was approximately equivalent to
that of naloxone at equieffective dose levels. These antagonist benzazepines
did not exhibit analgesic activity at doses significantly below those causing
other overt manifestations and thus resembled the pure antagonist, naloxone, rather than nalorphine. The data suggest that the benzazepine series
has the potential to provide a new source for useful narcotic antagonists
and analgesics.

INTRODUCTION

Elimination of ring fragments from morphine to form morphinans and
benzomorphans has been accomplished in the past without loss of analgesic
or narcotic antagonist activities (18). The bicyclic-ring system of the
1,2,4,5-tetrahydro-3H,3-benzazepines can be viewed as a further simplifi-

167

cation of the tricyclic benzomorphans with removal of the methylene-bridge carbon and contraction of the eight-membered azocine ring by one carbon. This view provides the rationale for synthesis of a series of benzazepines and subsequent evaluation for analgesic and narcotic antagonist activities. The present report describes the general synthesis and pharmacological characterization of some of these compounds, with primary emphasis on the properties of those which have been found to be active as narcotic antagonists.

METHODS

Chemical

Prior to the initiation of this work, few successful syntheses of 1,2,4,5-tetrahydro-3H,3-benzazepines had been reported. However, there are now several methods which offer alternative routes depending on the substituents desired on the aromatic and azepine rings (7, 8, 10, 14, 17, 19, 23). Two routes of synthesis, using readily available starting materials, were employed in our laboratory. The synthetic schemes are outlined in Fig. 1 and 2.

In the first scheme (Fig. 1), 4-methoxyphthalic acid (II) was obtained from 3,4-dimethylphenol (I) by treatment with dimethylsulfate and subsequent oxidation of the methyl ether with potassium permanganate. The acid (II) was reduced with lithium aluminum hydride to the diol which afforded 4-methoxy-α,α'-dibromo-o-xylene (III) on reaction with phosphorous tribromide. 4-Methoxy-o-phenylenediacetonitrile (IV) was obtained by reacting (III) with sodium cyanide in DMSO at 30 to 35°C. Catalytic reduction of (IV) over Raney-Nickel in 95% ethanol solution, afforded a mixture of primary and secondary amines which on fractional distillation gave 7-methoxy-1,2,4,5-tetrahydro-3H,3-benzazepine (V) in 30% yield. The amine (V) was obtained more readily by cyclization of the dinitrile (IV) with 32% hydrogen bromide in acetic acid (19) to form a mixture of the 7- and 8-methoxy derivatives of 2-amino-4-bromo-1H,3-benzazepine hydrobromide (VI), which were readily hydrolyzed by aqueous sodium acetate solution to the imide (VII). Reduction of (VII) with diborane afforded (V) in an overall yield of 50% from (IV).

The second scheme (Fig. 2) was used to prepare 8-methoxy-2,methyl-1,2,4,5-tetrahydro-3H,3-benzazepine (XII) in an overall yield of 35% from 2-(3-methoxyphenyl)-1-methylethylamine (VIII) by modification of known methods. Thus the amine (VIII) was mesylated, then the sulfonamide was

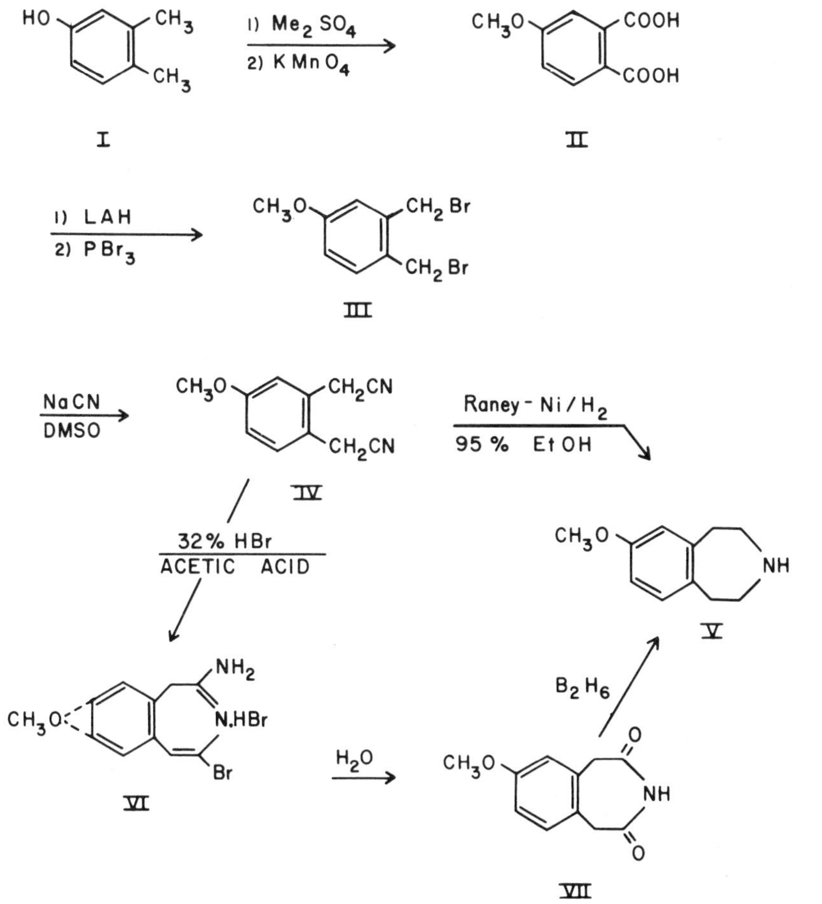

FIG. 1. Synthetic scheme for preparation of 1,2,4,5-tetrahydro-3H,3-benzazepines without the 2-methyl substituent.

reacted with ethyl bromoacetate and hydrolyzed to give the glycine (IX). Treatment of (IX) with thionyl chloride and cyclization under Friedel-Crafts conditions (23) with aluminum chloride in methylene dichloride at 10 to 15°C, afforded 3-methanesulfonyl-7-methoxy-4-methyl-1,2,4,5-tetra-hydro-3H,3-benzazepin-1-one (X) in 63% yield. The Friedel-Crafts reaction on the corresponding N-tosyl derivative gave only a 30% yield of ketone along with considerable quantities of the isoquinoline as a result of decarbonylation, even at −70°C (23). Reduction of the ketone (X) over palladium-

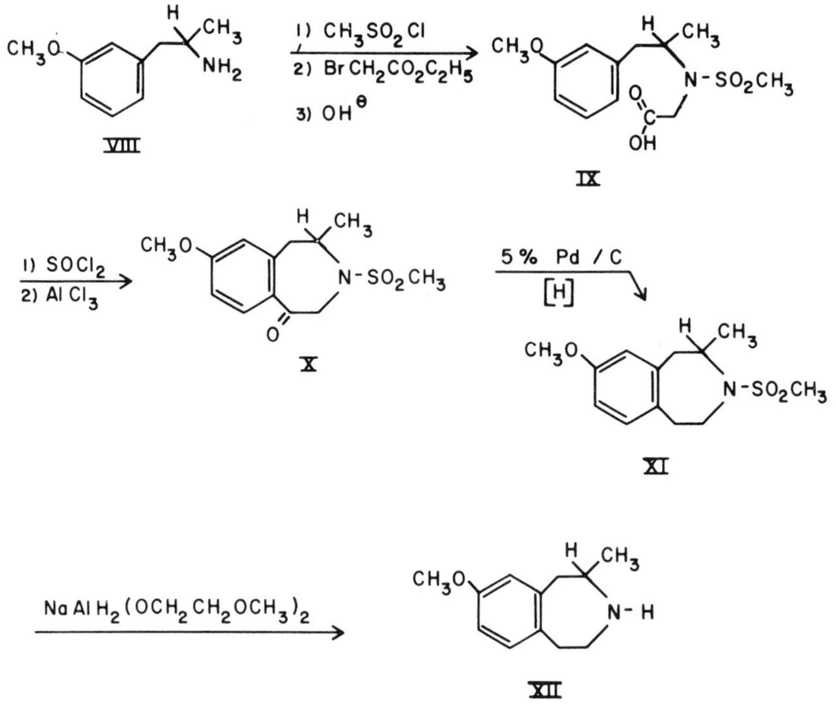

FIG. 2. Synthetic scheme for preparation of the 1,2,4,5-tetrahydro-3H,3-benzazepines with the 2-methyl substituent.

charcoal in acetic acid/hydrochloric acid gave the saturated benzazepine (XI), which was readily demesylated with sodium *bis*(2-methoxyethoxy)-aluminum hydride in benzene (85% yield).

Resolution of 8-methoxy-2-methyl-1,2,4,5-tetrahydro-3H,3-benzazepine (XI) was achieved by recrystallization of the D(+)- and (−)-tartaric acid salts. The nitrogen-substituted derivatives were prepared by standard methods such as direct alkylation or acylation followed by reduction with lithium aluminum hydride.

Pharmacological

All of the benzazepines except one (base of 701–086) were submitted for testing as the hydrochloride salts. The standard antagonists naloxone, nalorphine, and pentazocine, also as the hydrochloride salts, were used for comparison with the benzazepines. Oxymorphone hydrochloride and morphine sulfate were employed as agonists to elicit narcotic effects which could be reversed or reduced by an active antagonist. All doses of both the agonists and antagonists were calculated as the base.

With tests employing mice, male albino CF-1 (Carworth Farms, New City, New York) animals, body weight range of 18 to 24 g, were used. Female New Zealand white rabbits, weighing from 2.5 to 3.5 kg, were utilized for respiratory-depression determinations.

A battery of methods was used to evaluate the narcotic antagonist potential of benzazepine compounds. A rapid-screening test provided qualitative evidence of antagonist activity through use of the relatively long-lasting mydriatic response induced in mice by oxymorphone (4). Groups of mice were injected subcutaneously with 5 mg/kg of a solution containing 1 mg/ml of oxymorphone diluted with normal saline (0.9%). The volume injected was kept constant at 0.005 ml/g of body weight. Pupil diameter was measured with a binocular microscope equipped with a micrometer-disc eyepiece, and lighting conditions were kept constant. The diameter was recorded in each animal 10 min after an injection of oxymorphone that was followed immediately by intraperitoneal administration of saline or the test compound in logarithmically spaced dose levels. Pupil diameter was redetermined 15 min later. A compound was considered to be active if 50% or more of the treated animals showed a reduction of 0.2 units or greater in pupil diameter at a dose level significantly below that which caused overt signs of toxicity or secondary pharmacology. Compounds which caused pupil reduction in 50% of the animals, but at dose levels approaching toxicity, were classified as weakly active. If less than 50% of the mice exhibited reduced pupil size at doses causing manifestations of toxicity, the compound was interpreted to be inactive.

Respiratory depression, induced in unanesthetized rabbits by intravenous infusion of morphine, was used as a secondary test to confirm antagonist activity of benzazepine compounds. Rabbits, with a pneumograph around the thorax, were placed in restraining stocks. The pneumograph was attached to a strain-gauge coupler (Model 9803) contained in a two-channel recorder (Beckman Model RS Dynograph), for monitoring respiratory rate. The marginal ear vein was cannulated with a polyethylene catheter (PE 50) for infusion of morphine and antagonists. A Harvard infusion pump was set to deliver 0.2 ml/min and infusion of saline was initiated immediately upon insertion of the cannula to preserve patency of the vein and delivery system. Control respiratory rate was monitored for a 15-min equilibration period. A solution of morphine in saline, at a concentration of 1 mg/ml, was then infused at a rate of 1.23 ml/min. When respiratory rate decreased and stabilized at approximately 80 to 90% of the control rate, usually with a total dose of about 7 mg/kg of morphine, the delivery cannula was transferred to a 10-ml syringe containing a 0.1% solution of test compound, and infusion was reinstituted at a rate of 0.5 ml/min. The test compounds were infused until the respiratory rate returned to within 25 to 50% of control rate, or a dose of 7 mg/kg had been administered. Following cessation of compound infusion, respiration was monitored for 60 min to ascertain the approximate duration of antagonism. Experimental compounds were classified as having positive activity if the degree of reversal of respiratory depression, at a total dose less than 2 mg/kg, was 75 to 100%. This reversal was comparable to that obtained with nalorphine and naloxone. Weak activity was defined as less than 50%, but greater than 20%, and with reversal at dose levels between 2 and 7 mg/kg. Compounds were ranked as negative or inactive if the reversal achieved was less than 20% up to a dose of 7 mg/kg, or if the response was not dose related.

One of the active benzazepine compounds was evaluated further for ability to reverse or reduce the enhanced locomotor activity induced in mice by morphine (16, 24, 26). Locomotor activity was assessed in grouped mice by a modification of the method described by Dews (13) utilizing photocell activity cages (Woodard Research Corporation, Herndon, Virginia). Animals were placed in the cages and left undisturbed for 5 min after which pretreatment control activity was recorded over a period of 15 min. The groups of mice then received either 10 mg/kg of morphine subcutaneously and saline orally or subcutaneously as controls, morphine and various doses of the test compound, saline and test compound, or saline alone by the same routes used in control animals. Antagonist potency was determined from dose-response curves using accumulated counts over a 60-min session and is expressed as the dose of compound which reduced by 50% the locomotor response caused by 10 mg/kg of morphine.

Antagonism of analgesic activity was assessed in mice with the active benzazepine by use of the phenylbenzoquinone writhing test (27) and by the Nilsen method of electrical stimulation of the mouse tail (22). In both instances morphine was used as agonist. With the former test, relative oral and subcutaneous antagonist potency (AD_{50}) was determined as the dose of compound or standard causing 50% increase in the subcutaneous median effective dose (ED_{50}) of morphine administered 15 min after the antagonist. The latter test provided evidence of antagonism as reflected by the oral dose of a compound which was effective in causing 50% reduction in the electrical stimulation threshold achieved with 10 mg/kg of morphine administered subcutaneously 30 min after the antagonist.

Analgesic activities of the benzazepine and standard compounds were evaluated also through use of the phenylbenzoquinone method which has been reported (6) to detect analgesia of some narcotic antagonists. Median effective dose (ED_{50}) values were calculated by the method of Litchfield and Wilcoxon (20).

An additional test which was used to assess the selected representative benzazepine was the precipitation of the withdrawal-jumping reaction in morphine-dependent mice as described by Way et al. (29). Morphine dependence was produced according to the method of Saelens et al. (25). Antagonist activity was expressed as the median effective dose (ED_{50}), i.e., the dose of compound or antagonist, after intraperitoneal injection, required to cause 50% of a group of morphine-dependent mice to jump within 10 min.

Oral, intraperitoneal, intravenous, and subcutaneous, acute, lethal-toxicity values (48-hr postadministration) were determined for an active benzazepine compound and compared with naloxone, nalorphine, and pentazocine. Median lethal dose (LD_{50}) with 95% confidence limits was calculated also by use of the method of Litchfield and Wilcoxon. In addition, mice were observed following administration by these same routes of sublethal doses of the antagonists at 0.25 logarithmic intervals, and the highest dose which could be given without causing overt evidence of effects such as ataxia, depression, excitation was recorded. This dose is referred to as the highest nonsymptomatic dose (HNSD).

RESULTS

Twenty-four benzazepine derivatives were screened for narcotic antagonist activity by assessing their ability to reduce oxymorphone mydriasis and to reverse morphine respiratory depression. Qualitative results generated from these screening tests are correlated with structural modifications of the various derivatives in Table 1. Substitution on the nitrogen with hydrogen, methyl, ethyl, or propyl groups did not result in compounds with particularly strong narcotic antagonist properties. Unexpectedly, this was the case also for cyclopropylmethyl substitution. However, weak activity was observed with some N-substituted derivatives containing 7-hydroxy as opposed to 7-methoxy groups. Introduction of a methyl group in the 2-position did not alter the weak activity of the 7-hydroxy derivatives, nor did it impart activity to the 7-methoxy benzazepines.

Narcotic antagonist activity, within the range of that elicited by the standards nalorphine and naloxone, is signified in Table 1 by positive responses in both of the screening tests. In addition, the Straub tail phenomenon seems to be reduced or blocked by these compounds in mice receiving oxymorphone to elicit mydriasis. Structural modification of benzazepines

TABLE 1. Narcotic antagonist screening of 1,2,4,5-tetrahydro-3H,3-benzazepines

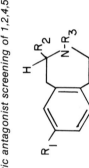

No.	R_1	R_2	R_3	Melting point[a] °C	Yield[c] %	Antagonist activity[d] versus	
						Oxymorphone mydriasis	Morphine respiratory depression
654–095	CH_3O	H	H	232–234	—	Neg.	Neg.
701–008	HO	H	H	249–251	—	Neg.	Neg.
701–077	CH_3O	H	CH_3	188–190	65	Neg.	Neg.
701–070	HO	H	CH_3	244–248	51	Neg.	Neg.
709–008	CH_3O	H	C_2H_5	219–221	62	Neg.	Neg.
709–002	HO	H	C_2H_5	247–250	68	Weak	Weak
727–915	CH_3O	H	nC_3H_7	208–210	43	Weak	Neg.
701–089	HO	H	nC_3H_7	221–223	52	Weak	Weak
701–038	CH_3O	H	△—CH_2	222–223	60	Neg.	Neg.
701–027	HO	H	△—CH_2	220–222	55	Neg.	Weak
795–209	CH_3O	CH_3	△—CH_2	150–155	50	Neg.	Neg.
807–607	HO	CH_3	△—CH_2	209–212	73	Neg.	Weak
727–051	CH_3O	H	$CH_2=CH—CH_2$	196–199	50	Pos.	Neg.
701–087	HO	H	$CH_2=CH—CH_2$	176–178	72	Pos.	Pos.
786–718	CH_3O	CH_3	$CH_2=CH—CH_2$	165–167	45	Neg.	Weak
727–941	CH_3O	H	$(CH_3)_2C=CH—CH_2$	204–206	35	Pos.[e]	Pos.
701–037	HO	H	$(CH_3)_2C=CH—CH_2$	254–256	50	Pos.[e]	Pos.
778–030	CH_3O	CH_3	$(CH_3)_2C=CH—CH_2$	165–168	35	Neg.	Weak
778–016	HO	CH_3	$(CH_3)_2C=CH—CH_2$	203–206	35	Pos.[e]	Pos.
795–229	HO	(+)CH_3	$(CH_3)_2C=CH—CH_2$	191–194	34	Neg.	Weak
795–232	HO	(−)CH_3	$(CH_3)_2C=CH—CH_2$	190–193	26	Pos.[e]	Pos.
727–052	CH_3O	H	$Ph—CH=CH—CH_2$	198–200	50	Weak	Neg.
786–796	CH_3O	CH_3	$Ph—CH=CH—CH_2$	184–186	50	Neg.	Weak
701–086	HO	H	$Ph—CH=CH—CH_2$	158–159[b]	71	Neg.	—
Naloxone						Pos.[e]	Pos.
Nalorphine						Pos.[e]	Pos.
Pentazocine						Pos.	Weak

[a] Melting points are for the recrystallized hydrochlorides.
[b] Melting point and yield are for the base.
[c] Yield of hydrochloride obtained from the unsubstituted methoxy or hydroxy precursor; not optimized.
[d] See "Methods" in text for explanation of activity designations; Positive (Pos.), Weak and Negative (Neg.).
[e] Effective in reversing oxymorphone induced Straub tail response.

175

to produce this degree of activity involved, primarily, dimethylallyl substitution on the nitrogen (701–037, 778–016, 795–232) and, to a lesser extent, was observed with an N-allyl derivative (701–087). As might be expected, the phenolic-hydroxy component, rather than a methoxy group in the 7-position, was essential for a high degree of antagonist activity.

Resolution of one of the active benzazepine antagonists, containing 2-methyl and N-dimethylallyl substituents (778–016), into its antipodes resulted in positive antagonist activity of the (−)-isomer but little or no effect from the (+)-antipode. This (−)-isomer (795–232) would appear to be of interest for further, more extensive evaluation as a narcotic antagonist and for comparison with the (+)-analog (795–229) and racemate.

In the case of the N-substituted phenylallyl derivatives, the phenyl group appeared to cause a decrease in antagonist activity as compared with unsubstituted allyl compounds.

The relative narcotic antagonism of three of the most active benzazepines (701–037, 701–087, 795–232) was compared further with that of naloxone and nalorphine utilizing morphine-induced respiratory depression in rabbits. Figure 3 provides a graphic representation of the results obtained. Morphine infusion caused marked reduction in respiratory rate from a control level of approximately 300 down to 50/min. Subsequent control infusion of 7 ml/kg of saline did not reverse respiratory depression and the morphine effect persisted for more than 60 min following cessation of this infusion. The doses of standard antagonists required for 50% reversal of respiratory depression were 0.1 mg/kg of naloxone and 0.2 mg/kg of nalorphine. Approximately comparable effect with the benzazepines was obtained with doses of 0.5, 0.75, and 0.4 mg/kg of 701–037, 701–087, and 795–232, respectively. It can be seen also in the figure that duration of antagonism with the benzazepines and standards did not persist, in most cases, beyond 60 min. When the antagonist action began to wane, respiratory rate reverted toward the depressed levels characteristic after morphine. The time after antagonist administration, when respiratory rate had again decreased to 50% of the control level, was close to 60 min for naloxone and nalorphine and approximately 40, 30, and 10 min for 701–037, 701–087, and 795–232 respectively. Thus, results of this comparison indicated that the benzazepine antagonists were slightly less potent and possessed shorter duration of action than the standards. However, it should be pointed out that the total doses of antagonists used in this experiment were not exactly equivalent from the standpoint of producing peak effects and therefore duration of action might have been influenced accordingly.

In the light of this point, a direct comparison was made of naloxone and compound 701–037 for duration of effects but at dose levels which were

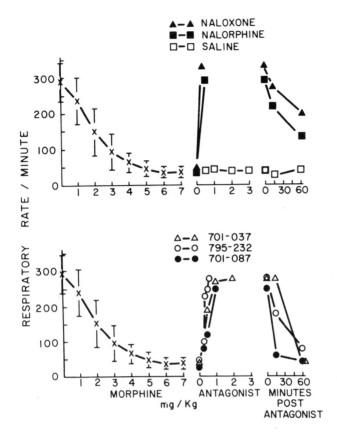

FIG. 3. Comparison of narcotic antagonist standards and benzazepines for ability to reverse morphine respiratory depression in rabbits. Vertical lines to points represent standard deviation. The points for morphine represent the mean values obtained with 25 rabbits. Points with antagonists are single determinations.

equivalent with respect to peak antagonist activity. The phenylbenzoquinone writing test was used for this comparison. Naloxone, 0.075 mg/kg, and 701–037, at a dose of 2.5 mg/kg, were administered subcutaneously to groups of 20 mice at various intervals between 15 and 120 min before subcutaneous injection of the ED_{90} dose (1.5 mg/kg) of morphine. It is evident from Fig. 4 that the duration of activity of naloxone and 701–037 did not differ significantly under these conditions. Both agents reduced the 90% analgesic effect of morphine to 35% and the duration of antagonism lasted for about 90 min in each instance. These results also indicate that compound 701–037 was less active than naloxone.

Table 2 provides a summary of antagonism obtained with compound

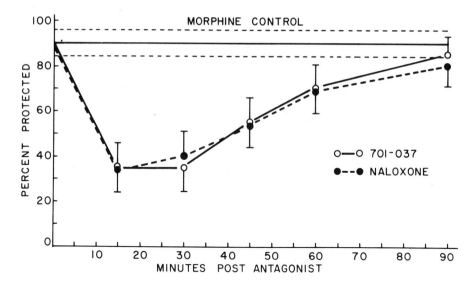

FIG. 4. Duration of antagonism with equieffective doses of naloxone and a benzazepine compound. Compound 701–037, 2.5 mg/kg; naloxone, 0.075 mg/kg; morphine ED_{90}, 1.5 mg/kg in phenylbenzoquinone writhing test. Each point represents the mean response from 20 mice. Vertical solid and broken horizontal lines indicate standard errors.

701–037 as compared with naloxone and nalorphine using several different morphine effects, including enhancement of locomotor activity and analgesia. In addition, ability to precipitate a withdrawal response in morphine-dependent mice was used. It should be pointed out that the time of administration of the antagonist relative to the agonist varied in the different tests. Therefore, comparisons can be made only within a single test procedure. As can be seen in the table, compound 701–037 was effective in antagonizing morphine-induced locomotor effects and analgesia. In addition, this benzazepine was highly active in precipitating the withdrawal-jumping response in morphine-dependent mice, an effect which is commonly associated with the more potent narcotic antagonists. Quantitatively, compound 701–037 was less active by the oral than the parenteral routes and was consistently less potent than naloxone by all of the routes tested. The order of difference ranged from approximately 20- to 200-fold depending upon route of administration and test method employed. Relative to nalorphine, the benzazepine compound was half as active or equipotent, again depending upon experimental conditions. It will become evident from consideration of toxicity data in a later section of this chapter that the effective antagonist dose levels of the benzazepine and standards were significantly below those causing toxicity or gross secondary pharmacological manifestations.

TABLE 2. Antagonism of various morphine effects by naloxone, nalorphine, and the benzazepine compound 701–037

Compound	Antagonism (AD_{50}) mg/kg				MTS Test[c] (p.o.)	ED_{50} mg/kg precipitated withdrawal[d] (i.p.)
	Locomotor Activity[a]		PBQ Test[b]			
	(p.o.)	(s.c.)	(p.o.)	(s.c.)		
701–037	140 (82–238)	2.3 (0.62–8.5)	22 (12.6–38.6)	1.6 (1.1–2.3)	23 (3.1–173)	6.4 (1.7–23.6)
Naloxone	6.9 (3.12–15.2)	0.14 (0.03–0.74)	0.31 (0.22–0.44)	0.0075 (0.004–0.016)	0.13 (0.0012–6.2)	0.3 (0.75–1.2)
Nalorphine	18.2 (14.3–26.2)	0.95 (0.24–3.80)	10.7 (0.95–12.1)	0.086 (0.041–0.182)	10.3 (8.6–12.4)	26.3 (10.5–65.9)

[a] Antagonist dose (AD_{50}) by the oral (p.o.) or subcutaneous (s.c.) routes to inhibit s.c. morphine effect on locomotor activity by 50%.
[b] Dose of antagonist by p.o. or s.c. routes to increase the s.c. median effective dose of morphine by 50% in the phenylbenzoquinone writhing test.
[c] Dose of antagonist p.o. to reduce by 50% the s.c. effect of 10 mg/kg morphine on electrical stimulation threshold in the mouse tail stimulation (MTS) test.
[d] Intraperitoneal (i.p.) dose of antagonist to precipitate withdrawal jumping in 50% of morphine-dependent mice.
( ) 95% confidence limits

Analgesic activity of the various benzazepine derivatives was compared with that of morphine, pentazocine, nalorphine, and naloxone, utilizing the phenylbenzoquinone writhing test. In order to characterize the benzazepines relative to these analgesic and antagonist standards, the doses causing analgesia, lethal toxicity, and nonlethal manifestations of secondary pharmacological or toxicological effects are compared in Table 3. Not included in the table are the benzazepines with hydrogen, methyl, ethyl, or propyl substituents on the nitrogen, but results of analgesic evaluation with these derivatives were comparable to effects obtained with compounds listed in the table. These benzazepine compounds and the pure antagonist, naloxone, did not exhibit analgesic activity at doses which were below the highest nonsymptomatic levels. Furthermore, with the exception of the N-phenylallyl derivatives, doses of the benzazepines required to produce positive analgesic effect in 100% of the animals (ED_{100}) also caused more than 10% mortality. In contrast to this relationship of analgesia to toxicity with the benzazepines and naloxone, effective analgesia was observed consistently with morphine, nalorphine, and pentazocine at doses considerably less than the highest nonsymptomatic levels. The slope of the nalorphine dose-response relationship for analgesia was relatively flat, however, and 10% mortality was evident in this case also at the ED_{100} level. Absence of analgesic activity, but presence of significant antagonism at dose levels below those producing signs of toxicity or secondary pharmacology, is considered evidence that the primary pharmacological action of some of these benzazepine compounds is narcotic antagonism.

Acute toxicity was determined in mice with the benzazepine compound 701–037, naloxone, nalorphine, and pentazocine administered by various routes. Table 4 shows that the benzazepine compound was significantly more toxic than nalorphine and naloxone when administered by all of the different routes but was approximately equivalent in toxicity to pentazocine. Death of animals was related to respiratory failure with all of these antagonists, and tonic-clonic convulsions and loss of righting-reflex preceded death. Some of the manifestations which occurred at sublethal dose levels included decreased motility, physical depression, ataxia, reduced respiratory function, and cyanosis. Qualitatively, major differences were not apparent in the type of effects seen with the antagonists.

Several other studies also were conducted to characterize the benzazepine compound 701–037. Physical-dependence capacity has been evaluated in monkeys (28) by a single-dose substitution test in morphine-dependent animals and by chronic administration every 6 hr for 33 days followed by abrupt withdrawal. Results showed that the benzazepine caused exacerbation of withdrawal in morphine-dependent monkeys, a characteristic of

TABLE 3. Comparison of analgesic activity and toxicity of benzazepines after subcutaneous administration to mice

Compound	Toxicity					Analgesia			
	HNSD[a] mg/kg	LD$_{10}$[b] mg/kg	LD$_{50}$ mg/kg	(95% C.L.)[c]	Slope (95% C.L.)	ED$_{50}$[d] mg/kg	(95% C.L.)	Slope	(95% C.L.)
701–038	60	200	260	(220–306)	1.24 (1.09–1.42)	93[e]	—	—	—
701–027	30	78	122	(100–149)	—	>75[e]	—	—	—
795–209	60	180	220	—	—	77[e]	—	—	—
727–051	30	160	>316	—	—	>100[e]	—	—	—
701–087	30	80	123	(101–149)	1.38 (0.6–3.17)	>60[e]	—	—	—
786–718	100	200	300	—	—	>100[e]	—	—	—
727–941	20	46	92	(61–139)	1.53 (1.20–1.94)	20.4[e]	—	—	—
701–037	30	120	198	(162–242)	1.36 (1.01–1.67)	77[e]	—	—	—
778–030	20	35	68	(51–89)	1.86 (0.84–4.13)	>20[e]	—	—	—
778–016	10	110	190	(143–252)	2.05 (1.21–3.49)	80[e]	—	—	—
795–229	20	72	145	(114–184)	1.73 (1.27–2.36)	70[e]	—	—	—
795–232	30	140	360	—	—	>56[e]	—	—	—
727–052	100	>316	>316	—	—	119	(76.7–185)	2.27	(1.42–3.62)
786–796	20	316	>316	—	—	34	(24.2–47.6)	1.96	(1.15–3.35)
Morphine	2	110	240	(200–288)	1.65 (1.32–2.60)	0.47	(0.29–0.75)	2.94	(1.51–5.74)
Pentazocine	30	140	180	(167–194)	1.23 (1.08–1.40)	2.0	(1.33–3.0)	2.24	(1.44–3.48)
Nalorphine	100	420	585	(509–674)	1.25 (1.08–1.45)	17.0[e]	(4.2–68)	10.8	—
Naloxone	30	210	252	(238–268)	1.10 (0.92–1.31)	84.0	(68.7–102)	1.37	(1.07–1.25)

[a] HNSD – Highest nonsymptomatic dose.
[b] LD$_{10}$ – Approximate lethal dose in 10% of the animals.
[c] 95% confidence limits.
[d] Median effective dose (ED$_{50}$) determined by use of the phenylbenzoquinone writhing test.
[e] The dose for analgesia in 100% of the animals (ED$_{100}$) exceeded the lethal dose 10% (LD$_{10}$).

181

TABLE 4. *Acute toxicity in mice of a benzazepine compound compared with narcotic antagonist standards*

Compound	Oral mg/kg LD_{50}[a] (95% C.L.)[b]	Oral mg/kg HNSD[c]	Intraperitoneal mg/kg LD_{50} (95% C.L.)	Intraperitoneal mg/kg HNSD	Subcutaneous mg/kg LD_{50} (95% C.L.)	Subcutaneous mg/kg HNSD	Intravenous mg/kg LD_{50} (95% C.L.)	Intravenous mg/kg HNSD
701–037[d]	270 (228–319)	100	96 (81.1–113)	31.6	198 (162–242)	31.6	32 (29.3–35.0)	–
Naloxone	>1000 –	316	350 (318–386)	56.2	252 (238–268)	31.6	99 (93.4–105)	17.8
Nalorphine	>1000 –	>1000	580 (504–668)	100	585 (509–674)	100	133 (120–148)	56.2
Pentazocine	345 (308–386)	56.2	107 (95.5–120)	31.6	180 (167–194)	31.6	25.2 (24.0–26.4)	5.62

[a] LD_{50} – median lethal dose determined 48 hr after administration of the compound or standard
[b] 95% confidence limits
[c] HNSD – highest nonsymptomatic dose. The dose which is 0.25 of a logarithmic interval below that causing overt signs of toxicity.
[d] 701–037 is 3-(3,3-dimethylallyl)-7-hydroxy-1,2,4,5-tetrahydro-3H,3-benzazepine.

narcotic antagonists, and did not substitute for morphine. Also, no distinct signs of an abstinence syndrome could be detected when 701–037 was discontinued after chronic injection. Nalorphine and naloxone were not effective in precipitating signs of abstinence in animals chronically treated with 701–037. These results support the conclusion that 701–037 is a narcotic antagonist and, in all probability, does not have physical dependence liability.

Subacute toxicity studies were performed in which 701–037 was injected intravenously daily for 30 days in rabbits and rhesus monkeys. Convulsions and disorientation were frequently evident with the highest dose administered in both rabbits and monkeys, but no gross tissue changes or significant histopathological, hematological, or clinical chemistry alterations were observed.

DISCUSSION

Analgesic antagonism has usually been associated with the N-allylation type of substitution in a given chemical series of strong analgesics (11). Thus, the polycyclic antagonists nalorphine, levallorphan, naloxone, and pentazocine are all derived from series in which the corresponding N-methyl compound is a strong analgesic, usually with a high physical dependence capacity. With the exception of naloxone, these antagonists also exhibit agonist activity, and all have significantly reduced physical dependence properties as compared with the N-methyl congeners. Naloxone is considered to be a pure antagonist (5) without agonist effect or physical dependence capacity. Manipulation of the 6,7-benzomorphan structure has produced compounds with varying degrees of agonist and antagonist actions (2, 3), and resolution of active racemates (1, 3, 21) has caused qualitative, as well as quantitative, separation of these actions. The phenolic-hydroxyl group has been essential for good activity in the polycyclic antagonists. In general, the order of antagonist potency, as related to N-substitution in various series, has been cyclopropylmethyl > allyl > dimethylallyl (2, 15). However, psychotomimetic and other side effects usually follow the same order.

In the benzazepine series as with the polycyclics, the phenolic-hydroxyl group is essential for good antagonism, and optical resolution causes quantitative separation of antagonist effect. Unlike the N-methyl-substituted polycyclic series, the N-methyl benzazepines are relatively weak or inactive as analgesics. However, compounds with potent analgesic activity but without significant antagonist action, as well as derivatives with both analgesic and antagonist activities, have been identified from the benzazepine series (12). The order of antagonist activity of the N-substituted benzazepines considered in this chapter is dimethylallyl > allyl > cyclopropylmethyl which is the reverse of that apparent with the polycyclic series.

Carabateas and Harris (9) reported that a group of 1,4-benzodiazepines, with various substituents on the aromatic and azepine rings, showed only antagonist activity when the 4-N-substituent was methyl, cyclopropylmethyl, or allyl. The general lack in this study of derivatives analagous to the benzazepines precludes direct comparison of structure-antagonist activity relationships. However, the absence of analgesia in the benzodiazepine derivatives is similar to that with corresponding benzazepines.

In consideration of structure-activity differences, it would appear that the benzazepines represent a novel class of antagonists with some properties resembling the pure antagonist, naloxone, rather than the agonist-antagonist compounds of the 6,7-benzomorphan class. The lack of physical dependence capacity in animals for several compounds tested from the series, both agonists and antagonists, provides further evidence that the benzazepines have potential as narcotic antagonists and analgesics.

CONCLUSIONS

A series of 1,2,4,5-tetrahydro-3H,3-benzazepines has been prepared by fully synthetic methods using readily available starting materials. Several compounds from this series have been found, in a variety of tests in animals, to possess narcotic antagonist activity. Relative to N-substitution, the order of activity of the phenolic-hydroxyl compounds in this series is dimethylallyl > allyl > cyclopropylmethyl. The antagonist benzazepines are weak or inactive as analgesics, even when tested by highly sensitive methods capable of detecting analgesia of agonist-antagonists. The results suggest, therefore, that some of these benzazepines have narcotic antagonism as their primary pharmacological action and, as such, might provide a new source for useful agents resembling the pure antagonist naloxone rather than the agonist-antagonists.

ACKNOWLEDGMENTS

The authors wish to express sincere appreciation to Mrs. Mary Stagnitto, Mrs. Rosemary Williams, and Messrs. Louis Freedman and William Kuipers for their capable technical assistance, to Mrs. Barbara Dow and Miss Judith Johnstone for expertise in organizing and typing of the manuscript and to Mr. James Rice for preparation of the figures.

REFERENCES

1. Ager, J. H., Jacobson, A. E., and May, E. L.: Separation of morphine-like effects by optical resolution. Levo isomers as strong analgetics and narcotic antagonists. J. Med. Chem. *12*:288–289, 1969.
2. Albertson, N. F., Archer, S., Bird, J. G., Harris, L. S., and Pierson, A. K.: Pentazocine. Strong analgesics and analgesic antagonists in the benzomorphan series. J. Med. Chem. *7*:123–127, 1964.
3. Albertson, N. F., Harris, L. S., Perry, R. L., Pierson, A. K., Soria, A. E., Tullar, B. F., and Wetterau, W. F.: Benzomorphans. Optically active and trans isomers. J. Med. Chem. *10*:383–386, 1967.
4. Beech, J. A., Stagnitto, M. L., and Giering, J. E.: A rapid screening method for narcotic antagonism in mice. *Unpublished observations.*
5. Blumberg, H., Dayton, H. B., George, M., and Rapaport, D. N.: N-allylnoroxymorphone: A potent narcotic antagonist. Fed. Proc. *20*:311, 1961.
6. Blumberg, H., Wolf, P. S., and Dayton, H. B.: Use of writhing test for evaluating analgesic activity of narcotic antagonists. Proc. Soc. Exp. Biol. Med. *118*:763–766, 1965.
7. Brossi, A., Percherer, B., and Sunbury, R. C.: The synthesis of some 7- and 7,8-substituted 2,3,4,5-tetrahydro-1*H*-3-benzazepines. J. Heterocyclic Chem. *8*:779–783, 1971.
8. Brossi, A., Pecherer, B., and Sunbury, R. C.: A novel synthesis of aromatic methoxy and methylenedioxy substituted 2,3,4,5-tetrahydro-1*H*-3-benzazepines. J. Heterocyclic Chem. *9*:609–616, 1972.
9. Carabateas, P. M., and Harris, L. S.: Analgesic antagonists. I. 4-Substituted 1-acyl-2,3,4,5-tetrahydro-1H-1,4-benzodiazepines. J. Med. Chem. *9*:6–10, 1966.
10. Chaykovsky, M., Tokuyama, T., Witkop, B., and Yonemitsu, O.: Photocyclizations of tyrosines, tyramines, catecholamines, and normescaline. J. Amer. Chem. Soc. *90*:776–784, 1968.
11. Clark, R. L., Pessolano, A. A., Pfister, K., 3rd, and Weijlard, J.: N-Substituted epoxymorphinans. J. Amer. Chem. Soc. *75*:4963–4967, 1953.
12. Davidson, T. A., Giering, J. E., and Shetty, B. V.: *Unpublished observations.*
13. Dews, P. B.: The measurement of the influence of drugs on voluntary activity in mice. Br. J. Pharmacol. Chemotherap. *8*:46–48, 1953.
14. Gardent, J., and Hazebroucq, G.: Sur quelques proprietes de l'amino-2-bromo-4 1H benzazepine-3 et de ses derives. Bull Soc. Chem. France, *2*:600–605, 1968.
15. Gates, M., and Montzka, T. A.: Some potent morphine antagonists possessing high analgesic activity. J. Med. Chem. *7*:127–131, 1964.
16. Goldstein, A., and Sheehan, P.: Tolerance to opioid narcotics. I. Tolerance to the "running fit" caused by levorphanol in the mouse. J. Pharmacol. Exp. Ther. *169*:175–184, 1969.
17. Halford, J. O., and Weissmann, B.: *o*-Phenylenediacetimide and other compounds related to 3,1*H*-benzazepine. J. Org. Chem. *17*:1646–1652, 1952.
18. Harris, L. S.: Structure activity relationships. In: Narcotic Drugs. Biochemical Pharmacology, edited by D. H. Clouet, pp. 89–98, Plenum Press, New York, 1971.
19. Johnson, F., and Nasutavicus, W. A.: Polyfunctional aliphatic compounds VI. The cyclization of dinitriles to benzazepines. J. Heterocyclic Chem. *2*:26–36, 1965.
20. Litchfield, J. T., Jr. and Wilcoxon, F.: A simplified method of evaluating dose-effect experiments. J. Pharm. Exp. Ther. *96*:99–113, 1949.
21. May, E. L., and Takeda, M.: Optical isomers of miscellaneous strong analgetics. J. Med. Chem. *13*:805–807, 1970.
22. Nilsen, P. L.: Studies on algesimetry by electrical stimulation of the mouse tail. Acta Pharmacol. et Toxicol. *18*:10–22, 1961.
23. Proctor, G. R., and Rehman, M. A.: Azabenzocycloheptencnes. Part VI. Preparation and some reactions of 1,2,4,5-tetrahydro-1-oxy-3-toluene-*p*-sulphonylbenz[d]azepine. J. Chem. Soc. (C) 58–61, 1967.

24. Rethy, C. R., Smith, C. B., and Villarreal, J. E.: Effects of narcotic analgesics upon the locomotor activity and brain catecholamine content of the mouse. J. Pharmacol. Exp. Ther. *176*:472–479, 1971.
25. Saelens, J. K., Granat, F. R., and Sawyer, W. K.: The mouse jumping test—a simple screening method to estimate the physical dependence capacity of analgesics. Arch. Intern. Pharmacodyn. *190*:213–218, 1971.
26. Shuster, L., Hannam, R. V., and Boyle, W. E., Jr.: A simple method for producing tolerance to dihydromorphinone in mice. J. Pharmacol. Exp. Ther. *140*:149–154, 1963.
27. Siegmund, E., Cadmus, R., and Lu, G.: A method for evaluating both nonnarcotic and narcotic analgesics. Proc. Soc. Exp. Biol. Med. *95*:729-731, 1957.
28. Villarreal, J. E.: Report on the physical dependence capacity of compound 701–037 (NIH 8376, UM 728). Single-dose suppression test and chronic administration. *Unpublished observations*.
29. Way, E. L., Loh, H. H., and Shen, F. H.: Simultaneous quantitative assessment of morphine tolerance and physical dependence. J. Pharmacol. Exp. Ther. *167*:1-8, 1969.

Narcotic Antagonists, edited by M. C. Braude, L. S. Harris, E. L.
May, J. P. Smith, and J. E. Villarreal. Advances in Biochemical
Psychopharmacology, Vol. 8. Raven Press, New York © 1974.

Perspectives in the Chemistry of Narcotic Antagonists

Arthur E. Jacobson and Everette L. May

National Institute of Arthritis, Metabolism, and Digestive Diseases, National Institutes of
Health, Bethesda, Maryland 20014

Research on narcotic antagonists has proceeded apace since the 1950's
from the classical N-allyl compounds of the morphine, morphinan, and
benzomorphan series to stronger, longer acting, orally effective substances
having groups such as cyclopropylmethyl, propyl, and furyl on nitrogen in
place of allyl. With these three polycyclic prototypes (in addition to the importance of the nitrogen substituent), a phenolic hydroxyl situated *meta*
to the quaternary carbon attachment is critical. Furthermore, activity is
improved by introduction of hydroxyl into position 14 of certain morphine
and morphinan types. A similar modification (OH in the 9-position, in this
instance) in the benzomorphan series will be of interest. Compounds, some
of radically different structure, have recently been synthesized and found
to exhibit exciting agonist-antagonist properties. These (benzazepines,
bridged aminotetralines, 2-hydroxymorphinans, etc.) add new dimensions
to the continuing research toward finding more useful drugs. Several of
these and newer "classical" types are suggested for future exploration in
man. Finally, another stratagem for the design of improved antagonists
and antagonist-agonists, one based on the use of regression analyses, is
suggested.

The tremendous surge in research on narcotic antagonists seen in the
last decade can be attributed largely to the discovery of nalorphine with
its peculiar variety of pharmacologic actions. From this (now classical)
antagonist have evolved *N-allyl compounds* in the morphinan, benzomorphan, and oxymorphone series, all characterized, in general, by a
relatively short duration of action, low oral effectiveness, and varying
degrees of agonistic effect.

After subsequent systematic studies with morphine, and later with
morphinan types, in respect to variations at nitrogen, antagonists have
been developed which exhibit vastly increased oral efficacy and duration of
action over the N-allyl prototypes. Probably the most important N-substituent to be used is cyclopropylmethyl which also almost invariably

187

confers strong analgesic, antagonistic, and dysphoric properties. Other N-substituents which have proved of interest are furyl radicals containing a strategically placed methyl group, especially in the benzomorphan series.

In addition, interesting new "nonclassical" structures have been synthesized, but these are still in early stages of evaluation. These include the bridged aminotetralines, N-substituted pyrrolidines, benzazepines, and the homobenzomorphans. Finally, it has been found that certain members of the benzomorphan series (particularly the N-methyl *levo*-isomers), morphine-like analgesics in their own right, can function as nalorphine-like antagonists in morphine-dependent monkeys, although they are much less potent than the classical type antagonists.

This wealth of structures with varying degrees of antagonistic and agonistic effect provides, it seems to us, a sound basis for further exploration not only into the mechanism of action of analgesics and antagonists but also for the synthesis of long-acting orally effective antagonists for deterrence of narcotic abuse. It is also possible, perhaps probable, that strategies involved in these researches will shed new light on tolerance and dependence phenomena and take us closer to the near-ideal analgesic — one with low or no abuse potential which is capable of relieving deep pain by either the oral or parenteral route of administration and which has negligible deleterious effects. It bears repeating that what progress has been made toward this goal has come about partly, perhaps largely, through pursuit of research on antagonists.

The structural features that are of most importance in the classical types of antagonists, those derived from morphine and congeners, the morphinans and the benzomorphans, are: (1) a phenolic hydroxyl situated *meta* to the quaternary carbon attachment; (2) an allyl, cycloalkylmethyl (especially cyclopropylmethyl), propyl, or propynyl group on the nitrogen; and (3) a 14-hydroxyl substituent on the morphine or morphinan molecule (this corresponds to the 9-position in the benzomorphan series). It is virtually impossible at this stage to sort out features that are important in the new structural types which have been discussed. Elsewhere in this volume are reports about efforts directed toward prolongation of the action of existing antagonists.

With regard to compounds now in various stages of the testing pipeline, we would like to suggest, perhaps redundantly, what appear to be the most promising candidates for further study not necessarily in the order of their importance. Morphine relatives of interest are diprenorphine and newer analogues and naltrexone. In the morphinan series, the *racemic* and *levo*-forms of 3,14-dihydroxy-N-cyclopropylmethyl morphinans, (−)-3-hydroxy-N-cyclopropylmethylmorphinan (cyclorphan), and *dextro*- and *levo*-2-

hydroxy-N-cyclopropylmethylmorphinans (the last two interesting from the standpoint of hydroxyl-group position) stand out. Benzomorphans of interest are L-cyclazocine, the N-furyl derivatives, and perhaps one 9,9-disubstituted compound. Of the new types, at least two representatives of the so-called bridged aminotetralins (very long-acting antagonists judging from monkey experiments), one from the benzazepine series, and at least one each of the pyrrolidines and homobenzomorphans mentioned here today, merit further attention.

May we also suggest that this might be an opportune time to begin examining the antagonistic activity of agonist-antagonists or the pure antagonists in a somewhat different way.

If accord could be reached among the various pharmaceutical and university groups to submit samples of their known antagonists for partition-coefficient determination, then perhaps application of the Hansch method might prove useful. Contract mechanisms might be employed to make these determinations as well as to perform appropriate regression analyses. The logic here would be to see if the antagonistic activity of these compounds, determined preferably in the same time-independent biological assay (again, perhaps, *via* a contract mechanism) could be correlated with some physical parameter of these compounds, including partition coefficients.

Further afield, perhaps, would be a molecular orbital study of these compounds using the well-known CNDO or, in some few instances, *ab initio* calculations. Such studies might also provide useful information for further work in synthesis.

We would be happy to join in such a theoretical effort to gain insight into the narcotic antagonists, and I am sure that others (notably Dr. Joyce Kaufman's group at Johns Hopkins) would be similarly interested. The Hansch type of analyses, could be undertaken by several groups, especially, of course, by Hansch's own team at Pomona College, or by Paul Craig of Craig Associates.

Narcotic Antagonists, edited by M. C. Braude, L. S. Harris, E. L. May, J. P. Smith, and J. E. Villarreal. Advances in Biochemical Psychopharmacology, Vol. 8. Raven Press, New York © 1974.

Predictive Value of Analgesic Assays in Mice and Rats

Robert I. Taber

Department of Pharmacology, Biological Research, Schering Corporation, Bloomfield, New Jersey 07003

The ultimate value of analgesic tests in animals is based on how well the results can be used to predict clinical therapeutic activity. To determine which assays permit the highest degree of predictive value, a comparison of the most common tests has been made using a rating scale for criteria of simplicity, reproducibility, and drug sensitivity. To be drug sensitive, a procedure should detect all the different classes of analgesics at doses and relative potencies comparable to those established in man. The three highest ratings were achieved by the mouse writhing, rat tail-flick, and rat paw yeast tests. Under well-defined conditions, all these tests have been shown to provide measures of analgesic activity for narcotic, non-narcotic anti-inflammatory, and narcotic antagonist analgesics. Experience with analgesic narcotic antagonists provides the most instructive example of the importance of data analysis and parametric studies to optimize sensitivity of predictive value. For example, pentazocine can be shown to be either ineffective, weakly effective, or equal in activity to morphine using three different statistical analyses of rat tail-flick data. A strategy of adjusting experimental parameters toward the objective of detecting activity at clinical dose levels is recommended as a means of enhancing the generality and predictive value of analgesic test procedures.

INTRODUCTION

The ultimate value of analgesic assays in animals is based on how well the results can be used to predict clinical therapeutic activity. Not only is this necessary for drug development but also for mechanism studies if the results are to have some relevance to understanding analgesia in man.

The development of the analgesic narcotic antagonists provides an object lesson in the importance of selecting and creating appropriate methods. The finding that nalorphine was nearly equivalent in clinical analgesic potency to morphine (48) was at first greeted with surprise because nalorphine was inactive in the animal analgesic assays, such as the hot-plate and tail-flick tests, commonly used at that time. In fact, nearly a decade later, *inactivity* in the mouse hot-plate test was a criterion employed in a strategy that led to the development of pentazocine, because activity in this test was thought to be more nearly related to addiction liability than to analgesic utility (1,2).

When our laboratory first became involved in testing analgesics, we were concerned about the reported inability of many of the standard methods to detect the activity of nalorphine and pentazocine. Although we were not interested in narcotic antagonists *per se,* we felt that the predictive value of animal analgesic tests would hinge on their ability to detect all agents with established clinical utility. We began to screen methods, rather than drugs, in the hope of finding one sensitive to the analgesic actions of the narcotic antagonists. The phenylquinone writhing test was tried first because it was known to be sensitive to both narcotic and non-narcotic drugs (37, 63). Nalorphine, pentazocine, and cyclazocine were all active at low doses and with the same order of potency as determined in man (64). Other groups came to the same conclusion at approximately the same time (7, 57).

Since then, a variety of tests have either been created or reexamined to demonstrate the analgesic action of narcotic antagonists. The experience with these drugs has helped spur the development of more predictive and relevant assays.

Methods for assessing analgesia have already been extensively reviewed (4, 13, 23, 26, 40, 44, 46, 53, 71, 74, 76). In this chapter I will try to identify those methods of proven value in detecting different classes of analgesics and to compare them according to criteria of simplicity, reproducibility, and drug sensitivity.

COMPARATIVE CRITERIA

For purposes of comparing the various methods, each of several criteria will be assigned point values. Obviously, the weighting of these various factors is arbitrary and different investigators might wish to place more emphasis on some characteristics than others. However, a rating scale can serve as a useful basis for discussing the degree to which the various procedures fulfill them.

1. Drug Sensitivity

Drug sensitivity is meant to be an all-inclusive term encompassing many of the quantitative characteristics desired in a potential test procedure. An ideal analgesic method would permit accurate determination of the nociceptive threshold and be sufficiently sensitive to discriminate between different intensities of stimulation, drugs of differing analgesic potencies, and low grades of analgesic activity. All these requirements are closely related and can be incorporated into the single term drug sensitivity, because no drug effects could be detected unless the method reflects small changes in the threshold and response to a painful stimulus. To be drug sensitive, *a procedure should detect all the different classes of analgesics in doses and relative potencies comparable to those established in man.* Ideally, it should be insensitive to drugs not analgesic in man. In addition, the establishment of a clear-cut relationship between stimulus intensity and response is highly desirable.

2. Simplicity

A procedure should be simple and economical; it should not require extensive technical expertise or sophisticated instrumentation. Biological variability is enough of a problem without compounding it by adding other variables. To require expensive equipment or a high level of technical sophistication would severely restrict the number of laboratories that might find these procedures feasible. Complicated methodology would not be useful in either the screening or the assays of structure activity relationships necessary for drug development.

TABLE 1. *Classification and dosage of clinical analgesics*

Drug class	Prototypes	Effective human dose (mg/kg)[a]	Route
Narcotic analgesics			
Strong narcotics	Morphine	0.2	s.c.
	Methadone	0.12	s.c.
Weak narcotics	Codeine	2.0	p.o., s.c.
	Meperidine	1.5	p.o., s.c.
Narcotic antagonist analgesics	Pentazocine	0.8	s.c.
	Nalorphine	0.2	s.c.
	Cyclazocine	0.06	s.c.
Anti-inflammatory analgesics	Aspirin	12.0	p.o.
	Aminopyrine	6.0	p.o.
	Paracetamol	12.0	p.o.
Neuroleptic analgesics	Methotrimeprazine	0.4	s.c.

[a] Dose based on 50-kg human body weight.

3. Reproducibility

A test procedure is not useful unless it can be replicated in more than one laboratory. The number of laboratories successfully using a technique is a good measure of its viability.

Classification and approximate clinical doses of established analgesics are listed in Table 1. A summary of the criteria discussed above and the point values assigned to them are listed in Table 2. In the next section, a number of widely used analgesic procedures will be discussed and compared with regard to how well they meet these criteria.

TABLE 2. *Analgesic method criteria rating scale*

Criteria	Score		
Sensitivity			
a. Is it sensitive to known analgesics?	1 for each class		4 (max. score)
b. How sensitive is it to doses in the clinical range?	Median of drug sensitivity		4 (max. score)
	No	*Questionable*	*Yes*
c. Is it insensitive to nonanalgesics?	0	1	2
d. Is there an established, clear-cut relationship between intensity and end point?	0	1	2
Simplicity	*Yes*	*Questionable*	*No*
a. Does it require technical expertise?	0	1	2
b. Does it require sophisticated instrumentation?	0	1	2
Reproducibility			
How many laboratories have successfully used the technique		0–4	4

ASSESSMENT OF EXISTING METHODS

1. Thermal Methods

Determination of drug-induced changes in reaction time of animals exposed to heat has served as the most widely employed measure of analgesic activity. All these methods owe their existence to the pioneering studies of Hardy, Wolff, and Goodell, who quantified the painful properties of radiant heat in man. Despite their widespread use, few drugs other than narcotic analgesics have been developed using them.

Of the thermal methods, the mouse hot-plate test (77) and the rat tail-flick test (16) have found the greatest use. These tests are easy to perform, require little instrumentation, and have a well-defined end point. In one case, the response is paw-licking, withdrawal, or escape attempts of mice when placed on a heated plate maintained at 55°C, and, in the other, the tail withdrawal of rats in response to radiant heat exposure. Repeated tests can be performed affording the advantages of using the animal as its own control and establishing time-response relationships in the same subjects. Generally, animals are tested at regular intervals before and after drug administration with a cut-off time ranging from 10 to 30 sec to prevent tissue damage. Results are analyzed by applying an all-or-none criterion or by using a graded response, such as measuring the area under the time-response curve.

Despite extensive modifications by various investigators, these tests have generally been shown to be robust and reproducible in determining relative potencies of narcotic analgesics at doses approximately 10 times higher than those used in man (43).

The mouse hot-plate test is only useful for narcotic analgesics. Aspirin-like drugs prolong hot-plate reaction times in mice only at near-toxic doses. One possible exception is aminopyrine, which is active in oral doses of approximately 100 to 200 mg/kg.

Nalorphine-like drugs also are ineffective in the mouse hot-plate test (19, 32, 48). When other classes of analgesics have demonstrated activity, the doses have been high and have borne little relationship to clinical relative potency.

In contrast, the rat tail-flick test has been shown to be capable of detecting both aspirin- and nalorphine-like drugs, although these findings are not consistent across all investigators. Relatively few have been able to detect aspirin in this test and the doses required were as high as 200 mg/kg, i.p. (8) and 350 mg/kg, p.o. (35). Winter et al. (73) found nalorphine to be approximately 1/10th as potent as morphine, whereas Harris and Pierson (32) could show no activity for nalorphine or pentazocine and found cyclazocine to be effective only at neurotoxic doses. In contrast, Hart and McCawley (34) found 1.5 mg/kg, s.c., of nalorphine to be equal in activity to 3.8 mg/kg, s.c., of morphine. Malis (49) has determined i.p. ED_{50} values of nalorphine and pentazocine to be 25 and 10 mg/kg, respectively; cyclazocine was inactive in his hands at an i.p. dose of 25 mg/kg. Hoffmeister (41), however, has found all three antagonist analgesics to be active with relative potencies comparable to clinical estimates. Carruyo et al. (11) have demonstrated unequivocal activity for pentazocine in s.c. doses ranging from 5.0 to 20.0 mg/kg. More recently, Gray et al. (27) found that the activity of pentazocine and, to a lesser degree, nalorphine could be demonstrated as a function of heat intensity.

The tail-flick test in mice has been used less frequently. As in the rat, aspirin-like drugs are only active at near-toxic dose levels. Nalorphine-like drugs show a transient effect only at high dose levels (33).

Of the other thermal methods, only one has been claimed to be capable of identifying and projecting the analgesic activity of all the major classes of analgesics. Grotto and Sulman (30), using the tail-withdrawal response of mice to hot water (58°C), have found aspirin, paracetamol, aminopyrine, codeine, *d*-propoxyphene, and pentazocine to have relative potencies comparable to those determined in man. These results have not yet been tested by others; however, a similar procedure employing rats has already been reported to be insensitive to both nalorphine and aspirin (45).

2. Mechanical Methods

Pressure-induced pain was used for analgesic testing before the advent of the thermal methods. In its simplest form (5, 31), pressure is applied to a rodent's tail with a forceps or artery clamp and the end point is the animal's biting, squeaking, or attempts to escape. This method has the twin drawbacks of lack of precision in measuring the amount of applied pressure and inability to use repeated stimuli because the tails become hypersensitive after relatively few tests. A means of calibrating the pressure generated by an artery clip has been suggested by Collier (13), and several newer methods have sought to gain more precision and repeatability by using a controlled gradual increase in pressure.

The simple mouse tail-pinch procedures do not detect either antagonist or anti-inflammatory analgesics alone (13); however, it has been claimed that nalorphine potentiates the activity of aminopyrine and antipyrine (42). Similarly, the pain evoked by applying a gradually increasing pressure to a rat's tail (17, 28) is also insensitive to nalorphine (29) and to most of the aspirin-type agents with the exception of aminopyrine and mefamic acid (72). Sensitivity to morphine-like drugs, on the other hand, is comparable to the thermal pain methods (28).

Enhanced sensitivity can be achieved by measuring the pressure-pain threshold of inflamed tissue. Hyperesthesia can be induced by inflaming a rat's paw with a subplantar injection of a yeast suspension (62). Comparing drug-induced alterations in the thresholds of the inflamed and normal paws was originally thought to provide a means of discriminating narcotic from anti-inflammatory analgesics. Narcotics would be expected to raise the threshold of both paws; anti-inflammatory analgesics would only affect the inflamed paw. The narcotic antagonists, however, have no anti-inflammatory activity, yet they too raise only inflamed paw thresholds (69, 74). Moreover, even aspirin-type drugs can produce analgesia in these tests under conditions in which their anti-inflammatory activity cannot be detected (24). If a nonsteroidal anti-inflammatory agent is given simultaneously, or following the phlogistic challenge, substantial increases in the inflamed paw pain thresholds are apparent in the absence of any diminution in edema.

The rat paw yeast test of Randall and Selitto (62) has been found to be useful in a number of laboratories. Usually, the drug is administered 1 hr after the yeast challenge and the pain thresholds determined at various intervals after treatment. A peg, either flattened or bullet-shaped, is used to apply pressure to the paw until the animal struggles or vocalizes. Several laboratories have described modifications in the instrumentation, end point, and position of the animal during threshold determinations (24, 74). Repeated determinations can be made at 1-hr intervals with little alteration in sensitivity; however, some have found it advisable to use only one determination per animal for greater precision (74).

3. Chemical Methods

Since the initial observation that an i.p. injection of a radio-opaque dye could elicit a syndrome characterized by squirming, stretching, cramping, or writhing which could be blocked by various analgesics (68), a wide variety of chemicals causing similar effects have been proposed as potential challenges for analgesic tests in mice and rats. Perhaps most widely used have been phenylquinone (63) and acetic acid (47). Other writhing agonists shown to be sensitive to analgesics in mice are bradykinin (14, 20), tryptamine, ATP, KCl, acetylcholine (14), epinephrine (51), oxytocin (54), and HCl (18). The various agents differ mainly in their time-response curves. For example, acetylcholine causes a low frequency of writhing with an onset of 30 sec and a duration of 2 to 5 min; acetic acid and phenylquinone evoke a high writhing frequency for 20 to 30 min with a 5-min delay, whereas bradykinin causes a low frequency of writhing after a delay of 20 min and lasts for approximately 1 hr. It should be noted that there exist considerable strain differences in mice in response to writhing agents. Some strains are insensitive and others extremely variable in their response (9).

Usually, potential analgesics are administered before the writhing agent, and either the number of animals writhing or the frequency of individual writhing episodes during the peak writhing time is used as a measure of activity. A writhe is commonly considered to represent a combination or a sequence of arching of the back, pelvic rotation, and hind-limb extension. Drug sensitivity can be enhanced if the data are analyzed on the basis of writhing frequency (37). When complete abolition of writhing is required as an all-or-none criterion, the potencies of drugs with relatively flat dose-response curves would either be grossly underestimated or go undetected. A combination of graded and quantal approaches wherein an animal is considered to show significant analgesia when its writhing frequency is 50% or less than the mean of that day's control group (7) may be useful because it can detect drugs such as nalorphine and aspirin and reduce the effect of day-to-day variations in control groups which can prove to be considerable with these procedures.

These tests are simple to perform and require no instrumentation. Their major drawback is that many drugs with no proven clinical analgesic activity may be detected as "false positives" (12, 37). Adrenergic blocking agents, antihistamines, cholinomimetics, muscle relaxants, psychomotor stimulants, serotonin antagonists, monoamine oxidase inhibitors, and neuroleptics have all been shown to be potent writhing inhibitors. This is not altogether surprising because autonomic changes can substantially alter pain responsiveness in man (4). Many of these false positives can be eliminated by a more careful scrutiny of the overt autonomic or neurological effects of these drugs at their antiwrithing doses. When rotarod-impairment of a group of non-analgesic writhing inhibitors was determined, it was found that all the drugs produced performance decrements at doses equal to, or less than, those blocking writhing. Only the analgesics were found to be selective writhing inhibitors (59, 60).

Writhing can be prevented by low dose levels of all the major classes of analgesics. Typical s.c. ED_{50} values versus phenylquinone obtained are morphine 0.5 mg/kg, nalorphine 1.0 mg/kg, and pentazocine 2.0 mg/kg (64). Three other laboratories have substantially replicated these results even though they used different data analyses and writhing-provoking agents (58). Oral doses ranging from 20 to 60 mg/kg of aspirin produce comparable effects depending on the writhing test used (14).

Rats have not been widely used for chemically induced nociception. Injection of bradykinin through an indwelling i.v. cannula produces an affective response which can be blocked by narcotic, narcotic antagonist, and anti-inflammatory analgesics (6). Recently, the abdominal constriction response to an i.p. injection of a hypertonic (4.0%) NaCl solution was used as part of a battery of tests to characterize useful narcotic antagonist analgesics (15). Pentazocine and cyclazocine were both effective. Nalorphine, levallorphan, and naloxone were not. However, cyclazocine, which is not a useful clinical analgesic because of side effects, would have been eliminated from consideration because it had reached a ceiling effect on abdominal constriction (no ED_{90} could be determined) and because it caused bizarre excitation at analgesic doses.

4. Electrical Methods

Although electric shock has been widely employed as a nociceptive stimulus in conditioning experiments in animals, it has found little use in analgesic screening tests in mice and rats until recently. This probably reflects the difficulty in maintaining adequate control of the electric shock. Even when voltage and amperage can be controlled, the impedance of biological tissues can be extremely variable. Other factors such as wave form and scrambling rates differ widely from laboratory to laboratory. Some of these difficulties in attaining consistent results with electric shock have been reviewed by Beecher (4) and Hill (38). With all these potential variables, the inconsistencies, difficulties, and insensitivities encountered by most investigators who have sought to measure analgesic effects in untrained animals shocked through their paws, tails, rectums, or scrotal sacs are not surprising (76).

Several procedures may be of potential importance. Two employ stepwise increments in electric shock to determine pain thresholds. In one, the successive intensities at which a rat first flinches and then jumps after its paws are shocked on a grid, serve as a measure of pain. No drugs affected the "flinch" threshold, but morphine, nalorphine, pentazocine, and aspirin all raise the "jump" threshold (21–23). The results with morphine, but not with the antagonist analgesics, have been confirmed by others (58). In the other procedure, successive thresholds for eliciting a motor escape response, vocalization, and vocalization that persists after termination of the stimulus are determined by shocking a rat's tail (10). The vocalization "after-discharge" threshold has been claimed to be most sensitive for detecting the activity of all but the aspirin class of analgesics (40). This method may offer some advantages in that the shock can be more reliably controlled by using electrodes on the tail and that the various thresholds have some theoretical value in describing the actions of these drugs at different levels of organization in the central nervous system. The usefulness of both techniques, however, must await further confirmation in other laboratories.

Recently, procedures using tail-shock-evoked vocalization in mice have been used with increasing frequency. By using the animals as their own controls to reduce individual variation and by implanting the electrodes subcutaneously to minimize impedance, more reproducible results have been obtained (36, 55, 56, 61). Even with these improvements, however, drug sensitivity is more nearly comparable to that observed with the thermal methods in mice. Narcotic analgesics are active in the tail-shock test at virtually the same doses as in the hot-plate tests. Aspirin-like drugs are only effective at near-toxic dose levels. The experience with narcotic antagonist analgesics has been mixed. Paalzow (56) found that i.v. administration of an emulsion of pentazocine was necessary to determine an ED_{50} value. Subcutaneous or oral administration gave a ceiling response of 40% at high doses. Similar ceiling effects have been observed with nalorphine, cyclazocine, and pentazocine by others (70). The same authors questioned the value of this test not only because drug effectiveness did not parallel clinical analgesic efficacy but also because transection studies seemed to indicate that tail-shock-induced vocalization was integrated at low brain-stem levels and that its inhibition by drugs did not necessarily require participation of higher neural levels.

In contrast, Perrine and his co-workers (61), in the NIH laboratory used as part of the NAS/NRC testing program, have reported the same three antagonist analgesics to be active with relative potencies similar to clinical estimates. These findings have been confirmed by unpublished observations in several pharmaceutical laboratories (52). An understanding of the reasons underlying these differences in results between laboratories might help to clarify the optimal conditions for this test and establish its validity as an analgesic testing procedure in mice.

5. Comparison of Methods by Rating Scales

The scoring of most of the major techniques according to the methods rating scales are listed in Table 3 and are meant to provide a summary of the foregoing discussion. Table 4 provides an example of the dose-sensitivity comparisons of several methods. Table 5 lists representative effective doses for standards in various analgesic assays. The three highest ratings went to the mouse writhing, rat tail-flick, and rat paw yeast tests (Table 3). The electrical tests, while promising, failed because they lack simplicity and reproducibility. The other tests scored low in terms of sensitivity. The area of drug sensitivity is where the greatest improvements can and should be made. The next section will review some factors to be considered when attempting to optimize drug sensitivity.

TABLE 3. *Comparison of analgesic tests by rating scale*

	Thermal			Mechanical	Chemical	Electric	
Criteria[a]	Mouse hot-plate	Rat tail-flick	Mouse tail-flick	Rat paw yeast	Mouse writhing	Rat flick-jump	Mouse tail-shock
Sensitivity							
a	2	4	2	4	4	4	3
b	2	2	1	3	4	3	3
c	2	1	2	1	0	2	1
d	1	2	0	2	2	2	2
Simplicity							
a	2	2	2	2	2	0	1
b	2	2	2	1	2	0	1
Reproducibility	4	4	4	4	4	1	2
Total Score	15	17	13	17	18	12	13

[a] See Table 2.

201

TABLE 4. *Analgesic activity versus different nociceptive stimuli*

	Thermal (rat tail-flick)	Mechanical (rat paw yeast)	Chemical (mouse phenylquinone writhing)	Electrical (mouse tail-shock)
Narcotics				
Morphine	3	3	4	4
Codeine	3	3	4	4
Narcotic antagonists				
Pentazocine	0–3	4	4	3
Nalorphine	0–3	4	4	3
Anti-inflammatory				
Aspirin	0–2	2	3	2
Aminopyrine	0–2	3	3	2
Neuroleptics				
Methotrimeprazine	3	–	4	–
Median Scores	2	3	4	3
Range	0–3	2–4	3–4	2–3

Legend: 1 = active at >125 × human dose
2 = active at 26 to 125 × human dose
3 = active at 6 to 25 × human dose
4 = active at 1 to 5 × human dose

202

TABLE 5. *Representative effective doses in various analgesic assays in rodents*

Test	Species	Dose (route)				
		Morphine	Codeine	Pentazocine	Nalorphine	Aspirin
Chemical						
Phenylquinone-writhing	Mouse	0.45 (s.c.)[14]	—	2.0 (s.c.)[64]	0.92 (s.c.)[64]	68.0 (p.o.)[37]
Aectic acid-writhing	Mouse	0.40 (s.c.)[65]	—	4.0 (s.c.)[66]	1.0 (s.c.)[65]	56.0 (p.o.)[66]
Acetylcholine-abdom. constriction	Mouse	0.52 (s.c.)[14]	3.9 (s.c.)[14]	2.7 (s.c.)[14]	1.9 (s.c.)[14]	54.6 (p.o.)[14]
Bradykinin-affective response	Rat	1.1 (s.c.)[6]	38.5 (s.c.)[6]	1.9 (s.c.)[6]	2.1 (s.c.)[6]	125 (i.p.)[6]
Hypertonic saline-abdom. constriction	Rat	0.9 (s.c.)[15]	—	5.5 (s.c.)[15]	not obtainable	—
Thermal						
Hot-plate	Mouse	1.2 (s.c.)[61]	7.5 (s.c.)[61]	12.3 (s.c.)[61]	36.3 (s.c.)[61]	—
Tail-flick	Rat	1.7 (I.M.)	—	7.2 (I.M.)[25]	6.2 (I.M.)[25]	—
Electrical						
Tail-shock	Mouse	0.8 (s.c.)[61]	4.5 (s.c.)[61]	4.7 (s.c.)[61]	4.8 (s.c.)[61]	—
Mechanical						
Paw yeast	Rat	1.0 (s.c.)[66]	5.0 (s.c.)[66]	4.0 (s.c.)[66]	2.0 (s.c.)[66]	225 (p.o.)[66]

Superscript numbers represent references.

203

SOME FACTORS AFFECTING DRUG SENSITIVITY

1. Data Analysis

One of the prime factors accounting for the dissimilarities in drug sensitivities of these procedures can be found in the varying forms of analyses applied to the data. In many cases, the experimental designs, end point, animals, and drugs are similar; however, analysis of the data differs widely, there being almost as many ways of interpreting results as there are investigators who use the method. In no way are the varying philosophies and styles of investigators better reflected than in the manner they decide what shall represent significance in their results and the importance of these dissimilarities cannot be overemphasized, because it determines not only quantitative but qualitative aspects of their work.

The widely divergent results obtained with the aspirin- or nalorphine-like drugs in the rat tail-flick test can serve as an instructive example. Those workers who fail to detect these drugs generally employ either stringent all-or-none criteria based on a doubling or tripling of reaction time or measure the area under the time-response curve. The effect of a short-acting drug that prolongs reaction time by only a few seconds would be either grossly underestimated or go undetected. Those employing less stringent, but nonetheless statistically valid criteria, have found both nalorphine and aspirin to be active. When the data of Hart and McCawley (34), Bonnycastle and Leonard (8), and Malis (49) are compared, their criteria for analgesia, although arrived at through different means, are found to be strikingly similar. All of them used a prolongation in reaction time of approximately 2.0 sec as an index of analgesia. One found nalorphine to be virtually equipotent to morphine (34), another found aspirin active and morphine to have an ED_{50} of 0.56 mg/kg, approximately one-fourth of the usual ED_{50} in this test (8), and the last found activity with both nalorphine and pentazocine (49).

Employing the same criteria, we have also found nalorphine, pentazocine, and cyclazocine to be active in this test in our laboratory. As an illustrative example of how these differences in data analyses can alter the magnitude of the drug response, we compared the activity of morphine and pentazocine in the rat tail-flick test. The time-response data show a small, but statistically significant, prolongation of reaction time with pentazocine (Fig. 1). In contrast, morphine shows a marked effect. If the area under the time-response curve were integrated, then pentazocine would be considered to be much less active than morphine. A comparison of three other

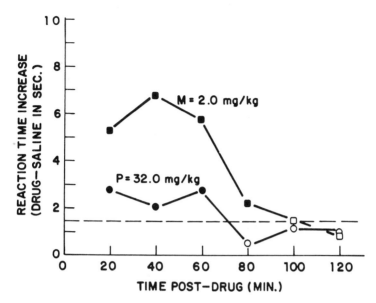

FIG. 1. Time response of morphine (M) and pentazocine (P) on rat tail-flick test. Each point represents the mean change in reaction time for groups of 10 rats at the indicated times after s.c. administration of drugs. Solid circles and squares denote significant differences from control. The dashed line represents the least significant difference from control as determined by analyses of variance.

analyses, all statistically valid, shows that pentazocine would be ineffective if the criterion was a doubling of reaction time, weakly effective if percentage of control response was used, and virtually equally effective to morphine when the number of animals showing a significant increase (2.0 sec) is the measure (Fig. 2).

Not all the discrepancies in the results with these drugs can be ascribed to data analysis, however, because some have failed to show activity using similar criteria (45) whereas others have observed strikingly large increments in reaction time with these same drugs (11, 41).

2. Pain Intensity

Too few attempts have been made to study drug sensitivity as a function of pain intensity. Generally, a relationship between pain intensity and end point is studied as the first phase in development of an analgesic method, but the purpose of these studies is usually to define an intensity at which variability is minimized. As a result, the possibility of enhancing drug

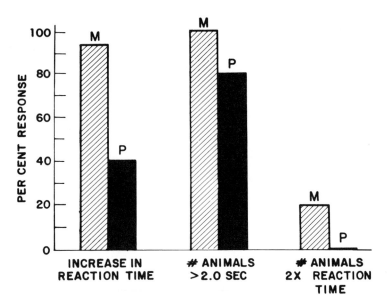

FIG. 2. Peak responses as a function of analgesic criteria. The peak responses shown in Fig. 1 were recalculated in three ways to show how differing data analyses yield different conclusions.

sensitivity by altering pain intensity is largely ignored. Martin (50), in his excellent review of the pharmacology of opioid antagonists, found that the analgesic activity of these drugs could only be demonstrated in procedures sensitive to 1.0 mg/kg or less of morphine. Perhaps a stratagem of determining optimal conditions under which low doses of analgesics can be reliably detected might improve not only the sensitivity but the generality of these methods.

The value of adjusting sensitivity by varying the intensity of the nociceptive stimulus is evident in the work of Gray and his co-workers (27). They demonstrated the activity of pentazocine to be most marked at low and intermediate levels of heat intensity in the rat tail-flick test. Higher intensity levels abolished the effect. Both the hot-plate (77) and tail-pinch (67) tests have also shown an inverse relationship between pain intensity and morphine sensitivity. It would be of interest to determine whether nalorphine and aspirin-like drugs would be active in these tests at lower grades of pain intensity. One potential problem is that variability will be greater at the lower intensities. An illustration of this relationship is seen in Fig. 3 where the tail-flick reaction times in the same mice were determined at five levels of heat intensity. The lowest levels had the highest degree of variability.

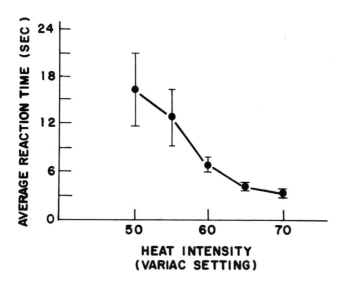

FIG. 3. Heat intensity versus tail-flick reaction time in mice. Each point represents the mean and standard error (*vertical line*) of reaction times of groups of 10 mice. Each animal was tested at each intensity level in a random sequence. Heat intensity was varied by changing the resistance to the heat lamp.

3. Route of Administration

Aside from the pharmacological implications, route of administration can be a complicating factor in analgesic studies. Intraperitoneal administration of irritants can produce analgesia (39, 75). Furthermore, the intraperitoneal route cannot be used in writhing studies because it may chemically antagonize the agent that provokes writhing or act as a local anesthetic. Striking species differences in intestinal absorption can diminish the relevance of studies employing the oral route. Recently, as an exercise, we compared the i.p. to p.o. LD_{50} values of a wide variety of drugs listed for mice and rats (3). In virtually every case, the p.o. to i.p. ratios for rats was more than double those found in mice, even though the actual i.p. doses were closely similar.

4. Strain, Sex, and Age Differences

These variables would be expected to account for large differences in drug sensitivity, yet few comparative studies of these factors are available. In those that are, striking differences in pain (55) and drug sensitivity (55, 67) have been observed as a function of strain, sex, and age. Another potentially useful strategy would test both sexes of a variety of inbred strains of rodents now available to determine those most sensitive to drug effects.

SUMMARY

Many testing procedures for analgesia have been compared as to how well they meet the criteria of drug sensitivity, simplicity, and reproducibility. The mouse-writhing, rat tail-flick, and rat paw yeast tests scored highest on the criteria rating scale. Several, but by no means all, of the factors affecting drug sensitivity are discussed. The relevance of these criteria and variables remains to be established by more intensive parametric studies.

REFERENCES

1. Archer, S., Harris, L. S., Albertson, N. F., Tullar, B. F., and Pierson, A. K.: Narcotic antagonists as analgesics—Laboratory aspects. Advances in Chemistry Series, 45:162–169, 1964.
2. Archer, S.: Biological activity: A medicinal chemist's view. In: Annual Reports in Medicinal Chemistry, 1967, edited by C. K. Cain, pp. vii–xxi. Academic Press, New York, 1968.
3. Barnes, C. D., and Eltherington, L. G.: Drug dosage in laboratory animals. University of California Press, Berkeley, 1965.
4. Beecher, H. K.: Measurement of pain. Pharmacol. Rev. 9:59–210, 1957.
5. Bianchi, C., and Francheschini, J.: Experimental observations on Haffner's method for testing analgesic drugs. Br. J. Pharmacol. Chemother. 9:280–284, 1954.
6. Blane, G. F.: Blockade of bradykinin-induced nociception in the rat as a test for analgesic drugs with particular reference to morphine antagonists. J. Pharm. Pharmacol. 19:367–373, 1967.
7. Blumberg, H., Wolf, P. S., and Dayton, H. B.: Use of writing test for evaluating analgesic activity of narcotic antagonists. Proc. Soc. Exp. Biol. Med. 118:763–766, 1965.
8. Bonnycastle, D. D., and Leonard, C. S.: An estimation of the activity of analgesic materials. J. Pharmacol. Exp. Ther. 100:141–145, 1950.
9. Brown, D. M., and Hughes, B. O.: Practical aspects of strain variation in relation to pharmacological testing. J. Pharm. Pharmacol. 14:399–405, 1962.
10. Carroll, M. N., Jr., and Lim, R. K. S.: Observations on the neuropharmacology of morphine and morphine-like analgesia. Arch. Int. Pharmacodyn. Ther. 125:383–403, 1960.
11. Carruyo, L., Florio, V., Longo, V. G., and Scotti de Carolis, A.: Effect of narcotics and narcotic-antagonists on the electrical activity of the brain: Its relationship with their pain-obtunding activity. In: Pain, edited by A. Soulairac et al., pp. 425–439. Academic Press, New York, 1968.
12. Chernov, H. I., Wilson, D. E., Fowler, F. and Plummer, A. J.: Non-specificity of the mouse writhing test. Arch. Int. Pharmacodyn. Ther. 167:171–178, 1967.
13. Collier, H. O. J.: Analgesics. In: Evaluation of drug activities: Pharmacometrics, Vol. 1, edited by D. R. Laurence and A. L. Bacharach, Chap. 8. Academic Press, New York, 1964.
14. Collier, H. O. J., Dinneen, L. C., Johnson, C. A., and Schneider, C.: The abdominal constriction response and its suppression by analgesic drugs in the mouse. Brit. J. Pharmacol. Chemother. 32:295–310, 1968.

15. Collier, H. O. J., and Schneider, C.: Profiles of activity in rodents of some narcotic and narcotic antagonist drugs. Nature *224*:610–612, 1969.
16. D'Amour, F. E., and Smith, D. L.: A method for determining loss of pain sensation. J. Pharmacol. Exp. Ther. *72*:74–79, 1941.
17. Eagle, E., and Carlson, A. J.: Toxicity, antipyretic and analgesic studies on 39 compounds, including aspirin, phenacetin and 27 derivatives of carbazole and tetrahydrocarbazole. J. Pharmacol. Exp. Ther. *99*:450–457, 1950.
18. Eckhardt, E. T., Cheplovitz, F., Lipo, M., and Govier, W. M.: Etiology of chemically induced writhing in mouse and rat. Proc. Soc. Exp. Biol. Med. *98*:186–188, 1958.
19. Eddy, N. B., and Leimbach, D.: Synthetic analgesics, Part II. Dithienylbutenyl- and dithienylbutylamines. J. Pharmacol. Exp. Ther. *107*:385–393, 1953.
20. Emele, J. F., and Shanaman, J.: Bradykinin writing: A method for measuring analgesia. Proc. Soc. Exp. Biol. Med. *114*:680–682, 1963.
21. Evans, W. O.: A new technique for the investigation of some analgesic drugs on a reflexive behavior in the rat. Psychopharmacologia *2*:318–325, 1961.
22. Evans, W. O.: A comparison of the analgesic potency of some analgesics as measured by the "flinch jump" procedure. Psychopharmacologia *3*:51–54, 1962.
23. Evans, W. O.: A critical review of some new methods in animal analgesiometry. J. New Drugs *4*:179–187, 1964.
24. Gilfoil, T. M., Klavins, I., and Grumbach, L.: Effects of acetylsalicylic acid on the edema and hyperesthesia of the experimentally inflamed rat's paw. J. Pharmacol. Exp. Ther. *142*:1–5, 1963.
25. Malis, J. L., and Gluckman, M. I.: Assaying narcotic antagonist drugs for analgesic activity in rhesus monkeys. *This Volume.*
26. Goetzl, F. R., Burrill, D. Y., and Ivy, A. C.: A critical analysis of algesimetric methods with suggestions for a useful procedure. Northwestern Med. School Quart. Bull. *17*:280–291, 1943.
27. Gray, W., Osterberg, A., and Scuto, T.: Measurement of the analgesic efficacy and potency of pentazocine by the D'Amour and Smith method. J. Pharmacol. Exp. Ther. *172*:154–162, 1970.
28. Green, A. F., Young, P. A., and Godfrey, E. I.: A comparison of heat and pressure analgesiometric methods in rats. Brit. J. Pharmacol. Chemother. *6*:572–585, 1951.
29. Green, A. F., Ruffell, G. K., and Walton, E. K.: Morphine derivatives with anti-analgesic actions. J. Pharm. Pharmacol. *6*:390–397, 1954.
30. Grotto, M., and Sulman, F. G.: Modified receptacle method for animal analgesimetry. Arch. Int. Pharmacodyn. Ther. *165*:152–159, 1967.
31. Haffner, F.: Experimentelle Prüfung schmerzstillender Mittel. Dtsch. Med. Wochenschr. *55*:731–733, 1929.
32. Harris, L. S., and Pierson, A. K.: Some narcotic antagonists in the benzomorphan series. J. Pharmacol. Exp. Ther. *143*:141–148, 1964.
33. Harris, L. S., Dewey, W. L., McMillan, D. E., and Nuite, J. A.: Personal communication as reported to 33rd Meeting, Committee on Problems of Drug Dependence, 1971.
34. Hart, E. R., and McCawley, E. L.: The pharmacology of n-allylnormorphine compared with morphine. J. Pharmacol. Exp. Ther. *82*:339–348, 1944.
35. Hart, E. R.: The toxicity and analgesic potency of salicylamide and certain of its derivatives as compared with established analgetic anti-pyretic drugs. J. Pharmacol. Exp. Ther. *89*:205–209, 1947.
36. Helsley, G., Richman, J., Lunsford, C., Jenkins, H., Mays, R., Funderburk, W., and Johnson, D.: Analgetics esters of 3-pyrrolidinemethanols. J. Med. Chem. *11*:472–475, 1968.
37. Hendershot, L. C., and Forsaith, J.: Antagonism of the frequency of phenylquinone-induced writhing in the mouse by weak analgesics and non-analgesics. J. Pharmacol. Exp. Ther. *125*:237–240, 1959.
38. Hill, H. E., Flanary, H. G., Kornetsky, C. H., and Wikler, A.: Relationship of electrically induced pain to the amperage and the wattage of shock stimuli. J. Clin. Invest. *31*:464–472, 1952.

39. Hitchens, J. T., Goldstein, S., Shemano, I., and Beiler, J. M.: Analgesic effects of irritants in three models of experimentally-induced pain. Arch. Int. Pharmacodyn. Ther. *169*:384–393, 1967.
40. Hoffmeister, F.: Tierexperimentelle Unterschunger über den Schmerz und seine pharmakologische Beeinflussung, edited by K. G. Cantor. Aulendorf i. Württ, 1968.
41. Hoffmeister, F.: Personal communication, 1968.
42. Imukai, T., and Takaji, H.: Potentiation by nalorphine of the analgesic effect of aminopyrine and antipyrine. Jap. J. Pharmacol. *16*:481–482, 1966.
43. Janssen, P. A. J., and Jageneau, A. H.: Dextro 2:2-diphenyl-3-methyl-4-morpholino-butyrylpyrrolidine and related amines, Part I. Chemical structure and pharmacological activity. J. Pharm. Pharmacol. *9*:381–400, 1957.
44. Janssen, P. A. J.: Synthetic analgesics – Part I. Diphenylpropylamine. *In:* International Series of Monographs on Organic Chemistry, edited by D. H. R. Barton and W. Doerig pp. 7–12. Pergamon Press, New York, 1960.
45. Janssen, P. A. J., Niemegeers, C. J. E., and Dony, J. G. H.: The inhibitory effect of fentanyl and other morphine-like analgesics on the warm-water induced tail withdrawal reflex in rats. Arzneim. Forsch. *13*:502–507, 1963.
46. Keath, E. F.: Evaluation of analgesic substances. Amer. J. Pharm. *132*:202–230, 1960.
47. Koster, R., Anderson, M., and DeBeer, E. J.: Acetic acid for analgesic screening. Fed. Proc. *18*:412, 1959.
48. Lasagna, L., and Beecher, H. K.: The analgesic effectiveness of nalorphine and nalorphine-morphine combinations in man. J. Pharmacol. Exp. Ther. *112*:356–363, 1954.
49. Malis, J.: Personal communications, 1968.
50. Martin, W. R.: Opioid antagonists. Pharmacol. Rev. *19*:463–522, 1967.
51. Matsumoto, C., and Nickander, R.: Epinephrine-induced writhing in mice. Fed. Proc. *26*:619, 1967.
52. May, E.: Personal communication, 1972.
53. Miller, L. C.: A critique of analgesic testing methods. Ann. N.Y. Acad. Sci. *51*:34–50, 1948.
54. Murray, W. J., and Miller, J. W.: Oxytocin-induced "cramping" in the rat. J. Pharmacol. Exp. Ther. *128*:372–379, 1960.
55. Nilsen, P.: Studies on algesimetry by electrical stimulation of the mouse tail. Acta Pharmacol. Toxicol. *18*:10–22, 1961.
56. Paalzow, L.: An electrical method for estimation of analgesic activity in mice. Acta Pharm. Suec. *6*:207–226, 1969.
57. Pearl, J., and Harris, L. S.: Inhibition of writhing by narcotic antagonists. J. Pharmacol. Exp. Ther. *154*:319–323, 1966.
58. Pearl, J., Harris, L. S., and Fitzgerald, J. J.: Effects of analgesic-antagonists on vocalizing and jumping of rats to electric shock. Arch. Int. Pharmacodyn. Ther. *161*:359–363, 1966.
59. Pearl, J., Aceto, M. D., and Harris, L. S.: Prevention of writhing and other effects of narcotics and narcotic antagonists in mice. J. Pharmacol. Exp. Ther. *160*:217–230, 1968.
60. Pearl, J., Stander, H., and McKean, D.: Effects of analgesics and other drugs on mice in phenylquinone and rotarod tests. J. Pharmacol. Exp. Ther. *167*:9–13, 1969.
61. Perrine, T., Atwell, L., Tice, I., Jacobson, A., and May, E.: Analgesic activity as determined by the Nilsen method. J. Pharm. Sci. *61*:86–88, 1972.
62. Randall, L. O., and Selitto, J. J.: A method for measurement of analgesic activity on inflamed tissue. Arch. Int. Pharmacodyn. Ther. *111*:409–419, 1957.
63. Siegmund, E., Cadmus, R., and Lu, G.: A method for evaluating both non-narcotic and narcotic analgesics. Proc. Soc. Exp. Biol. Med. *95*:729–731, 1957.
64. Taber, R. I., Greenhouse, D. D., and Irwin, S.: Inhibition of phenylquinone induced writhing by narcotic antagonists. Nature *204*:189–190, 1964.
65. Taber, R. I., Greenhouse, D. D., Rendell, J. K., and Irwin, S.: Agonist and antagonist interactions of opioids on acetic acid-induced stretching in mice. J. Pharmacol. Exp. Therap. *169*:29–38, 1969.
66. Taber, R. I.: Unpublished data, 1972.

67. Takagi, H., Inukai, T., and Nakama, M.: A modification of Haffner's method for testing analgesics. Jap. J. Pharmacol. *16*:287–294, 1966.
68. Vander Wende, C., and Margolin, S.: Analgesic tests based upon experimentally induced acute abdominal pain in rats. Fed. Proc. *15*:494, 1956.
69. Ward, J. W., Foxwell, M., and Funderburk, W. H.: The detection of analgesia produced by morphine antagonists in laboratory animals. Pharmacologist *7*:163, 1965.
70. Weller, C., and Sulman, F.: Drug action on tail shock-induced vocalization in mice and its relevance to analgesia. Eur. J. Pharmacol. *9*:227, 234, 1970.
71. Winder, C. V.: Aspirin and algesimetry. Nature *184*:494–497, 1959.
72. Winder, C. V., Wax, J., Scotti, L., Scherrer, R. A., Jones, E. M., and Short, F. W.: Anti-inflammatory, antipyretic and antinociceptive properties of N(2,3-xylyl)-anthranilic acid (mefenamic acid). J. Pharmacol. Exp. Ther. *138*:405–413, 1962.
73. Winter, C. A., Orahovats, P. D., and Lehman, E. G.: Analgesic activity and morphine antagonism of compounds related to nalorphine. Arch. Int. Pharmacodyn. Ther. *110*:186–201, 1957.
74. Winter, C. A., and Flataker, L.: Reaction thresholds to pressure in edematous hind paws of rats and responses to analgesic drugs. J. Pharmacol. Exp. Ther. *150*:165–171, 1965.
75. Winter, C. A., and Flataker, L.: Nociceptive thresholds as affected by parenteral administration of irritants and of various antinociceptive drugs. J. Pharmacol. Exp. Ther. *143*:373–379, 1965.
76. Winter, C. A.: The physiology and pharmacology of pain. *In:* Analgetics, edited by G. de Stevens, pp. 10–75. Academic Press, New York, 1965.
77. Woolfe, G., and MacDonald, A. D.: The evaluation of the analgesic action of pethidine hydrochloride (Demerol). J. Pharmacol. Exp. Ther. *80*:300–307, 1944.

Narcotic Antagonists, edited by M. C. Braude, L. S. Harris, E. L.
May, J. P. Smith, and J. E. Villarreal. Advances in Biochemical
Psychopharmacology, Vol. 8. Raven Press, New York © 1974.

Reversal by Narcotics and Narcotic Antagonists of Pain-Induced Functional Impairment

R. Rodríguez and E. G. Pardo

Instituto Miles de Terapeutica Experimental, México 22, D. F. México

Reversal by narcotics and narcotic antagonists of pain-induced functional impairment. The antinociceptive activity of the narcotic antagonists
nalorphine and pentazocine and the narcotic analgesics morphine, meperidine, and codeine was determined in dogs using the pain-induced functional impairment procedure. Nalorphine, 0.56 and 1.0 mg/kg, pentazocine, 3.1 and 5.6 mg/kg, morphine, 0.31 and 0.56 mg/kg, and codeine and
meperidine 3.1 and 5.6 mg/kg, restored the motor behavior disrupted by
the nociceptive stimulus. In all cases the effect was proportional to drug
dose. Potency estimates based on "total" effects during the 150 min of
observation indicate nalorphine and pentazocine to be 0.620 and 0.097,
respectively, as potent as morphine. Meperidine and codeine were found
to be 13 times less potent than the standard analgesic.

INTRODUCTION

Many methods have been developed for the assessment of analgesic
activity in animals (2, 9, 35). Whereas some of these methods reflect the
clinical potency of narcotics fairly well, they tend to be insensitive to other
analgesics of the non-narcotic or opioid antagonist type (5, 6, 12, 14, 36).
On the other hand, procedures that detect the activity of such drugs respond
nonspecifically to other classes of agents besides analgesics (16). Perhaps
one reason for the lack of correlation with clinical data is that whereas the
current animal methods measure the capacity of the drug to increase the
minimal stimulus required to elicit a nociceptive response, clinically, the
efficacy of drugs is measured in terms of their ability to reduce the effects
of suprathreshold painful stimulation. Considering this basic difference, a
method was developed in 1966 for assessing the antinociceptive action of
drugs in experimental conditions more closely related to the clinical situation. In earlier reports the method was shown to be sensitive to relatively
low oral doses of aspirin-type analgesics and narcotics (24, 27, 28) and to

detect the activity of certain psychotropic drugs (25) claimed to influence pain in man (4, 29, 37).

The present study was undertaken to ascertain whether the procedure could also detect the activity of narcotic antagonists and to determine their potency as related to various narcotic analgesics.

METHODS

The procedure employed was essentially that previously described (28). A total of 37 adult mongrel dogs were trained to walk on a treadmill running at a speed of 3 mph. Training sessions consisted of 20 2-min periods of walking on the band, with an interval of 5 min between each period. Sessions were repeated on from 5 to 8 days. At the time of the experiment, a properly conformed strain gage transducer was glued to the shaved skin of the flexor aspect of the ankle joint on the hind limb to which the nociceptive stimulus (formalin injection) was to be applied. The attachment of the transducer to the skin was strengthened with adhesive tape. Animals were then made to walk on the band twice for 20 sec at 5-min intervals. Recordings of hind limb ambulatory activity were made through the strain gauge into two channels of a Grass polygraph. In one, the standard record of activity was taken and in another, the pen point was widened to give a solid ink recording which, when cut and weighed, represented an approximate integrated measurement of ambulatory activity. After control recordings, an injection of 0.5 ml of a 5% formalin solution was made intra-articularly in the knee joint of the limb on which the transducer had been fixed. Recordings of ambulatory activity were taken immediately after injection and at 15-min intervals over a 150-min observation period. Immediately after the recording taken 15 min after the injection of formalin, compounds to be tested or saline were administered. In 23 dogs two successive experiments were carried out, one on each hind limb, with an interval of at least 1 week between experiments. In the other 14 animals only a single experiment was performed.

Ten experiments were carried out to determine the time course of recovery of ambulatory activity with the formalin-injected limb in animals receiving saline. The influence of nalorphine hydrochloride, morphine sulfate, codeine sulfate, meperidine hydrochloride, and pentazocine at two dose levels on the time course of recovery was evaluated in 50 other experiments, 10 for each drug. Compounds were dissolved in distilled water and administered intravenously in a volume of 5 ml. Stated dosages refer to the free base. Data were transformed and analyzed as previously described (28).

RESULTS

Tracings of ambulatory activity as recorded through a transducer placed in the flexor aspect of the ankle joint were very uniform for any given animal in the course of the 20-sec walking time on the band, and were not different from those taken when the animal was circling a walkway (28). The appearance of such records in different animals is exemplified in the top segment of each of the columns shown in Fig. 1. In all animals the injection of formalin elicited a behavioral reaction characterized by barking, mydriasis, salivation, and sometimes biting of the restraining chain and aggressive growling. This reaction lasted in most cases no more than 3 min and was followed by persisting flexion of the injected limb. When the animals were required to walk on the band they did so on three legs. Figure 1 illustrates several points. The nonparticipation of the injected limb for ambulation is demonstrated in the second and third recordings of each of the experiments shown in this figure. In addition, the spontaneous recovery of the injected limb in a control animal can be seen. In this animal, some participation of the affected limb in ambulation was recorded at 120 min and there was almost complete recovery 150 min after the injection (Column A). Finally, the intravenous injection of 5.6 mg/kg of pentazocine, 1.0 mg/kg of nalorphine, 5.6 mg/kg of codeine, 5.6 mg/kg of meperidine, and 0.56 mg/kg of morphine restored the motor performance disrupted by the nociceptive stimulus (Columns B, C, D, E, F).

The reproducibility and stability of the motor impairment induced by the formalin injection is demonstrated by the time-recovery curve of the saline-treated controls shown in Fig. 2. The mean effects for the two doses of morphine, nalorphine, and pentazocine on recovery from pain-induced functional impairment are plotted in Figs. 2–4, and provide time-effect curves for these drugs. The curves for codeine and meperidine were quite similar to that for pentazocine. Peak activity after the two doses of both drugs occurred 15 min after administration and some decrement in the effect was apparent between 30 and 75 min after drug injection. Student's t test (30) indicated significant ($p<0.05$) acceleration of recovery for the two doses of morphine, nalorphine, codeine, and meperidine and for the high dose of pentazocine (5.6 mg/kg). For calculation of relative potencies, the acceleration of recovery attributable in each animal to the drug used was determined by substracting the mean area under the time-recovery curves of the control animals from the corresponding area of each treated animal. This difference in area was considered a measure of the total effect of each dose over the entire period of observation. Dose-effect curves based on data of total effects for each drug treatment are presented in Fig. 5. It is

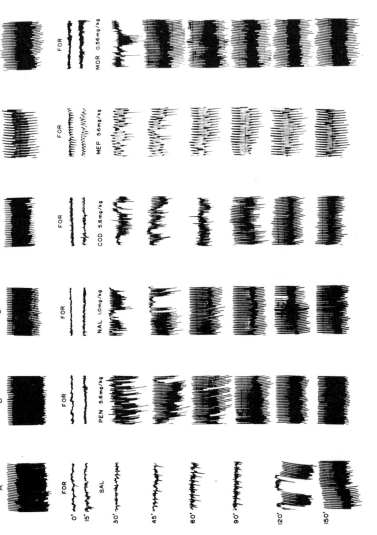

FIG. 1. Impairment of ambulatory activity of dogs by injection of formalin (FOR) into the knee joint of one of the hind limbs, spontaneous recovery from the pain-induced impairment, and recovery following the intravenous administration of drugs under study. Polygraph records of ambulatory movements taken through strain gage pickups from hind limbs of six dogs are compared. Segments in column A are from a saline-treated animal; those in columns B through F are from dogs receiving pentazocine (PEN), nalorphine (NAL), codeine (COD), meperidine (MEP), and morphine (MOR) at the doses indicated. In each case the top segment is a control record of ambulatory movements; the next two are records immediately and 15 min after the intraarticular injection of 0.5 ml of 5% formalin; the following segments record ambulatory movements at different times, up to 150 min after injection of formalin. Test drugs were administered immediately after the 15-min recording.

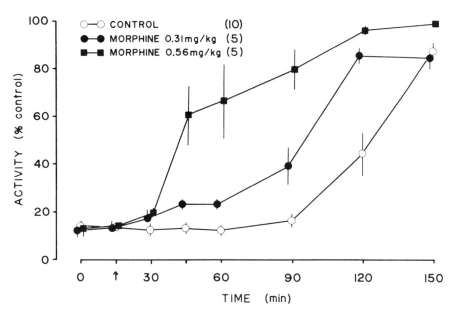

FIG. 2. Influence of morphine on the recovery from pain-induced functional impairment. Data from 10 saline-treated control animals are compared with data from groups of five animals receiving 0.31 and 0.56 mg/kg of morphine intravenously. For construction of this graph, ambulatory activity in walking on a treadmill at the rate of 3 mph was integrated and the values obtained were transformed to percent of control activity for each animal. Each point on the graph represents the mean from the animals in the corresponding group; the vertical lines are standard errors. Abscissas represent time after formalin injection into the joint; ordinates, ambulatory activity. Arrow indicates drug administration.

apparent that pentazocine, meperidine, and codeine are of approximately equal potency, that all are nearly 10 times less potent than morphine, and that nalorphine is approximately one-half as potent as morphine. The relative potencies of different compounds, estimated by the four-point assay (8), are summarized in Table 1.

Low doses of all drugs tested produced salivation in some animals. The higher doses of morphine, nalorphine, meperidine, and codeine (0.56, 1.0, 5.6, 5.6 mg/kg, respectively) caused salivation, irregular and periodic breathing, and sedation. Muscle jerks and increased muscular tone were seen in some animals after the large dose of pentazocine (5.6 mg/kg). None of the side effects described for any drug was of sufficient intensity to prevent the animals from walking on the band as required.

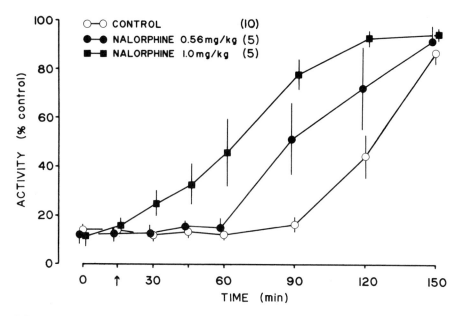

FIG. 3. Influence of nalorphine on the recovery from pain-induced functional impairment. Data from 10 saline-treated control animals are compared with data from groups of five animals receiving 0.56 and 1.0 mg/kg of nalorphine intravenously. Details as in Fig. 2.

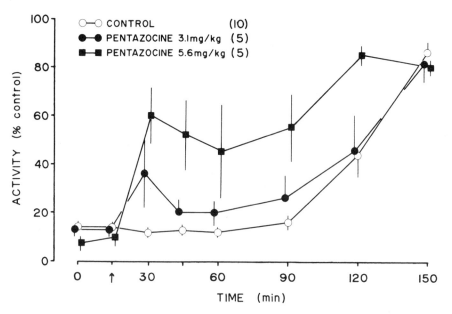

FIG. 4. Influence of pentazocine on the recovery from pain-induced functional impairment. Data from 10 saline-treated control animals are compared with data from groups of five animals receiving 3.1 and 5.6 mg/kg of pentazocine intravenously. Details as in Fig. 2.

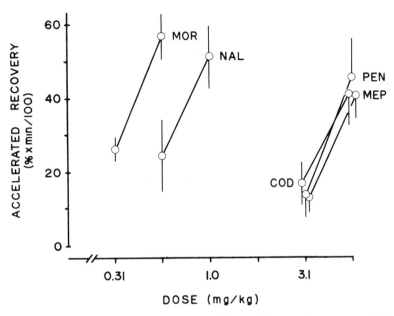

FIG. 5. Dose-effect curves for morphine, nalorphine, codeine, pentazocine, and meperidine. Data from individual experiments were transformed to percent-minutes of accelerated recovery. Each point represents the mean of five experiments; vertical lines are standard errors. Abscissas represent doses of test compounds in mg/kg; ordinates, accelerated recovery percent × min/100, as calculated from areas between the line representing average recovery in controls and that representing recovery in any individual drug experiment.

TABLE 1. *Potency of drugs tested relative to morphine*

Drugs	Potency (Morphine = 1)	Confidence limits ($p = 0.05$)
Nalorphine	0.620	0.490–0.780
Pentazocine	0.097	0.079–0.120
Meperidine	0.074	0.061–0.090
Codeine	0.070	0.063–0.092

DISCUSSION

The present results indicate that pain-induced functional impairment is influenced by narcotic antagonists and confirm the sensitivity of the method to the effects of narcotic analgesics. Thus, nalorphine, pentazocine, morphine, codeine, and meperidine restored the motor performance disrupted by the nociceptive stimulus in a dose-dependent fashion. The method was capable of detecting the effect of doses of morphine as low as 0.31 mg/kg and permitted discrimination between relatively small differences in doses (0.25 log). Its sensitivity is comparable only to that of the phenylquinone writhing test (3) and of the chronic spinal dog (22), which can measure the effect of morphine at doses of less than 1 mg/kg. In other animal-testing procedures such as the tail-flick (5), radiant heat (7), hot-plate (36), and tail-pressure (10), the minimal detectable doses of morphine typically run into several mg/kg.

The activity of narcotic antagonists which are analgesics in man is of particular interest because commonly used techniques can usually demonstrate little or no activity for these agents (11, 15, 32, 33). There are, however, procedures in which narcotic antagonists produce measurable activity. A large group of narcotic antagonists, including nalorphine and pentazocine, have been found to be active in the phenylquinone writhing test in mice (3, 26, 31). Nalorphine and cyclazocine depress spinal cord reflexes in the chronic spinal dog (23). Pentazocine, nalorphine, cyclazocine, and N-cyclopropylmethylnormorphine, have been reported to raise the pain threshold in the yeast-inflamed paw of the rat (34). Pentazocine, but not nalorphine, was also found to increase the aversive threshold level in monkeys (32).

In this study nalorphine was found to be two-thirds as potent as morphine. This estimate agrees well with clinical data. Lasagna and Beecher (20) first reported that nalorphine at dose levels of 10 and 15 mg produced relief of postoperative pain comparable to that produced by 10 mg of morphine. These findings were confirmed by the work of Keats and Telford (17). Clinical investigators' estimates of the analgesic potency of pentazocine have varied considerably from one-sixth as potent (1) to almost equipotent to morphine (18), the most rigorous study showing that 60 mg of pentazocine is equivalent to 10 mg of morphine in patients with pain due to cancer (1). In the present study pentazocine was found to be only $\frac{1}{10}$ as potent as morphine, thus underestimating the potency of the drug. This discrepancy may be simply due to the fact that in clinical studies, the activity of a morphine salt, generally the sulfate, is compared with the activity of the free base of pentazocine. The sulfuric acid residue represents approximately 25% of the total molecular weight of the salt. The discrepancy could also be attributed to the fact that, in the dog, pentazocine appears to have a shorter duration of action than morphine, as judged by the configuration of the time-effect curves. This phenomenon, observed also in man, could become more apparent when the intravenous route is used. The present data also underestimate somewhat the potency of meperidine and codeine.

Codeine by injection, in 60-mg doses, approaches but does not equal 10 mg of morphine as analgesic (21), whereas 100 mg of meperidine has been reported to be only slightly more effective than 10 mg of morphine (19). Present results indicate both drugs to be 13 times less potent than morphine. The above arguments could also account for this difference.

These data and those previously reported indicate the usefulness of the technique used in this chapter for evaluating analgesic compounds. The degree of motor impairment is a dependable and sensitive indicator of the effects of compounds which have been otherwise established as analgesics. On the other hand, the method is reasonably specific for analgesics, since among a number of compounds of different pharmacological classes, such as sympathomimetics, antihistaminics, CNS estimulants, hypnotics, neuroleptics, steroids, anticholinergics, alpha adrenergic blockers, and antihypertensive agents, only chlorpromazine and amphetamine accelerated recovery from motor impairment (25). It should be pointed out, however, that drugs of this type have been claimed to possess analgesic properties in man (4, 29, 37), although this contention has been denied by others (13). In addition to the above, other drugs may influence the rate of recovery from pain-induced functional impairment, but the fact that they do so only at doses producing obvious side effects allows differentiation of such false positive results.

It may be that the sensitivity of the method to analgesic agents and the significance of its results in terms of the analogy of the rank order of potency with clinical data is due to the utilization of an experimental situation closely analogous to clinical conditions in which analgesics are used. In contrast to standard analgesic tests, which measure fundamentally the ability of drugs to elevate the threshold to the nociceptive stimulus, this procedure measures the antinociceptive activity of drugs in terms of their capacity to restore a motor behavior disrupted by a nociceptive stimulus. In the clinical situation the criterion of effectiveness is based on the ability of the drug to relieve the effects on continuous suprathreshold painful stimuli. The fact that even powerful narcotic analgesics are neither capable of consistently and significantly elevating experimental pain threshold in man nor of adequately controlling sudden and fleeting pain of pathological origin (2), yet are universally found to be effective in relieving apparently persistent pain, indicates that the ability to elevate threshold and the capacity to relieve pain may be two different pharmacological properties underlying different mechanisms of analgesic action.

On the other hand, the principal drawback of this procedure is the fact that it is laborious and time consuming. It takes a long time to train an animal so that its ambulatory activity can be properly recorded, and an equally long time to perform a complete quantitative study of a single drug. Furthermore, the relatively large amount of compound needed for the test makes its routine use as a screening procedure impossible.

CONCLUSIONS

Data presented here show that the pain-induced functional impairment procedure is sensitive to the antinociceptive activity of narcotic antagonists.

The sensitivity of the procedure to the action of narcotic analgesics and narcotic antagonists is similar to that reported for the phynylquinone-induced writhing test and for the chronic spinal dog, but greater than that of other animal tests.

As determined by this method, the potency of nalorphine in relationship to morphine correlates fairly well with clinical data. The method underestimates somewhat the potency of pentazocine, meperidine, and codeine.

The technique offers an interesting change from the commonly used tests in that it takes advantage of an experimental situation analogous to clinical conditions in which analgesics are used, and considers the degree of utilization of the affected limb in ambulation as a nonverbal statement of the degree of pain or its suppression by analgesic agents.

REFERENCES

1. Beaver, W. T., Wallenstein, S. L., Houde, R. W., and Rogers, A.: A comparison of the analgesic effects of pentazocine and morphine in patients with cancer. Clin. Pharmacol. Ther. 7:740–751, 1966.
2. Beecher, H. K.: The measurement of pain. Pharmacol. Rev. 9:59–209, 1957.
3. Blumberg, H., Wolf, P. S., and Dayton, H. B.: Use of the writing test for evaluating analgesic activity of narcotic antagonists. Proc. Soc. Exp. Biol. Med. 118:763–766, 1965.
4. Cass, L. J., and Frederik, W. S.: Clinical evaluation of aletamine as an analgesic. J. New Drugs 6:96–104, 1966.
5. D'Amour, F. E., and Smith, D. L.: A method for determining loss of pain sensation. J. Pharmacol. Exp. Ther. 72:74–79, 1941.
6. Eddy, N. B., and Leimbach, D.: Synthetic analgesics. II. Dithienylbutenyl- and dithienylbutylamines. J. Pharmacol. Exp. Ther. 107:385–393, 1953.
7. Ercoli, N., and Lewis, M. N.: Studies on analgesics. I. The time-action curves of morphine, codeine, dilaudid and demerol by various methods of administration. II. Analgesic activity of acetylsalicylic acid and aminopyrine. J. Pharmacol. Exp. Ther. 84:301–317, 1945.
8. Finney, D. J.: Statistical Method in Biological Assay. Charles Griffin & Co., London, 1952.
9. Goetzl, F. R., Burrill, D. Y., and Ivy, A. C.: A critical analysis of algesimetric methods with suggestions for a useful procedure. Quart. Bull. Northw. Univ. Med. Sch. 17:280–291, 1943.
10. Green, A. F., Young, P. A., and Godfrey, E. I.: A comparison of heat and pressure analgesiometric methods in rats. Brit. J. Pharmacol. Chemother. 6:572–585, 1951.
11. Green, A. F., Ruffell, G. K., and Walton, E.: Morphine derivatives with antianalgesic action. J. Pharm. Pharmacol. 6:390–397, 1954.
12. Haffner, F.: Experimentelle Prüfung schemerzstillender Mittel. Dtsch. Med. Wschr. 55:731–733, 1929.

13. Houde, R. W.: On assaying analgesics in man. *In*: Pain, edited by R. S. Knighton and P. R. Dumke, pp. 183–196. Little, Brown and Co., Boston, 1966.
14. Hardy, J. D., Wolff, H. G., and Goodell, H.: Studies on pain. A new method for measuring pain threshold: Observations on spatial summation of pain. J. Clin. Invest. *19*:649–657, 1940.
15. Harris, L. S., and Pierson, A. K.: Some narcotic antagonists in the benzomorphan series. J. Pharmacol. Exp. Ther. *143*:141–148, 1964.
16. Hendershot, L. C., and Forsaith, J.: Antagonism of the frequency of phenylquinone-induced writhing in the mouse by weak analgesics and nonanalgesics. J. Pharmacol. Exp. Ther. *125*:237–240, 1959.
17. Keats, A. S., and Telford, J.: Nalorphine, a potent analgesic in man. J. Pharmacol. Exp. Ther. *117*:190–199, 1956.
18. Keats, A. S., and Telford, J.: Studies of analgesic drugs. VIII. A narcotic antagonist analgesic without psychotomimetic effects. J. Pharmacol. Exp. Ther. *143*:157–164, 1964.
19. Lasagna, L., and Beecher, H. K.: The analgesic effectiveness of codeine and meperidine (Demerol). J. Pharmacol. Exp. Ther. *112*:306–311, 1954.
20. Lasagna, L., and Beecher, H. K.: The analgesic effectiveness of nalorphine and nalorphine-morphine combinations in man. J. Pharmacol. Exp. Ther. *112*:356–363, 1954.
21. Lasagna L.: The clinical evaluation of morphine and its substitutes as analgesics. Pharmacol. Rev. *16*:47–83, 1964.
22. Martin, W. R., Eades, C. G., Fraser, H. F., and Wikler, A.: Use of hindlimb reflexes of the chronic spinal dog for comparing analgesics. J. Pharmacol. Exp. Ther. *144*:8–11, 1964.
23. McClane, T. K., and Martin, W. R.: Effects of morphine, nalorphine, cyclazocine and naloxone on the flexor reflex. Int. J. Neuropharmacol. *6*:89–97, 1967.
24. Pardo, E. G., and Rodríguez, R.: Reversal by acetylsalicylic acid of pain induced functional impairment. Life Sci. *5*:775–781, 1966.
25. Pardo, E. G., and Rodríguez, R.: The use of pain induced functional impairment for assessing analgesic action. *In*: Pharmacology of Pain, edited by R. K. S. Lim, D. Armstrong, and E. G. Pardo, pp. 101–111. Pergamon Press, Oxford, 1968.
26. Pearl, J., and Harris, L. S.: Inhibition of writhing by narcotic antagonists. J. Pharmacol. Exp. Ther. *154*:319–323, 1966.
27. Rodríguez, R., and Pardo, E. G.: Drug reversal of pain induced functional impairment. Fed. Proc. *25*:501, 1966.
28. Rodríguez, R., and Pardo, E. G.: Drug reversal of pain induced functional impairment. Arch. Int. Pharmacodyn. Thér. *172*:148–160, 1968.
29. Sigwald, J., Bouttier, D., and Solignag, J.: Essai de traitements de la nevralgie essentielle du trijumeau par la lévomépromazine. Presse Med. *67*:349–353, 1957.
30. Snedecor, G. W., and Cochran, W. G.: Statistical Methods. Iowa State University Press, Iowa City, 1967.
31. Taber, R. I., Greenhouse, D. D., and Irwin, S.: Inhibition of phenylquinone-induced writhing by narcotic antagonists. Nature *204*:189–190, 1964.
32. Weiss, B., and Laties, V. G.: Analgesic effects in monkeys of morphine, nalorphine, and a benzomorphan narcotic antagonist. J. Pharmacol. Exp. Ther. *143*:169–173, 1964.
33. Winter, C. A., Orahovats, P. D., and Lehman, E. G.: Analgesic activity and morphine antagonism of compounds related to nalorphine. Arch. Int. Pharmacodyn. Thér. *110*:186–202, 1957.
34. Winter, C. A., and Flataker, L.: Reaction thresholds to pressure in edematous hindpaws of rats and responses to analgesic drugs. J. Pharmacol. Exp. Ther. *150*:165–171, 1965.
35. Winter, C. A.: The physiology and pharmacology of pain and its relief. *In*: Analgetics, edited by G. deStevens, pp. 9–74. Academic Press, New York and London, 1965.
36. Woolfe, G., and MacDonald, A. O.: The evaluation of the analgesic action of pethidine hydrochloride (Demerol). J. Pharmacol. Exp. Ther. *80*:300–307, 1944.
37. Zeh, W.: Die reine Megaphenbehandlung vegetativer Schmerzzustände, insbensondere der Trigeminusneuralgien. Dtsch. Med. Wschr. *80*:689–693, 1955.

Narcotic Antagonists, edited by M. C. Braude, L. S. Harris, E. L. May, J. P. Smith, and J. E. Villarreal. *Advances in Biochemical Psychopharmacology, Vol. 8.* Raven Press, New York © 1974.

Assaying Narcotic-Antagonist Drugs for Analgesic Activity in Rhesus Monkeys

Jerry L. Malis and Melvyn I. Gluckman

Wyeth Laboratories, Inc., Research Division, Radnor, Pennsylvania 19087

Male rhesus monkeys, seated in primate chairs, were trained to regulate the intensity of 60-Hz current applied to their legs. The animals could respond by pressing a lever attached to their chairs. In the absence of a response, solid state programming equipment automatically increased the shock intensity every 2 sec in steps of approximately .15 mA. Both shock increases and the animal's responses were graphically recorded, thus providing ongoing threshold base lines which were quite stable over time. In drug-testing sessions the animals were placed in sound-deadening chambers and base line data were collected over a 30- to 60-min period. Drugs were administered intramuscularly, no animal receiving more than one dose every 7 days. Since each animal served as its own control, the effects of each dose of drug could be independently evaluated. In addition to changes in thresholds, the animals were evaluated for respiratory depression, sedative or excitant effects, and for changes in pupil size. Analgesic dose-response curves were obtained for pentazocine, cyclazocine, and a new 2-amino-bridged tetralin compound, Wy-14,910. Changes in threshold have also been observed with nalorphine. The analgesic effect of pentazocine, cyclazocine, Wy-14,910, and nalorphine was reversed by naloxone. Nalorphine partially reversed the effects of both pentazocine and Wy-14,910.

INTRODUCTION

We have previously reported on the use of the monkey shock titration procedure in assessing the analgesic activity of a wide range of narcotic and non-narcotic agents (4, 5). The present study will present data obtained by this procedure on the analgesic properties of cyclazocine, pentazocine, and a new agonist-antagonist agent, Wy-14,910 (2). In addition, shock titration changes after nalorphine are reported.

Antagonism of the agonist effect of cyclazocine, pentazocine, Wy-14,910, and nalorphine were also demonstrated using the shock titration procedure.

METHODS

Male rhesus monkeys, seated in primate chairs, were trained to regulate the intensity of 60-Hz current applied to their feet, through aluminum foil boots. In the absence of response by the animal, solid state programming equipment automatically increased the shock intensity every 2 sec in steps of approximately 0.15 mA. There were 32 steps from 0 to maximum intensity. Each response by the monkey reduced the intensity by one step. Both shock increases and the animal's responses were graphically recorded, thus providing an ongoing threshold base line. Figure 1 shows a section of the graphic record with an enlarged insert showing the relationship between shock step increases and responses by the animal. Once threshold base lines were established, they were quite stable over long periods of time, both within sessions and from session to session. Figure 2 shows two sections of an animal's record, the first portion taken at 30 min after the start and the second portion taken 8 hr later. In drug-testing sessions the animals were placed in sound deadening chambers and baseline data were collected over a 30- to 60-min period. The animals were under constant surveilance by closed circuit television. Drugs were administered i.m. as base, no animal receiving more than one dose every 7 days. After drug administration, the testing

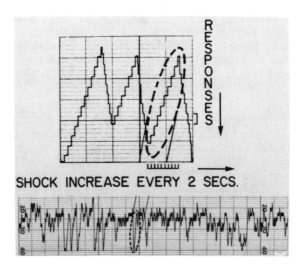

FIG. 1. The bottom trace is a section of behavioral recording from the monkey foot shock titration procedure. The upper trace is an enlarged section, indicated by the dashed circle, showing both shock increases (upward step function) and responses by the animal (downward rapid steps).

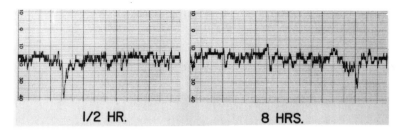

FIG. 2. Shock titration behavioral records showing threshold stability. The first section was taken 30 min after the beginning of the test session. The second section was taken 8 hr later during a continuous session.

session continued until the animals returned to predrug base line levels. The shock level at which the analgesic effect reached a plateau was used to calculate dose-response curves. Results were expressed as the average number of steps over the control threshold level.

RESULTS AND DISCUSSION

Cyclazocine, pentazocine, and Wy-14,910 produced dose-related increases in shock thresholds. A typical set of behavioral records is shown in Fig. 3. The onset of analgesia after cyclazocine and Wy-14,910 was rapid, usually within 2 to 8 min. Pentazocine-treated animals took longer (21 to 45 min) to show analgesic effects. Although the full duration of effects is not shown in Fig. 3, pentazocine was the shortest lasting of the three compounds with a range of duration from 2 to $3\frac{1}{2}$ hr. Both cyclazocine and Wy-14,910 were longer acting with significant activity still present, in most cases, at 6 hr after administration.

Since the animal's precision in regulating shock intensity is sensitive to disruption by stimulant, depressant, or psychotomimetic side effects, the dose levels that produce such disruption can be compared with the maximum nondisruptive doses and give a measure of a compound's range of utility. Both pentazocine and cyclazocine had limited utility ranges. At doses just twice those shown in Fig. 3, animals treated with cyclazocine or pentazocine showed marked disruptive effects which limited their upper dose analgesic effectiveness. These effects were not seen with Wy-14,910, even at a dose 10 times that shown in Fig. 3.

Dose-response curves from the shock titration procedure are shown in Fig. 4. The curve for morphine is included for potency comparisons. With the exception of Wy-14,910 the curves in Fig. 4 indicate, at the highest doses shown, the maximum level of analgesia the compounds could produce

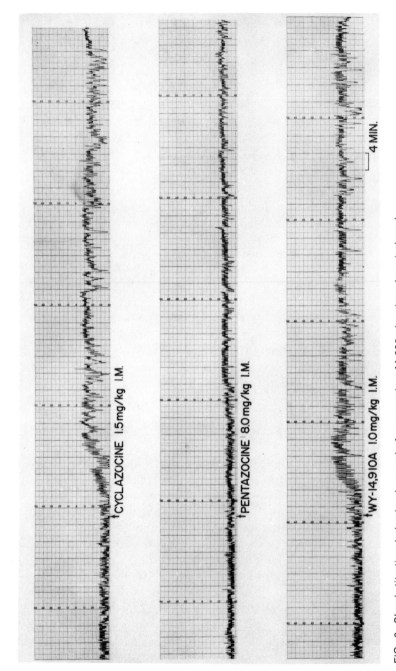

↑CYCLAZOCINE 1.5mg/kg I.M.

↑PENTAZOCINE 8.0mg/kg I.M.

↑WY-14,910A 1.0mg/kg I.M.

4 MIN.

FIG. 3. Shock titration behavioral records from monkey M-002 showing drug induced increases in threshold levels. Arrows indicate time of injection.

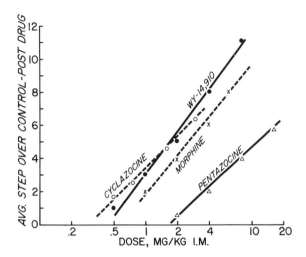

FIG. 4. Dose-response curves from the monkey shock titration procedure. Each point on the graph is the mean response of at least three animals.

without totally disrupting the monkey's ability to regulate shock intensity.

The potency relationships in Fig. 4 for cyclazocine, morphine, and pentazocine are very similar to those found in man (1). Since no human potency data are yet available for Wy-14,910, confirmation of the monkey data will have to await the outcome of clinical studies. It would appear, however, that the shock titration procedure has good predictive ability for human potency of the agonist-antagonist compounds.

As we have previously shown (5), the shock titration procedure also allows one to make rather precise measurements of antagonism of analgesic effect. These effects can also be shown on the agonist effect of the agonist-antagonist compounds. A series of records showing antagonism by nalorphine and naloxone are shown in Fig. 5. The analgesic effect of cyclazocine (*top tracing*) was unaffected by nalorphine but completely antagonized by naloxone. Nalorphine partially antagonized the agonist effects of pentazocine and Wy-14,910. We define partial antagonism as either one, or both, of the two following conditions, not related to the dose of the antagonist: 1) lack of complete return to predrug base line; 2) not all animals tested showed angagonism of analgesia.

In subsequent experiments, naloxone totally antagonized the analgesic effects of pentazocine and Wy-14,910. High doses (up to 8 mg/kg) of nalorphine, however, still produced only a partial antagonistic effect on pentazocine and Wy-14,910.

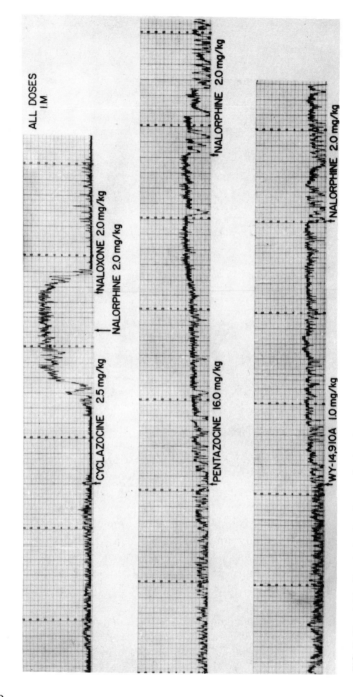

FIG. 5. Shock titration behavioral records showing antagonism by naloxone or nalorphine of the analgesic effects of cyclazocine, pentazocine, and Wy-14,910.

230

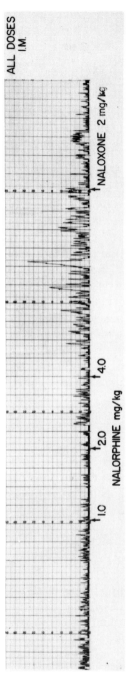

FIG. 6. Shock titration record showing the effects of cumulative doses of nalorphine and the antagonism of the agonist effect by naloxone.

Nalorphine has been reported to have analgesic effects in man (3), but has been reported to have no analgesic effect in monkeys (5, 6). With our present test system, we have been able to show, in preliminary experiments, threshold increases after the administration of nalorphine. A record showing serial injections of nalorphine is shown in Fig. 6. Although a slight increase in threshold was obtained after a cumulative dose of 3 mg/kg, the addition of 4 mg/kg (cumulative 7 mg/kg) produced a definite and sustained increase in shock threshold. Naloxone at 2 mg/kg antagonized the agonist affect of nalorphine.

Three factors may possibly be involved in the initial inability to show the agonist effect of nalorphine in monkeys. The first factor is the size of the current steps. Our early studies were done with current steps approximately twice the 0.15 mA we now use. This did tend to lower markedly the sensitivity of the assay. The second factor to be considered is the animal itself. Two distinct groups exist within our rhesus monkey population; the first, we call high-shock monkeys. These animals are relatively insensitive to shock current and require high doses of drug to produce threshold changes. These animals make up approximately 40% of our population. The second group, and the animals we now use for drug testing, are low-shock monkeys. These animals respond consistantly to low-shock intensities and are quite sensitive to drug-induced threshold changes.

The third possible factor which could affect the response to nalorphine may be related to the lowering of the threshold base line that is seen after the administration of cyclazocine, pentazocine, and nalorphine before the onset of their analgesic effects (see Fig. 5 and 6). This increase in lever pressing may be associated with "pain" on the injection of these agents, or, more likely in the case of nalorphine, with the possibility of aversiveness of the psychotomimetic properties of the compound. Examples of the former, would tend to argue against the demonstration of analgesic effects with all three compounds, wheras the latter example could be made specific for nalorphine by nature of its agonist-antagonist ratio and its high incidence of "unpleasant" side effects in man (3).

CONCLUSIONS

The monkey leg shock titration procedure has been shown to be an accurate, sensitive method for measuring the agonist effect of agonist-antagonist compounds. In addition to duration of action, antagonism of agonistic effect can also be measured. It would appear, from our data, that this method has good predictive ability of human agonist effects. In addition, the agonist properties of nalorphine and the ability of naloxone to antagonize them have been demonstrated. A possible set of conditions which may have contributed to the early negative findings on the agonist effects of nalorphine on the titration procedure has been discussed.

REFERENCES

1. Beaver, W. T.: The pharmacological basis for the choice of an analgesic. Pharmacol. Physicians 4, No. 10, 1970.
2. Freed, M. E., Potoski, J., Freed, E. H., Malis, J. L., and Gluckman, M. I.: 2-amino bridged tetralins. *This volume.*
3. Lasagna, L., and Beecher, H. K.: The analgesic effectiveness of nalorphine and nalorphine-morphine combinations in man. J. Pharmacol. Exp. Ther. *112*:356–363, 1954.
4. Malis, J. L.: Effects of drugs on the regulation of an aversive stimulus in the monkey. Fed. Proc. *21*:327, 1962.
5. Malis, J. L.: Analgesic testing in primates. *In:* Agonist and Antagonist Actions of Narcotic Analgesic Drugs, edited by H. W. Kosterlitz, J. O. H. Collier, and J. E. Villarreal. Macmillan, London, *in press.*
6. Weiss, B., and Laties, V. G.: Analgesic effects in monkeys of morphine, nalorphine and a benzomorphan narcotic antagonist. J. Pharmacol. Exp. Ther. *143*:169–173, 1964.

Narcotic Antagonists, edited by M. C. Braude, L. S. Harris, E. L.
May, J. P. Smith, and J. E. Villarreal. *Advances in Biochemical
Psychopharmacology, Vol. 8.* Raven Press, New York © 1974.

What Is Analgesia?

P. B. Dews

*Laboratory of Psychobiology, Department of Psychiatry, Harvard Medical School,
Boston, Massachusetts 02115*

It has not been proved that morphine selectively attenuates the behavioral effects of painful stimulation in either experimental subjects or
clinical situations. Morphine affects the behavior of experimental subjects in situations involving painful stimulation and in situations not involving painful stimulation. Morphine attenuates distress in acutely dis-
tressed patients whether the distress arises from painful stimulation or
from nonpainful causes. Even the familiar effect of morphine on distress
may derive its apparent specificity from the selected clinical population on
whom the observations are made. Analgesic assays have been contrived
to detect activity in drugs called analgesic drugs in the clinic and to differentiate them from drugs called nonanalgesic in the clinic. The assays have
proved their value in guiding programs of organic synthesis to valuable new
drugs. The assays cannot illuminate the whole behavioral pharmacology of
morphine.

Before the significance of analgesia test procedures can be assessed,
"analgesia" must be defined. An analgesic drug is a drug that selectively
attenuates pain. Unfortunately, we must now define pain, and here begins
trouble. Beecher (2) asked Gasser, Bishop, Adrian, and Wikler and considered the writings of T. Lewis in seeking a definition of pain, but failed to
find a satisfactory one. Perhaps he was not really trying since he had concluded at the beginning that "pain is a universal experience of mankind and
everybody knows what is meant by it." Part, but only part, of the difficulty
results from analogical extensions of the meaning of the word pain in expressions such as "his indifference pained me" and "a pain in the neck."
It would be manifestly absurd to expect a mere drug to track the vagaries
of the evolution of the English language and to attenuate all those phenomena we have chosen to refer to as pain while leaving, more or less unmodi-
fied, similar phenomena that we do not relate verbally to pain.

It is easier to define painful stimulation than it is to define pain, since we
can invoke physiology to limit the meaning of the former: painful stimulation
is stimulation that leads to excitation of the ubiquitous system of nerve

endings we call, for short, pain endings but which can be recognized as the receptors of the nociceptor system without reference to pain. Let us accept this system as a specific system carrying information relating to actual or physically impending tissue damage, on the basis of the sort of evidence presented by Sweet (14). Does a typical analgesic drug, say, morphine, selectively attenuate the effects of painful stimulation, selectively in the sense that the effects of painful stimulation are attenuated by morphine more, or at lower dose, than the effects of other kinds of stimuli, and that morphine is different in this regard from nonanalgesic drugs?

The effects of painful stimulation are first the initiation of impulses in the nociceptor system: there is no evidence that morphine interferes here. There is considerable evidence, however, that acetylsalicylic acid does interfere with the chemical mediation of the effects of painful stimulation on the nerve endings, at least in some places (7, 15). The selectivity, however, seems to depend on prostaglandin participation and so other functions involving prostaglandins and having nothing to do with painful stimulation, such as temperature regulation, are equally affected by acetylsalicylic acid. Nevertheless, few people would dispute that the effect of acetylsalicylic acid on prostaglandin excitation of nociceptor fibers satisfactorily defines acetylsalicylic acid as an analgesic. Unfortunately, this definition does not help us understand what is meant when it is said that morphine is an analgesic drug, since morphine does not have an effect on nociceptor excitation.

The initiation of impulses in the nociceptor system, their conduction to the central nervous system, and their subsequent transmission in ascending pathways up at least to the lemniscus have not been shown convincingly to be selectively reduced by morphine (13). Neuropharmacological studies, by which I mean direct recording of the effects of drugs on neural tissues, have not provided us with widely accepted criteria by which we could say that morphine is an analgesic whereas pentobarbital or chlorpromazine is not. The analgesic assays in use today are almost exclusively behavioral assays, having a behavioral end point or dependent variable. Does morphine selectively attenuate the behavioral effects of painful stimulation?

Painful stimulation, like other stimulation modes, affects behavior in a variety of ways. Only two will be discussed. First, painful stimulation can elicit simple behavioral responses such as reflex responses. An open minded review of the literature does not yield a strong conviction that the analgesic effects of morphine in man are tied in with the attenuation of simple behavioral responses to painful stimulation, a negative conclusion that is in accord with the neuropharmacological findings. Nevertheless, some of the best assays we have for detecting morphine-like activity and distinguishing such activity from barbiturate-like or chlorpromazine-like activity are tests using the flick of the tail of rats or mice in response to applied heat or strong pressure, or simple responses of mice on a hot plate; responses which are simple elicited responses. But the assays that show the selectivity have survived for that very reason. In developing an analgesic assay, investigators have first decided on some means of inflicting pain on subjects—they have decided whether to burn them, shock them, squeeze them hard, or irritate them chemically. Then they selected a flinch or other simple behavioral change to record. Then they have seen how morphine performed in the test. If morphine has shown good attenuation of the response, they have then looked for selectivity by trying pentobarbital or chlorpromazine or some other nonanalgesic drugs. If selectivity was shown, fine, the assay was ready for use. If not, the end point, the conditions, or the mode of stimulation were modified until selectivity was achieved. In other words, the assays have been contrived and selected to differentiate morphine from nonanalgesic drugs. No disparagement of the tests is intended; on the contrary, they have performed admirably, providing us with excellent new drugs such as meperidine and methadone and a wealth of valuable information, well represented in the pages of the present volume. In seeking a general appreciation of the behavioral pharmacology of morphine, however, a broader perspective is needed than can be provided by the deliberately biased analgesic assays.

Interestingly, analgesic assays in man have been viewed in a different light. When Keats and Beecher (5) reported that small doses of barbiturates had analgesic activity comparable to morphine, people did not say "What a poor analgesic assay"; they said rather "What a surprise, barbiturates being such good analgesics, and we never suspected it." Of course, the new information did not change the prescribing practices of physicians because barbiturates are not, in fact, effective in the vast majority of painful situations in which morphine and its congerers are so helpful. It is worthy of comment that some anesthesiologists use the term analgesia to include reduction in reflex response to skin incision and other forms of painful stimulation even when the drug has rendered the subject unconcious. Ether, chloroform, and nitrous oxide are said to have, and halothane not to have, analgesic properties (11). Is this a different use of the term? Occasionally, people working with animal subjects have come to take their analgesic assays seriously as indicators of specific analgesia and so have reported as analgesic drugs a whole variety of substances from physostigmine and epinephrine through amphetamine and barbiturates to chlorpromazine and methotrimeprazine. Fortunately, most such claims are either ignored or soon forgotten.

When investigators have started with a plausible model of a human painful condition, morphine has tended not to look different from non-analgesic drugs. For example, Gasserian ganglion stimulation has been studied as a model of trigeminal neuralgia. Morphine attenuates the behavioral response to the stimulation, but so do chlorpromazine, pentobarbital, and methamphetamine (16). Again, stimulation of tooth pulp to mimic toothache yields a response that is also attenuated by morphine; but again, the response is also attenuated by chlorpromazine although not by nalorphine (10).

When people have been primarily interested in the behavioral consequences of painful stimulation, drug studies have given results still more at variance with popular beliefs. Take for example, the effects of punishment. When a painful stimulus is made consequent upon an already occurring behavioral response, under a whole variety of schedules, the rate of responding, not surprisingly, tends to go down. Morphine has no tendency to attenuate the effects of the painful stimulation, that is, to restore the rate of responding toward the levels prevailing before the punishment was imposed (6). But barbiturates do, and so do meprobamate and chlordiazepoxide, but not chlorpromazine or amphetamine (3, 6). Finally, as McMillan reminds us in the present volume, morphine is as highly effective in attenuating behavioral responses related to food (and no pain) as it is in any situation relating to painful stimulation. The attacking behavior evoked by painful stimulation in a variety of species (1) has been considered by pharmacologists as "aggressive behavior" rather than as behavior resulting from pain, so morphine has not been studied; here is a glaring example of the constraint to thinking imposed by simplistic stereotype notions of behavioral phenomena and of drug effects.

It has been recognized for a long time, of course, by many authors both clinical and experimental that the effects of morphine are not confined to a simple uniform reduction in all behavioral responses to all painful stimulation. It is also generally recognized that the strength of behavioral response to painful stimulation is not a simple monotonically increasing function of the intensity of painful stimulation; the relationship is much more complicated. Evidently great painful stimulation, as in battle wounded, may evoke little behavioral response, whereas a little twinge, as down the medial aspect of the left arm of a middle-aged cardiologist, may evoke profound behavioral effects. If behavioral response is poorly related to intensity of painful stimulation, how can we expect the change due to morphine to be consistent? Paradoxically, in clinical usage, morphine is an extremely reliable drug, producing the desired response in a very large proportion of those to whom it is given. How can we account, on the one hand, for the poor relationship between intensity of painful stimulation and strength of behavioral response and, on the other hand, for the consistency of the clinical response to morphine?

We have discussed first how painful stimulation elicits behavioral responses directly; a second way painful stimulation modulates behavior is as a discriminative stimulus. A discriminative stimulus controls behavior because of the past associations, directly or indirectly, of the stimulus with circumstances of behavioral significance. For example, in animal experiments, when a response of a food-deprived animal is followed by food only when a particular light is present, then characteristically the light comes to control the occurrence of the response; the light is a discriminative stimulus, controlling responding because of past association with a program of food delivery. A discriminative stimulus derives its power from what it has been associated with rather than by what it is. In general, there is only an ill-defined relationship between the increasing physical intensity of a discriminative stimulus and the strength of its control over behavioral responding. If past associations are with a particular physical intensity of the stimulus, both greater and lesser intensities may exert less control; therefore, above a certain value, increasing intensity may lead to less powerful control. There is no doubt that painful stimulation can function as a discriminative stimulus (8); in so far as the behavioral response is controlled by the painful stimulation functioning in a discriminative mode, the behavioral response may not be related to the intensity of stimulation as a monotonically increasing function. The intense stimulation of the battle wounded is associated with escape from the horror of the battle whereas the radiating twinge in the cardiologist is associated with myocardial ischemia likely to lead to disability and proximate death. The behavioral responses correspond to the informational content rather than the intensity of stimulation. We could, therefore, account for the disparities between evident intensity of painful stimulation and behavioral response on well-established behavioral principles. If the effect of morphine were to attenuate the discriminative control of painful stimulation, the effect of morphine could be consistent even if the relationship of painful stimulation and behavioral response were not.

Unfortunately, there is no substantive evidence that the effects of morphine can be consistently ascribed to selective attenuation of discriminative control by painful stimulation, and clinical impression is against such selectivity. Morphine is extremely effective in acute pulmonary edema and preoperatively even in patients free from pain; in such cases, painful stimulation is absent so the effect of morphine cannot be to attenuate its effects. What the two situations have in common is not painful stimulation but that in both (as with painful stimulation) the subject is in distress; and morphine attenuates the distress. We are back where we started; incredibly, morphine does seem to attenuate clinically what we call pain and suffering, whether or not specific stimulation of pain pathways is involved. Before we enshrine the generalization as a great unifying principle, remember that at least a component of the relief by morphine of the distress of acute pulmonary edema is due to the shift to the right of the curve relating pulmonary ventilation to alveolar pCO_2, an effect that cannot account for the preoperative usefulness of morphine. The physiological and behavioral effects of morphine are too various to be subsumed by a single simple principle.

Even as a descriptive generalization, the notion that morphine is the great attenuator of distress has the weakness of being based exclusively on clinical experience, that is, based on responses of patients. Patients are an unrepresentative sample of the general population at a given time; being generally ill and usually in bed. Patients given morphine are even more unrepresentative since, in addition to the other pecularities of patients, they are almost always in acute distress. That such patients given morphine have their distress alleviated is poor grounds for postulating a selective effect of morphine on distress. Patients given morphine therapeutically have a much lower incidence and even a different type of side effect from other members of the population (2). In patients in distress, distress is the dominant feature of their situation. If morphine alleviates the distress, then such alleviation will be the dominant effect of the drug in that situation; but it does not follow that alleviation of distress is the only or even the main characteristic of the behavioral pharmacology of morphine. If the behavioral effects of morphine in experimental animals are considered without prejudice, the usual effect would be said to be reduction in output of behavior. Morphine, consequently, has been, generally, a dull drug to work with in behavioral pharmacology. We can perhaps convince ourselves that the dominant effect of morphine in addicts is also to reduce behavioral output generally. Morphine is the surrogate for action. Morphine does maintain self-administration behavior, but it does so much less easily than does cocaine, as though direct pharmacological effects were opposing the reinforcing effects of the drug. In devising tests of analgesia, perhaps we are mostly selecting situations in which pentobarbital and chlorpromazine do not suppress whereas morphine does.

And yet, there are reports of morphine enhancing behavior. Wikler and his colleagues (4) reported attenuation of conditioned suppression and Rodriguez and Pardo (12) now report restoration of induced functional impairment in dogs. Even food-maintained behavioral output can be enhanced over a narrow dose range (9). There are glimpses of a truly interesting behavioral pharmacology of morphine waiting to be explored. The identification of morphine as an analgesic has suggested that there is some recognizable specific pharmacological effect — analgesia — and that it is the job of the pharmacologist to measure it. The obsession with analgesia has prevented pharmacologists from studying systematically the behavioral effects of morphine. To give a single example, a nonanalgesia so-called soporific component to the effects of morphine has been long recognized, but it has been scarcely studied and not at all analyzed; even the similarities and differences of morphine from barbiturates as a soporific have not been explored. Yet, who is to say that the "soporific" component is not as important in many of the therapeutic uses and in the abuse of morphine as the so-called analgesic component?

It is not my intention to convince you that morphine is not an analgesic drug but rather to persuade you that the term analgesia is inconsistently defined and loosely used and, more importantly, that the evidence is inadequate to establish that the dominant behavioral effect of morphine is particularly related to pain and that morphine differs from nonanalgesic drugs particularly in respect to pain; inadequate by the standards of other branches of science and other branches of pharmacology. Morphine can be shown to have behavioral effects clearly different from those of other classes of drugs, and, less decisively, drug effects on pain-related behavior can be shown to differ from the effects on other varieties of behavior, but it has not been proved in any single situation that morphine differs from nonanalgesic drugs *and* that the difference is based on the contribution of pain to the situation. Surely, morphine attenuates distress in subjects under painful stimulation, but it equally attenuates distress in subjects under nonpainful stimulation. It also attenuates satisfactions from food and fluid ingestion, from work, from sex, and more or less from all social factors. Having a nice, socially accepted term such as analgesia for ill-understood phenomena is dangerous. If you study drug effects on patterns of responding under fixed interval, and people ask what you are finding and you give a simple descriptive answer, they make it clear that they are not satisfied, and you are impelled to explore the context and try to develop some more general and satisfying conclusions. If, however, you say you are measuring analgesic activity, they go away satisfied, thinking you have said something and soon you, too, come to think you have said something meaningful. To paraphrase Karl Marx, names are the opiate of the pharmacologist. In the past when morphine was largely confined to clinical use, the question of whether the effect of morphine on distress was selective was largely academic. But this volume is in response to the widespread use of morphine and its congerers in a more or less normal population and it behooves us to be concerned to get a balanced view of morphine.

In conclusion, although an important contribution of studies in animals is prediction of clinical therapeutic activity, it is not the only contribution. Animal studies are essential for the exploration of the behavioral pharmacology of morphine. We need broad studies, unfettered by prejudice based on the names of supposed effects. We need to know the relevant characteristics of situations in which morphine, pentobarbital, and chlorpromazine are similar and of situations in which they differ. We need to develop an understanding of the relevant situational and behavioral factors that influence the behavioral effects of morphine, so that, eventually, we can make some general statements about the effects. The term analgesia will either be discarded or its definition made apparent quite incidentally, just as we discarded the term cardiac sedative (for digitalis because it often slowed the heart rate) and redefined parasympathetic paralysis (for atropine) when we came to know enough about the relevant pharmacology.

As to the significance of analgesic assays, the tests are, simply, no more than they pretend to be: screening tests, valuable for guiding programs of organic synthesis toward substances with desired attributes. They cannot illuminate the whole behavioral pharmacology of morphine.

ACKNOWLEDGMENT

Studies leading to the point of view expressed in this chapter have been supported by U.S. Public Health Service grant MH 02094 from the National Institute of Mental Health.

REFERENCES

1. Azrin, N. H., Hutchinson, R. R., and Salley, R. D.: Pain aggression toward inanimate objects. J. Exp. Anal. Behav. 7:223–228, 1964.
2. Beecher, H. K.: Measurements of Subjective Responses, pp. 5–8. Oxford University Press, New York, 1959.
3. Geller, I., Kulak, J. T., Jr., and Seifter, J.: The effects of chlordiazepoxide and chlorpromazine on a punishment discrimination. Psychopharmacologia 3:374–385, 1962.
4. Hill, H. E., Kornetsky, C. H., Flanary, H. G., and Wikler, A.: Studies on anxiety associated with anticipation of pain. I. Effects of morphine. Arch. Neurol. and Psychiatr. 67:612–619, 1952.
5. Keats, A. S., and Beecher, H. K.: Pain relief with hypnotic doses of barbiturate and a hypothesis. J. Pharmacol. Exp. Ther. 100:1–13, 1950.
6. Kelleher, R. T., and Morse, W. H.: Escape behavior and punished behavior. Fed. Proc. 23:808–817, 1964.
7. Lim, R. K. S., Guzman, F., Goto, K., Braun, C., and Rodgers, D. W.: Evidence establishing central and peripheral sites of action for narcotic and non-narcotic analgesics respectively. Fed. Proc. 22:248, 1963.
8. McMillan, D. E., and Morse, W. H.: Schedules using noxious stimuli. II. Low intensity electric shock as a discriminative stimulus. J. Exp. Anal. Behav. 10:109–118, 1967.

9. McMillan, D. E., and Morse, W. H.: Some effects of morphine and morphine antagonists on schedule-controlled behavior. J. Pharmacol. Exp. Ther. *157*:175–184, 1967.
10. Mitchell, C. L.: The effect of drugs on the latency for an escape response elicited by electrical stimulation of the tooth pulp in cats. Arch. Int. Pharmacodyn. Ther. *164*:427–434, 1966.
11. Price, H. L., and Dripps, R. D.: General anesthetics. *In:* The Pharmacological Basis of Therapeutics, edited by L. S. Goodman and A. Gilman, pp. 79, 83, 85, 94. Macmillan Company, New York, 1970.
12. Rodríguez, R., and Pardo, E. G.: *This volume.*
13. Sinitsin, L. N.: Effect of morphine and other analgesics on brain evoked potentials. Int. J. Neuropharmacol. *3*:321–327, 1964.
14. Swett, W. H.: Pain. *In:* Handbook of Physiology, Section 1: Neurophysiology, Vol. 1, edited by J. Field, American Physiological Society, Washington, D.C., 1959.
15. Vane, J. R.: Prostaglandins and aspirin-like drugs. Proc. V International Cong. Pharmacol., *in press.*
16. Weitzman, E. D., and Ross, G. S.: A behavioral method for the study of pain perception in the monkey. Neurology *12*:264–272, 1962.

Narcotic Antagonists, edited by M. C. Braude, L. S. Harris, E. L. May, J. P. Smith, and J. E. Villarreal. *Advances in Biochemical Psychopharmacology, Vol. 8.* Raven Press, New York © 1974.

Assays for Narcotic Antagonist Activity in Rodents

Anne K. Pierson

Sterling-Winthrop Research Institute, Rensselaer, New York 12144

Laboratory testing for determination of narcotic antagonist activity has been traced from early, strictly qualitative detection procedures to the present state of the art. Currently useful assay procedures which have been described and discussed are the rat tail-pressure test, rat tail-flick test, rat narcosis-counteraction test, and mouse Straub tail test. It is concluded that the clinical potency of the narcotic antagonists may be predicted with a high degree of accuracy from rodent assay techniques.

INTRODUCTION

Narcotic antagonist activity is easily detected and quantified in the laboratory. Anyone who has ever observed the effect of a narcotic antagonist on an animal which has received a large dose of opiate never forgets the remarkable normalization that takes place. Although the effect is most dramatic in larger experimental animals, many of the early observations were made on rodents, and most of the current assay procedures are performed on rats and mice. Early studies providing yes or no qualitative answers in regard to the presence of this pharmacological property will be cited in this chapter, and it is hoped that a chronological resume of some of the major contributions in the area will illustrate the procedural development which has led to our present state of the art. Currently used assay techniques will be described and discussed. Tests performed on rabbits will be included since (a) lagomorphs were for many years classified as rodents (7) and (b) they are unlikely to be included in subsequent reports dealing with dogs and primates.

In all cases the ability of the test agent to prevent or abolish an opiate agonist effect is determined and the test situation should be one in which the narcotic antagonists do not exert an agonist effect.

245

HISTORICAL

Tests versus Opiate-induced Respiratory Depression

The first disclosure of specific narcotic antagonist activity was made in 1915 by Pohl (44), who reported that N-allylnorcodeine completely prevented or abolished the respiratory depression usually seen with morphine and heroin in rabbits. This observation was based upon recordings of respiratory rate and relative minute volume. Apparently pharmacologists were not particularly intrigued by this disclosure for it was at least 25 years before the next significant published work in this area appeared. Hart (28–30) confirmed the antimorphine properties of N-allylnorcodeine and concluded that the newly synthesized N-allylnormorphine also antagonized the depressant effects of morphine on the respiratory mechanism of unanesthetized rabbits. During this period Unna (49) also demonstrated the antimorphine activity of nalorphine while recording the respiratory rate of anesthetized rabbits. In 1952 the ability of levallorphan to antagonize respiratory depression induced by morphine and Dromoran® (3-hydroxy-N-methylmorphinan) in unanesthetized rabbits was reported by Fromherz and Pellmont (18) and Benson et al. (8). The latter authors monitored minute volume exchange as well as respiratory rate. This effect of levallorphan in unanesthetized rabbits was further investigated by Miller et al. (41), who found that it antagonized, further depressed, or stimulated the respiration of morphine-treated animals depending on the relative and absolute doses used. In their study postmedication volumes were expressed as a percentage of control values. Winter et al. (53) studied the reversal by nalorphine of meperidine-induced respiratory depression in anesthetized rabbits; a 1954 publication presented numerical data from individual animals on minute volume before meperidine, before nalorphine, and after nalorphine. Estimates of narcotic antagonist relative potency derived from measurements of respiratory parameters were reported by Blumberg and co-workers beginning in 1961 (10–12). These investigators found naloxone to be 10 to 15 times as powerful as nalorphine and two to three times as powerful as levallorphan as an antagonist of oxymorphone or morphine-induced respiratory depression in unanesthetized rabbits. No ED_{50} values were reported and the potency estimates were apparently based on relative amounts of drug necessary to return depressed parameters to normal levels. From another study in unanesthetized rabbits in which Rubin et al. (46) reported molar ratios of morphine to agent needed to return depressed minute volume to control levels, the potencies of levallorphan and other antagonists relative to nalorphine could be estimated.

The ability of antagonists to prevent or reverse opiate-induced respiratory depression in rats has also been studied. Smith et al. (47) stated that N-allylnormorphine prevented the respiratory depression obtained from injecting morphine, methadone, and methadone derivatives into rats, and Costa and Bonnycastle (16), using nalorphine and levallorphan, determined for several opiates the ratios of opiate to antagonist needed to return 50% depressed minute volumes to control levels in unanesthetized rats.

Tests versus Opiate-induced Analgesia

Antagonism of opiate effects in analgesic tests was demonstrated in 1943 by Unna (49), who found that N-allylnormorphine, given 20 min before morphine, prevented the analgesic effect of the latter. Also the antagonist, given 40 min after morphine, abolished its analgesic effect. These observations were made in mice by determining the threshold for pain perception in the abdominal skin following electrical shocks of known voltage. Almost a decade later Fromherz and Pellmont (18) and Benson et al. (8), utilizing thermal stimulus techniques in rats, reported that levallorphan antagonized the analgesic action of morphine and morphine-like compounds. The tail-flick test in rats was used by Orahovats et al. (42) to show degrees of reduction of opiate analgesia obtained by the administration of small doses of nalorphine. The work of Winter et al. (53, 54) was a major step forward in the quantitation of narcotic antagonist activity. In 1954 they constructed a dose-response curve using various doses of nalorphine against a standard dose of morphine in the rat tail-flick test. Nearly complete antagonism was obtained, and the linear relationship of dose to antagonist activity was clearly shown. A few years later, in a comprehensive study involving 70 N-substituted compounds related to morphine and to similar alkaloids, these investigators reported relative antimorphine activity estimates for several active drugs. Although no ED_{50} values were reported, dose-response slopes were determined for the active compounds and were compared with that obtained for nalorphine. Thus, these were probably among the first valid relative potency estimates for narcotic antagonists to be recorded.

In 1961 Blumberg et al. (11) stated that naloxone was seven times more active than nalorphine in blocking oxymorphone analgesia on the mouse hot-plate test but details for arriving at this relative potency estimate were not given. Qualitative antagonism of ED_{70} doses of several opiates by nalorphine was reported by Weinstock (50), who also used the hot-plate test in mice. In the mid 1960's Kugita and co-workers (34, 35) reported that certain N-allylphenylpiperidine derivatives could antagonize the effect of a standard dose of morphine on the pain response to a clamp placed on the tail of mice [Haffner method (23)]. Actual reductions in the % analgesia were determined after two doses of test drugs and, for comparison, after the same two doses of nalorphine.

Tests versus Opiate-induced Lenticular Opacities

According to Weinstock et al. (51), lenticular opacities in mice which were found to occur following the administration of several opiate analgesics were prevented by the simultaneous injection of small doses of nalorphine. Furthermore, if the effect had already developed, nalorphine caused it to disappear in less than one-fifth of the normal time. Cloudiness produced by cocaine was not antagonized. Further evidence of a qualitative nature regarding the specificity of this antagonism was presented in a later publication (50).

Tests versus Opiate Mortality

Unna (49) observed that prior administration of N-allylnormorphine made mice more resistant to the toxic effects of morphine since 250 mg/kg, s.c., of the antagonist raised the s.c. LD_{50} of morphine from 660 to 820 mg/kg. Furthermore, smaller divided doses given after a lethal dose of morphine markedly reduced mortality. This protective effect was also studied by Hart and McCawley (30), who constructed dose-mortality curves from fixed ratios of nalorphine and morphine. Some of the curves of the mixtures were not only horizontally displaced but also had slopes which were markedly different from the morphine slope. Prevention of opiate mortality in rodents is probably not a suitable method for quantitating narcotic antagonism since the antagonists do not prevent lethal opiate effects of a stimulant nature (55). Nevertheless, Blumberg et al. (11) have reported that naloxone was approximately three times as active as nalorphine in reducing mortality in mice from oxymorphone overdosage.

ASSAY PROCEDURES

Currently used assay techniques in rodents are described and discussed in the following sections. These procedures yield ED_{50} values and slopes of the regression lines; thus they are amenable either to rough estimates of relative potency on a screening basis or to calculation of a more precise relative potency estimate with appropriate confidence limits when concurrent assays are performed.

DESCRIPTION

Assays versus Opiates in Analgesic Tests

A. *Tail-Pressure Test—Rat*

In this technique originally described by Green et al. (20), pressure applied to the tail as previously described (21) constitutes the nociceptive stimulus and threshold pressures for the squeak-struggle response are determined 30 min after medication. A quantal interpretation of results is used based on a criterion for analgesia of a postmedication threshold at least two times the mean value of a control group. Antagonist activity is determined by injecting the test agent s.c. at the same time as morphine sulfate, 10 mg/kg, s.c. This dose of morphine is approximately four times its analgesic ED_{50} and at least twice the amount necessary to double the pain threshold in all rats. In other words, it is a supra-ED_{100} dose of morphine in this test. The antagonist ED_{50} of a test agent is the dose required to reduce the incidence of doubling of the pain threshold to 50%, as estimated by probit analysis of tests in which at least three doses of test agents are administered to groups of 10 rats each.

Masson and Stephenson (38) studied narcotic antagonism with this basic test but treated their data in a quantitative manner as described by Millar and Stephenson (40). In this modification an index of analgesia was determined for each group and plotted against the dose of drug:

$$\text{Index of analgesia} = \frac{\text{threshold pressure before drug}}{\text{threshold pressure after drug}}$$

If a rat did not squeak with a pressure four times the control figure, the index was arbitrarily taken as 0 and was included in calculating a mean value for a group. Thus, an average graded agonist effect ranging from 1.0 (no analgesia) to 0 (complete analgesia) was obtained and a reduction of agonist effect by antagonists could be observed.

Blane and Dugdall (9) have published antagonist data on several of the newer antagonists using the method as originally described (20).

B. *Tail-Flick Test—Rat*

Green et al. (20) also quantitated narcotic antagonist activity by measuring reaction times to a thermal stimulus applied to rat tails. Their criterion for analgesia and procedure for determination of the antagonist ED_{50} are the same as described for the tail-pressure test.

Harris and Pierson (25) have reported a method for evaluating narcotic antagonist activity based on graded reaction times for the tail-flick response of rats. Average premedication reaction times (set at 2 to 4 sec) and average 30-min postmedication reaction times are determined for groups of 18 rats per treatment. The maximum exposure to the stimulus is 20 sec and

$$\% \text{ agonism} = \left(\frac{\text{avg. reaction time after drug} - \text{avg. reaction time before drug}}{20 - \text{avg. reaction time before drug}} \right) \times 100$$

Agents to be tested for antagonist activity are administered s.c. 10 min before meperidine hydrochloride (60 mg/kg), morphine sulfate (15 mg/kg), or phenazocine hydrobromide (0.5 mg/kg) s.c. These doses of opiates produce approximately an 80% agonist effect as determined above. Narcotic antagonists cause a dose-dependent reduction in the expected 80% effect of the narcotic and

$$\% \text{ antagonism} = 100 - \frac{\% \text{ agonism of narcotic} + \text{test agent}}{0.80}$$

The AD_{50} of a test agent is the dose causing a 50% decrease in the effect of an approximate ED_{80} of opiate and is obtained by the method of Litchfield and Wilcoxon (36) from a plot of percent antagonism versus log-dose on probit paper for at least three dose levels of antagonist. Estimates of the narcotic antagonist activity of numerous compounds, as determined by this method, have appeared in the literature (2–6, 25, 27, 48). This method has been modified for use in mice by Harris et al. (24) and others (45, 52).

A most thorough and theoretically significant study of the antagonist action of nalorphine and levallorphan against several opiates was conducted in rats by Grumbach and Chernov (22). These investigators utilized the tail-flick test as a quantal system. Their criterion for analgesia is the failure of a rat to respond during a 20-sec exposure to the stimulus, and the agonist effect is the percentage of animals per treatment not responding 30 min after drug administration. Agents to be tested for narcotic antagonist activity are administered s.c. 5 min before a s.c. approximate ED_{80} dose of opiate, and animals receiving saline as a pretreatment serve as controls.

$$\% \text{ antagonism} = 100 \left(1 - \frac{\% \text{ rats to cut-off with } ED_{80} + \text{antagonist}}{\% \text{ rats to cut-off with } ED_{80} + \text{saline}} \right)$$

The AD_{50} of the test agent is determined either from plots of percent antagonism versus log-dose of drug or from probit analysis of data from three dose levels.

Assay versus Opiate Narcosis

Narcotic antagonist potency has been estimated by the counteraction of oxymorphone narcosis in rats by Blumberg et al. (10–15). Animals are injected s.c. with oxymorphone hydrochloride, 1 mg/kg, and narcosis with loss of righting reflex is observed within 20 min. Presumably this is at least an ED_{100} of the opiate. The test agent is injected s.c. 30 min after the opiate injection and, if the rat regains its righting reflex within 10 min, the narcosis is considered to be counteracted. The antagonist ED_{50} is determined by the method of Litchfield and Wilcoxon (36) from plots of percent counteraction versus log-dose for three dosage levels with 10 rats per level.

The Blumberg group (12) has also reported potency estimates for narcotic antagonists from a method requiring complete counteraction of narcosis induced in rats by oxymorphone hydrochloride (1 mg/kg), morphine sulfate (15 mg/kg), or meperidine hydrochloride (50 mg/kg) s.c.

Assay versus Straub Phenomenon

Prevention of the opiate-induced Straub tail in mice was used by Aceto et al. (1) to demonstrate narcotic antagonist activity. In their procedure the test agent is given in at least three doses s.c. immediately before meperidine (64 mg/kg), morphine (16 mg/kg), or phenazocine (1.0 mg/kg) s.c. These doses of opiates are approximate ED_{84}, ED_{88}, and ED_{100} agonist doses respectively. Groups of animals receiving distilled water as a pretreatment serve as controls, and treatment groups consist of 15 or 25 animals. The Straub reaction is defined as elevation of the tail at angles greater than 45° and the number of animals showing the reaction from 15 to 25 min after injection is tabulated. Aceto and co-workers recommend that the experiment be conducted in a sound-attenuated room to minimize the effects of noise on the reaction. The antagonist ED_{50} is the dose of test agent at which only 50% of the mice exhibit the reaction and is estimated according to the method of Litchfield and Wilcoxon (36).

Blumberg et al. (14) reported somewhat earlier on the potency of a test agent relative to nalorphine in preventing the oxymorphone-induced mouse Straub tail, but no details of the procedure were given.

Assay versus Opiate Respiratory Depression

Matsumoto et al. (39) have reported a method for estimating narcotic antagonist potency by measuring the reversal of respiratory depression produced in unanesthetized rabbits by morphine. Minute volume and rate are recorded, and all drugs are administered intravenously. Various doses of the test agent are given 10 min after a depressant dose of morphine and the degree of antagonism is recorded 5 min later. The AD_{50}, or 50% antagonizing dose, is calculated by the method of Litchfield and Wilcoxon (36).

DISCUSSION

A summary of relative potencies for several narcotic antagonists is presented in Table 1; an effort was made to include as many compounds in as many test situations as possible. In some cases the relative potencies were taken directly from statements in published sources; in other cases I derived them from ED_{50} values in published sources. It should be understood that in most instances these potencies are rough estimates and were obtained without concurrent assays of standard and test agent, or other possible control conditions. Actually, the rat tail-flick AD_{50} values upon which the potency estimates from the Sterling-Winthrop group are based were determined in the course of routine screening over a number of years. Nevertheless there is amazingly good overall agreement among the various techniques, although a few minor exceptions can be noted.

It was the general impression of Archer and Harris (4) that the Winter method (54) tends to minimize differences between active drugs. I am inclined to agree with that impression and suggest that the inclusion of the "duration factor" in this technique may be at least partially responsible since various combinations of peak potency and duration of antagonists could result in similar reductions in minute-seconds of analgesia.

Blumberg et al. (10–12, 15) have studied the ability of narcotic antagonists to reverse oxymorphone-induced narcosis in rats by means of two criteria. When return of the righting reflex was observed the potencies of levallorphan and naloxone relative to nalorphine were 3.4 and 11 to 19 respectively. When complete counteraction of narcosis was required, the potencies of levallorphan and naloxone relative to nalorphine were eight and 48 respectively. When the relative potency estimates for levallorphan and naloxone in all procedures are considered, the complete counteraction test appeared to overestimate the potency of these two drugs. On the other hand, in the righting reflex test the relative potencies of cyclazocine and cyclorphan appear to be somewhat underestimated. There is evidence that they are more potent than levallorphan (2, 19, 25, 32). This discrepancy may be an artifact related to the discoordinative muscle-relaxant and polyneuronal-blocking properties of the two N-cyclopropylmethyl compounds (25, 27, 43). The antagonist ED_{50} values for cyclazocine and cyclorphan are 0.45

TABLE 1. *Potency of antagonists relative to nalorphine in rodent assays*

Drug	Versus analgesia		Versus narcosis	Versus Straub tail	Versus respiratory depression
	Tail flick, rat[a]	Tail pressure, rat[b]	Rat[c]	Mouse[a]	Rabbit[d,e]
N-Allylnorcodeine	0.4 (54)	0.02 (20)	—	—	—
Nalorphine	1	1	1	1	1
Levallorphan	0.7 (54) 2.5[f] (2) 3 (22)	1.6 (9)	3.4 (12, 15) 8[g] (12)	4.7 (1)	4–5 (10–12) 3 (46)
Pentazocine	0.03[f] (25)	0.016 (9)	0.05 (12, 15)	0.05 (1)	—
Cyclazocine	7[f] (25)	—	1.8 (12, 15)	6.3 (1)	—
Cyclorphan	3.8[f] (19, 27)	—	2.0 (12, 15)	4.0 (1)	
Naloxone	32[f] (1, 6)	—	11–19 (10–12, 15) 48[g] (12)	16 (1)	10–15 (10–12) 7,12,61[h] (39)

[a] versus meperidine; [b] versus morphine; [c] versus oxymorphone; [d] versus oxymorphone and/or morphine; [e] drugs given i.v., all others given s.c.; [f] test performed at S.W.R.I. by H. Lawyer; [g] criterion for antagonism = complete counteraction, others in column = return of righting reflex; [h] versus different morphine doses, see text for explanation.

and 0.40 mg/kg s.c., respectively (see Table 3, second column from right). The discoordinative ED_{50} doses, as reported by Pearl et al. (43) in the mouse rotorod test, are 1.58 and 1.56 mg/kg s.c., respectively, or roughly three to four times the antagonist ED_{50}'s.

The naloxone relative potency estimate from the tail-flick test seems to be a little high in comparison with those obtained from the other tests.

The relative potency estimates for naloxone- versus morphine-induced respiratory depression derived from the work of Matsumoto et al. (39) require further clarification. AD_{50} values for nalorphine and naloxone were calculated versus three doses of morphine (Table 2). Increasingly larger doses of naloxone were required to antagonize the larger morphine doses, but the AD_{50} doses of nalorphine remained relatively constant. Therefore, the potency of naloxone relative to nalorphine appears to decrease as the standard dose of morphine is increased. These findings may reflect a problem inherent in any attempt to evaluate narcotic antagonism in a system where drugs such as nalorphine are capable of exerting an agonist effect. The ability of similar doses of nalorphine to antagonize the larger doses of morphine may reflect its greater efficacy in the presence of severe respiratory depression. Since naloxone is apparently devoid of agonist activity as a respiratory depressant (37), the proportionately larger AD_{50} values obtained versus the higher doses of morphine are most likely indicative of a pure competitive antagonism situation. The complex interactions occurring between opiates and antagonists which are also partial agonists (37) probably militate against the use of respiratory depression tests when accurate, quantitative, relative potency estimates are desired. Nevertheless it must be admitted that the estimates which Blumberg et al. (10–12) have reported from respiratory depression studies in unanesthetized rabbits, using one standard dose of opiate, are in good agreement with the others.

The antagonist ED_{50} values for several antagonists in the rat and mouse tests are listed in Table 3. The mg/kg doses versus meperidine, 60 mg/kg

TABLE 2. *Nalorphine and naloxone versus morphine-induced respiratory depression (unanesthetized rabbit)*

Drug	AD_{50}[a], mg/kg i.v. versus morphine HCl		
	4 mg/kg, i.v.	16 mg/kg, i.v.	32 mg/kg, i.v.
Nalorphine	0.36	0.36	0.54
Naloxone	0.0059	0.031	0.077

[a] From Matsumoto et al., 1972 (39).

TABLE 3. Antagonist ED_{50}'s (mg/kg, s.c.) in rodent assays

Drug	Tail-flick, rat versus meperidine (60 mg/kg, s.c.)	Tail-pressure, rat versus morphine (10 mg/kg, s.c.)	Narcosis[a], rat versus oxymorphone (1.0 mg/kg, s.c.)	Straub tail, mouse versus meperidine (64 mg/kg, s.c.)
Nalorphine	0.13[c] (25) 0.112[b] (22)	0.79 (20) 0.48 (9)	0.81 (15)	0.094 (1)
Levallorphan	0.052[c] (2) 0.035[b] (22)	0.30 (9)	0.24 (15)	0.020 (1)
Pentazocine	3.9[c] (25)	≈30 (9)	16 (15)	1.9 (1)
D-Pentazocine	14[c] (48)	—	—	8.8 (1)
L-Pentazocine	0.9[c] (48)	—	—	0.66 (1)
Cyclazocine	0.019[c] (25)	—	0.45 (15)	0.015 (1)
D-Cyclazocine	2.5[c] (48)	—	—	3.0 (1)
L-Cyclazocine	0.006[c] (48)	—	—	0.006 (1)
Cyclorphan	0.034[c] (19,27)	—	0.40 (15)	0.024 (1)
Naloxone	0.004[c] (1,6)	—	0.045 (15) 0.1[d] (12)	0.006 (1)

[a] criterion = return of righting reflex; [b] versus meperidine, 120 mg/kg, s.c.; [c] test performed at S.W.R.I. by H. Lawyer; [d] criterion = complete counteraction.

255

s.c., in the rat tail-flick test and the mg/kg doses versus meperidine, 64 mg/kg s.c., in the mouse Straub tail test are remarkably similar. Also, the actual 50% effective antagonist doses of nalorphine and levallorphan obtained by Harris and Pierson (25) using a graded response for the tail flick are almost identical to those of Grumbach and Chernov (22), who used a quantal response. Generally, the 50% effective doses of antagonists in the rat tail-pressure test and the rat narcosis-counteraction test were approximately 10 times the ED_{50} doses in the other two tests. This is not surprising since, in the tests requiring larger doses of antagonists, supra-ED_{100} doses of opiate are employed to produce the agonist effect. Likewise, the amount of naloxone needed to completely counteract oxymorphone narcosis was nearly double the amount needed to return the righting reflex.

In spite of the overall excellent agreement among the various techniques for the estimation of antagonist relative potency it is wise to obey the rules for proper experimental design when precise relative potency estimates are desired or required. A case in point is the potency of L-cyclazocine relative to DL-cyclazocine. It has previously been reported (4, 5) that the L-isomer was approximately four times as active as the racemate versus meperidine in the rat tail-flick test. This estimate was based on assays conducted at different points in time. Table 4 contains data on cyclazocine and its L-isomer versus phenazocine in the tail-flick test. When the AD_{50} of DL-cyclazocine obtained in 1962 is compared with the AD_{50} of L-cyclazocine obtained in 1965 the L-isomer appears to be nearly five times as active as the racemate. However, when concurrent assays of the drugs were performed in 1971, the potency ratio of the L-form to the racemate was closer to the expected 2:1. According to Jasinski (31), L-cyclazocine is twice as potent as cyclazocine in precipitating abstinence in human subjects dependent on morphine, 240 mg/day.

For a number of years the Sterling-Winthrop group routinely used meperidine as the agonist in the rat tail-flick test when screening for narcotic antagonist activity. In the course of our experience it was noted that oc-

TABLE 4. *Antagonist activity of cyclazocine and L-cyclazocine*

Drug	AD_{50}[a], mg/kg, s.c. versus phenazocine HBR, 0.5 mg/kg, s.c.	
Cyclazocine	0.028[b]	0.007[d]
L-Cyclazocine	0.0055[c]	0.0025[d]

[a] All tests performed at S.W.R.I. by H. Lawyer; [b] test performed in 1962; [c] test performed in 1965; [d] test performed in 1971, concurrent assays.

casionally a test compound displayed what we initially considered to be atypical narcotic antagonist activity. The compound appeared to be active to some extent, e.g., 50 to 60% antagonism might be observed at a particular dose or doses, but complete antagonism of the standard dose of meperidine was not achieved even when the dose of test compound was increased severalfold. In addition, when subsequently the compound was tested versus morphine or phenazocine, negative results were obtained. While filling out profiles of activity for various drugs with other CNS properties, it was found that diazepam (Valium®) was such a compound (see Table 5). Some data indicative of antagonism of meperidine were obtained at doses from 1.25 to 80 mg/kg s.c., but a complete dose response could not be obtained, and no antagonism of morphine or phenazocine was observed. These and other data have suggested to us that, for some as yet undefined reason, it is possible to obtain false positive results when meperidine is used as the agonist in the rat tail-flick test. When chlordiazepoxide (Librium®) was tested at several doses ranging from 0.05 to 80 mg/kg s.c. versus meperidine, most treatments were inactive but some apparent antagonism ($\leq 30\%$) was noted at 5.0 and 10 mg/kg s.c. The observations on diazepam and chlordiazepoxide were made in our laboratory in 1966. A few years later reports of morphine-antagonist activity in laboratory animals associated with these two drugs appeared in the literature (45, 52). Weiss (52), using a mouse tail-flick test, showed an atypical, biphasic dose response for chlordiazepoxide with a peak antagonistic effect of nearly 80% at approximately 50 mg/kg s.c. The fixed dose of morphine HCl (5 mg/kg s.c.)

TABLE 5. *Narcotic antagonist activity of diazepam in rats*

Dose of diazepam (mg/kg, s.c.)	Versus meperidine HCl (60 mg/kg s.c.)		Versus morphine SO₄ (15 mg/kg s.c.)		Versus phenazocine HBr (0.5 mg/kg s.c.)	
	No. of Rats	% Antagonism[a]	No. of Rats	% Antagonism[a]	No. of Rats	% Antagonism[a]
80	6	34	6	0	6	9
40	6	27	6	6	—	—
20	6	44	—	—	—	—
10	18	56	6	0	6	0
5.0	18	59	6	0	6	0
2.5	18	39	6	16	—	—
1.25	18	45	—	—	—	—
1.0	6	13	6	2	6	0
0.625	18	10	—	—	—	—
0.1	6	0	6	7	6	0

[a] Calculated according to the Harris and Pierson method, 1964 (25)

used in this experiment resulted in only 40 to 50% analgesia, a factor probably contributing bias in favor of demonstration of antagonism. However, Randall et al. (45), using a standard 10 mg/kg s.c. dose of morphine SO_4 and a mouse tail-flick test, confirmed the Weiss observation and reported an antagonist ED_{50} of 4.5 mg/kg s.c. for chlordiazepoxide. These authors also reported diazepam to be active in the range of chlordiazepoxide with an antagonist ED_{50} of 2.1 mg/kg s.c., but they commented that this effect could be demonstrated only in a very narrow dose range. Since they did not fully describe the antagonist dose responses for these drugs or compare them with the dose response of a typical narcotic antagonist such as nalorphine in their test system, it is difficult to reach a conclusion as to the significance of these findings. Their significance is truly questionable when one considers that narcotic antagonism has not been observed with these drugs clinically, and it seems highly improbable that this pharmacological property could have gone unrecognized, particularly in view of their frequent administration in conjunction with opiate therapy.

At the Sterling-Winthrop laboratory, where the rat tail-flick test has been used for more than 10 years, the following conditions have been found to contribute to the specificity of the test: (a) The thermal stimulus is of such an intensity that *only* opiates can cause the maximum possible agonist effect. (b) A test compound must demonstrate a full-scale antagonism dose-effect relationship against a dose of opiate which customarily produces 80 to 90% of the maximum possible agonist effect, to be considered a narcotic antagonist. (c) Phenazocine is now routinely used as the agonist in screening tests and the presence of narcotic antagonist activity may be confirmed in tests versus morphine and/or meperidine.

The utility of a laboratory procedure is to a great extent dependent upon the accuracy with which clinical efficacy can be predicted from laboratory results. Table 6 presents potency estimates relative to nalorphine for four narcotic antagonists based on results from assay procedures in which an agonist effect of a standard dose of morphine is prevented, together with potency estimates of the drugs as precipitants of abstinence in human subjects dependent on morphine, 240 mg/day (32). Potency estimates for two of the drugs as antagonists of opiate-induced respiratory depression in surgical patients (17) are available and are also included. It is obvious that the potency estimates obtained in the laboratory with these techniques, even rough estimates from routine screening tests, correlate very well with potency estimates obtained in human studies. Therefore, currently used rodent assay procedures for narcotic antagonist activity do predict clinical narcotic antagonist efficacy with a high degree of accuracy.

TABLE 6. *Potency of antagonists relative to nalorphine versus morphine: laboratory assays and man*

	Rat		Mouse	Man
Drug	Tail flick versus morphine (15 mg/kg, s.c.)	Tail pressure versus morphine (10 mg/kg, s.c.)	Straub tail versus morphine (16 mg/kg, s.c.)	Abstinence precipitation versus morphine (240 mg/day, s.c.)
Nalorphine	1	1	1	1
Levallorphan	3.3 (26)	1.6 (9)	3.7 (1)	1.9 (32)
				5ᵃ (17)
Pentazocine	0.014 (25)	0.016 (9)	0.07 (1)	0.02 (33)
Cyclazocine	4.5 (25)	—	5.6 (1)	5.5 (32)
Naloxone	32 (26)	—	16 (1)	7 (32)
				30ᵃ (17)

ª Versus opiate-induced respiratory depression in surgical patients.

REFERENCES

1. Aceto, M. D., McKean, D. B., and Pearl, J.: Effects of opiates and opiate antagonists on the Straub tail reaction in mice. Brit. J. Pharmacol. *36*:225–239, 1969.
2. Archer, S., Albertson, N. F., Harris, L. S., Pierson, A. K., and Bird, J. G.: Pentazocine. Strong analgesics and analgesic antagonists in the benzomorphan series. J. Med. Chem. *7*:123–127, 1964.
3. Archer, S., Albertson, N. F., Harris, L. S., Pierson, A. K., Bird, J. G., Keats, A. S., Telford, J., and Papadopoulos, C. N.: Narcotic antagonists as analgesics. Science *137*:541–542, 1962.
4. Archer, S., and Harris, L. S.: Narcotic antagonists. *In:* Progress in Drug Research, edited by E. Jucker, pp. 261–320, Birkhäuser Verlag, Basel, 1965.
5. Archer, S., Harris, L. S., Albertson, N. F., Tullar, B. F., and Pierson, A. K.: Narcotic antagonists as analgesics; laboratory aspects. *In:* Molecular Modification in Drug Design, Advances in Chemistry Series No. 45, edited by R. F. Gould, pp. 162–169, American Chemical Society, Washington, D.C., 1964.
6. Archer, S., Pierson, A. K., Pittman, K., and Aceto, M.: Laboratory and clinical studies with pentazocine and related compounds. *In:* Pain, edited by R. Janzen, W. D. Keidel, A. Herz, C. Steichele, J. P. Payne, and R. A. P. Burt, pp. 282–288, Georg Thieme, Stuttgart, and Churchill Livingstone, London, 1972.
7. Arrington, L. R.: Introductory Laboratory Animal Science. The Interstate Printers and Publishers, Inc., Danville, Illinois, 1972.
8. Benson, W. M., O'Gara, E., and Van Winkle, S.: Respiratory and analgesic antagonism of Dromoran by 3-hydroxy-N-allyl morphinan. J. Pharmacol. Exp. Ther. *106*:373, 1952.
9. Blane, G. F., and Dugdall, D.: Interactions of narcotic antagonists and antagonist-analgesics. J. Pharm. Pharmacol. *20*:547–552, 1968.
10. Blumberg, H., Dayton, H. B., and George, M.: Combinations of the analgesic oxymorphone with the narcotic antagonist N-allylnoroxymorphone. Fed. Proc. *21*:327, 1962.
11. Blumberg, H., Dayton, H. B., George, M., and Rapaport, D. N.: N-allylnoroxymorphone: A potent narcotic antagonist. Fed. Proc. *20*:311, 1961.
12. Blumberg, H., Dayton, H. B., and Wolf, P. S.: Narcotic antagonist activity of naloxone. Fed. Proc. *24*:676, 1965.

13. Blumberg, H., Dayton, H. B., and Wolf, P. S.: Analgesic and narcotic antagonist properties of noroxymorphone derivatives. Toxicol. Appl. Pharmacol. *10*:406, 1967.
14. Blumberg, H., Dayton, H. B., and Wolf, P. S.: Analgesic properties of the narcotic antagonist EN-2234A. Pharmacologist *10*:189, 1968.
15. Blumberg, H., Wolf, P. S., and Dayton, H. B.: Use of writing test for evaluating analgesic activity of narcotic antagonists. Proc. Soc. Exp. Biol. Med. *118*:763–766, 1965.
16. Costa, P. J., and Bonnycastle, D. D.: The effect of levallorphan tartrate, nalorphine HCl and Win 7681 (1-allyl-4-phenyl-4-carbethoxypiperidine) on respiratory depression and analgesia induced by some active analgetics. J. Pharmacol. Exp. Ther. *113*:310–318, 1955.
17. Foldes, F. F., Lunn, J. N., Moore, J., and Brown, I. M.: N-allylnoroxymorphone: A new potent narcotic antagonist. Amer. J. Med. Sci. *245*:23–30, 1963.
18. Fromherz, K., and Pellmont, B.: Morphinantagonisten. Experientia *8*:394–395, 1952.
19. Gates, M., and Montzka, T. A.: Some potent morphine antagonists possessing high analgesic activity. J. Med. Chem. *7*:127–131, 1964.
20. Green, A. F., Ruffell, G. K., and Walton, E.: Morphine derivatives with antianalgesic action. J. Pharm. Pharmacol. *6*:390–397, 1954.
21. Green, A. F., and Young, P. A.: A comparison of heat and pressure analgesiometric methods in rats. Brit. J. Pharmacol. *6*:572–587, 1951.
22. Grumbach, L., and Chernov, H. I.: The analgesic effect of opiate-opiate antagonist combinations in the rat. J. Pharmacol. Exp. Ther. *149*:385–396, 1965.
23. Haffner, F.: Experimentelle prüfung schmerzstellender mittel. Deut. Med. Wochenschr. *55*:731–733, 1929.
24. Harris, L. S., Dewey, W. L., Howes, J. F., Kennedy, J. S., and Pars, H.: Narcotic-antagonist analgesics: Interactions with cholinergic systems. J. Pharmacol. Exp. Ther. *169*:17–22, 1969.
25. Harris, L. S., and Pierson, A. K.: Some narcotic antagonists in the benzomorphan series. J. Pharmacol. Exp. Ther. *143*:141–148, 1964.
26. Harris, L. S., and Pierson, A. K.: *Unpublished observations.*
27. Harris, L. S., Pierson, A. K., Dembinski, J. R., and Dewey, W. L.: The pharmacology of (−)-3-hydroxy-N-cyclopropylmethylmorphinan (cyclorphan). Arch. Int. Pharmacodyn. Ther. *165*:112–126, 1967.
28. Hart, E. R.: N-Allyl-norcodeine and N-allyl-normorphine, two antagonists to morphine. J. Pharmacol. Exp. Ther. *72*:19, 1941.
29. Hart, E. R.: Further observations on the antagonistic actions of N-allylnormorphine against morphine. Fed. Proc. *2*:82, 1943.
30. Hart, E. R., and McCawley, E. L.: The pharmacology of N-allylnormorphine as compared with morphine. J. Pharmacol. Exp. Ther. *82*:339–348, 1944.
31. Jasinski, D. R.: Studies in man of optical isomers of some opioid antagonists. Fifth International Congress on Pharmacology, Satellite Symposium on Narcotics Research. July 29, 1972.
32. Jasinski, D. R., Martin, W. R., and Haertzen, C. A.: The human pharmacology and abuse potential of N-allylnoroxymorphone (Naloxone). J. Pharmacol. Exp. Ther. *157*:420–426, 1967.
33. Jasinski, D. R., Martin, W. R., and Hoeldtke, R. D.: Effects of short- and long-term administration of pentazocine in man. Clin. Pharmacol. Ther. *11*:385–403, 1970.
34. Kugita, H., Inoue, H., Oine, T., Hayashi, G., and Nurimoto, S.: 3-Alkyl-3-phenylpiperidine derivatives as analgesics. J. Med. Chem. *7*:298–301, 1964.
35. Kugita, H., Oine, T., Inoue, H., and Hayashi, G.: 3-Alkyl-3-phenylpiperidine derivatives as analgesics. II. J. Med. Chem. *8*:313–316, 1965.
36. Litchfield, J. T., and Wilcoxon, F.: A simplified method of evaluating dose-effect experiments. J. Pharmacol. Exp. Ther. *96*:99–113, 1949.
37. Martin, W. R.: Opioid antagonists. Pharmacol. Rev. *19*:463–521, 1967.
38. Masson, A. H. B., and Stephenson, R. P.: Antagonism of pethidine by levallorphan in rats. Anaesthesia *14*:345–348, 1959.
39. Matsumoto, S., Oka, T., Takemori, A. E., and Hosoya, E.: Comparative studies on the

antagonism of naloxone and nalorphine to the morphine-induced respiratory depression in rabbits. Jap. J. Pharmacol. *22*:Suppl. 89, 1972.

40. Millar, R. A., and Stephenson, R. P.: Analgesic action in a series of N-substituted ethyl 4-phenylpiperidine-4-carboxylates. Brit. J. Pharmacol. *11*:27–31, 1956.

41. Miller, J. W., Gilfoil, T. M., and Shideman, F. E.: The effects of levallorphan tartrate (levo-3-hydroxy-N-allylmorphinan tartrate) on the respiration of rabbits given morphine. J. Pharmacol. Exp. Ther. *115*:350–359, 1955.

42. Orahovats, P. D., Winter, C. A., and Lehman, E. G.: Pharmacological studies of mixtures of narcotics and N-allylnormorphine. J. Pharmacol. Exp. Ther. *112*:246–251, 1954.

43. Pearl, J., Aceto, M. D., and Harris, L. S.: Prevention of writhing and other effects of narcotics and narcotic antagonists in mice. J. Pharmacol. Exp. Ther. *160*:217–230, 1968.

44. Pohl, J.: Ueber das N-allylnorcodein, einen antagonisten des morphins. Z. Exp. Path. Ther. *17*:370–382, 1915.

45. Randall, L. O., Scheckel, C. L., and Pool, W.: Pharmacology of medazepam and metabolites. Arch. Int. Pharmacodyn. Ther. *185*:135–148, 1970.

46. Rubin, A., Chernov, H. I., Miller, J. W., and Mannering, G. J.: Antagonism of morphine-induced respiratory depression and analgesia and inhibition of narcotic N-demethylation in vitro by N-substituted analogues of L-3-hydroxymorphinan and by N-allyl-normorphine. J. Pharmacol. Exp. Ther. *144*:346–353, 1964.

47. Smith, C. C., Lehman, E. G., and Gilfillan, J. L.: Antagonistic action of N-allyl-normorphine upon the analgetic and toxic effects of morphine, methadone derivatives and isonipecaine. Fed. Proc. *10*:335–336, 1951.

48. Tullar, B. F., Harris, L. S., Perry, R. L., Pierson, A. K., Soria, A. E., Wetterau, W. F., and Albertson, N. F.: Benzomorphans. Optically active and trans isomers. J. Med. Chem. *10*:383–386, 1967.

49. Unna, K.: Antagonistic effect of N-allyl-normorphine upon morphine. J. Pharmacol. Exp. Ther. *79*:27–31, 1943.

50. Weinstock, M.: Similarity between receptors responsible for the production of analgesia and lenticular opacity. Brit. J. Pharmacol. *17*:433–441, 1961.

51. Weinstock, M., Stewart, H. C., and Butterworth, K. R.: Lenticular effect in mice of some morphine-like drugs. Nature *182*:1519–1520, 1958.

52. Weis, J.: Morphine antagonistic effect of chlordiazepoxide (Librium®). Experientia *25*:381, 1969.

53. Winter, C. A., Orahovats, P. D., Flataker, L., Lehman, E. G., and Lehman, J. T.: Studies on the pharmacology of N-allylnormorphine. J. Pharmacol. Exp. Ther. *111*:152–160, 1954.

54. Winter, C. A., Orahovats, P. D., and Lehman, E. G.: Analgesic activity and morphine antagonism of compounds related to nalorphine. Arch. Int. Pharmacodyn. Ther. *110*:186–202, 1957.

55. Woods, L. A.: The pharmacology of nalorphine (N-allylnormorphine). Pharmacol. Rev. *8*:175–198, 1956.

Narcotic Antagonists, edited by M. C. Braude, L. S. Harris, E. L. May, J. P. Smith, and J. E. Villarreal. *Advances in Biochemical Psychopharmacology, Vol. 8.* Raven Press, New York © 1974.

Narcotic-Antagonist Assay Procedures in Dogs

William L. Dewey

Department of Pharmacology, Medical College of Virginia, Richmond, Virginia 23219, and Department of Pharmacology, School of Medicine, University of North Carolina, Chapel Hill, North Carolina 27514

Dogs have not been widely used to screen for analgesic or analgesic-antagonist activity for a number of reasons. An inability to quantitate the response in this species and the high cost of animals are paramount among them. However, anesthetized dogs have been used to test for the ability of compounds to antagonize the respiratory depression produced by narcotic analgesics. There is a correlation between the activity of antagonists in reversing respiratory depression caused by opiates in dogs and their potency in reversing many of the effects of opiates in man. Physical dependence on narcotic analgesics can be produced in dogs by a 1-day intravenous infusion of an opiate. This model can be used for studying addiction liability of an unknown compound or for the ability of the pretreatment of an antagonist to inhibit dependence development. The advantages and shortcomings of each of these types of experiments are discussed.

Certain criteria are necessary for a particular test procedure to be useful as a bioassay procedure for determining relative potencies of drugs. First, the results obtained from such an assay should allow potency predictability in man. That is, the potency and duration of action of each of a series of compounds as narcotic antagonists in the dog should correlate with their potency and duration of action as narcotic antagonists in man. Secondly, the test procedure must yield reproducible results. Ideally the procedure should be relatively easy to run, not be costly nor too time consuming, and the data should be amenable to strict statistical analysis. A considerable amount of work has been done with narcotic antagonists in dogs. This review will attempt to summarize the information obtained from these studies and to evaluate the merits of the use of dogs to assay for narcotic-antagonist activity. The criteria mentioned above will be used as a guideline in the evaluation procedure.

OVERT BEHAVIOR IN DOGS

A number of techniques have been used to determine the narcotic-antagonist potency of a compound in dogs. One method which has been used (4) is to induce overt behavioral changes in unanesthetized dogs by injecting a narcotic analgesic such as morphine or meperidine and once ataxia, sedation, loss of postural reflex, vomiting, defecation, and salivation are observed, the purported antagonist is given by the intravenous route of administration. A qualitative estimate of the antagonism is made 5 to 10 min after the intravenous injection. The best one can do with an overt behavioral test of this nature is set an arbitrary scale to determine if the antagonism is poor, fair, or good for each dose of the drug tested. Using this type of procedure, known narcotic antagonists such as nalorphine produce significant antagonism within this time period.

Table 1 contains a list of many of the effects produced in dogs by an injection of a narcotic analgesic. Each of these effects has been prevented or reversed by an injection of a narcotic antagonist. The first report of narcotic-antagonist activity appeared in 1943. Unna reported that 10 or 20 mg/kg nalorphine given either 20 or 60 min prior to the injection of 5 or 10 mg/kg morphine blocked the vomiting, drowsiness, and ataxia usually observed with these doses of the narcotic (13). He also reported that nalorphine could reverse the drowsiness induced by a previous injection of 5 mg/kg morphine in dogs. The specificity for the narcotic-antagonist effect of nalorphine was evident when this drug did not inhibit the vomiting induced in dogs by apomorphine. Furthermore, as subsequently demonstrated (7), nalorphine also could antagonize the effects of a number of other narcotics. The intravenous administration of 20 mg/kg nalorphine blocked the lethal respiratory depression in dogs produced by high doses of codeine, dilaudid, metapon, or methadone but not that of meperidine. The same dose of nalorphine given 30 sec after respiration had stopped following an injection of a lethal dose of codeine, dilaudid, metapon, or methadone restored the respiration to normal values, although it did not reverse the lethal respiratory depression produced by meperidine (7). In another study (12) nalorphine reversed the miosis, hypothermia, respiratory depression, and

TABLE 1. *Effects of narcotic analgesics in dogs which have been either blocked or reversed by narcotic antagonists*

Analgesia	Miosis
Ataxia	Salivation
Loss of postural reflex	Vomiting
Marked sedation	Bradycardia
Narcosis	Hypotension
Respiratory depression	Increased intestinal tone
Hypothermia	

bradycardia produced in dogs by morphine, methadone, heptazone, acetyl-DL-methadol, or isonipecaine.

It has been shown by Heng and Domino (6) that an intravenous injection of 2 mg/kg morphine significantly increased the threshold voltage which could be applied to dog tooth pulp. This apparent analgesic effect of morphine was antagonized by 1 mg/kg nalorphine. The difficulty in handling dogs for this type of procedure and the irreproducibility of the measurements obtained with tooth pulp stimulation experiments in the guinea pig and rabbit suggest that this procedure is not a feasible bioassay for narcotic-antagonist activity.

Orahovats and his colleagues (11) have shown that one can inhibit the emesis and respiratory effects of 2 mg/kg morphine if this narcotic is given in combination with 0.15 mg/kg nalorphine. They also observed a decrease but not a complete reversal in the hypothermia, miosis, and bradycardia produced by morphine when the antagonist was also given.

Harris (3) has shown that the potent narcotic-antagonist cyclazocine produces a good antagonism of the behavioral effect of either morphine or meperidine in dogs. Pentazocine, which has relatively weak narcotic-antagonist activity in the rodent tests also, did not produce a good reversal of the effects of either morphine or meperidine in dogs. As a matter of fact, some evidence of an additive effect was observed between the weak antagonists and the narcotics. This was particularly true at higher doses of the antagonist. A number of deaths occurred with these combinations. In essence, this study showed that the potency of four benzomorphans and nalorphine in antagonizing the effects of narcotics in dogs was similar to their potency in producing narcotic antagonism in the rodent analgesic procedures.

Gray (2) has studied the ability of the narcotic antagonists nalorphine and levallorphan to antagonize the increased intestinal tone produced by a number of narcotic analgesics. Due to the fact that the analgesics do not produce data amenable to a dose-response analysis on intestinal tone, an all or none response was used. The criterion for the antagonism studies was complete prevention of the visible change in tone produced within 5 min after administration of the narcotic.

In the reversal studies when the antagonist was given after the narcotic, the return of the intestine to its normal tone was a positive response. Both levallorphan and nalorphine antagonized the actions of the analgesics in this procedure. However, the amount of antagonist needed for prevention or reversal of the increased tone was quite constant regardless of the dose of analgesic that was used. The effective dose of levallorphan was between 0.01 and 0.05 micromoles/kg and for nalorphine between 0.015 and 0.075

micromoles/kg. The lack of dose-response effect for the antagonists makes this a very poor preparation for assay of narcotic antagonists.

Dayton and Blumberg (1) have reported that naloxone at the small dose of 0.04 mg/kg given either subcutaneously, intramuscularly, or intravenously antagonized the depression in dogs produced by meperidine, morphine, fentanyl, or oxymorphone. Repeated administrations of the relatively pure antagonist, naloxone to nonpretreated dogs did not produce a decrease in minute volume as was observed with repeated administrations of equiantagonistic doses of nalorphine.

In summary, these studies on the effects of narcotic antagonists on the overt behavioral effects of the potent analgesics show that all the antagonists tested will prevent or inhibit the effects of each of the analgesics. It appears that nalorphine is not a good antagonist to the effects of meperidine but this phenomenon also appears in man (1a). The order of potency for antagonistic activity in dogs correlates well with the order of potency for the antagonism seen in rodent tests or in man. Although this is the main criteria for a good assay procedure, the dog test is less than an ideal screen due to the subjectiveness of the observations (double-blind experiments and semiquantitative worksheets would be helpful), the cost of the experiments, and the time necessary to test each animal. It appears, therefore, that the reversal of overt behavior in dogs has no advantages over the less expensive and faster techniques used in rodents.

REVERSAL OF RESPIRATORY AND CARDIOVASCULAR DEPRESSION

Another assay of narcotic-antagonistic activity is performed to determine the ability of a compound to reverse the respiratory and cardiovascular depression produced by narcotic analgesics in anesthetized dogs. Mongrel dogs of either sex are used in these studies and anesthetized with an intravenous injection of 15 mg/kg sodium thiopental followed immediately with 250 to 300 mg/kg sodium barbital. This barbiturate combination is recommended for these experiments because a deep level of anesthesia is obtained which lasts for at least 6 hr. Therefore, there are no changes in respiratory or cardiovascular parameters due to a lightening of the anesthesia during the experiment. Blood pressure, heart rate, pulmonary ventilation rate, and percent CO_2 in expired air are measured throughout the experiment. Once each of these parameters has stabilized, an injection of a narcotic analgesic is administered which causes a depression of the cardiovascular and respiratory systems as indicated by these measurements. The purported narcotic antagonist is then injected intravenously and the degree of antagonism is measured 5 min later. This technique has been used to determine parameters of narcotic-antagonistic activity for new compounds (4) and also in the search for compounds which might be useful in reversing cardiovascular and, even more importantly, the respiratory depression which can be seen in some patients given the narcotic-antagonist analgesic pentazocine (3).

The ability of nalorphine, cyclazocine, and pentazocine to antagonize the respiratory and cardiovascular depression produced by meperidine is shown by the data presented in Table 2. In general, the activity of these compounds versus morphine-induced depression of these systems is similar to that observed versus meperidine-induced depression. From these data, pentazocine would appear to be only slightly less potent than nalorphine. However, it should be pointed out that higher doses of pentazocine did not produce greater antagonism and in some instances were additive with the narcotics.

A series of experiments were run in dogs in which the ability of naloxone to reverse the depression of respiration and the cardiovascular system caused by the intravenous administration of pentazocine was investigated. Once a steady state was obtained following anesthesia, pentazocine was administered and, 20 min later, when these systems were depressed, nalxone was administered by the intravenous route. Blood pressure, heart rate, percent CO_2 in the expired air, and pulmonary ventilation rate were determined as described above.

TABLE 2. *The effect of nalorphine, cyclazocine, and pentazocine on the depressant effects of 25 mg/kg i.m. meperidine in dogs*

Parameter	Drug	Dose (mg/kg)	Pre-mep.	Post-mep.	Post-ant.
Blood pressure	Nalorphine (3)	1.0	130	58	78
(mm Hg)	Cyclazocine (3)	0.015	133	68	96
	Pentazocine (2)	1.25	136	81	112
Heart rate	Nalorphine (3)	1.0	151	125	127
(beats/min)	Cyclazocine (3)	0.015	149	128	137
	Pentazocine (2)	1.25	118	94	104
Pulmonary venti-	Nalorphine (3)	1.0	2.05	1.24	2.29
lation rate	Cyclazocine (3)	0.015	1.98	1.24	1.47
(1/min)	Pentazocine (2)	1.25	1.94	0.71	1.02
Percent CO_2	Nalorphine (3)	1.0	4.9	7.6	6.3
	Cyclazocine (3)	0.015	4.4	5.5	5.2
	Pentazocine (2)	1.25	4.1	6.0	6.0

Numbers in parentheses after drugs are dogs used.

TABLE 3. *Naloxone reversal of Pentazocine depression in dogs*

| Parameter | Direction and percent change from preinjection value | | | |
	Pentazocine (15 mg/kg)		Naloxone (0.5 mg/kg)	
Blood pressure (mm Hg)	Decrease	$13.6 \pm 4.4^*$	Increase	11.6 ± 4.8
Heart rate (beats/min)	Decrease	9.5 ± 5.7	Increase	4.9 ± 2.5
Pulmonary ventilation rate (1/min)	Decrease	26.8 ± 9.7	Increase	40.6 ± 6.2
pCO_2	Increase	40.6 ± 9.0	Decrease	15.4 ± 5.0
Percent CO_2	Increase	52.4 ± 17.5	Decrease	12.8 ± 2.4
Respiration rate (resp/min)	Decrease	64.9 ± 5.9	Increase	42.4 ± 11.2
pO_2	Decrease	30.6 ± 2.6	Increase	30.9 ± 3.4

* Average $\pm$ SE for five dogs. Naloxone alone at 0.5 or 1.0 mg/kg caused minimal changes.

The effects of naloxone on the respiratory and cardiovascular depression induced by pentazocine are presented in Table 3. Although the doses of pentazocine used (10 and 15 mg/kg) produced a slight cardiovascular and a moderate respiratory depression, naloxone at a dose of 0.5 mg/kg produced a pronounced reversal of these depressed functions. Twice this dose of naloxone had little effect in anesthetized dogs not previously treated.

TABLE 4. *The dose-response reversal of cyclorphan on meperidine-induced respiratory depression in dogs*

| Parameter | Dose of cyclorphan (mg/kg, i.v.) | Percent change from preinjection value | |
		Meperidine (25 mg/kg, i.m.)	Cyclorphan (i.v.)
Respiratory rate (resp/min)	0.48	−54	+40
	0.12	−69	+52
	0.03	−59	+41
Pulmonary ventilation rate (1/min)	0.4	−34	+49
	0.12	−54	+58
	0.03	−47	+50
Percent CO_2 in expired air	0.4	+30	+ 9
	0.12	+27	−10
	0.03	+16	−20

Clearly, the narcotic antagonists are capable of reversing the respiratory depression induced by the potent analgesics in the dog. However, smooth dose-response functions are not always obtained. A number of doses of cyclorphan, the N-cyclopropylmethyl analogue in the morphinan series, have been tested for their ability to antagonize the respiratory depression induced by meperidine in anesthetized dogs. This work has been reported previously by Harris and his colleagues (5) and portions of it are presented in Table 4. Very small doses of cyclorphan were inactive but, as the dose was increased, an active dose was found which reversed the meperidine-induced depression almost completely and, therefore, higher doses of cyclorphan were not more active. In other words, the response was for practical purposes of the all-or-none type.

STUDIES IN CHRONIC SPINAL DOGS

A number of studies have been performed which have shown that the chronic spinal dog is a useful model for predicting analgesic dependence propensity and analgesic antagonist activity for a new compound. Wikler and Frank (15) reported that in dogs which had been subjected to spinal transection at either D-10 or D-12, a marked depression of the ipsilateral flexor and crossed extension reflexes was observed following an injection of morphine or methadone. Tolerance developed to these depressant effects and when chronic treatment with either morphine or methadone was terminated, a significant increase in these reflexes was observed and was interpreted as withdrawal. The peak of this syndrome was observed approximately 24 hr after the last methadone injection and 3 or 4 days after the last injection of morphine. This syndrome of "hyperreflexia" lasted for nearly 2 weeks. It was later shown (14) that N-allynormorphine could precipitate this withdrawal syndrome when injected to chronic spinal dogs who had been given injections of morphine every 6 hr. The intensity of the syndrome depended on the dose of nalorphine used and the duration of the morphine addiction. The hyperreflexia observed following nalorphine in the morphine-dependent dogs was greater than that produced by nalorphine in chronic spinal dogs who were not dependent on morphine. As a matter of fact, nalorphine resembled morphine in that it depressed the ipsilateral flexor and crossed extensor reflexes in the drug-naive chronic spinal dog. It was shown in subsequent experiments (9) that nalorphine precipitated abstinence signs in acutely and chronically, physically dependent dogs with low (T-10) or high (C5-C6) spinal transection.

Cyclazocine, a narcotic-antagonist analgesic, depresses the flexor reflex of a chronic spinal dog similarly to morphine, methadone, and nalorphine

(10). These agonistic effects of cyclazocine can be reversed by the relatively pure narcotic antagonist naloxone. The naloxone reversal of cyclazocine's effects as well as the reversal of the depression of the reflex induced by morphine occurs at doses of naloxone which are not stimulatory in chronic spinal dogs who have not received prior drug treatment. Thebaine, a morphine analogue which is devoid of analgesic activity also will reverse the depressant effects produced by morphine. However, this effect of thebaine is observed only at doses which cause an increase in the reflex in non-pretreated dogs. It appears that naloxone antagonism and nalorphine antagonism are examples of a pharmacological antagonism whereas the antagonism produced by thebaine is due to its stimulant properties.

The chronic spinal dog offers good promise as a preparation for bioassay of antagonistic activity of unknown compounds. The results reported to date suggest that new compounds with narcotic-antagonist activity would produce abstinence signs of "hyperreflexia" in the chronic spinal dog. Other signs of opiate withdrawal, such as mydriasis, running movements, hyperthermia, and increased respiratory rate, which are seen in spinal cord intact dogs, are also observed in the chronic spinal dog.

A continuous intravenous infusion of 3 mg/kg/hr of morphine sulfate produced a rapid tolerance to the depressant effects of this narcotic on spinal reflexes. Tolerance was observed to the depression of withdrawal reflexes, to miosis, to the depression of the skin-twitch response, and to behavioral depression. A subcutaneous administration of 20 mg/kg nalorphine soon after the infusion was terminated produced defecation, lacrimation, tremors, apprehension, rhinorrhea, salivation, vomiting, mydriasis, and tachycardia (8). These effects of nalorphine are not observed in a drug naive dog and do resemble those observed when nalorphine was administered to dogs injected chronically with morphine. This behavioral syndrome seen after nalorphine injection subsequent to morphine infusion indicates that the dogs were physically dependent on the opiate. This type of procedure might be useful in determining the duration of action of purported narcotic antagonists.

CONCLUSIONS

It is concluded from this review of the literature that the assay of antagonists against the overt behavioral effects or respiratory depression produced by narcotic analgesics in dogs is useful in predicting narcotic-antagonist activity in man. A good correlation exists between potency in the dog assays and potency as antagonists in man. The assays in dogs produce data which are reproducible although they are time-consuming and, therefore, expensive. It is difficult to quantitate the overt behavioral effects; a fact which precludes the use of parametric statistical analysis for this assay procedure. Although a good correlation exists between the ability of a compound to reverse narcotic-induced respiratory depression in the anesthetized dog and potency as a narcotic antagonist in man, respiratory depression is a side effect of the narcotics and not the therapeutic intent for these drugs.

The chronic spinal dog is a promising preparation for the study of analgesics and antagonists. Either agonist or antagonist actions of the narcotic-antagonist analgesics can be demonstrated. Tolerance and physical dependence can also be produced in this preparation.

The techniques in dogs are especially useful for studying mechanisms of action of narcotics and narcotic antagonists but have little advantage for screening purposes over the quicker, less expensive, and more quantitative rodent tests described in the previous chapter.

ACKNOWLEDGMENTS

The preparation of this manuscript was supported in part by U.S. Public Health Service grant No. MH19759.

REFERENCES

1. Dayton, H. B., and Blumberg, H.: Studies on the narcotic antagonist activity of naloxone in dogs. Fed. Proc. *30*:278, 1971.
1a. Drill, V. A. (editor): *Pharmacology in Medicine,* McGraw-Hill, New York, p. 255, 1971.
2. Gray, G. W.: Some effects of analgesic and analgesic-antagonist drugs on intestinal motility. J. Pharmacol. Exp. Ther. *124*:165–178, 1958.
3. Harris, L. S.: Narcotic antagonists in the benzomorphan series. Respiratory, cardiovascular and behavioral effects in dogs. Arch. Exp. Pathol. Pharmakol. *248*:426–436, 1964.
4. Harris, L. S., Dewey, W. L., Howes, J. F., Voyda, C., Kennedy, J. S., Nuite, J. A., Snyder, J. W., and Porter, J. F. Studies of narcotic-antagonist analgesics. Comm. on Prob. Drug Depend.: 5366–5375, 1968.
5. Harris, L. S., Pierson, A. K., Dembinski, J. R., and Dewey, W. L.: The pharmacology of (−)-3-hydroxy-N-cyclopropylmethylmorphinan (cyclorphan). Arch. Int. Pharmacodyn. *165*:112–126, 1967.
6. Heng, J. E., and Domino, E. F.: Effects of morphine and nalorphine upon tooth pulp thresholds of dogs in the alert and drowsy state. Psychopharmacologia *1*:433–436, 1960.
7. Huggins, R. A., Glass, W. G., and Bryan, A. R.: Protective action of N-allyl-normorphine against respiratory depression produced by some compounds related to morphine. Proc. Soc. Exp. Biol. and Med. *75*:540–541, 1950.
8. Martin, W. R., and Eades, C. G.: Demonstration of tolerance and physical dependence in the dog following a short-term infusion of morphine. J. Pharmacol. Exp. Ther. *133*:262–270, 1961.
9. Martin, W. R., and Eades, C. G.: A comparison between acute and chronic physical dependence in the chronic spinal dog. J. Pharmacol. Exp. Ther. *146*:385–394, 1964.

10. McClane, T. K., and Martin, W. R.: Antagonism of the spinal cord effects of morphine and cyclazocine by naloxone and thebaine. Int. J. Neuropharmacol. *6*:325–327, 1967.
11. Orahovats, P. D., Winter, C. A., and Lehman, E. G.: Pharmacological studies of mixtures of narcotics and N-allylnormorphine. J. Pharmacol. Exp. Ther. *112*:246–251, 1954.
12. Smith, C. C., Lehman, E. G., and Gilfillan, J. L.: Antagonistic action of N-allyl-normorphine upon the analgetic and toxic effects of morphine, methadone derivatives and isonipecaine. Fed. Proc. *10*:335–336, 1951.
13. Unna, K.: Antagonistic effect of N-allyl-normorphine upon morphine. J. Pharmacol. Exp. Ther. *79*:27–31, 1943.
14. Wikler, A., and Carter, R. L.: Effects of single doses of N-allylnormorphine on hindlimb reflexes of chronic spinal dogs during cycles of morphine addiction. J. Pharmacol. Exp. Ther. *109*:92–101, 1953.
15. Wikler, A., and Frank, K.: Hindlimb reflexes of chronic spinal dogs during cycles of addiction to morphine and methadone. J. Pharmacol. Exp. Ther. *94*:382–400, 1968.

Narcotic Antagonists, edited by M. C. Braude, L. S. Harris, E. L. May, J. P. Smith, and J. E. Villarreal. *Advances in Biochemical Psychopharmacology, Vol. 8.* Raven Press, New York © 1974.

The Actions of Narcotic Antagonists in Morphine-Dependent Rhesus Monkeys

Julian E. Villarreal* and Michael G. Karbowski

Department of Pharmacology, University of Michigan, Ann Arbor, Michigan 48106

The use of morphine-dependent organisms as pharmacologic preparations for the study of other drugs was originally intended for the identification of substances with morphine-like physical dependence capacity. However, the introduction of nalorphine and other derivatives of narcotics that possess morphine-antagonist properties quickly led to the recognition that morphine-dependent organisms respond in a very unique and sensitive way to the narcotic antagonists. The injection of nalorphine-like antagonists to rhesus monkeys or men physically dependent on morphine is followed within a few minutes by a dramatic series of gross behavioral and physiologic disturbances closely resembling the disturbances occurring after withdrawal of morphine (11, 27). This syndrome of "precipitated abstinence" has been extensively used as a pharmacologic end point to characterize the actions of a large series of narcotic antagonists in morphine-dependent rhesus monkeys at the University of Michigan. This chapter is a brief review of these studies. The main issues discussed here are: 1) the methodologies for identification of narcotic antagonists and for the assessment of their relative potencies and durations of action; 2) the most salient principles relating chemical structure with the capacity to precipitate abstinence in the monkey; 3) the predictive value for man of findings in the monkey for the various chemical classes of antagonists.

GENERAL PROCEDURE

Details of the procedures for drug testing in monkeys maintained on a stable level of morphine dependence have been published elsewhere (4, 10, 18). Briefly, monkeys housed in groups in large cages are maintained on 3 mg/kg of morphine sulfate injected subcutaneously every 6 hr, around the clock, 7 days a week. Special care is taken to train the monkeys on a chain of behaviors that generates injection and handling routines which are smooth and stable. When fully trained, the monkeys come out of their

---

* Present address: Instituto Miles de Terapeutica Experimental, Mexico City, Mexico.

home cage, one by one, and climb to a spot on one of the screen walls of an aisle in the room. At the injection spot, the monkeys present their backs to the experimenter and receive their injection while this person holds the animal lightly with one hand. Once trained for injections, the monkeys are also trained on a handling routine in which they again are made to come out to their injection spot but instead of receiving an injection they get their abdomens squeezed by the experimenter. With fully trained monkeys maintained on morphine, the abdomen-squeezing maneuver easily allows the experimenter to compress the anterior abdominal wall all the way back to the spinal column with minimal or no resistance by the animal.

The entire system just described is designed to maximize the number of behavioral signs that can be identified during abstinence (Table 1). Thus, observations can be made of individual behavior in the home cage, of social interactions, and of behavior during the handling routine.

Monkeys trained as described above and maintained on morphine for

TABLE 1. *Signs for point-score assessment of abstinence severity in morphine-dependent rhesus monkeys*

General behavior in home cage	Trunk and extremities
Restlessness-pacing	Shivering
Restlessness-crawling and rolling	Piloerection
Avoidance of contact with other monkeys	Holding of abdomen
Screaming when provoked	Tremors
Unprovoked screaming	Rigidity in extremities
Moaning and groaning	Spasticity
Attacking when provoked	
Unprovoked attacking	Autonomic signs
Contact-elicited attacking	
Lying on side or abdomen	Coughing
	Tachypnea
Face	Dyspnea
	Retching
Grimacing to observer or other monkeys	Vomiting
Dysphoric facies	Erection and masturbation
Yawning	Loose stools
Sweating face	
Pallor	Signs during handling routine
Perinasal redness	
Perioral redness	Vocalization
Salivation	Piloerection
Rhinorrhea	Twitches in abdominal muscles
Lacrimation	Generalized defense reaction in abdomen
Miosis	Attempts to scratch or bite handler
	Hesitation to come out of cage
	Will not come out of cage
	Will not climb to handling place

at least 90 days are used for studies with other drugs in two test procedures. The first is the single-dose suppression test, in which the ability of a drug to suppress morphine abstinence is determined in monkeys deprived of morphine for 14 hr. Morphine-like narcotics suppress abstinence and narcotic antagonists exacerbate the severity of the syndrome. Compounds thought to have narcotic-antagonist properties because of their effects on suppression tests are then evaluated in acute precipitation studies. In these studies the drug is administered to nonwithdrawn monkeys and then observations are made to determine whether or not an acute abstinence syndrome is precipitated.

THE SYNDROME OF PRECIPITATED ABSTINENCE

In the full-blown syndrome of antagonist-precipitated abstinence there is a rapid mobilization of a multitude of response systems — behavioral, neurological, and autonomic — producing a very striking and characteristic condition. In Table 1 there are 42 overt signs of abstinence as they can be observed in the Michigan routine. A minute or two after a subcutaneous injection of 0.1 mg/kg of naloxone, the dependent monkey shows a marked increase in locomotor activity (fast pacing in the cage), increased respiration

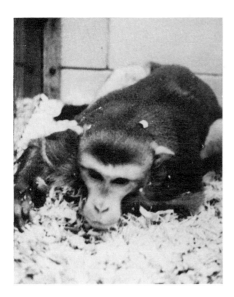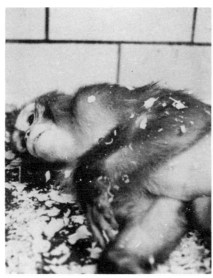

FIG. 1. A morphine-dependent rhesus monkey in the depressed phase of nalorphine-precipitated abstinence. Photographs by S. Todokoro.

rate, and bouts of coughing and retching. This is soon followed by a rapid increase in the overall severity of the syndrome, with the autonomic signs listed in Table 1 appearing in rapid succession within 15 to 20 min after the naloxone injection. The animal's behavior is frantic during this period but afterward it changes to dejected restlessness (Fig. 1), with the animal

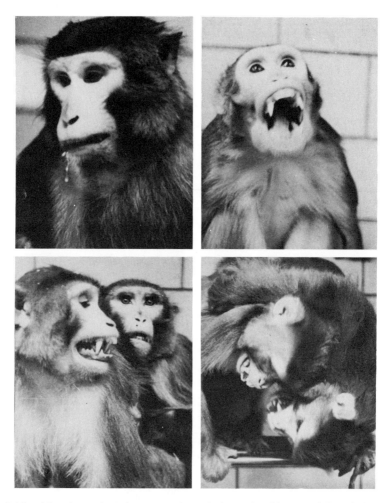

FIG. 2. Morphine-dependent rhesus monkeys during nalorphine-precipitated abstinence. *Upper left:* dysphoric facies and salivation; *upper right:* yawning; *lower left:* contact-induced aggression; *lower right:* a vicious cycle of contact-induced aggression. Photographs by S. Todokoro.

spending most of its time lying on the cage floor and wearily crawling and rolling from one end of the cage to the other. During abstinence the monkeys become very sensitive to physical contact so that touching or other forms of bodily contact with other monkeys readily elicit biting attacks (Fig. 2). Much of the quarreling observed in severe abstinence seems analogous to pain-induced aggression (2). Fighting during abstinence most frequently consists of quick biting responses to physical contact and it generally lacks the elements of long-lasting pursuit.

Another sign always observed in abstinence is the grimacing response to the approach of other monkeys or experimenters. Here, the teeth are bared with the jaws closed and with a marked retraction of the angles of the mouth, giving the face a wry expression. Hinde and Rowell (8) have described the same type of facial expression in small or in sick monkeys responding to the approach of a large monkey. They refer to this response as the "appeasement" grimace.

The handling routine is the most sensitive means of identifying low levels of abstinence. Even with minimal observable signs in the home cage, monkeys in mild abstinence show disruptions in their behavior during the handling routine, with prolonged hesitation to come out of their cages and failure to climb to their established handling spots. The abdomen-squeezing maneuver produces high-pitched vocalizations, piloerection, attempts to scratch the handler, and other defensive reactions. The abdominal wall is found to be hard as in the defense response of peritoneal inflammatory reactions.

QUANTITATIVE ASSESSMENTS OF ABSTINENCE

It is impossible to obtain a single formal measure of abstinence on a "ratio scale" (17) that would encompass everything that happens to the abstinent animal. However, two ordinal scale systems have been successfully used in the monkey to measure abstinence for the purposes of obtaining relative potencies or durations of action of drugs. In one of these systems, different levels of abstinence are defined by groups of signs that tend to occur in clusters that clearly correspond to different rank orders of overall abstinence severity. One such scale, routinely used at Michigan, is an eight-grade scale developed by Deneau (4) which is based on Seevers' (16) original classification of morphine abstinence signs in the rhesus monkey. The data presented in Fig. 3 were obtained with Deneau's system.

Another system, a point-score scale, was developed by the present authors to obtain greater accuracy at the lower levels of abstinence. This

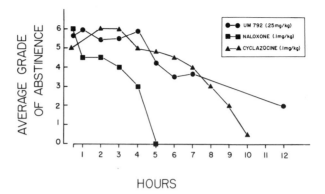

FIG. 3. Time-action curves for precipitated abstinence by three narcotic antagonists in morphine-dependent monkeys. The maintenance dose of morphine (3 mg/kg) was injected 2 hr before the antagonists, and again at 4 and 10 hr after the antagonist.

scale is more exact but, like other point-score systems, it can be misleading if used injudiciously. Each of the 42 signs of abstinence listed in Table 1 are given a score of 0, 1, 2, or 3, according to the intensity with which the sign is observed (intensity is magnitude and/or frequency according to the nature of the sign). Observations are made continuously during a single 30- to 60-min period after the injection of the antagonist. A total score is

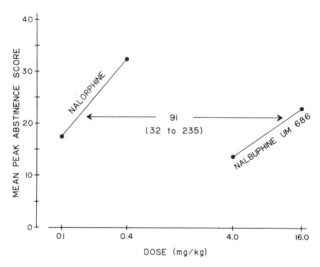

FIG. 4. Bioassay of the relative abstinence-precipitating potency of nalbuphine with nalorphine as standard. Numbers in parenthesis represent 95% confidence limits of the relative potency estimate.

then obtained by adding up all the scores for the individual signs. It should be noted that the list in Table 1 contains signs that are mutually incompatible (e.g., restlessness-pacing and lying on the side). Therefore, this point-score system can only be properly used when the total score is a cumulative measure of everything that happens in the transition from the baseline state to the peak of abstinence. Otherwise, if this scoring system is used on a time-sampling format, the points from the milder signs may simply be replaced by the points of more severe signs without altering the total score. The cumulative elements in this system make it useful to deal with low levels of abstinence in which many signs can be observed in succession but in which discrimination of different overall degrees of severity is difficult.

This point-score system has been used in instances where precise estimates of relative abstinence-precipitating potency are desired, particularly with weak antagonists. The data presented in Fig. 4 were obtained with this system. This figure shows the results of a study of the relative potency of nalbuphine, with nalorphine as reference standard. A "symmetrical pairs" design was employed for the bioassay (7a).

DURATION OF ACTION

The precipitation of abstinence by antagonists presents a unique opportunity to determine the duration of their antimorphine effects in single experiments. In contrast, determinations of duration of antimorphine actions in nondependent animals require multiple challenges with a narcotic agonist in multiple experimental groups at different times after the administration of the antagonist. Figure 3 presents time-action curves for the abstinence-precipitating effects of equivalent doses of three narcotic antagonists. In these experiments, the antagonists were injected subcutaneously 2 hr after one of the maintenance doses of morphine. The regular schedule of morphine injections remained in effect throughout the experiments. Therefore, the monkeys received morphine at 4 and 10 hr after the injection of antagonist. The effects of naloxone (Fig. 3) were short-lived and the administration of morphine at the 4th hour brought the animals back to baseline. The effects of cyclazocine and UM792 (naltrexone) lasted for more than twice as long.

CRITERIA FOR THE IDENTIFICATION OF COMPOUNDS WITH MORPHINE-ANTAGONIST PROPERTIES

Some parts of the syndrome of precipitated abstinence can be reproduced with the administration of compounds that do not have narcotic-antagonist properties; e.g., emetics and muscarinic agonists. Also, different narcotic antagonists produce acute syndromes of abstinence which differ somewhat from the syndromes precipitated by nalorphine or naloxone. To deal with the problem of specificity of these effects, the following criteria have been adopted as the minimum requirements to judge a compound as capable of precipitating abstinence: 1) the compound must produce a majority of the signs of behavioral hyperirritability listed in Table 1, plus a positive abdominal defense reaction, and bodily postures indicative of general malaise; 2) the severity of the syndrome of precipitated abstinence must be dose related over at least a fourfold range of doses; 3) the various signs corresponding to the different degrees of abstinence severity must be present in roughly the same proportions as they occur after nalorphine administration or during morphine deprivation. The presence of autonomic signs greatly strengthens the evidence for the identification of a compound as a narcotic antagonist. Yet, since the autonomic signs are not all invariably produced by weak antagonists, they cannot be used as exclusive criteria.

STRUCTURE-ACTIVITY RELATIONSHIPS

Accounts of the relationships between chemical structure and biologic activity for the narcotic antagonists must consider at least the following three types of pharmacologic activities: 1) antimorphine properties; 2) morphine-like agonist actions; 3) cyclazocine-like agonist actions. Very few narcotic antagonists possess antimorphine properties in pure form; most of them have agonist actions of one or both of the types mentioned (12a, 14). Thus, descriptions of the effects of structural changes on the biologic activity of these drugs can only be regarded as reasonably complete when such effects are expressed as changes not only in overall potency but also as changes in the relative proportions of the three types of properties listed above. Studies with narcotic agonist-antagonist drugs in morphine-dependent monkeys are of special value because these pharmacologic preparations allow not only the evaluation of antimorphine properties but also the identification of morphine-like and cyclazocine-like agonist actions. Unfortunately, a review of the structural determinants of the three kinds of activity is far beyond the scope of this chapter. Details of the analysis of the agonist properties of narcotic antagonists are discussed elsewhere (21). The present section will deal primarily with the features of chemical structure that confer the capacity to precipitate acute abstinence syndromes in the morphine-dependent monkey and the transitions to compounds that behave predominantly as agonists.

A further factor to be borne in mind when drawing inferences from the effects of drugs that precipitate acute abstinence is the contribution of the recently identified "abstinoid" actions of narcotic antagonists (21, 26). These are direct actions of the antagonists, apparently distinct from their competitive antimorphine properties; actions that are short-lived, that reproduce the signs of narcotic abstinence even in normal organisms, and that are greatly exaggerated by chronic narcotic treatment. Consequently, it seems quite possible that the antagonist-precipitated abstinence syndrome is a result of the combined effects of the abstinoid plus the competitive antimorphine actions of the antagonists. It is too early to assign relative roles to the contributions which these two actions make to overall effects of antagonists. Yet, since the early part of the antagonist-precipitated syndrome is resistant to reversal by morphine, it is conceivable that this early part is to a significant extent determined by the abstinoid actions. The intervention, or lack of it, of the abstinoid actions may account for some discrepancies between findings on precipitating potency and antinarcotic potency in nondependent animals for some antagonists.

Twenty-one of the compounds tested in the morphine-dependent monkey precipitate abstinence with a potency as great or greater than nalorphine. All of these substances possess structures that contain the complete morphine skeleton or a substantial fraction of it. Thus, they all belong to one of the following families: oripavines, thebaines, morphine, morphines, morphinones, morphinans, and 6,7-benzomorphans. Some of these potent antagonists are shown in Figs. 5 and 6. The N-substituents of these 21 compounds are either 3-carbon straight-chain groups, allyl or propyl, or cyclopropylmethyl. Departures from this type of N-substituent lead to pronounced decreases in abstinence-precipitating potency (Fig. 5).

The structural requirements for abstinence-precipitating activity are much more strict than the requirements for morphine-like activity in abstinence-suppression tests. The fact that a substantial representation of the basic morphine skeleton is not necessary for full morphine-like activity has been demonstrated by the wide diversity of synthetic chemicals which suppress morphine abstinence specifically (20). In these synthetic chemicals, however, the replacement of N-methyl by N-allyl does not yield compounds with strong abstinence-precipitating effects. N-Allyl substituted analogues of meperidine suppress abstinence instead of precipitating it (5, 24). One N-cyclopropylmethyl substituted 4-carbomethoxypiperidine precipitates abstinence in the monkey, but it has only $\frac{1}{100}$th of the potency of nalorphine (24). One 3-phenylpiperidine with an allyl group on the nitrogen also precipitates abstinence, but its potency is only $\frac{1}{12}$th of that of nalorphine (7).

All these findings give evidence of a general correspondence between the

ANTAGONISTS

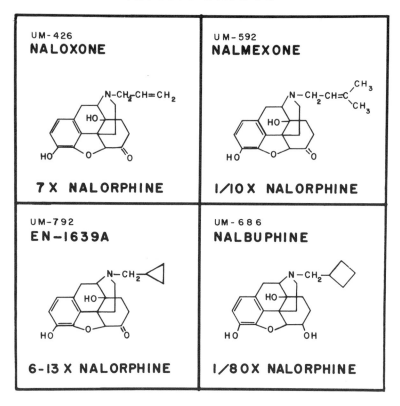

FIG. 5. Compounds possessing different side chains which precipitate acute abstinence syndromes in morphine-dependent monkeys.

structural characteristics that impart abstinence-precipitating activity and the characteristics imparting antinarcotic activity in nondependent animals (1, 13).

The precipitating effects of most of the antagonists tested in the monkey are of short duration. The exceptions are the antagonists with N-cyclopropylmethyl substituents. These compounds consistently precipitate abstinence lasting between 10 and 24 hr. The structures of some such antagonists, along with their corresponding durations of action, are shown in Fig. 6.

Abstinence-precipitating activity is readily reduced or eliminated by minor modifications on the N-substituent or on other parts of the molecule.

ANTAGONISTS

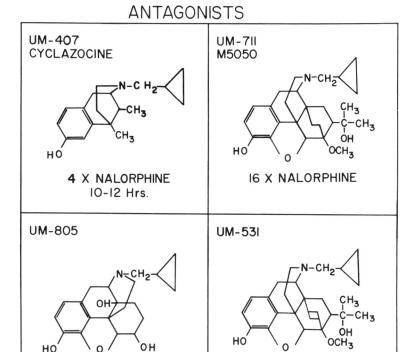

FIG. 6. Compounds possessing N-cyclopropylmethyl side chains which precipitate acute abstinence syndromes in morphine-dependent monkeys. Numbers below each relative potency estimate express the duration of precipitated abstinence when the magnitude of effect corresponded to a grade 5 or 6 of peak severity.

The chemical modifications sometimes result in a simple loss of potency but they often produce switchings of activity yielding compounds that behave predominantly as agonists. As in nalmexone (Fig. 5) and pentazocine, the addition of two methyl groups to allyl to produce 3,3-dimethylallyl N-substituents causes a marked fall in precipitating potency, which can be several hundredfold in magnitude.

Interestingly, several compounds with N-3,3-dimethylallyl chains have been found to suppress abstinence in the monkey: (-)-3-hydroxy-N-(3,3-dimethylallyl)-morphinan; (-)-3-nicotinyloxy-N-(3,3-dimethylallyl)-morphinan; N-(3,3-dimethylallyl)-5-methyl-dihydromorphinone; and N-(3,3-

dimethylallyl)-6,14-endoetheno-7-(2-hydroxy-2-pentyl)-tetrahydronororipavine. The latter suppressed abstinence with a potency six times greater than morphine.

The change from N-cyclopropylmethyl to N-cyclobutylmethyl also produces a drastic fall in abstinence-precipitating potency. This simple addition of a carbon atom produces drops in potency of 400- to 800-fold (18). Elsewhere (20), it has been pointed out that the switch from N-cyclopropylmethyl to N-cyclobutylmethyl causes the transformation of a potent precipitating compound into a potent morphine agonist for two antagonists of the morphinan family.

Modifications in parts of the molecule other than the side chain on the nitrogen also produce marked changes in biological activity. The abstinence-precipitating potency of oripavine antagonists is markedly reduced with a change from 3-hydroxy to 3-methoxy (20, 24). Here again, this simple change has been found to transform a potent precipitating drug into a potent morphine agonist: N-cyclopropylmethyl-7-(2-hydroxybutyl)-6,14-endoethenotetrahydronorthebaine, which is approximately equipotent with morphine in suppressing abstinence.

The effects of substituents on position 7 of compounds of the oripavine-thebaine families have been systematically explored by the group of Lewis, Bentley, and Cowan (13). Many of these compounds have been tested in the morphine-dependent rhesus monkey. Compounds of high precipitating potency are obtained when there are N-allyl or N-cyclopropylmethyl substituents and the group on position 7 is small (2-hydroxy-2-propyl). Increments in the size of the group attached on 7 reduce precipitating potency and bring out predominant agonist activity. In some cases, this agonist activity is of the morphine type, as in N-allyl-6,14-endoetheno-7-(1-hydroxy-1-cyclohexylethyl)-tetrahydronororipavine (7). In other cases, the agonist activity is of the cyclazocine type as in the N-cyclopropylmethyl analogue of the above compound (7) or in N-cyclopropylmethyl-7-(2-hydroxy-5-methyl-2-hexyl)-6,14-endoetheno nororipavine (24).

In an earlier review on narcotic antagonists (1) Archer and Harris noted that the replacement of N-methyl by N-allyl in potent morphine-like narcotics yielded potent antagonists. There was a correlation between the potency of the parent narcotic with the potency of the corresponding antagonist. Exceptions to this rule have been discovered more recently (13). Several compounds have been mentioned in the present review which possess strong morphine-like activity in spite of the fact that they have N-allyl or N-cyclopropylmethyl substituents. Other drugs that suppress morphine abstinence specifically and that have these same N-substituents are: N-allyl-7-(2-hydroxy-4-phenylbutyl)-6,14-endoethenonortetrahydrothebaine (24) and N-cyclopropylmethyl-7-(2-hydroxy-2-butyl)-6,14-endoethenonortetrahydrothebaine (25).

It is clear, therefore, that abstinence-precipitating and antimorphine activities cannot be obtained be merely taking a strong narcotic and providing it with an allyl or cyclopropylmethyl group on its nitrogen. Abstinence-precipitating and antimorphine actions have structure-activity characteristics which are substantially different from the characteristics for agonist actions either of the morphine type or of the cyclazocine type. The characteristics for antagonism deserve a thoroughly systematic experimental analysis. The evidence at hand, however, strongly suggests a different structure of receptor for antagonist action. Thus, it is quite conceivable that the "morphine receptor" is a polymer complex made up of several different subspecies of monomers. Some of the monomers would initiate agonist actions after binding with the different chemical classes of agonists in slightly different modes (see 3 and 15). Different monomers would bind with antagonists so as to allosterically cancel the consequences of agonist interactions and also to produce abstinoid effects.

CORRELATIONS WITH OTHER SPECIES

In general, the estimates of relative potency for antagonists show good agreement across species and across different preparations. Table 2 presents a comparison of potency estimates for eight well-known antagonists. The figures obtained in morphine-dependent monkeys closely parallel the figures obtained in morphine-dependent humans, nondependent rodents, and the isolated ileum. One compound, however, stands out because its precipitating potency in the monkey is quite out of line with the estimates of its potency in the other preparations. This compound is nalbuphine, N-cyclobutylmethyl-7,8-dihydro-14-hydroxynormorphine. This anomaly in the dependent monkey may indicate that this species underreacts to the precipitating effects of compounds with N-cyclobutylmethyl side chains. Other compounds with N-cyclobutylmethyl side chains capable of suppressing morphine abstinence in the monkey were previously mentioned.

Another group of compounds for which the monkey shows a deviation from the responses obtained in other species is made up of a series of N-methyl substituted 6,7-benzomorphans. The actions of these drugs in the monkey have been reviewed in detail elsewhere (19). The behavior of the monkey with regard to the 6,7-benzomorphan analgesics is in general anomalous (20). The monkey tends to underestimate the morphine-like agonist actions of this family of drugs. Some N-methyl 6,7-benzomorphans were resolved into their optical isomers. As with other analgesics, the *levo* iso-

TABLE 2. *Relative potencies of antagonists in different species relative to nalorphine**

Drug	Man[a]	Monkey[b]	Rodent[c]	Guinea pig[d] ileum
Nalorphine	1	1	1	1
Levallorphan	2–5	4	2–5	4
Naloxone	7	7	7	3–4
Cyclazocine	6	4–5	4–6	3
Profadol	1/40–1/50	1/80	–	1/70
Nalbuphine	1/4	1/90	1/2–1/6	1/2
M5050	–	16	160	35
UM 792; EN 1639 A; Naltrexone	17	6–13	14	1–2

[a] Precipitation of morphine abstinence
[b] Precipitation of morphine abstinence
[c] Prevention of analgesia or narcosis
[d] Blockade of morphine. Inhibition of elicited twitch.
* Information on the effects in monkeys was obtained from work at the University of Michigan reported annually in the Proceedings of the Committee on Problems of Drug Dependence, NAS-NRC, Washington. Information on effects in man was taken from references 7a, 11a, 11b, and 14a; effects in rodents from 1, 2a, 2b, 2c, and 3a; and effects in guinea pig ileum from 12a.

mers were found to be more potent than their *dextro* counterparts in mouse analgesia tests. In the dependent monkey, however, the *levo* isomers precipitated abstinence whereas most of the *dextro* antipodes suppressed abstinence. More recently, the same pattern of effects has been reported for isomers in the phenylmorphan class (25). The data presented in Figs. 7 and 8 show that this separation of effects for optical isomers was not limited to gross behavioral signs. The figures show that a *dextro* isomer, GPA1658, readily reverses the hypothermia of the dependent monkey, whereas the *levo* compound, GPA1657, not only fails to reverse hypothermia but also blocks the effects of morphine. Two of the *levo* 6,7-benzomorphans that precipitated abstinence in the monkey have been tested in man. Both of them were found to be predominantly morphine-like in their effects (12, 19). The findings in the monkey have been interpreted as evidence that these N-methyl compounds have "intrinsic activities" slightly lower than those of classical narcotics (19). This intrinsic agonistic activity is low enough to lead to abstinence in the monkey, which is relatively insensitive to the agonistic actions of the 6,7-benzomorphans. However, this low intrinsic agonistic activity is not enough to produce the same result in the human, which is highly sensitive to this family of analgesics. Therefore, findings with the 6,7-benzomorphans in the monkey have to be considered with great reservation if attempts are made to extrapolate them to man. Never-

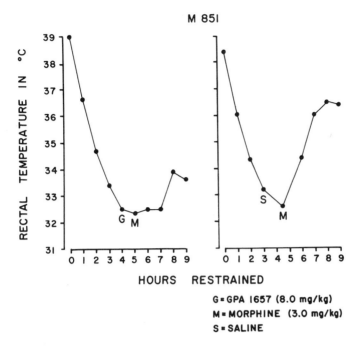

FIG. 7. Effects of GPA1657, morphine, and saline on restraint-induced hypothermia (9) in morphine-dependent monkeys. GPA1657 does not reverse hypothermia but it blocks the effects of morphine. (Unpublished, Holtzman and Villarreal.)

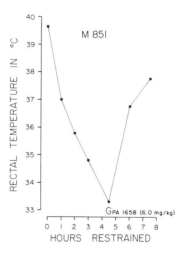

FIG. 8. Effects of GPA1658, the *dextro* isomer of GPA1657, on restraint-induced hypo-thermia in morphine-dependent monkeys. Like morphine (Fig. 7), GPA1658 reverses retraint-induced hypothermia. (Unpublished, Holtzman and Villarreal.)

theless, it must be recognized that, with the *levo* N-methyl compounds, the monkey has allowed the identification of another channel of investigation for the separation of dependence from analgesic activity.

ACKNOWLEDGMENTS

The studies reviewed in this chapter have been part of the activities of a research program directed by M. H. Seevers in the Department of Pharmacology of the University of Michigan, supported by grants from the Committee on Problems of Drug Dependence of the National Research Council, Washington, D.C. This review covers not only studies carried out by the present authors but also by other associates of M. H. Seevers, especially G. A. Deneau. The results of studies with individual compounds have been published annually as addenda to the minutes of the meetings of the above committee.

REFERENCES

1. Archer, S., and Harris, L. S.: Narcotic antagonists. *In:* Progress in Drug Research, edited by E. Jucker, pp. 261–320. Birkhauser Verlag, Basel, 1965.
2. Azrin, N. H., Hutchinson, R. R., and Hake, D. F.: Pain-induced fighting in the squirrel monkey, J. Exp. Analysis Behav. 6:620, 1963.
2a. Blane, G. F., and Boura, A. L. A.: On the mode of action of morphine antagonist analgesics. Proc. Committee on Problems of Drug Dependence, Appendix 11, 1968.
2b. Blumberg, H., Dayton, H. B., George, M., and Rapaport, D. N.: N-Allylnoroxymorphone: A potent narcotic antagonist. Fed. Proc. 20:311, 1961.
2c. Blumberg, H., Dayton, H. B., and Wolf, P. S.: Analgesic and narcotic antagonist properties of noroxymorphone derivatives. Toxicol. Appl. Pharmac. 10:406, 1967.
3. Casy, A.: Analgesics and their antagonists: Recent developments. *In:* Progress in Medicinal Chemistry, edited by G. P. Ellis and G. B. West, pp. 229–284. Appleton-Century-Crofts, New York, 1970.
3a. Costa, P. J., and Bonnycastle, D. D.: The effect of levallorphan tartrate, nalorphine HCl, and Win 7681 (1-allyl-4-phenyl-4-carbethoxypiperidine) on respiratory depression and analgesia induced by some active analgesics. J. Pharmac. Exp. Ther. *113*:310, 1955.
4. Deneau, G. A.: An analysis of factors influencing the development of physical dependence to narcotic analgesics in the rhesus monkey with methods for predicting physical dependence liability in man. Doctoral Dissertation, University of Michigan, 1956.
5. Deneau, G. A., and Seevers, M. H.: Evaluation of morphine-like physical dependence in the rhesus monkey (*Macaca mulatta*). Proc. Committee on Drug Addiction and Narcotics, 23rd meeting, Addendum, 1962.
6. Deneau, G. A., and Seevers, M. H.: Evaluation of new compounds for morphine-like physical dependence capacity in the rhesus monkey. Proc. Committee on Problems of Drug Dependence, 26th meeting, Addendum, 1965.
7. Deneau, G. A., Villarreal, J. E., and Seevers, M. H.: Evaluation of new compounds for morphine-like physical dependence in the rhesus monkey. Proc. Committee on Problems of Drug Dependence, 27th meeting, Addendum, 1966.
7a. Emmens, C. W.: *Principles of Biological Assay.* Chapman & Hall Ltd., London, 1948.
8. Hinde, R. A., and Rowell, T. E.: Communication by postures and facial expressions in the rhesus monkey (*Macaca mulatta*). Proc. Zool. Soc. Lond. *138*:1–21, 1962.

9. Holtzman, S. G., and Villarreal, J. E.: Morphine dependence and body temperature in rhesus monkeys. J. Pharmac. Exp. Ther. *166*:125–133, 1969.

10. Irwin, S.: Characteristics of depression, antagonism and development of tolerance, physical dependence and neuropathology to morphine and morphine-like agents in the monkey. Doctoral Dissertation, University of Michigan, 1953.

11. Irwin, S., and Seevers, M. H.: Comparative study of regular and N-allylnormorphine-induced withdrawals in monkeys addicted to morphine, 6-methyldihydromorphine, Dromoran, methadone and ketobemidone. J. Pharmac. Exp. Ther. *106*:397, 1952.

11a. Jasinski, D. R., Martin, W. R., and Haertzen, C. A.: The human pharmacology and abuse potential of N-allylnoroxymorphone (naloxone). J. Pharmac. Exp. Ther. *157*:420–426, 1967.

11b. Jasinski, D. R., and Mansky, P. A.: Evaluation of nalbuphine for abuse potential. Clin. Pharmac. Ther. *13*:77–90, 1971.

12. Jasinski, D. R., Martin, W. R., and Hoeldtke, R.: Studies of the dependence-producing properties of GPA-1657, profadol, and propiram in man. Clin. Pharmac. Ther. *12*:613–649, 1971.

12a. Kosterlitz, H. W. *This Volume.*

13. Lewis, J. W., Bentley, K. W., and Cowan, A.: Narcotic analgesics and antagonists. Ann. Rev. Pharmac. *11*:241–270, 1971.

14. Martin, W. R.: Opioid antagonists. Pharmac. Rev. *19*:463–521, 1967.

14a. Martin, W. R., Jasinski, D. R., and Mansky, P. A.: Characteristics of the blocking effects of EN 1639A (N-cyclopropylmethyl-7,8-dihydro-14-hydroxynormorphinone HCl). Proc. Committee on Problems of Drug Dependence, 32nd meeting, 1971.

15. Portoghese, P. S.: A new concept on the mode of interaction of narcotic analgesics with receptors. J. Med. Chem. *8*:609–616, 1965.

16. Seevers, M. H.: Opiate addiction in the monkey. I. Methods of study. J. Pharmac. Exp. Ther. *56*:147–156, 1936.

17. Stevens, S. S.: On the theory of scales of measurement. Science *103*:677–680, 1946.

18. Villarreal, J. E.: Pharmacologic characterization of morphine-antagonists in the rhesus monkey. Doctoral Dissertation, University of Michigan, 1969.

19. Villarreal, J. E. Recent advances in the pharmacology of morphine-like drugs. *In:* Advances in Mental Science, Vol 2, Drug Dependence, edited by R. T. Harris, C. R. Schuster, and D. McIsaac, pp. 83–116. University of Texas Press, Houston, 1970.

20. Villarreal, J. E.: The effects of morphine agonists and antagonists on morphine-dependent rhesus monkeys. *In:* The Pharmacology of Morphine Agonists and Antagonists, edited by H. W. Kosterlitz, H. O. J. Collier, and J. E. Villarreal, McMillan, London, 1972.

21. Villarreal, J. E.: The pharmacology of narcotic antagonists. *Unpublished.*

22. Villarreal, J. E.: Assessment of the dependence capacity of narcotic antagonists in the rhesus monkey. *Unpublished.*

23. Villarreal, J. E., and Seevers, M. H.: Evaluation of new compounds for morphine-like physical dependence in the rhesus monkey. Proc. Committee on Problems of Drug Dependence, 30th meeting, Addendum, 1969.

24. Villarreal, J. E., and Seevers, M. H.: Evaluation of new compounds for morphine-like physical dependence in the rhesus monkey. Proc. Committee on Problems of Drug Dependence, 31st meeting, Addendum, 1970.

25. Villarreal, J. E., and Seevers, M. H.: Evaluation of new compounds for morphine-like physical dependence in the rhesus monkey. Proc. Committee on Problems of Drug Dependence, 33rd meeting, Addendum, 1972.

26. Villarreal, J. E., and Dummer, G.: Separation of the dependence-producing from the direct actions of narcotics. Fed. Proc. (*in press*), 1973.

27. Wikler, A., Fraser, H. F., and Isbell, H.: N-allylnormorphine: Effects of single doses and precipitation of "abstinence syndromes" during addiction to morphine, methadone or heroin in man (post-addicts). J. Pharmac. Exp. Ther. 109:8, 1953.

Narcotic Antagonists, edited by M. C. Braude, L. S. Harris, E. L. May, J. P. Smith, and J. E. Villarreal. *Advances in Biochemical Psychopharmacology, Vol. 8.* Raven Press, New York © 1974.

Assays of Antagonistic Activity of Narcotic Antagonists in Man

Charles W. Gorodetzky

National Institute of Mental Health, Addiction Research Center, Lexington, Kentucky 40507

This chapter reviews the methods which have been developed and briefly summarizes the results which have been obtained for evaluation of the antagonistic actions of narcotic antagonists in man over approximately the last 10 years at the NIMH Addiction Research Center. The major assay procedure is the precipitation test. Single doses of narcotic antagonist are administered to subjects dependent on 60 or 240 mg of morphine per day, and abstinence is quantitatively evaluated over the next 3 hr using a modification of the method of Himmelsbach. By using two doses each of a standard antagonist (nalorphine) and a test antagonist, relative potency for precipitation of abstinence can be determined using the design and statistics for a four-point parallel line bioassay. Relative potencies published to date (expressed as mg = 1 mg of nalorphine) have been determined as follows: 1) using subjects dependent on 240 mg/day morphine: naloxone, 0.14; cyclazocine, 0.18; levallorphan, 0.52; nalorphine, 1.00; profadol, 43.5; pentazocine, 51.2; propiram, 192; 2) using subjects dependent on 60 mg/day morphine: naloxone, 0.10; nalorphine, 1.00; nalbuphine, 3.7. To evaluate duration of action, a single dose of narcotic antagonist (or placebo) is administered at various intervals prior to a standard test dose of morphine, the effects of which are measured on pupillary diameter and parameters of the standard single-dose opiate questionnaire. Published results have shown antagonistic actions of naloxone to last at least 9 hr and cyclazocine for 12 to 24 hr.

To assess the antagonistic actions of narcotic antagonists during their chronic administration, single test doses of opiate have been administered prior to and then during chronic antagonist administration. In addition, during chronic antagonist administration, morphine at 240 mg/day has been chronically administered, then abruptly withdrawn under double-blind conditions, and abstinence quantitatively evaluated by the method of Himmelsbach. Results have shown that chronically administered narcotic antagonists maintain their ability to block the effects of single doses of narcotic analgesics and to antagonize the development of physical dependence on chronically administered morphine.

To evaluate narcotic antagonists for their possible therapeutic use in the treatment of narcotic addiction in man it is necessary to determine their antagonistic potency, duration of antagonistic effect, and antagonistic action during chronic administration. This chapter reviews those methods which have been developed and briefly summarizes the results which have been obtained for the measurement of these parameters over approximately the last 10 years at the NIMH Addiction Research Center. Three general test procedures will be discussed: (1) the precipitation test for determination of antagonistic potency; (2) evaluation of duration of antagonistic action of single doses of narcotic antagonists; and (3) evaluation of antagonistic actions of chronically administered narcotic antagonists.

THE PRECIPITATION TEST

The precipitation test as a bioassay for relative antagonistic potency was described by Jasinski and colleagues in 1967 (5). All subjects who participated in these studies were federal prisoner volunteers incarcerated at the Addiction Research Center. All had long histories of opiate abuse, were in good health, and had no major psychiatric illness.

Groups of six to seven subjects are first made physically dependent on morphine at maintenance dose levels of 60 or 240 mg/day administered subcutaneously in four equal doses at 6:00 A.M., 10:00 A.M., 4:00 P.M., and 10:00 P.M. On the day of the precipitation test, predrug control observations are made at 8:00 and 8:30 A.M., and a single dose of narcotic antagonist is administered at 9:00 A.M., 3 hr following the last morphine maintenance dose. Observations are repeated at 15 min, 30 min, 1 hr, 2 hr, and 3 hr following administration of the antagonist. Observations include measurement of pupillary diameter, respiratory rate, systolic blood pressure, and rectal temperature, as well as the notation of the presence or absence of specified signs of opiate abstinence. Pupillary diameter is measured by a photographic technique utilizing an especially modified Polaroid close-up camera (4). At each of the five observation times, an abstinence score is calculated according to a modification of the method of Himmelsbach as shown in Table 1. Points are assigned for the presence of the abstinence signs as noted; physiologic measures are evaluated in comparison to the mean of the two pre-drug control measures. Summation of points gives an abstinence score at each observation. The abstinence scores for the five observations may then be summed for each subject to give a total 3-hr abstinence score.

Bioassay experiments are run in a randomized, full-crossover design, usually utilizing two doses of nalorphine as the standard drug, two doses of the test drug, and a saline placebo. Precipitation tests are run at weekly intervals, and all drugs are administered under double-blind conditions. A

TABLE 1. *Source of points*
for abstinence score

Observation	Value
Yawning	1
Lacrimation	1
Rhinorrhea	1
Perspiration	1
Goose flesh	3
Tremor	3
Restlessness	5
Emesis	5
Each 0.1 mm dilation of pupil	1
Each increase in respiratory rate	1
Each 2 mm increase in systolic blood pressure	1
Each 0.1°C rise in body temperature	1

mean total abstinence score is determined for each antagonist dose, and relative potencies and confidence limits are determined using the nalorphine response as the standard. The validity of the assay is determined by an analysis of variance for a parallel line bioassay (1). For an assay to be valid, there must be significant regression, no significant deviation from parallelism or differences between preparations, and, when more than two points are used for each drug, no significant deviation from linearity.

Table 2 shows a summary of the results of precipitation tests published by Jasinski and colleagues (3, 5–7). All antagonists in these studies were

TABLE 2. *Relative potency of narcotic antagonists for precipitation*
of abstinence in morphine-dependent subjects

Daily morphine maintenance dose	Antagonist	Relative potency (95% confidence limits) (no. mg = 1 mg nalorphine)	Reference
240 mg	Naloxone	0.14 (0.12–0.20)	(5)
(60 mg. q.i.d.)	Cyclazocine	0.18	(5)
	Levallorphan	0.52 (0.38–0.73)	(5)
	Nalorphine	1.00	(5–7)
	Profadol	43.5 (32.8–52.6)	(7)
	Pentazocine	51.2 (34.3–96.3)	(6)
	Propiram	192 (127–503)	(7)
60 mg	Naloxone	0.10 (0.06–0.16)	(7)
(15 mg. q.i.d.)	Nalorphine	1.00	(3, 7)
	Nalbuphine	3.7 (2.4–5.5)	(3)

administered subcutaneously, and they are listed in order of decreasing potency in each group. No confidence limits were calculated for cyclazocine because the assay was not valid; there were significant and widely divergent differences between preparations. In some of these studies the nature of the precipitated abstinence syndrome elicited by the test drug was compared to that elicited by nalorphine (6, 7). The sources of points making up the abstinence scores from nalorphine and the test drug were examined, and each source was ranked according to the relative magnitude of its contribution to the total abstinence score from each drug. Spearman rank-order correlation coefficients were significantly positive in all cases, indicating a close similarity in the nature of the precipitated abstinence syndromes.

It should be noted that this test procedure has been used for purposes other than the assay of relative antagonistic potency. For example, in several studies nalorphine or naloxone precipitation tests were used to demonstrate the development of physical dependence on a test drug which was being administered chronically (3, 6, 7). Data from precipitation tests have also been used to explore the theoretical concepts of drug-receptor interactions of opiates and opiate antagonists (3, 6, 7).

DURATION OF ACTION OF SINGLE DOSES
OF NARCOTIC ANTAGONISTS

Evaluation of the duration of action of single doses of narcotic antagonists has been reported in two papers (5, 10). Although the details of the procedures differ somewhat, in general a single dose of narcotic antagonist is administered from 1 to 24 hr prior to subcutaneous administration of a 25 to 30 mg/70 kg test dose of morphine. After the test dose is given, pupillary diameter is measured by a standard photographic technique, and the single-dose opiate questionnaire for both subjects and observers described by Fraser et al. (2) is administered at hourly intervals for 5 or 6 hr. Mean hourly scores are then determined for miosis, opiate signs, opiate symptoms, liking "subjects," and liking "observers"; a total 5- or 6-hr score for each parameter may also be calculated. The time-action curves for the morphine test dose administered at various intervals after a single dose of antagonist may then be examined and compared to the time action curves for the same test dose administered at one of the time intervals following a saline placebo. Similarly, the mean total 5- or 6-hr scores for the test dose given after antagonist may be statistically compared to the scores for the test dose following placebo by a paired data *t*-test to demonstrate antagonistic activity. Experiments are run under double-blind conditions at weekly intervals in a randomized, full-cross-over design.

In a study by Jasinski et al. (5), the duration of antagonistic action of 15 mg/70 kg of naloxone administered subcutaneously was studied. A 30 mg/70 kg morphine test dose was administered subcutaneously 1, 2, and 4 hr after the naloxone dose and also 4 hr after a saline placebo. Parameters as described above were evaluated for 5 hr after the morphine test dose. Naloxone showed significant antagonistic action at all time intervals studied, and, for most parameters, the degree of antagonism decreased with increasing intervals between naloxone and the morphine test dose. The fifth hourly observation on the test dose administered 4 hr after naloxone indicates that at this dose naloxone shows antagonistic activity for at least 9 hr.

In another study (10), the duration of action of cyclazocine was investigated. Cyclazocine (0.6 mg/70 kg) was administered subcutaneously at 4, 12, and 24 hr prior to a 25 mg/70 kg test dose of morphine. A significant antagonistic effect was demonstrated for 12 to 24 hr following the antagonist.

ANTAGONISTIC ACTIONS OF CHRONICALLY ADMINISTERED NARCOTIC ANTAGONISTS

The antagonistic actions of chronically administered narcotic antagonists have been studied with both single and chronic doses of narcotics. In the evaluation of antagonistic actions to single doses of opiate during chronic antagonist administration, the procedure is analogous to that described in the duration-of-action studies. Single doses of opiate at one or more dose levels are administered prior to initiation of chronic antagonist administration. After stabilization at peak levels of the antagonist, single test doses of opiate at equal or higher dose levels than in the control conditions are again administered. After the test opiate doses, hourly observations are made of pupillary diameter and the single-dose opiate questionnaire for subjects and observers is administered. Assessment of antagonistic activity is made by comparison of the effects of the opiate test doses before and during chronic antagonist administration.

Antagonistic actions to single doses of narcotics have been reported during chronic administration of nalorphine (9), cyclazocine (10), and naloxone (5). During chronic nalorphine administration at 240 mg/70 kg/day subcutaneously (40 mg every 4 hr), there was almost complete blockade of the effects of a 16 mg/70 kg morphine test dose compared to the same test dose given prior to initiation of chronic nalorphine administration. Chronic cyclazocine administration was investigated at two stabilization levels. During chronic administration of 1 mg/70 kg orally twice daily, test doses of 30 and 60 mg/70 kg morphine produced effects less than test doses of 10 and 30 mg/70 kg of morphine, respectively, administered during the pre-drug control period. At levels of chronic cyclazocine administration of 2 mg/70 kg orally twice daily, test doses of 60 and 120 mg/70 kg of morphine produced effects less than or equal to the control test doses of 10 and 30 mg/70 kg of morphine. Also at the high level of chronic administration, 60 mg/70 kg of heroin administered intravenously had less effect than the control test dose of 30 mg/70 kg subcutaneously administered morphine. A 90 mg/70 kg morphine test dose during chronic naloxone administration (15 mg/70 kg subcutaneously every 4 hr) produced effects less than or equal to morphine doses of 10 mg/70 kg administered during the control period.

The antagonistic actions to chronic morphine administration have been studied during chronic administration of cyclazocine (10). Subjects receiving chronic cyclazocine (2 mg/70 kg orally twice daily), were given morphine subcutaneously four times per day. The initial morphine dose of 10 mg was rapidly increased so that a 60 mg dose was attained in 11 days. This level was maintained four times per day for 9 days, at which time the morphine was abruptly withdrawn by double-blind substitution of saline. Abstinence scores were calculated daily for the next 10 days by the method of Kolb and Himmelsbach (8) from observations made three times daily for the presence of abstinence signs and measurement of vital signs, body weight, and caloric intake which had been made routinely during the entire study. When the morphine was abruptly withdrawn, an abstinence syndrome was observed. A mean peak abstinence score ($\pm$ SE) of 12.2 $\pm$ 2.6 was measured on the second day. The mean 10-day-area abstinence score was 70.8 $\pm$ 11.0. The abstinence syndrome was judged to be mild, and two of six subjects did not recognize that they were undergoing opiate abstinence. For comparison, in a study by Fraser et al. (2), subjects were maintained on morphine 60 mg four times daily administered subcutaneously for 10 days then abruptly withdrawn under double-blind conditions. The mean peak abstinence score (also seen on the second day) was 36.8 $\pm$ 2.7 and the mean 10-day-area abstinence score was 198.1 $\pm$ 16.3. It was concluded that chronic adminis-tration of cyclazocine significantly antagonized the development of physical dependence on morphine.

SUMMARY

This chapter has briefly reviewed the methods which have been developed at the Addiction Research Center to evaluate the antagonistic actions of narcotic antagonists in man. The major assay procedure is the precipitation test which allows determination of the relative potency of narcotic antagonists for the precipitation of abstinence in subjects physically dependent on morphine. Evaluation of the duration of action of single doses of narcotic antagonists has demonstrated antagonistic actions of naloxone for at least 9 hr and of cyclazocine for 12 to 24 hr. Methods to assess the antagonistic actions of narcotic antagonists during their chronic administration have shown that they maintain their antagonistic effects and continue to block the effects of single doses of narcotics and that they antagonize the development of physical dependence on chronically administered morphine.

REFERENCES

1. Finney, D. J.: Statistical Methods in Biological Assay. Hafner Publishing Co., New York, 1964.
2. Fraser, H. F., Van Horn, G. D., Martin, W. R., Wolbach, A. B., and Isbell, H.: Methods for evaluating addiction liability. (A) "Attitude" of opiate addicts toward opiate-like drugs. (B) A short-term "direct" addiction test. J. Pharmacol. Exp. Ther. *133*:371–387, 1961.
3. Jasinski, D. R., and Mansky, P. A.: Evaluation of nalbuphine for abuse potential. Clin. Pharmacol. Ther. *13*:78–90, 1972.
4. Jasinski, D. R., and Martin, W. R.: Evaluation of a new photographic method for assessing pupil diameters. Clin. Pharmacol. Ther. *8*:271–272, 1967.
5. Jasinski, D. R., Martin, W. R., and Haertzen, C. A.: The human pharmacology and abuse potential of N-allylnoroxymorphone (naloxone). J. Pharmacol. Exp. Ther. *157*:420–426, 1967.
6. Jasinski, D. R., Martin, W. R., and Hoeldtke, R. D.: Effects of short- and long-term administration of pentazocine in man. Clin. Pharmacol. Ther. *11*:385–403, 1970.
7. Jasinski, D. R., Martin, W. R., and Hoeldtke, R.: Studies of the dependence-producing properties of GPA-1657, profadol, and propiram in man. Clin. Pharmacol. Ther. *12*:613–649, 1971.
8. Kolb, L., and Himmelsbach, C. K.: Clinical studies of drug addiction. III. A critical review of the withdrawal treatments with method of evaluating abstinence syndromes. Amer. J. Psychiat. *94*:759–797, 1938.
9. Martin, W. R., and Gorodetzky, C. W.: Demonstration of tolerance to and dependence on N-allylnormorphine (nalorphine). J. Pharmacol. Exp. Ther. *150*:437–442, 1965.
10. Martin, W. R., Gorodetzky, C. W., and McClane, T. K.: An experimental study in the treatment of narcotic addicts with cyclazocine. Clin. Pharmacol. Ther. *7*:455–465, 1966.

Narcotic Antagonists, edited by M. C. Braude, L. S. Harris, E. L. May, J. P. Smith, and J. E. Villarreal. *Advances in Biochemical Psychopharmacology, Vol. 8.* Raven Press, New York © 1974.

Potential Usefulness of Single-Dose Acute Physical Dependence on and Tolerance to Morphine for the Evaluation of Narcotic Antagonists

J. J. C. Jacob, Colette D. Barthelemy, Evelyne C. Tremblay, and Marie-Claude L. Colombel

Laboratory of Pharmacology and Toxicology, Pasteur Institute, F 75015 Paris, France

The purpose of this work was to check the validity of a single morphine injection procedure for the quantitative assessment of naloxone potencies in precipitating abstinence, antagonizing precipitated abstinence, and antagonizing acute tolerance to the antinociceptive effect of morphine. The experimental animal was the mouse; the responses studied were jumping for precipitated abstinence and licking (hot plate technique) for antinociceptive action. Precipitated jumping occurred, and, when measured either quantally or by the mean numbers of jumps, this was in direct relation to the naloxone dose and most often but not always to the morphine dose, which also influenced the time course of the phenomenon underlying this kind of abstinence. Naloxone-precipitated jumping was inhibited by previous administration of naloxone, this antagonism being directly related to the (preventive) dose of naloxone and inversely to that of morphine. Single-dose morphine tolerance was also antagonized by naloxone given either before or after morphine: when given before, complete antagonism was obtained and dose-effect relations were the same as for antagonism of precipitated abstinence; when given after, antagonism was incomplete and curious relations to the dose of morphine were observed. The new facts are outlined and the mechanisms, specificity, and relevance of such acute "abstinence" and tolerance are discussed. The conclusion is reached that the morphine single-dose technique is, in some specified conditions, potentially valid for quantitative comparisons of potencies of antagonists in precipitating abstinence and in preventing it, antagonisms of tolerance being less accurately quantifiable. Limitations and advantages of such procedures are briefly discussed.

INTRODUCTION

This chapter deals with the assessment of three properties of narcotic antagonists: precipitation of abstinence and antagonism of precipitated abstinence and of tolerance in acute experiments.

299

Evaluation of the abstinence-precipitating potencies in chronically morphinized animals and human beings is a standard procedure discussed elsewhere in this volume. Antagonism of precipitated abstinence or of tolerance has most often been described in chronic experiments with agonist-antagonist mixtures, where quantification of the results is not an easy task (in rat 24, rabbit 30, monkey 27).

Several techniques have been developed which cause, in animals, states of dependence (or hyperexcitability) and tolerance with a single or several injections. These include, for example, in mice the techniques of morphine pellet implantation (19, 29), of a few opioid injections (18, 21, 25) or of a single injection (2, 4, 11, 15, 28); in rats the techniques of slow intravenous infusion (6), of reservoir implantation (8), and of a single injection of a sustained-release preparation (5); in dogs, the technique of slow intravenous infusion (23).

In general [an exception being a study by Huidobro and Maggiolo (12)] these techniques have been used in experiments designed to study not antagonists but agonists either for comparison of their tolerance or dependence potential or for attempts to elucidate mechanisms of actions. This is also the case for our experiments wherein only one antagonist (naloxone) was studied.

However, the results obtained suggest that these techniques might be of value for the quantitative assessment of the three above-cited activities of antagonists. Those reported here will focus mainly on the conclusions regarding the potential usefulness of the single morphine injection technique in the mouse; fundamental aspects of the problems will be discussed insofar as they are pertinent to the validity and limits of this acute model.

METHODS

Male Swiss Albino mice (CNRS—Orléans) weighing 18 to 24 g were used.

Precipitated Abstinence

It was measured by recording the number of jumps during 15 min after naloxone injection. Results are expressed by mean numbers of jumps (with their standard errors; a cut-off value of 40 jumps was used) and by the proportions of mice jumping once. Median effective doses (ED_{50}) and their fiducial limits ($p = 0.05$) were calculated with the classical Litchfield and Wilcoxon graphic procedure.

The experimental animals received a single dose of morphine and thereafter naloxone; three control groups received saline instead of morphine, or naloxone, or morphine and naloxone.

Antagonism of Precipitated Abstinence

The experimental animals received, successively, naloxone (antagonistic dose), morphine 15 min later, and then naloxone (precipitating dose). Concomitantly, a control group receiving saline instead of the antagonistic dose of naloxone was always run, and often another one receiving only the "precipitating" dose of naloxone. In one experiment morphine injection was followed by two separate injections of naloxone.

Antagonism of Single-Dose Tolerance

The procedure to produce single-dose tolerance in mice has been described (15). Briefly, a first (desensitizing) dose of morphine is injected followed by a second (test) one. The antinociceptive effect of morphine is determined with a modification of the hot plate method (16); the mice are exposed only once, 30 min after having received the test dose. Licking reaction times are measured (cut-off time 45 sec).

Control groups are injected with saline instead of the desensitizing dose, the test dose, or both doses. The effects of the test dose of morphine in normal or in tolerant mice are expressed by the mean increases of licking times as compared with the licking times of their respective controls (i.e., normal or tolerant mice receive saline instead of the morphine test dose).

In these antagonist experiments, naloxone was administered either before or after the desensitizing dose of morphine. Controls were a) mice injected with saline instead of naloxone, b), c), and d) treated as a), b), and c) above, and e) receiving naloxone, saline and the morphine testing dose to ascertain that the antagonist did not itself inhibit the effect of the testing dose.

Experimental groups were of at least 10 or, more often, 20 animals. The size of some control groups was reduced when accumulation of data had been obtained.

All injections were given subcutaneously. Morphine and naloxone hydrochlorides were used. Doses are expressed in milligrams per kilogram of body weight; they refer to the morphine base or to the naloxone salt.

RESULTS

Precipitated Abstinence

The intensity of naloxone-induced jumping in mice having received one single dose of morphine was related to the dose of both drugs and was a function of the time interval between the two injections.

The major influences of these different parameters are shown in Fig. 1, illustrating the effects of graded doses of naloxone administered at different times after either 15 or 200 mg/kg of morphine. For each dose of morphine, the intensity of the phenomenon increases with the naloxone doses, until a ceiling effect is reached for the higher doses (when injected at the optimal

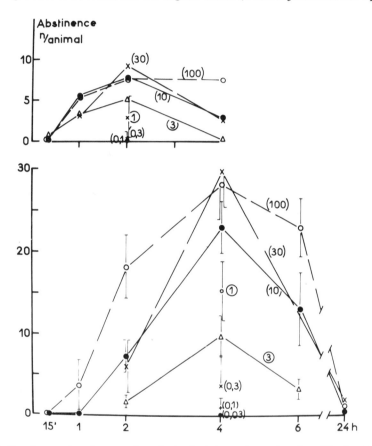

FIG. 1. Development and regression of physical dependence in mice. Effects of graded doses of naloxone injected at different intervals after a single dose of morphine. *Abscissa:* Time of the naloxone injection in (hr) (0 is time of morphine injection). *Ordinate:* Mean number of jumps per animal. The single dose of morphine was 15 mg/kg s.c. in the upper graph and 200 mg/kg s.c. in the lower graph. Numbers in parentheses indicate doses of naloxone in mg/kg s.c. Separate groups of mice (usually 20, sometimes 10) were used for each dose-time schedule. Bars represent SEM.

Mean numbers of jumps for control mice treated with naloxone alone were: 0.03 after a dose of 0.03 mg/kg (N = 30); 0 after 0.1 mg/kg (N = 25) and 0.3 mg/kg (N = 25); 0.1 after 1 mg/kg (N = 20) and 3 mg/kg (N = 20); 0.06 after 10 mg/kg (N = 135); 0.09 after 30 mg/kg (N = 35); 0.08 after 100 mg/kg (N = 50). Other controls did not jump.

time interval). Also, it is usually far more pronounced with the higher than with the lower dose of morphine. The time course of its development and of its decay depends on the morphine dosage: with the lower dose, very small effects were already noticed after 15 min, and a maximum was reached after 2 hr. With the higher dose, no effect was observed after 15 min.; it was clear-cut and significant after 1 hr, reached a maximum after 4 hr, and then declined and became very small 24 hr after the morphine injection.

The results of the same experiments together with those performed with other morphine dosages are more thoroughly analyzed in Figs. 2 and 3. It may be noticed that these two analyses are not equivalent; in particular, mean numbers of jumps make it possible to estimate variations in the phenomenon when all mice or a great proportion of mice are jumping, whereas percentages of mice jumping just once represent the less pronounced effects.

When the time interval was 4 hr (i.e., the optimal time for the mice receiving 100 and 200 mg/kg of morphine), a family of curves (Fig. 2) was obtained showing clearly the increase in the mean numbers of jumps with increasing doses of morphine and naloxone (in the dosage ranges of 15 to 200 mg for morphine, of 0.03 to 100 mg for naloxone). It may be noticed that the maximal effects, i.e., those obtained with the highest dose of naloxone used (100 mg/kg) (still higher ones have been observed by Villarreal to have clear-cut detrimental actions), are also different for the different morphine doses, a fact which argues in favor of the limiting influence of the morphine doses. The quantal representation again demonstrates the influence of the naloxone dose (Fig. 3) but allows only a distinction-limiting influence of the morphine dose.

The same conclusions hold when the curves which have been obtained for the optimal times are compared, i.e., 2 hr for 15 mg/kg of morphine, 4 hr for 50, 100, and 200 mg/kg. With the shorter time intervals (1 and 2 hr), the increase of the effect with increasing doses of naloxone was generally still observed, exceptions being represented by ceiling effects. However, the rate of increase of the effects (mean numbers of jumps) varied with the morphine doses used. For the low dose (15 mg/kg), it was slow up to a "ceiling" value; for the higher doses (100 and 200 mg/kg), it was at first only somewhat faster but with larger doses of naloxone the effects increased rapidly (2-hr interval).

The relations between mean numbers of jumps and morphine doses were no more univocal. In most cases, there was no relation at all or an inverse one (Fig. 4); a direct relation is obtained only with the high dose of naloxone (100 mg/kg) administered 2 hr after morphine. Quantal representations indicate direct variation only with the dose of naloxone and an inverse re-

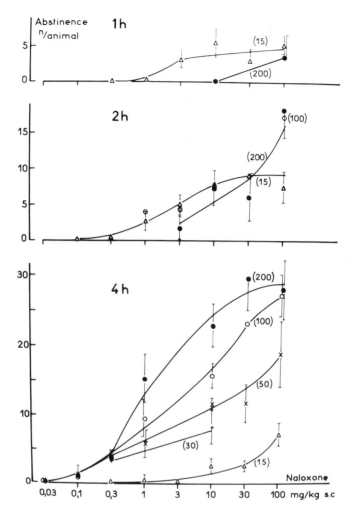

FIG. 2. Relations between precipitated abstinence and naloxone doses (graded response plot). *Abscissa:* Naloxone doses (log scale). *Ordinates:* Mean number of jumps per mouse. The time intervals between the morphine and the naloxone injections were: upper graph, 1 hr.; middle, 2 hr.; lower, 4 hr. The numbers in parentheses indicate morphine doses (mg/kg s.c.). The curve for 100 mg/kg of morphine and a 2-hr interval (open circle) has been omitted so as not to obscure the figure; it coincides with that for 15 mg/kg of morphine up to 30 mg/kg of naloxone and thereafter with the curve for 200 mg/kg of morphine.

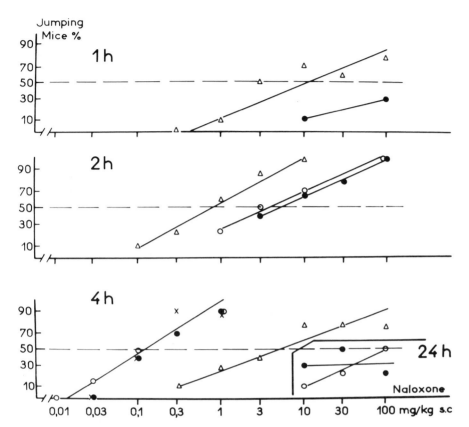

FIG. 3. Relations between precipitated abstinence and naloxone dose (quantal response plot). *Abscissa:* Naloxone doses (log scale). *Ordinate:* Percent of jumping mice (probit scale). The time intervals between the morphine and naloxone injections were: upper graph, 1 hr; middle, 2 hr; lower, 4 hr; insert, 24 hr. Morphine doses (mg/kg): △ 15; × 50; ○ 50; ● 200. Numbers of jumping mice when treated with naloxone alone were: 0.03 mg/kg, 1/30; 0.1 mg/kg, 0/30; 0/3 mg/kg, 0/25; 1 mg/kg, 1/20; 3 mg/kg, 1/20; 10 mg/kg, 4/135; 30 mg/kg, 2/35; 100 mg/kg, 1/50.

lation with the dose of morphine. Thus, complex interplays between naloxone and morphine are disclosed at these time intervals.

Table 1 summarizes the results of this section in terms of the ED_{50} values of naloxone.

Antagonism of Precipitated Jumping

Graded (antagonistic) doses of naloxone were injected 15 min before morphine (10 to 50 or 100 mg/kg) and a precipitating dose (10 mg/kg) was

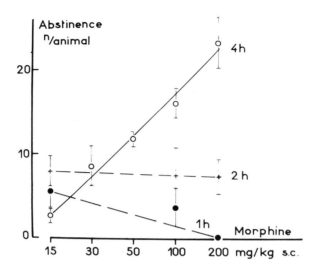

FIG. 4. Relations between precipitated abstinence and morphine dose. *Abscissa:* Morphine doses (log scale). *Ordinate:* Mean numbers of jumps. The precipitating naloxone dose was 10 mg/kg in these experiments. Number of animals as in Figs. 2 and 3.

TABLE 1. *Naloxone-precipitated abstinence after single doses of morphine*

Morphine dose (mg/kg s.c.)	ED_{50} and slope	Intervals between morphine and naloxone injections					
		15 min	1 hr	2 hr	4 hr	6 hr	24 hr
15	ED_{50} (mg/kg)	>100[a]	10 (5–20)[b]	0.95 (0.5–2)	6.5 (3.3–12.7)		
	slope		7.3	5.8	9.7		
50	ED_{50} (mg/kg)	>10[a]			0.13 (0.06–03)		
	slope				3.6		
100	ED_{50} (mg/kg)	>10[a]	≈10		0.13 (0.06–0.3)	≈10[a]	≈100[a]
	slope				3.6		
200	ED_{50} (mg/kg)	>100[a]	>100[a]	5 (3–8.3)	0.13 (0.06–0.3)	0.65 (0.3–2.3)	≈100[a]
	slope			3.6	3.6	12.3	

[a] Highest dose studied.
[b] Fiducial limit for $p = 0.05$.

given either 2 hr (for the morphine dose of 10 mg/kg) or 4 hr (for the morphine doses of 50 and 100 mg/kg) later (Fig. 5). These schedules were
chosen because controls, treated with saline instead of the naloxone antagonistic dose, responded to the precipitating dose in a proportion of 90 to
100%.

Clear-cut antagonisms were observed, which varied directly with the
preventive dose of naloxone and made possible the calculation of a median
antagonistic dose. These values of the median antagonist doses (mg/kg)
were related to the morphine dose: they were 0.14 (fiducial limits 0.05 and
0.39), 38 (f.l. 12–122), and 65 (f.l. 34–124) for 10, 50, and 100 mg/kg of
morphine, respectively.

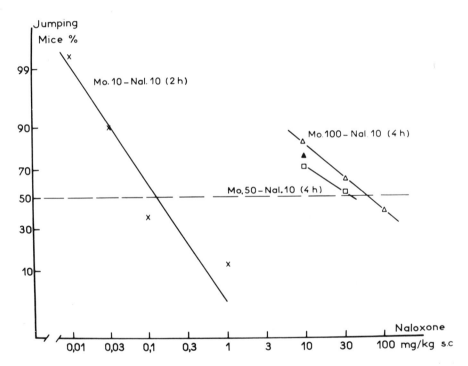

FIG. 5. Antagonism of precipitated jumping. Naloxone "antagonizing" doses were injected 15 min before morphine. The naloxone "precipitating" dose was 10 mg/kg. *Abscissa:* Naloxone antagonistic doses (log scale). *Ordinate:* Percent of jumping mice
(probit scale). × Morphine (Mo) 10 mg/kg; naloxone (Nal) precipitating dose injected 2 hr
later (groups of 10 mice). □ and △ Morphine 50 and 100 mg/kg, respectively; precipitating dose of naloxone injected 4 hr later; groups of 10 and 20 mice, respectively ▲ The
"antagonizing" dose of naloxone was injected 2 hr after morphine and 2 hr before the
"precipitating" dose of naloxone. For the controls receiving no naloxone pretreatment,
the numbers of jumping mice were 18/20, 18/20, and 49/50.

The difference in the time interval between the antagonistic (preventive) and the precipitating doses of naloxone probably contributes to the difference in antagonistic potencies existing when the lower and higher doses of morphine were used. This was indicated by the results of another series of experiments in which this time interval was kept the same for the two doses of morphine (100 and 15 mg/kg), but sound statistical evaluation was not possible as the controls responded with too low a frequency (60%). Some, but not significant, increase in protection was also observed when the antagonistic dose was given not before the dose of morphine (100 mg/kg) but 2 hr later (i.e., 2 hr before the challenging dose of naloxone). It is to be noticed that, in this experiment in which the "antagonistic" dose also precipitated jumping in some mice, there was no relation between this precipitated jumping and the protection observed afterwards: the protected mice were in equal numbers, animals which had jumped before or not.

Antagonism of Single-Dose Tolerance

Two series of experiments were performed: in the first one, graded doses of naloxone were injected 15 min before the dose of morphine (50, 100, or 200 mg/kg) which caused desensitization; in the second, naloxone was administered 4 hr after the dose of morphine. The testing dose of morphine (15 mg/kg) was injected either 24 or 28 hr after the desensitizing dose. This change was designed to avoid the morning-afternoon variations in reaction times, whereas it did not materially modify the effects of the testing dose in the control desensitized mice which, expressed in prolongation of licking times, were for 24 and 28 hr, respectively: after 50 mg/kg of morphine, 12.4 ± 1.2 sec (40 mice) and 11.1 ± 0.8 sec (65 mice); after 100 mg/kg of morphine, 8 ± 0.8 sec (70 mice) and 7.3 ± 0.7 sec (60 mice); and after 200 mg/kg of morphine 5.2 ± 0.6 sec (70 mice) and 5.8 ± 0.6 sec (75 mice). At 24 and 28 hr, the proper antinociceptive effects of the desensitizing dose had vanished and, as shown in Figs. 6 and 7, naloxone, at any dose used, did not modify the effect of the testing dose of morphine in nontolerant mice. This was not the case when the time interval between the administration of naloxone (10 or 30 mg/kg) and the testing dose of morphine was reduced to 4 hr, a time schedule which would have otherwise allowed for more precise determination; the effect of morphine was then inhibited by 66%.

Antagonism by Naloxone Injected Before Morphine

Antagonism of tolerance induction was produced by naloxone in proportion with its dose (Fig. 6). When the desensitizing doses of morphine were 50 or 100 mg/kg, the antagonism was significant with a dose of 0.3

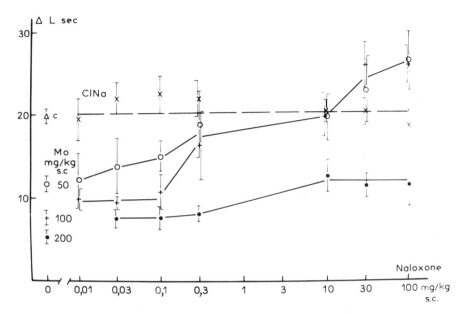

FIG. 6. Antagonism of naloxone before morphine. Naloxone was injected 15 min before the desensitizing dose of morphine. The challenging dose of morphine (15 mg/kg s.c.) was injected 24 hr after the desensitizing one. *Abscissa:* Naloxone dose (log scale). *Ordinate:* Increase in licking times (sec) induced by the challenging dose of morphine. △ Normal controls (200 mice); × naloxone controls (mice having not received the desensitizing dose of morphine, each group 20 mice); ○, +, and ● mice having received desensitizing doses of morphine (Mo) of 50, 100, and 200 mg/kg, respectively. Desensitized controls (100, 130, and 140 animals) correspond to the 0 on the abscissa. Experimental groups included 10 animals, except for the combination of the highest doses of naloxone with the highest dose of morphine (20 animals).

mg/kg naloxone and complete with 10 mg/kg; tolerance was even reversed to moderate potentiation with 30 and 100 mg/kg. With doses of naloxone lower than 0.3 mg/kg, naloxone apparently antagonized tolerance more readily when induced by 50 than by 100 mg/kg of morphine, but the differences cannot be considered significant.

When the morphine desensitizing dose was 200 mg/kg, the antagonism increased very slowly with the naloxone dose and remained very partial (but significant) even for doses of 10 to 100 mg/kg of naloxone. Antagonism appears then more clearly related in an inverse manner to the desensitizing dose of morphine.

Antagonism by Naloxone Injected After Morphine

Antagonism caused by naloxone injected after morphine was observed but was never complete (Fig. 7). After a small dose of morphine, the

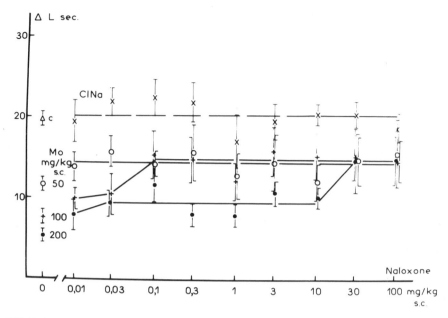

FIG. 7. Antagonism of naloxone injected after morphine. Naloxone was injected 4 hr after the desensitizing dose of morphine and the challenging dose of morphine (15 mg/kg) 24 hr after that. Abscissa, ordinate, and symbols as in Fig. 6. Experimental groups of 10 mice.

antagonism was slight and nonsignificant when calculations were done with the values of each experimental group separately, but highly so ($p < 0.01$) when they were done with those of all groups combined. After the dose of 100 mg/kg of morphine, the antagonism was more marked and clearly related to the dose of naloxone (0.01 to 0.1 mg/kg); it was significant for 0.1 mg/kg but did not increase further with higher doses of naloxone. After the dose of 200 mg/kg of morphine, the antagonism was poor up to 10 mg/kg of naloxone but clear-cut and significant when 30 and 100 mg/kg of naloxone was used.

Curiously, the part of tolerance which cannot be antagonized (as expressed by the difference between the effect of the testing dose of morphine in normal mice and the maximal effects observed in naloxone-treated tolerant mice) was the same for the three desensitizing doses of morphine. This was observed for seven pairs of values obtained from mice injected with 50 and 100 mg/kg of morphine and for two triplets with the three doses; such multiple congruence increases the likelihood of the phenomenon which otherwise would have been doubtful.

In this connection it should be mentioned that the common maximal partial antagonism was obtained with doses of naloxone which had to be increased as the doses of morphine were increased. It might be noticed that, at the time when naloxone was injected, the desensitizing dose of morphine still had some antinociceptive effect (as measured on independent groups of mice) which slowed prolongations of licking times of 2.6 to 3.2 and 9.5 sec after 50, 100, and 200 mg/kg of morphine, respectively. Some tolerance had already developed also (effects of the testing dose in independent groups of mice, which showed values of 6, 6.8, and 13.5 sec instead of 20 sec in nonmorphinized controls).

DISCUSSION

That narcotic antagonists precipitate abstinence in mice which have received a single dose of a narcotic analgesic has already been reported by Huidobro (9), Cheney and Goldstein (4), and Villarreal (28), and in a preliminary note of this laboratory (2); these authors used nalorphine-morphine, naloxone-levorphanol, and naloxone-morphine, respectively. The most extensive investigation was that of Villarreal who studied the effects of several doses of both agonists and antagonists, administered with different time schedules and furthermore investigated the effects of naloxone injected after codeine or pentazocine. The sign of abstinence was jumping, except in Huidobro's observations.

Our experiments confirm that the effect of the antagonist is related to its dose, a relation also observed with short-term repeated injections (20) or pellet implantation techniques (14, 29). Villarreal (28), however, pointed out that this relationship no longer applied for doses of naloxone higher than 100 mg/kg, probably because of interfering toxic effects; similarly, Huidobro, Maggiolo, and Contreras (14) found that large doses of nalorphine (e.g., 100 mg/kg) were less effective than lower ones, and had depressive actions.

Likewise, confirmation was obtained of the generally direct relationship between precipitated abstinence and the morphine dose (also established with the short-term techniques) and of the time course of the phenomenon (physical dependence?) underlying it. As in Villarreal's experiments, a maximum was reached 2 to 4 hr after morphine administration, and slight effects were still elicited 1 day after large morphine doses. Huidobro (9) also found some nonquantifiable signs 2 or even 4 days after morphine injections. The time course after levorphanol was seemingly somewhat different: the maximum was reached later (8 hr), and recovery was said to be complete after 16 hr (4).

Our results stressed the earliness of this phenomenon, as threshold jumping could already be induced 15 min or 1 hr after administration of morphine, depending on its dose. They also disclosed that with some schedules the relation between jumping and morphine dosages was no longer a direct one. Particularly relevant were the following facts. When naloxone was injected 2 hr after morphine, a low dose of naloxone was more effective after a low (15 mg/kg) than after a high dose of morphine (200 mg/kg) whereas the converse was true for a high (100 mg/kg) dose of naloxone. Furthermore, the curve relating the number of jumps to the log dose of naloxone, which rose slowly up to a moderate effect for the low doses, did rise slowly at first for the high doses also but later very abruptly. The simplest interpretation of these facts might be that 2 hr after the injection of morphine, high but not low doses still have a depressant effect which can be observed for the jumping behavior when a modification of the hot plate procedure is used (17). This action would balance the effect of naloxone until the dosage of this latter drug is high enough to overcome it. With a longer time interval (4 hr), between morphine and naloxone injections, any residual depressant action of morphine should be so slight that very low doses of naloxone would already overcome it. This does not mean that the antagonism of this depressant effect of morphine is the only action of naloxone to be taken into account (see below).

Antagonism of naloxone-precipitated jumping by naloxone itself, as well as antagonism of tolerance to morphine by naloxone, has not to our knowledge been described before with techniques using single injection of an opioid in mice. Using the technique of implantation of morphine pellets, Huidobro and co-workers (13, 14) obtained results which were interpreted by Martin (22) as indicating antagonism of both tolerance and physical dependence by repeated injections of nalorphine. More recently, Huidobro (9) described a moderate antagonism of tolerance by nalorphine injected in mice (implanted for 7 days) and an acceleration of the dissipation of tolerance in mice implanted for 14 days. Kaneto (18), using five morphine injections at 1-hr intervals, observed that naloxone, given simultaneously with each injection, prevented the development of acute tolerance and of naloxone-induced jumping but not the protracted tolerance which was tested 3 days later.

Our experiments show that a single injection of naloxone can antagonize precipitated jumping and tolerance obtained after a single injection of morphine. When naloxone was injected before morphine, the antagonism was directly related to the dose of naloxone and adversely related to the dose of morphine. With this latter schedule, naloxone curiously antagonized tolerance much more readily (completely overcome with 10 mg/kg naloxone) than it antagonized precipitated jumping (incompletely overcome with 100 mg/kg). Furthermore, the anti-"abstinence" action was seemingly of shorter duration than the anti-tolerance one. These facts raise again the problems of the intimate relations between the mechanisms of tolerance and physical dependence, which will not be discussed here.

Another observation was that naloxone was less effective in antagonizing tolerance when injected 4 hr after morphine than when injected 15 min before morphine. In the latter case, a ceiling residual tolerance remained which, when expressed in absolute terms (i.e., in differences of prolongations of licking times induced by the testing dose of morphine in nontolerant and tolerant mice), was the same for the three doses of morphine. The influences of the morphine dose were twofold: this ceiling effect was obtained with doses of naloxone which had to be raised when the doses of morphine were increased, and that part of tolerance which can be antagonistic was also directly related to the amount of morphine injected.

On the other hand, this "antagonizable" part of tolerance was also related to the residual effect of the desensitizing doses of morphine at the time when naloxone was administered. It would be tempting to consider that the antagonism of these residual effects by naloxone is at the origin of the partial antagonism of tolerance, an interpretation which would strengthen the view that tolerance to an effect of morphine is intimately linked to the elicitation of this very effect. However, this relation is not firmly established. Other interpretations might be relevant: for example, time (in these experiments 4 hr) might be the preponderant factor either for a binding of a given amount of morphine with some receptors (not necessarily the antinociceptive receptors) or for the development of biochemical events (e.g., protein synthesis) which, once started, would not be controlled by naloxone.

As to the mechanism of naloxone-precipitated jumping, it would appear that neither an unmasking of a stimulatory effect of the narcotic analgesic [by postulated selective antagonism of a depressant action (16, 22)] nor an "abstinoid" effect of naloxone (28) might *alone* account for the phenomenon.

The unmasking of such an effect of morphine is unlikely because administration of naloxone before morphine not only did not induce jumping but antagonized naloxone-precipitated jumping. This latter should, on the contrary, have been enhanced by cumulation of the antidepressant actions of the two naloxone doses. As seen above, this antagonism *per se* plays, nevertheless, some role manifest in particular schedules. An "abstinoid" effect of naloxone, which, as Villarreal (28) showed, accounts entirely for the contraction of the isolated gut after administration of a single dose of morphine, does not account for precipitated jumping, the importance of which is related to the amount of the single dose of morphine.

Both *a state of hyperexcitability* [as postulated by Seevers and Deneau (26, 27)], induced by morphine, possibly but not necessarily favored by naloxone and some abstinoid effects of naloxone, should be implied, the former potentiating the latter, as postulated by Villarreal (28) for repeated injections. Evidence for a very slight "abstinoid" jumping effect of naloxone is given by the rare occurrence of this phenomenon in mice treated with naloxone alone and also, indirectly, by the fact that naloxone shortens the jumping times of mice put for the first time on a hot plate (65°C) (unpublished experiments of our laboratory). This concept leads us to question the specificity of the jumping test with regard to the excitatory state induced by morphine and the "abstinoid" effect of naloxone. Amphetamine has been shown to precipitate some jumping in morphinized mice (28); it also shortens the time to jumping of mice on a hot plate [so, too, do several central anticholinergic (1, 3) agents]. Nevertheless, the naloxone-precipitated jumping after morphine is specific insofar as it is antagonized by naloxone, i.e., a drug considered as a specific antagonist.

This concept, however, does not account for the fact that Way, Loh, and Shen (29) observed withdrawal jumping after repeated injections of morphine or 2 days after pellet implantation. This indicates that an "abstinoid" effect of an antagonist is not indispensable, unless one assumes that a metabolite of morphine might play this role, the effect being then not an "abstinoid" one but abstinence itself.

Thus, the relevance of precipitated jumping after a single dose of morphine to chronic dependence cannot be settled yet, nor can that of acute single-dose tolerance to chronic tolerance. In short-term experiments, Villarreal (28) has shown that subacute "dependence" on morphine is built up by summation or potentiation of acute ones; similarly, Goldstein and Sheehan (7) gained evidence for levorphanol, and Jacob and Barthelemy (15) for morphine, that subacute tolerance is probably the result of summation processes. However, protracted dependence and tolerance have been described in a variety of animal species and in man, the mechanisms of which may involve other factors. Needless to say, much more experimental work is needed to outline which factors may be common in acute and chronic dependence and tolerance.

CONCLUSIONS

Quantitative Assessment of the Potency of an Antagonist to Precipitate Abstinence

The results obtained justify the conclusion that the morphine single-injection procedure will be adequate provided a suitable single dose of morphine (50, 100, or 200 mg/kg) and time interval (4 hr) between its injection and that of the antagonist are used. In such conditions, the ED_{50}

of naloxone is 0.13 mg/kg s.c. (95% C.L., 0.06 and 0.13); these values make possible valid comparisons of potencies of different antagonists. Plotting mean numbers of jumps versus log doses of the antagonist appears to be useful in obtaining additional information. Marshall and Graham-Smith (20) commented about the relative sensitivities of the two plotting procedures. In our experiments, it was found that, as might be anticipated on theoretical grounds, the quantal procedure was particularly suitable for quantifying the progression of low effects whereas the second procedure can satisfactorily assess further increases in effects when high percentages of mice are responding, i.e., when, as is well known, the probit method fails. Thus, a more complete survey of the evolution of effects as related to doses can be gained which might uncover, for example, complexities caused by mixed agonist-antagonist properties. With the strain of mice used here, we also found that groups of 10 mice may be insufficient for establishing the reliability of some potentially relevant differences.

Our experiments do not make it possible to draw conclusions on the validity of the technique with regard to the assessment of the duration of precipitated abstinence, which is brief with naloxone. This is also true for procedures involving short-term repeated administration of morphine or implantation. Owing to its great importance in preclinical studies, this parameter should be further investigated by comparing different antagonists.

Potencies of Drugs That Antagonize Precipitated Abstinence

It is recognized that too few drug combinations and insufficient numbers of animals have so far been studied. Nevertheless, satisfactory probit-log dose regression lines were obtained and median antagonistic doses with reasonable fiducial limits were calculated when protective single doses of naloxone were injected 15 min before the morphine dose. The median antagonistic dose of naloxone was 0.14 mg/kg (0.05 to 0.39) versus 10 mg/kg of morphine and 65 mg/kg (34 to 124) versus 100 mg/kg of morphine when a precipitating dose of 10 mg/kg of naloxone was injected 2 or 4 hr after morphine. Thus, the procedure promises to be useful for comparing both potencies and durations of action. For the study of curative antagonism, which is obtained in mice pretreated with morphine, its practical, but not theoretical, interest might be less, especially as the duration of a sufficiently developed dependence state is rather short, even after high morphine doses.

Potencies of Drugs That Antagonize Tolerance

The quantitative assessment of the potencies of drugs that antagonize tolerance was poor. The principal reason was that, with the time interval used (chosen because naloxone did not itself antagonize the effect of the testing doses of morphine), tolerance was still moderate even after the highest desensitizing dose of morphine. The ED_{50} values of morphine, determined in other experiments, were 33 mg/kg (26 to 42) in tolerant mice and 12 mg/kg (9.6 to 15) in nontolerant mice. Other reasons included a possibly poor choice of the testing dose which was selected for practical purposes or variability of responses inherent in the hot plate method. No sound quantal treatment of tolerance antagonism was possible in such conditions. Way et al. (29), with the technique of pellet implantations and the tail-flick test, obtained ED_{50} values of morphine that were increased by a factor of approximately five in tolerant animals and had narrow fiducial limits. These authors, however, stated that the pellet technique would be difficult to apply for the study of naloxone, which might not be the case for antagonists with long duration of action. Nevertheless, in addition to the theoretical interest indicated in the Discussion, the single-dose procedure, as it stands, might be useful for screening.

From a more general point of view, the single-dose procedure as presented here has some important limitations. Only one sign of abstinence and tolerance to only one effect of morphine has been studied. This limitation will be best met by extending the investigation to other animal species which have a richer semeiology and respond to single injections or similar short-term administrations of morphine [rat (5), dog (23)] or which will be found to do so. This procedure will also meet the requirement that preclinical studies should be performed in more than one animal species.

The specificity of the naloxone jumping test and the relevance of acute dependence and tolerance to the corresponding chronic conditions have already been considered in the Discussion. At present, acute studies are nevertheless the only ones that permit practical investigations of the posological variables necessary for sound comparisons of the properties of narcotic antagonists considered in this chapter with their various other acute effects. The results of such investigations would help in designing and restricting the indispensable but much more expensive chronic experiments. Finally, the validity of these conclusions must be checked by comparative studies of other antagonists.

ACKNOWLEDGMENTS

This work was supported by grants of the Institut National de la Santé et de la Recherche Médicale (Director, C. Burg) and the Direction des Recherches et des Moyens d'Essais (Director, Pr. J. E. DuBois).

Naloxone hydrochloride was a gift of Endo Laboratories (Dr. M. J.

Ferster). We also thank the Head of the Service Central de la Pharmacie (Ministry of Health) for the authorization to use morphine. The aid of M. Ch. Suaudeau and Miss D. Drouot in preparing the manuscript is also acknowledged.

REFERENCES

1. Barthelemy, C., and Jacob, J.: Réactivité nociceptive de souris de diverses souches. Sélection pour la recherche d'effets facilitateurs. J. Pharmacol. (Paris) *3*:199–209, 1972.
2. Barthelemy, C., and Jacob, J.: Naloxone precipitated abstinence after one simple injection of morphine and effects of naloxone on single dose tolerance to morphine. J. Pharmacol. (Paris) *3*:C$_2$, 1972.
3. Barthelemy, C., Tremblay, E., and Jacob, J.: Effets de divers anticholinergiques sur la motricité et sur des réactions nociceptives chez la Souris. J. Pharmacol. (Paris) *2*:35–52, 1970.
4. Cheyney, D. L., and Goldstein, A.: Tolerance to opioid narcotics: Time course and reversibility of physical dependence in mice. Nature, *232*:477–478, 1971.
5. Collier, H. O. J., Francis, D. L., and Schneider, C.: Modification of morphine withdrawal by drugs interacting with humoral mechanisms: Some contradictions and their interpretation. Nature, *237*:220–223, 1972.
6. Cox, B. M., Ginsburg, M., and Osman, O. H.: Acute tolerance to narcotic analgesic drugs in rats. Br. J. Pharmacol. Chemother. *33*:245–256, 1968.
7. Goldstein, A., and Sheehan, P.: Tolerance to opioid narcotics. 1. Tolerance to the "running fit" caused by levorphanol in the mouse. J. Pharmacol. Exp. Ther. *169*:175–184, 1969.
8. Goode, P. G.: An implanted reservoir of morphine solution for rapid induction of physical dependence in rats. Br. J. Pharmacol. *41*:558–566, 1972.
9. Huidobro, F.: Some relations between tolerance and physical dependence to morphine in mice. Europ. J. Pharmacol. *15*:79–84, 1971.
10. Huidobro, F., and Contreras, E.: Studies on morphine. II. Repeated administration of nalorphine to white mice chronically treated with pellets of morphine. Arch. Int. Pharmacodyn. *144*:206–213, 1963.
11. Huidobro, J. P., and Huidobro, F.: Kinetics of morphine tolerance development in mice. Fifth Int. Congress on Pharmacol., San Francisco, July 23–28, 1972,) Abstract 654.
12. Huidobro, F., and Maggiolo, C.: Studies on morphine. V. Effects of various antimorphine compounds and of normorphine on mice implanted with pellets of morphine. Arch. Int. Pharmacodyn. *149*:78–89, 1964.
13. Huidobro, F., and Maggiolo, C.: Studies on morphine. IX. On the intensity of the abstinence syndrome to morphine induced by daily injections of nalorphine in white mice. Arch. Int. Pharmacodyn. *158*:97–112, 1965.
14. Huidobro, F., Maggiolo, C., and Contreras, E.: Studies on morphine. I. Effects of nalorphine and levallorphan in mice implanted with pellets of morphine. Arch. Int. Pharmacodyn. *144*:196–205, 1963.
15. Jacob, J. C., and Barthelemy, C. D.: Single dose and repeated dose tolerance to the antinociceptive effect of morphine in mice. As reported to the 34th meeting of The Committee on Problems of Drug Dependence, 1972, pp. 592–606.
16. Jacob, J., and Blozovski, M.: Actions de divers analgésiques sur le comportement de souris exposées à un stimulus thermoalgésique. 1. Technique rapide de sélection et de caractérisation. Arch. Int. Pharmacodyn. *122*:287–299, 1959.
17. Jacob, J., and Blozovski, M.: Actions de divers analgésiques sur le comportement de souris exposées à un stimulus thermoalgésique. 2. Apprentissage nociceptif d'urgence. Actions différentielles de substances psychoactives sur les réactions de léchement et de bond. Arch. Int. Pharmacodyn. *133*:296–309, 1961.

18. Kaneto, H.: Dissociation of analgesic effect from tolerance or physical dependence liability of morphine in mice. Fifth Int. National Congress on Pharmacol., San Francisco, July 23–28, 1972. Abstract 712.

19. Maggiolo, C., and Huidobro, F.: Administration of pellets of morphine to mice. Abstinence syndrome. Acta Physiol. Lat. Am. *11*:70–78, 1961.

20. Marshall, I., and Grahame-Smith, D. G.: Evidence against a role of brain 5-hydroxytryptamine in the development of physical dependence upon morphine in mice. J. Pharmacol. Exp. Ther. *173*:634–641, 1971.

21. Marshall, I., and Weinstock, M.: A quantitative method for the assessment of physical dependence on narcotic analgesics in mice. J. Pharmacol. *37*:505–506P, 1969.

22. Martin, W. R.: Opioid antagonists. Pharmacol. Rev. *19*:463–521, 1967.

23. Martin, W. R., and Eades, C. G.: Demonstration of tolerance and physical dependence in the dog following a short-term infusion of morphine. J. Pharmacol. Exp. Ther. *133*:262–270, 1961.

24. Orahovats, P. D., Winter, C. A., and Lehman, E. G.: The effect of N-allylnormorphine upon the development of tolerance to morphine in the albino rat. J. Pharmacol. Exp. Ther. *109*:413–416, 1953.

25. Saelens, J. K., Granat, F. R., and Sawyer, W. K.: The mouse jumping test. A simple screening method to estimate the physical dependence capacity of analgesics. Arch. Int. Pharmacodyn. *190*:213–218, 1971.

26. Seevers, M. H., and Deneau, G. A.: A critique of the "dual action" hypothesis of morphine physical dependence. Arch. Int. Pharmacodyn. *140*:514–520, 1962.

27. Seevers, M. H., and Deneau, G. A.: Physiological aspects of tolerance and physical dependence. *In* Pharmacological Pharmacology, edited by W. S. Root and F. G. Hofmann, *1*:565–640. Academic Press, New York, 1963.

28. Villarreal, J. E.: Pharmacologic analysis of the dependence-producing actions of narcotic analgesics. Communication to Bayer Symposium IV: Psychic dependence – Definition, Assessment in Animal and Man; Theoretical and Clinical Implications, Grosse Ledder, Sept. 27-Oct. 1, 1972.

29. Way, E. L., Loh, H. H., and Shen, F.: Simultaneous quantitative assessment of morphine tolerance and physical dependence: J. Pharmacol. Exp. Ther. *167*:1–8, 1969.

30. Yim, G. K. W., Keasling, H. H., and Gross, E. G.: Simultaneous respiratory minute volume and tooth pulp threshold charges following chronic administration of levorphan and a levorphan-levallorphan mixture in rabbits. J. Pharmacol. Exp. Therap. *118*:193–197, 1956.

Narcotic Antagonists, edited by M. C. Braude, L. S. Harris, E. L. May, J. P. Smith, and J. E. Villarreal. *Advances in Biochemical Psychopharmacology, Vol. 8.* Raven Press, New York © 1974.

Assessment of the Agonist and Antagonist Properties of Narcotic Analgesic Drugs by Their Actions on the Morphine Receptor in the Guinea Pig Ileum

H. W. Kosterlitz, Angela A. Waterfield, and Valerie Berthoud

Department of Pharmacology, University of Aberdeen, Aberdeen, AB9 2ZD, Scotland

Agonist potencies of narcotic analgesic drugs are determined by their depressant effects on the contractions of the longitudinal muscle of the isolated guinea pig ileum; the contractions are evoked by coaxial electrical stimulation. Antagonist potencies are determined by interaction with the depressant effects of morphine or normorphine. The agonist potencies of narcotic analgesic drugs can be satisfactorily predicted by this method. The antagonist potencies of narcotic analgesic drugs determined on the guinea pig ileum correlate well with the antagonist potencies determined in morphine-dependent monkeys. The ratio of the antagonist and agonist potencies of a narcotic analgesic drug appears to be of greater predictive value for its clinical usefulness than its absolute agonist and antagonist potencies. Such a ratio can be readily obtained on the guinea pig ileum but requires carefully chosen methods in rodents. In compounds with powerful agonist activity (e.g., cyclorphan and ketocyclazocines), the relatively weak antagonist activity is difficult to discern by the standard assay on the guinea pig ileum. An increase in the concentration of naloxone, which is required to antagonize the agonist effects of these drugs, may be due to their antagonist activity.

INTRODUCTION

Agonist and antagonist potencies of narcotic analgesic drugs can be assayed *in vivo* by several methods which, for reasons not fully understood, do not always yield results in agreement with each other. Other chapters in this volume deal with this particular problem.

Assay techniques which are based on isolated tissues examined *in vitro* have certain advantages. Effects of absorption, distribution, biotransformation, and excretion of the drugs are almost completely excluded. Moreover, it is possible to study the effects of a drug immediately after its addition to the bath fluid whereas in the whole animal secondary effects during the first few minutes after injection of the drug may complicate the interpretation of the results.

It would, therefore, be desirable to assay drugs on relatively simple systems which have more or less homogeneous neuron pools, with a majority of morphine-sensitive synaptic junctions. Such a situation would make possible the estimation of some of the kinetic parameters of the interaction of drug and receptor. Ideally, one should examine neuron pools that mediate analgesia but such an approach is at present impossible.

There are in the peripheral autonomic nervous system neuroeffector junctions which in some species, but not in others, are morphine sensitive. For instance, transmission from the myenteric plexus to the longitudinal muscle is depressed by morphine in the guinea pig but not in the rabbit or rat (22) whereas transmission from the vagus nerve to the sinoatrial node is morphine sensitive in the rat and rabbit but not in the guinea pig (19). As far as adrenergic autonomic junctions are concerned, the nictitating membrane of the cat and the vas deferens of the mouse, but not of the rabbit and guinea pig, are morphine sensitive (4, 14, 31).

So far only the junction from the myenteric plexus to the longitudinal muscle of the guinea pig ileum has been investigated systematically as to its suitability for the assay of narcotic analgesic drugs (18, 20).

METHODS

The experimental procedure has already been described (20). In principle, a segment of guinea pig ileum is taken from 10 to 15 cm above the ileocecal junction and suspended in modified Krebs solution; it is stimulated coaxially (24, 25) by rectangular pulses of 0.5 msec duration, supramaximal strength, and a frequency of 0.1 Hz. The twitch-like contractions of the longitudinal muscle are recorded isometrically.

Assessment of Agonist and Antagonist Activity

The following parameters have been chosen: (1) the concentration of the drug which causes 50% inhibition of the evoked contraction of the longitudinal muscle (ID_{50}), to characterize agonist activity; (2) the dissociation or equilibrium constant (K_e) to characterize antagonist activity; (3) the effective antagonist potency, P_a, which is the ratio ID_{50}/K_e, to characterize the relative agonist and antagonist activities; (4) the rate of recovery (K_r) or its half-time (T_r), to characterize duration of action.

In this chapter, particular attention will be paid to the assessment of relative agonist and antagonist potencies, and, therefore, parameters 1, 2, and 3 will be discussed in more detail.

ID_{50} as Parameter of Agonist Activity

Tachyphylaxis to agonist activity occurs with all narcotic analgesic drugs whether they are predominantly of an agonist or antagonist nature. For this reason, it may be difficult to determine ID_{50} from dose-response curves ("multiple-dose" method). Reproducible dose-response curves can be obtained for morphine when the dose interval is 15 to 20 min (11) and for normorphine when the dose interval is 10 min (18). With compounds of considerable antagonist activity the dose interval may have to be extended to 1 to 2 hr which makes it impracticable to use the multiple-dose method. On the other hand, the fact that with a dose cycle of 20 min a shallow dose response curve may be obtained is useful additional information.

When the "single dose" method is used, the preparation is set up and stimulated for 1 hr at 0.1 Hz. Then a dose-response curve for morphine is constructed with dose intervals of 20 min or for normorphine with a dose interval of 10 min; morphine and normorphine are equipotent in this preparation (18). It is advantageous to repeat the dose-response curve to test the preparation for stability. Forty-five min after the last dose of morphine or normorphine has been washed out, the compound to be tested is added. The dose will vary according to its agonist activity; an amount is chosen to give a depression of the twitch of preferably 30 to 40% (Fig. 1). The ID_{50}

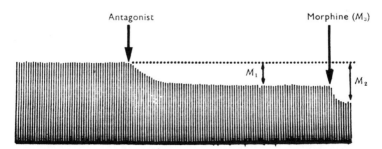

FIG. 1. Measurement of the antagonist activity of a partial agonist by determination of its equilibrium constant, K_e. Guinea pig isolated ileum. Isometric recording of the contractions of the longitudinal muscle induced by electrical coaxial stimulation. At the arrow marked antagonist, the partial agonist was added and produced a depression of the twitch equal to a depression caused by morphine in concentration M_1. Morphine was added 20 min later to give a concentration M_3; the total depression was equal to a reduction in the height of the twitch caused by morphine in a concentration M_2 in the absence of the antagonist. $DR = M_3/(M_2 - M_1)$. Reproduced, with permission, from Kosterlitz and Watt (20).

value is then extrapolated by assuming that the slopes of the dose-response curves of morphine or normorphine, on the one hand, and of the test substance, on the other, do not differ significantly.

Because the slopes of the dose-response curves of compounds with significant antagonist activity are likely to be less steep than that of morphine or normorphine, the ID_{50} values obtained with the single-dose method may be expected to be too low, i.e., the agonist potency will be overestimated. On the other hand, the values obtained with the multiple-dose method will underestimate agonist activity because of interaction between doses. Experience has shown that the ID_{50} values obtained with the multiple-dose method may be twice those obtained with the single-dose method.

The single-dose assay is the method of choice, but it is advisable to examine more fully the dose relationship of any new drug in order to determine whether the slope of the curve is shallow and also whether a depression of at least 50% is obtainable.

K_e as Parameter of Antagonist Activity

K_e is the dissociation or equilibrium constant; it is determined by estimating the dose ratio at a given concentration of antagonist: $K_e = a/DR - 1$, where a is the molar concentration of the antagonist and DR the ratio of the concentrations of agonist required to give the same depression of the twitch in the presence and absence of the antagonist (26, 30).

In the estimations of K_e, morphine or normorphine is used as the agonist, for which a dose-response curve has been constructed 45 min before exposure of the ileum to the antagonist. An objection to this estimation is the fact that morphine has itself agonist and weak antagonist actions (11). Normorphine appears to be a better agonist but is not free from self-antagonist effects (18). The absence of a pure agonist makes the estimation of K_e somewhat unreliable, particularly for compounds with strong agonist and relatively weak antagonist properties.

Because the great majority of narcotic analgesic drugs exhibit both agonist and antagonist actions, the following method has been adopted for the estimation of K_e. After the ileum has been exposed to the antagonist, as already described for the single-dose method for the determination of ID_{50} (Fig. 1), the concentration of morphine or normorphine (M_1) that would have been expected to produce the same depressant effect on the twitch is read off the dose-response curve already constructed for morphine or normorphine. After the ileum has been exposed to the antagonist for 20 min, morphine or normorphine in a concentration M_3 is added to depress the twitch further. The morphine or normorphine concentration (M_2) which would have a depressant effect equal to the combined actions of the antagonist and the morphine or normorphine present in the bath is read off the dose-response curve for morphine or normorphine. The dose ratio is then $DR = M_3/(M_2 - M_1)$. M_3 should reduce the residual contraction by at least 20% and the total inhibition should not be more than 80%.

After the antagonist has been washed out, the sensitivity of the preparation to a test concentration of morphine or normorphine increases again. When there is no further increase in sensitivity, another dose-response curve for morphine or normorphine is constructed. It is desirable that the ID_{50} values before and after the exposure of the ileum to the antagonist should not differ by more than 30%.

K_e represents the concentration of the antagonist in moles per liter at which the concentration of the agonist has to be doubled in order to have the same depressant effect on the twitch as in the absence of the antagonist. pA_2, which is often used to characterize antagonist potency, equals $-\log_{10}K_e$.

Effective Antagonist Potency

This term (P_a) takes into account the relative agonist and antagonist activities and is expressed as follows: $P_a = ID_{50}/K_e$. $P_a = DR - 1$ when the drug is used in the concentration which has an agonist effect equal to ID_{50}. P_a is related to efficacy, e (30), since $P_a = 1/(e - 1)$.

The method used for the assessment of K_e and P_a is valid only if the antagonism between morphine or normorphine and the antagonist is competitive. So far it has been possible to prove this for the antagonism by naloxone of the agonist effects of morphine, normorphine, levorphanol, codeine, phenoperidine, etorphine, 1-diethylamino-ethyl-2-*p*-methoxy-benzyl-5-nitrobenzimidazole, ketocyclazocine, and nalorphine (15, 17; *unpublished observations*).

RESULTS

Agonist Activity

The rank order of the agonist potencies of a wide range of compounds agrees well with the findings in man (Table 1). The absolute values may differ by a factor of up to three but this finding is not altogether surprising when one considers the uncertainties of the assays in the isolated ileum and even more in man. Two compounds show a much more marked discrepancy. The first is codeine which is less active in the guinea pig ileum than would be expected from its analgesic potency in man. The discrepancy is probably

TABLE 1. *Comparison of agonist potencies in man and guinea pig ileum*

Drug	Potency (morphine = 1)	
	Man	Guinea pig ileum
Codeine	0.08[a]	0.007[j]
Nalmexone	0.13[b]	0.17[k]
Pentazocine	0.3[c]	0.27[j]
Profadol	0.3[d,e]	0.2[j]
Nalorphine	1.0[a]	2.8[j]
Levallorphan	1.0[f]	16[j]
Nalbuphine	1.2[g]	0.5[l]
Diamorphine	3[a]	2[j]
Levorphanol	5[a]	7[j]
Dextromoramide	4[h]	10[j]
Cyclazocine	30[c]	19[j]
Cyclorphan	75[c]	240[l]
Etorphine	200[i]	700[l]

The values obtained in the guinea pig are always calculated on a molar basis and those found in man, monkey, or rodent on a weight basis, except in Table 7.
[a] (8); [b] N-dimethylallylnoroxymorphone (9); [c] (21); [d] (17); [e] (29); [f] (27); [g] N-cyclobutylmethyl-7,8-dihydro-14-hydroxymorphine (16); [h] (15); [i] (2); [j] (20); [k] (18); [l] *unpublished observations.*

due to biotransformation of codeine to morphine in man but not in the guinea pig isolated ileum. The second discrepancy cannot be explained at present. Levallorphan is a potent agonist in the guinea pig ileum although the dose-response curve is shallow as is the case with all partial agonists which have a strong antagonist component. In man, however, the agonist potency of levallorphan is very difficult to determine and is at most equal to that of morphine and nalorphine. The most plausible explanation is rapid self-antagonism. In the guinea pig ileum the agonist activity is determined much more rapidly after administration, namely within the first 2 min of addition of the drug to the organ bath. A second dose given 20 min later is considerably less effective so that the dose response of levallorphan is much shallower than that of morphine.

Antagonists with Negligible Agonist Activity

As far as compounds with predominant antagonist and only little agonist effects are concerned, their classification is readily obtained (Table 2). Three

TABLE 2. *Antagonists with little or no agonist activity*

Drug	Antagonist potency (naloxone = 1)	Agonist potency (morphine = 1)
(−)-β-5-phenyl-9-methyl-2'-hydroxy-6,7-benzomorphans[a]		
N-Propargyl (GPA 2163)	0.04	0
N-3-Chloro-2-propenyl (GPA 1894)	0.05	0
N-Allyl (GPA 1843)	0.06	0
(±)-α-5,9-Dimethyl-2'-hydroxy-6,7-benzomorphan[b]		
N-Furylmethyl (Mr 1256-MS)	0.18	0.35[c]
Noroxymorphone[a]		
N-Allyl (naloxone)	1.0	<0.001
N-Cyclopropylmethyl (EN 1639A)	3.1	<0.08[c]

[a] (15); [b] *unpublished observations;* [c] *shallow dose-response curves (15 and unpublished observations)*

derivatives of the β-5-phenyl-9-methyl-2'-hydroxy-6,7-benzomorphan series are devoid of an agonist component but, unfortunately, have only a weak antagonist effect. Naloxone has only negligible agonist effect whereas EN-1639A and, even more, Mr 1256-MS have agonist actions, but the dose-response curves in the guinea pig ileum are very shallow. It is probably for this reason that their agonist effects are scarcely noticeable in the whole animal (3, 23).

Comparison of Antagonist Activity in Monkey and Guinea Pig Ileum

If the antagonist activity in the guinea pig ileum (K_e) is compared with that observed in morphine-dependent monkeys, good agreement is found for compounds with varying relative agonist and antagonist properties (Table 3). Discrepancies are found with compounds which are more potent antagonists than nalorphine. The guinea pig ileum method gives higher values for cyclazocine and diprenorphine whereas naloxone and (±)-N-cyclopropylmethyl-3,14-dihydroxymorphinan (BC-2605) appear to be more active in the dependent monkey.

Antagonists with Definite Agonist Activity

In contrast to the compounds listed in Table 2, most antagonists exhibit agonist activity in the guinea pig ileum. In Table 4 such compounds are arranged in ascending order of antagonist potency, calculated from the values of their dissociation constants (K_e), and expressed as multiples of the K_e

TABLE 3. *Comparison of antagonist potencies determined in morphine-dependent monkeys and in the guinea pig ileum*

Drug	Antagonist potency (nalorphine = 1)	
	Monkey	Guinea pig ileum
Pentazocine	0.03[a,b]	0.03[h]
Nalmexone	0.1[b]	0.1[i]
(−)-β-2-Propargyl-5-phenyl-9-methyl-2'-hydroxy-6,7-benzomorphan (GPA 2163)	0.18[c]	0.14[i]
(±)-α-2-(3-Furylmethyl)-5,9-dimethyl-2'-hydroxy-6,7-benzomorphan (Mr 1256)	0.5[d]	0.66[j]
Cyclazocine	3.5[a]	3.0[h]
Levallorphan	3.5[a]	4.0[h]
Naloxone	7[e]	3.7[h]
(±)-N-Cyclopropylmethyl-3,14-dihydroxymorphinan (BC 2605)	8[d]	2.7[j]
N-Cyclopropylmethylnoroxymorphone (EN 1639A)	6–13[f]	11.5[i]
Diprenorphine	16[g]	34[h]

[a] (5); [b] (7); [c] (32); [d] (35); [e] (6); [f] (34); [g] (33); [h] (20); [i] (18); [j] *unpublished observations.*

TABLE 4. *Antagonists with definite agonist activity*

Drug	Antagonist potency (nalorphine = 1)	Agonist potency (morphine = 1)	Effective antagonist potency (ID_{50}/K_e)
Profadol[a]	0.015	0.16	1.4
Pentazocine[a]	0.03	0.27	1.7
Nalmexone[b]	0.1	0.17	9.3
Nalorphine[a]	1.0	2.8	5.4
Cyclazocine[a]	3.0	19	2.4
Levallorphan[a]	4.0	16	3.8
(−)-N-cyclopropylmethyl-morphinans			
3,14-dihydroxy (BC 2605)[c]	5.2	27	3.0
3-nicotinoyl-14-hydroxy[c] (BC 2888)	6.3	16	6.0
Diprenorphine[a]	34	100[d]	5.2

[a] (20); [b] (18); [c] *unpublished observations;* [d] shallow response curve.

of nalorphine. The agonist potencies of these compounds are of a quite different order. Therefore the rank order of their effective antagonist potencies would appear to be as follows: nalmexone > BC 2888, nalorphine, diprenorphine > levallorphan, BC 2605 > cyclazocine > pentazocine, profadol. It is by no means certain how far effective antagonist potency, as determined in the guinea pig ileum, correlates with useful antagonist potency in the whole animal or man.

Assessment of Antagonist Activity in Compounds with High Agonist Activity

When a compound with high agonist activity is used, the contraction of the longitudinal muscle is depressed by very low concentrations. If its antagonist potency is relatively weak in comparison with its agonist potency, the concentration of the compound in the bath fluid would have to be raised beyond the point at which complete suppression of the longitudinal contraction is obtained. Table 5 illustrates this situation for three compounds. Their agonist activity rises in the following order: isocyclorphan < diprenorphine < cyclorphan; on the other hand, their antagonist potency is arranged in a different order: isocyclorphan < cyclorphan < diprenorphine. For this reason, the effective antagonist potency, P_a, of diprenorphine is approximately five but that of cyclorphan and isocyclorphan is below one. The dose ratios caused by the two latter drugs are just above unity. The criteria which are applied to compounds with less agonist potency would lead to the conclusion that neither cyclorphan nor isocyclorphan have significant antagonist properties. And yet, in the tail-flick test, it has been shown that cyclorphan and isocyclorphan have antagonist properties (10, 13).

TABLE 5. *Assessment of agonist and antagonist activities of cyclorphan, isocyclorphan, and diprenorphine*

Drug	ID_{50} (nM)	K_e (nM)	P_a (ID_{50}/K_e)	Agonist potency (morphine = 1)
Cyclorphan (4)	0.283 ± 0.035	0.606 ± 0.332	0.5	240
Isocyclorphan (4)	1.01 ± 0.13	2.40 ± 0.77	0.4	68
Diprenorphine[a](6)	0.68 ± 0.07	0.13 ± 0.02	5.2	100

The values are the means with their standard errors; the number of observations are given in brackets. The dose ratios for morphine or normorphine concentrations which cause inhibition of the twitch by 30 to 60% were as follows: cyclorphan 2.03 ± 0.47 (4) and isocyclorphan 1.49 ± 0.15 (4).

[a] (20).

To solve this dilemma, two possible approaches are being explored. It is known that, under certain circumstances, even compounds with preponderant agonist activity, such as morphine, show self-antagonism in the guinea pig ileum (11). If in the construction of a dose-response curve for morphine the dose interval is reduced below 10 to 15 min, the slope of the regression line is shallower than with the optimum dose interval of 15 to 20 min. Compounds with relative strong antagonist properties will give shallow dose-response curves or at least dose-response curves with varying slopes in different experiments. Such an observation has been made with diprenorphine (ID_{50} = 0.68) and ($\pm$)-α-2-furfuryl-5,9-dimethyl-2'hydroxy-6,7-benzomorphan (Mr 1029-MS, ID_{50} = 10.6). It has not been possible, so far, to examine systematically the relationship between the slope of the dose-response curve and the relative antagonist potency of a compound.

Another approach is based on the observation that a higher concentration of naloxone is required to antagonize the agonist effects of partial agonists with high effective antagonist potency (e.g., nalorphine, levallorphan, and diprenorphine) than the agonist effect of a compound with negligible antagonist properties (18, 20). The values of K_e are the molar concentration of naloxone at which twice the concentration of the agonist is required to depress the longitudinal contraction to the same extent as in the absence of naloxone; pA_2 is the negative logarithm of K_e. These K_e values do not differ significantly for a number of agonists of widely differing potency and structure (18).

Two new compounds have recently been sent to us by Dr. S. Archer, ketocyclazocine and its congener which has an ethyl group instead of a methyl group in position 5 of the benzomorphan ring. They are both very potent agonists in the writhing test. Ketocyclazocine is inactive as an agonist in the tail-flick test but shows weak antagonist action. In the tail-flick test the ethyl derivative has a weak agonist action which requires a high concentration of naloxone for antagonism (1). In the guinea pig ileum both compounds are very potent agonists, the ethyl derivative more so than ketocyclazocine; the dose-response curves have normal slopes. The (−)-isomers have about twice the agonist potency of the racemates. Neither compound shows antagonist activity, the dose ratio at 30 to 60% inhibition being close to unity (Table 6).

In contrast to these findings, both compounds require high concentrations of naloxone to reverse their agonist effects (Fig. 2). If the assumption is correct that compounds with antagonist properties require high concentrations of naloxone to antagonize their agonist actions, then it would appear that ketocyclazocine and its ethyl congener have antagonist properties which cannot be shown in the guinea pig ileum by the single-dose method.

TABLE 6. *Assessment of α-2-cyclopropylmethyl-8-keto-5-R-9-methyl-2'-hydroxy-6,7-benzomorphans (Sterling-Winthrop) (1)*

R	ID_{50} (nM)	ID_{50} Normorphine (nM)	Agonist potency (Normorphine = 1)	Potency ratio (±)/(−)
(±)-Methyl (ketocyclazocine)	2.11 ± 0.19(5)	68.7 ± 9.2	32.5 ± 3.8	−
(−)-Methyl	0.77 ± 0.06(9)	51.8 ± 3.9	68.5 ± 4.3	0.475
(±)-Ethyl	0.469 ± 0.050(6)	103.1 ± 18.2	213 ± 30	−
(−)-Ethyl	0.181 ± 0.024(7)	63.8 ± 5.4	397 ± 43	0.535
(+)-Ethyl	infinite (5)	67.5 ± 11.8	0	−

The values are the means with their standard errors; the numbers of observations are given in parentheses. The dose ratios for normorphine produced by test drug concentrations which cause inhibition of the twitch by 30 to 60% were as follows: (−)-methyl compound, 1.09 ± 0.14(6) and (−)-ethyl compound, 1.78 ± 0.36(5). The (+)-ethyl compound, which has no agonist activity, gave in concentrations of 500 to 1,000 nM a dose ratio of 1.35 ± 0.08(5).

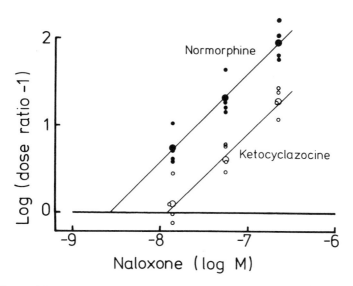

FIG. 2. Competitive antagonism by naloxone of the depressant effects of normorphine, (±)-α-2-cyclopropylmethyl-8-keto-5,9-dimethyl-2'-hydroxy-6,7-benzomorphan (ketocyclazocine), and (±)-α-2-cyclopropylmethyl-8-keto-5-ethyl-9-methyl-2'-hydroxy-6,7-benzomorphan. Individual observations are given by the small symbols and mean values by the large symbols. The lines are drawn from the regression equations, log $(DR − 1) = 1.01$ (log naloxone + 8.57) for normorphine (●) and log $(DR − 1) = 0.98$ (log naloxone + 7.94) for ketocyclazocine (○). The individual observations and the regression line for the 5-ethyl compound, log $(DR − 1) = 1.04$ (log naloxone + 7.83), are not shown because the regression line almost coincides with that for ketocyclazocine. The pA_2 values 8.57, 7.94, and 7.83 correspond to K_e values of 2.7, 11.4, and 14.8 nM, respectively.

This view has support by the observation that both compounds have no or only little agonist action in the tail-flick test (1).

DISCUSSION

There is little doubt that the assay of the agonist potencies of narcotic analgesic drugs by the guinea pig ileum method can predict their analgesic potencies in man. This agreement is satisfactory for compounds with mainly agonist activity and also for compounds with strong antagonist properties.

Often, the guinea pig ileum method gives somewhat higher values for agonist potency than is found in man. This finding may be due partly to the fact that, in the guinea pig ileum, the agonist activity is measured immediately after addition of the drug to the organ bath whereas in man a considerable time elapses after administration before analgesia is assessed. There may be a loss in agonist effectiveness with time; such an observation has been made with the writhing test where the agonist effectiveness of compounds also having antagonist properties declines rapidly whereas the potency of preponderantly agonist drugs changes very little (Table 7) (28). The values determined 10 to 15 min after injection of the analgesic drugs agree better with the values obtained on the guinea pig ileum than the values determined 25 to 30 min after injection. The potency ratio for levallorphan, however, is much lower in the mouse writhing test than in the guinea pig ileum.

TABLE 7. *Comparison of agonist potencies assayed by the guinea pig ileum test, and by the mouse writhing test at different intervals after administration of the narcotic analgesic drug*

	Agonist potency (morphine = 1)		
	Mouse writhing test[a]		
	After injection of analgesic		
Drug	(10 to 15 min)	(25 to 30 min)	Guinea pig ileum[b]
Pentazocine	0.41	0.09	0.3
Nalorphine	2.5	0.10	2.8
Levallorphan	0.57	0.04	16
Cyclazocine	12.6	4.9	35
Phenazocine	7.6	6.0	—

[a] Recalculated on a molar basis from Pearl et al. (28); the values for pentazocine are for the racemate and those for cyclazocine for the (−)-isomer. The ED_{50} values for morphine were 1.4 mg/kg at 10 to 15 min and 1.1 mg/kg at 25 to 30 min.

[b] (18, 20). The value for pentazocine is for the racemate and that for cyclazocine for the (−)-isomer.

There are two drugs where the agreement between analgesia in man and the potency as assessed by the guinea pig ileum is not good. The first compound is codeine which is less potent in the guinea pig ileum than in man; in the section on results it was suggested that this may be due to the absence of biotransformation to morphine in the guinea pig ileum. The other compound is levallorphan which has a higher potency in the guinea pig ileum than it has in man or in the mouse writing test. No explanation can be offered for this discrepancy.

The antagonist potency of compounds with negligible agonist properties can be readily predicted by the guinea pig ileum. When the antagonist potencies of compounds with or without definite agonist potencies are compared with the values obtained on the morphine-dependent monkey, the agreement is satisfactory.

From clinical experience it would appear that compounds with strong agonist and antagonist properties are liable to produce dysphoria and other psychomimetic symptoms. For this reason, the estimation of the relative agonist and antagonist properties of new compounds would appear to be of considerable importance. In the guinea pig ileum method this relationship is measured by the effective antagonist potency ($P_a = ID_{50}/K_e$). In tests on rodents a similar assessment can be made by relating the antagonist potency, as measured by the rat tail-flick test, to the agonist potency, as measured by the mouse writing test. Although the values are obtained from two species, the results are interesting (Table 8). Since the rat tail-flick test is insensitive to the agonist activity of compounds which also have strong antagonist properties (12, 13), values obtained by this test do not take into account agonist potency. It is probable for this reason that cyclorphan appears as a highly potent antagonist. However, if the agonist properties are also taken into account, the ratio of writing ED_{50} to tail-flick ED_{50} is only a little higher than that of pentazocine and much lower than the ratios for cyclazo-

TABLE 8. *Measurement of relative agonist and antagonist*
potencies in rodents[a]

Drug	Mouse writing test ED_{50} (mg/kg)	Rat tail-flick test ED_{50} (mg/kg)	Ratio writing/ tail flick
(±)-Pentazocine	7.5	3.9	1.9
(±)-Cyclorphan	0.12	0.034	3.5
(±)-Cyclazocine	2.32	0.019	122
Levallorphan tartrate	46	0.052	890

[a] calculated from Pearl et al. (27).

cine, levallorphan, and nalorphine. In other words, the simultaneous consideration of agonist and antagonist potencies gives results showing much less discrepancy from the values obtained on the guinea pig ileum which measures agonist and antagonist potency in one and the same assay.

From the results presented in this chapter it is clear that with the guinea pig ileum method it is difficult to detect antagonist activity when this is small compared with the agonist activity of the compound. No antagonist effect can be detected in the guinea pig ileum when concentrations that would be large enough to show an antagonist effect are such as to completely suppress the contractile response to electrical stimulation. In these circumstances, no estimate of antagonist activity can be made. The antagonist effect of such highly agonist compounds may or may not be of practical importance.

A possible approach to this problem is based on the observation that nalorphine, levallorphan, and diprenorphine require a higher concentration of naloxone to antagonize their agonist activities than is needed to antagonize the agonist activity of morphine and other more or less pure agonist compounds. It is hoped that this observation, which also holds for the monkey and man, may be helpful in unmasking antagonist activity in compounds with high agonist potency. Such compounds would possibly be cyclopropylmethyl derivatives of morphinans and benzomorphans, e.g., cyclorphan, isocyclorphan, ketocyclazocine, and the 5-ethyl congener of ketocyclazocine. The latter two compounds have weak antagonist action and none or only little agonist action in the rat tail-flick test. In the guinea pig ileum they behave as powerful agonists, but in both rodents and the guinea pig ileum they require high concentrations of naloxone for the antagonism of their agonist action.

SUMMARY

Agonist potency of narcotic analgesic drugs can be satisfactorily predicted by assay on the guinea pig ileum. Antagonist potency of narcotic analgesic drugs determined on the guinea pig ileum correlates well with the antagonist potency determined in morphine-dependent monkeys.

The ratio of the antagonist and agonist potencies of a narcotic analgesic drug appears to have greater value for its clinical usefulness than its absolute agonist and antagonist potencies. Such a ratio can be readily obtained on the guinea pig ileum but requires carefully chosen methods in rodents.

In compounds with powerful agonist activity (cyclorphan, isocyclorphan, and ketocyclazocines) any relatively weak antagonist activity is difficult to discern by the standard assay on the guinea pig ileum. An increase in the concentration of naloxone required to antagonize the agonist effects of these drugs seems to be due to their masked antagonist action.

ACKNOWLEDGMENTS

Support by the Committee on Problems of Drug Dependence, NAS-NRC is gratefully acknowledged.

We are much indebted for the supply of the following drugs: to Boehringer-Ingelheim for Mr 1029-MS and Mr 1256-MS, to Bristol Laboratories for BC 2605 and 2888, to Endo Laboratories for nalbuphine, nalmexone, naloxone, and EN 1639A, to Dr. M. D. Gates for cyclorphan and isocyclorphan, to Geigy Pharmaceuticals for GPA 1843, 1894, and 2163, to Parke, Davis & Co. for profadol, to Reckitt & Colman for etorphine and diprenorphine, to Sterling-Winthrop for pentazocine, cyclazocine, ketocyclazocine, and the 5-ethyl derivative of ketocyclazocine.

REFERENCES

1. Archer, S., and Pierson, A. K.: Ketocyclazocines. *Personal communication,* 1972.
2. Blane, G. F., and Robbie, D. S.: Trial of etorphine hydrochloride (M99 Reckitt) in carcinoma pain: Preliminary report. Brit. J. Pharmacol. *39*:252–253P, 1970.
3. Blumberg, H., and Dayton, H. B.: Naloxone and related compounds. *In*: Agonist and Antagonist Actions of Narcotic Analgesic Drugs, edited by H. W. Kosterlitz, H. O. J. Collier, and J. E. Villarreal, pp. 110–119. London: Macmillan, 1972.
4. Cairnie, A. B., Kosterlitz, H. W., and Taylor, D. W.: Effect of morphine on some sympathetically innervated effectors. Brit. J. Pharmacol. *17*:539–551, 1961.
5. Deneau, G. A., and Seevers, M. H.: Evaluation of morphine-like physical dependence in the rhesus monkey (*Macaca mulatta*). Bull. Drug Addiction and Narcotics *24*:Addendum 2, 1–26, 1962.
6. Deneau, G. A., and Seevers, M. H.: Evaluation of morphine-like physical dependence on the rhesus monkey (*Macaca mulatta*). Bull. Drug Addiction and Narcotics *25*:Addendum 1,1–25, 1963.
7. Deneau, G. A., Villarreal, J. E., and Seevers, M. H.: Evaluation of new compounds for morphine-like physical dependence in the rhesus monkey. Bull. Problems Drug Dependence *28*:Addendum 2, 1–15, 1966.
8. Eddy, N. B., Halbach, H., and Braenden, O. J.: Synthetic substances with morphine-like effect. Clinical experience: Potency, side-effects, addiction liability. Bull. World Health Organ. *17*:569–863, 1957.
9. Forrest, W. H., Shroff, P. F., and Mahler, D. L.: Analgesic and other effects of nalmexone in man. Clin. Pharmacol. Ther. *13*:520–525, 1972.
10. Gates, M. D.: Antagonist properties of isocyclorphan. *Personal communication,* 1972.
11. Gyang, E. A., and Kosterlitz, H. W.: Agonist and antagonist actions of morphine-like drugs on the guinea-pig isolated ileum. Brit. J. Pharmacol. *27*:514–527, 1966.·
12. Harris, L. S., and Pierson, A. K.: Some narcotic antagonists in the benzomorphan series. J. Pharmacol. Exp. Ther. *143*:141–148, 1964.
13. Harris, L. W., Pierson, A. K., Dembinski, J. R., and Dewey, L.: The pharmacology of (−)-3-hydroxy-N-cyclopropylmethylmorphinan (cyclorphan). Arch. Int. Pharmacodyn. *165*:112–126, 1967.
14. Henderson, G., Hughes, J., and Kosterlitz, H. W.: A new example of a morphine sensitive neuro-effector junction: Adrenergic transmission in the mouse vas deferens. Brit. J. Pharmacol. *46*:764–766, 1972.

15. Janssen, P. A. J.: A review of the chemical features associated with strong morphine-like activity. Brit. J. Anaesth. *34*:260–268, 1962.
16. Jasinski, D. R., and Mansky, P. A.: Evaluation of nalbuphine for abuse potential. Clin. Pharmacol. Ther. *13*:78–90, 1972.
17. Jasinski, D. R., Martin, W. R., and Hoeldtke, R.: Studies of the dependence-producing properties of GPA-1657, profadol, and propiram in man. Clin. Pharmac. Ther. *12*:613–649, 1971.
18. Kosterlitz, H. W., Lord, J. A. H., and Watt, A. J.: Morphine receptor in the myenteric plexus of the guinea-pig ileum. *In:* Agonist and Antagonist Actions of Narcotic Analgesic Drugs, edited by H. W. Kosterlitz, H. O. J. Collier, and J. E. Villarreal, pp. 45–61. London: Macmillan, 1972.
19. Kosterlitz, H. W., and Taylor, D. W.: The effect of morphine on vagal inhibition of the heart. Brit. J. Pharmacol. *14*:209–214, 1959.
20. Kosterlitz, H. W., and Watt, A. J.: Kinetic parameters of narcotic agonists and antagonists, with particular reference to N-allylnoroxymorphone (naloxone). Brit. J. Pharmacol. *33*:266–276, 1968.
21. Lasagna, L.: Drug interaction in the field of analgesic drugs. Proc. Roy. Soc. Med. *58*:978–983, 1965.
22. Lees, G. M., Kosterlitz, H. W., and Waterfield, A. A.: Characteristics of morphine-sensitive release of neuro-transmitter substances. *In:* Agonist and Antagonist Actions of Narcotic Analgesic Drugs, edited by H. W. Kosterlitz, H. O. J. Collier, and J. E. Villarreal, pp. 142–152. London: Macmillan, 1972.
23. Merz, H., Langbein, A., Stockhaus, K., and Wick, H.: Novel opioid antagonists of the 2'-hydroxy-6,7-benzomorphan series. *Personal communication,* 1972.
24. Paton, W. D. M.: The response of the guinea-pig ileum to electrical stimulation by coaxial electrodes. J. Physiol. *127*:40–41P, 1955.
25. Paton, W. D. M.: The action of morphine and related substances on contraction and acetylcholine output of coaxially stimulated guinea-pig ileum. Brit. J. Pharmacol. *12*:119–127, 1957.
26. Paton, W. D. M.: A theory of drug action based on drug-receptor combination. Proc. Roy. Soc. B. *154*:21–69, 1961.
27. Pearl, J., Aceto, M. D., and Harris, L. S.: Prevention of writhing and other effects of narcotics and narcotic antagonists in mice. J. Pharmacol. Exp. Ther. *160*:217–230, 1968.
28. Pearl, J., Stander, H., and McKean, D. B.: Effects of analgesics and other drugs on mice in phenylquinone and rotarod tests. J. Pharmacol. Exp. Ther. *167*:9–13, 1969.
29. Pearson, J. W., Lasagna, L., and Laird, R. D.: Analgesic activity of oral and intramuscular profadol. Clin. Pharmacol. Ther. *12*:683–690, 1971.
30. Stephenson, R. P.: A modification of receptor theory. Brit. J. Pharmacol. *11*:379–393, 1956.
31. Trendelenburg, U.: The action of morphine on the superior cervical ganglion and on the nictitating membrane. Brit. J. Pharmacol. *12*:79–85, 1957.
32. Villarreal, J. E., and Seevers, M. H.: Evaluation of new compounds for morphine-like physical dependence in the rhesus monkey. Bull. Problems Drug Dependence *30*:Addendum 2, 1–15, 1968.
33. Villarreal, J. E., and Seevers, M. H.: Evaluation of new compounds for morphine-like physical dependence in the rhesus monkey. Bull. Problems Drug Dependence *31*:Addendum 2, 1–12, 1969.
34. Villarreal, J. E., and Seevers, M. H.: Evaluation of new compounds for morphine-like physical dependence in the rhesus monkey. Bull. Problems Drug Dependence *32*:Addendum 1, 1–18, 1970.
35. Villarreal, J. E., and Seevers, M. H.: Evaluation of new compounds for morphine-like physical dependence in the rhesus monkey. Rep. Problems Drug Dependence *34*:Addendum 7, 1040–1053, 1972.

Narcotic Antagonists, edited by M. C. Braude, L. S. Harris, E. L. May, J. P. Smith, and J. E. Villarreal. *Advances in Biochemical Psychopharmacology, Vol. 8.* Raven Press, New York © 1974.

Determination of Pharmacological Constants: Use of Narcotic Antagonists to Characterize Analgesic Receptors

A. E. Takemori

Department of Pharmacology, University of Minnesota, Health Sciences Center, Medical School, Minneapolis, Minnesota 55455

The concept of pA_x (17) has been used mostly with isolated tissue preparations to identify agonists which act on similar receptors. In recent years our group has applied the concept of pA_x to data obtained in intact animals for the characterization of analgesic receptors. The definition of the apparent pA_2 *in vivo* then becomes the negative logarithm of the molar dose of the injected antagonist which reduces the effect of a double dose of an agonist to that of a single dose. The concentration of the antagonist at the receptor site is unknown but it is assumed to be proportional to the dose. Although pA_2 is regarded as equal to the log of the affinity constant (K_B) of the antagonist for the receptor, this is not entirely true *in vivo*. However, the "K_B" *in vivo* should be proportional to the real K_B if the above assumption about the antagonist concentration is correct. Aside from the theoretical implications of "pA_2" *in vivo*, the procedure offers a means to summarize a large amount of quantitative data on competitive drug antagonism as well as a standard method to compare antagonists. Our group has used this procedure for the characterization of receptors interacting with narcotic and narcotic-antagonist analgesics, for the comparison of the type of narcotic-receptor interaction involved in various analgesic assays, and for the comparison of the potencies of certain narcotic antagonists. The concept of pA_x has also been used to gather evidence that morphine causes a structural change in analgesic receptors.

INTRODUCTION

Clark and Raventos (5) suggested a method to study the potency of antagonists whereby the concentration of an antagonist, which would alter by a certain proportion (e.g., 10-fold) the concentration of the agonist required to produce a selected effect, would be determined. This suggestion is the basis for the concept of pA_x which Schild (14) has introduced as a

335

convenient and quantitative measure of drug antagonism. Schild's method is used to study competitive antagonists and the assumption is made that equal responses by agonists are produced by occupation of equal fractions of receptors. In subsequent papers (2, 15, 16), the usefulness of this method for the identification of agonists which act on the same receptor population was described. Schild (14) defined the pA$_x$ as pA$_x = -\log$ [B] where [B] is the molar concentration of the antagonist which necessitates an increase of the original agonist concentration by X-fold to produce the original effect. Arunlakshana and Schild (2) employed the following equation to determine the values for K_B: $\log (X - 1) = \log K_B - n\mathrm{pA}_x$ where $X =$ dose ratio $\left[\dfrac{\text{agonist dose in presence of antagonist}}{\text{agonist dose in absence of antagonist}}\right]$ and $K_B =$ affinity constant of the antagonist for the receptor. When $X = 2$, pA$_2 = \log K_B$. If $\log (X - 1)$ is plotted against $-\log$ [B], a straight line with a slope (n) of -1.0 should result if the antagonism is competitive and the intercept would equal the pA$_2$ or the logarithm of the affinity constant. This method does not depend on any assumptions about the relationship between the pharmacological response and the proportion of receptors occupied by the antagonist since the responses are kept equal. It follows that if a combination of a single antagonist with several agonists have pA$_2$ values that are the same, then it is quite possible the receptors which are involved in the responses are the same.

The concept of pA$_x$ is used primarily with isolated tissue preparations where the concentrations of antagonists and agonists in the bath can be well controlled. However, Cox and Weinstock (6) have estimated the equivalent of a pA$_2$ in intact mice. *In vivo*, the apparent pA$_2$ then becomes the negative logarithm of the molar dose of the injected antagonist which reduces the effect of a double dose of an agonist to that of a single dose. The antagonism by nalorphine of analgesia and lenticular opacity produced in mice by a number of narcotics was investigated by these authors, and the apparent pA$_2$ values were found to be quite similar. The authors suggested that these drugs may combine with the same receptors and that the receptors for analgesia and lenticular opacity are of the same type. Since this initial study of "pA$_2$" *in vivo*, Green and Fleming (10) have used "pA$_2$" values *in vivo* to study adrenergic receptors of the nictitating membrane of cats, and Blane et al. (3) have used "pA$_2$" values to compare receptors associated with morphine and etorphine in rats. In the past several years, my colleagues and I have been involved in the characterization of analgesic receptors by using the concept of pA$_x$ in intact animals, and these studies will be described herein.

METHODS

Analgesic Assays

The acetic acid writhing assay is described by Hayashi and Takemori (11), the hot-plate assay by Eddy and Leimbach (8), and the tail-flick assay by D'Amour and Smith (7).

Determination of the Apparent pA$_2$ Value

Dose-response curves for an analgesic alone and in combination with three increasing doses of an antagonist are determined in mice using one of the analgesic assays. Usually the writhing assay is used where both the narcotic and narcotic-antagonist type of analgesics are employed. A parallel shift of the dose-response curve to the right in the presence of the antagonist is presumptive evidence that the antagonism is of the competitive type. The dose ratios (ED$_{50}$ with antagonist/ED$_{50}$ without antagonist) are then calculated and log (dose ratio -1) is plotted against $-$log (dose of antagonist in moles/kg). The intercept is the apparent pA$_2$ value. An example of this type of plot can be seen in the paper by Hayashi and Takemori (11).

Statistics and Calculations

The results are analyzed statistically by the parallel line assay described by Finney (9). The values for apparent pA$_2$ are estimated as described previously (18). All statistical analyses and calculations are performed with the aid of a computer program.

APPARENT pA$_2$ AS A PHARMACOLOGIC CONSTANT

In order to utilize meaningfully the apparent pA$_2$ value as a pharmacologic constant, one must be able to reproduce this value consistently. The values of apparent pA$_2$ for morphine-naloxone which have been determined in six separate studies are recorded in Table 1. The writhing assay was used in all studies but different nociceptive agents were used. Various strains of mice were employed and different personnel performed the assays in these studies. In spite of these variables, the apparent pA$_2$ of morphine-naloxone was the same in all six studies. This finding attests to the utility of pA$_2$ values derived *in vivo* as a pharmacologic constant.

TABLE 1. *The apparent pA$_2$ of morphine-naloxone in different studies using the writing analgesic assay*

Assayer	Writhing agent	Mouse strain	Apparent pA$_2$ of morphine-naloxone (95% confidence interval)	Reference
Takemori-Kupferberg	benzoquinone	Swiss-Webster (Simonsen)	7.01 (6.90–7.12)	20
Smits	phenylbenzoquinone	Swiss-Webster (Simonsen)	7.08 (6.86–7.29)	18
Hayashi-Takemori	acetic acid	CD-1 (Charles River)	7.00 (6.86–7.14)	12
Hayashi	acetic acid	Swiss-Webster (Simonsen)	7.07 (6.96–7.16)	19
			7.05 (6.95–7.15)	11
Oka-Nishiyama	acetic acid	ICR-JCL (Nihon Clea, Japan)	6.96 (6.81–7.11)	21

USE OF APPARENT pA$_2$ VALUES

Characterization of Analgesic Receptors

Apparent pA$_2$ values have been employed to determine if narcotic and narcotic-antagonist analgesics interact with similar receptors (18). The writhing assay and the antagonist naloxone were used to obtain *in vivo* equivalents of pA$_2$ values since the analgesic activity of both types of analgesics can be detected by this assay and naloxone antagonizes the action of both types. The apparent pA$_2$ values were similar when the narcotic agents morphine, levorphanol, or methadone were tested; the mean ± SE of the values was 6.98 ± 0.06. The apparent pA$_2$ values among the narcotic-antagonist analgesics pentazocine, nalorphine, and cyclazocine were also the same, with a mean of 6.32 ± 0.11. The two groups of analgesics had significantly different apparent pA$_2$ values. It was concluded that the narcotic and narcotic-antagonist analgesics interact either with two different receptors or with the same receptor in a different manner.

Quantitative Comparison of Antagonists

Potency of competitive antagonists can be quantitated and the use of apparent pA$_2$ offers a standard method to compare antagonists. The potencies of the antagonists naloxone and diprenorphine in antagonizing the analgesic action of etorphine have been compared (19). A comparison between these two antagonists in antagonizing three different agonists is shown in Table 2. Inspection of the apparent pA$_2$ values and the potency ratios indicate that on a molar basis diprenorphine is 6.6 times more potent than naloxone in antagonizing the actions of etorphine and pentazocine and is 4.5 times more potent than naloxone in antagonizing the actions of mor-

TABLE 2. *Comparison of the potencies of naloxone and diprenorphine by use of apparent pA$_2$ values*

Agonist	Antagonist	Apparent pA$_2$	Potency ratio[a]
Morphine	naloxone	7.07	4.5
	diprenorphine	7.73	
Etorphine	naloxone	6.58	6.6
	diprenorphine	7.40	
Pentazocine	naloxone	6.45	6.6
	diprenorphine	7.27	

[a] Antilog [pA$_2$ − pA$_2'$] where pA$_2$ = apparent pA$_2$ of agonist diprenorphine, and pA$_2'$ = apparent pA$_2$ of agonist naloxone.

phine. The data also indicate that the interactions between the receptor(s) and the three analgesics may differ.

Receptors Involved in Various Analgesic Assays

The analgesic activity of the narcotic analgesics but not those of the narcotic-antagonist analgesics can be assessed readily by the hot-plate or tail-flick assays. On the other hand, the writing assay can be used to assess both types of analgesics. The question arises as to whether the types of analgesic-receptor interactions which are measured by these assays differ. This question is important to answer since these assays are frequently used to assess the degree of tolerance development. It would be of interest if tolerance data collected from the use of one assay can be compared to those gathered by employing a different assay. We addressed ourselves to these questions and determined the apparent pA_2 values of morphine-naloxone using the writing, hot-plate, and tail-flick assays (11). The apparent pA_2 values of morphine-naloxone were 7.10 for the tail-flick assay, 7.27 for the hot-plate assay, and 7.05 for the writing assay; the values are not significantly different from each other. According to Arunlakshana and Schild (2), tissues with similar receptors would be expected to give similar pA_2 values with a given antagonist. Analogously these data suggest that in the case of morphine, the three analgesic assays are probably measuring similar analgesic-receptor interactions. Thus, tolerance data involving morphine which are obtained by using the three analgesic assays can probably be compared meaningfully.

Qualitative Changes in Analgesic Receptors

Green and Fleming (10) employed apparent pA_2 values to show that qualitative changes in the adrenergic receptors do not occur after various drugs and treatments to produce supersensitive nictitating membranes in cats.

In another application of apparent pA_2 values, we have shown that morphine induces some type of qualitative change in analgesic receptors (21). Mice were pretreated with a dose of morphine larger than ED_{99}, and, after 2 hr when the analgesic effect of morphine was no longer evident, dose-response curves for morphine with and without naloxone were determined. Naloxone shifted the dose-response curves much more to the right in pretreated than in non-pretreated or control mice. The apparent pA_2 value also changed significantly from 6.96 to 7.30. This means that the "affinity constant" of the naloxone for the analgesic receptor more than doubled when mice were exposed to one acute injection of morphine. This was interpreted to mean that morphine causes a structural change in the analgesic receptors such that the affinity of the receptors for narcotic antagonists is increased. This alteration may last for as long as 4 days. The narcotic-antagonist analgesic pentazocine did not cause these changes in naloxone sensitivity. The possible relationship of this change in receptors to the phenomena of tolerance and physical dependence is discussed elsewhere (21).

LIMITATIONS OF APPARENT pA$_2$ VALUES

Concentrations of Agonists and Antagonists at the Receptor Site

Aside from the several problems encountered in kinetic studies of drug action *in vitro* (4), the variables encountered in studies *in vivo* may seem insurmountable. However, by definition, pA$_x$ is independent of the agonist concentration. Also, the method of determining pA$_2$ values makes no assumptions about the relationship between the pharmacological responses and the proportion of receptors occupied because this is a null method and the response is kept constant. The actual concentration of antagonist at the receptor site is unknown but it is assumed to be proportional to the dose of the injected antagonist. Since the apparent pA$_2$ values for a variety of narcotic analgesics were so similar, it would appear that this assumption is justified. Even in isolated tissue preparations, it is usually assumed that the concentration of a drug at the receptor site is equal to that of the medium. The apparent pA$_2$ value is not the affinity constant (K_B) but should be proportional to the K_B if the antagonist concentration at the receptor site is indeed proportional to the injected dose of the antagonist.

Noncompetitive Antagonists

The use of pA$_x$ is limited to antagonists of the competitive type, and the pA$_2$ value is constant only if the shift in the dose-response curves due to the antagonist is parallel. Ariëns and van Rossum (1) have used pD$_2'$ values for noncompetitive or nonequilibrium competitive antagonists. The pD$_2'$ value is defined as the negative logarithm of the molar concentration of an antagonist which reduces the maximal effect of an agonist to 50% of its initial value. Green and Fleming (10) have successfully used pD$_2'$ values in experiments *in vivo*. Other methods for studying these antagonists such as those discussed by Mackay (13) should be explored.

Situations Where the Slope of the pA_x Plot Is Greater Than Unity

For competitive antagonism, the curve of the pA_x plot is a straight line with a slope of -1.0 (2). Slopes greater than -1.0, however, have been encountered in our studies, especially with the narcotic-antagonist analgesics and with etorphine (18, 19). Arunlakshana and Schild (2) have attributed a slope greater than unity in the pA_x plot either to the failure of drugs to attain equilibrium with the receptors or to paradoxical potentiating effects of the antagonist. The latter explanation would not apply to our studies since neither naloxone nor diprenorphine had analgesic effects in the dosages employed. The difficulty in obtaining pA_2 values using the antagonist nalorphine, which has considerable agonistic activity, has been shown by Takemori et al. (20). The possibility that the drugs are not in equilibrium with the receptors cannot be excluded. However, analgesic measurements were always carefully made at peak effects of both the agonist and antagonist, and this would be the time at which the drugs would be most likely to be in equilibrium. The importance of making measurements at peak effects has been discussed by Takemori et al. (19).

Alternative explanations for an anomalous slope of the pA_x plot have been proposed (18, 19). In Schild's analysis it is assumed that both agonist and antagonist combine with receptors according to the Langmuir equation. If narcotic-antagonist analgesics and etorphine did not obey the Langmuir equation but followed instead some steeper binding function, then the anomalous slope could be accounted for. For example, $\log (X - 1) = \log K_B - npA_x$ in the usual pA_x concept, where X = dose ratio, B = antagonist concentration, and n and K_B = constants. The slope of the pA_x plot is represented by n and is usually unity when dealing with competitive antagonism; the law of mass action is assumed in the interaction of the receptors with the agonist and the antagonist. However, for some agonists the relationship of $\log (X^n - 1) = \log K_B - pA_x$ has been considered and the possibility that $\log K_B$ may be equal to "pA_2" when $X^n = 2$ instead of when $X = 2$ has been discussed and exemplified by Takemori et al. (19).

With the narcotic-antagonist analgesics, another explanation for anomalous pA_x plots may apply. It is conceivable that the narcotic-antagonist analgesics and the antagonist used to determine pA_x may exert synergistic antagonistic actions. Such an effect would result in self-antagonism of the narcotic-antagonist analgesic and in a greater than expected increase in the antagonism produced by increasing doses of the antagonist. This would result in a pA_x plot which would become steeper with increasing doses of the antagonist. This possibility has also been discussed by Takemori et al. (19).

CONCLUSIONS

The pA$_x$ concept has been applied in intact animals to study analgesic receptors, and the apparent pA$_2$ value has been shown to be a reliable pharmacologic constant. Some of the practical uses of this pharmacologic constant have been described, and it is shown that much information about analgesic receptors can be acquired by use of the constant. Aside from the theoretical implications of "pA$_2$" *in vivo*, the method offers a means to summarize a vast amount of quantitative data on competitive drug antagonism and a standard method to compare antagonists.

ACKNOWLEDGMENT

I wish to thank my many colleagues who made these studies possible. The studies described herein were supported mainly by the U.S. Public Health Service Grant GM 15477 and partly by Research Funds of the Graduate School of the University of Minnesota, U.S. Public Health Service Grant NB05171, China Medical Board of New York, Inc., and Japan Society for the Promotion of Science.

REFERENCES

1. Ariëns, E. J., and van Rossum, J. M.: pD, pA$_x$ and pD$_x$' values in the analysis of pharmacodynamics. Arch. Int. Pharmacodyn. Ther. *110*:275–299, 1957.
2. Arunlakshana, O., and Schild, H. O.: Some quantitative uses of drug antagonists. Brit. J. Pharmacol. *14*:48–58, 1959.
3. Blane, G. F., Boura, A. L. A., Fitzgerald, A. E., and Lister, R. E.: Actions of etorphine hydrochloride (M99): A potent morphine-like agent. Brit. J. Pharmacol. *30*:11–22, 1967.
4. Clark, A. J.: *The Mode of Action of Drugs on Cells*. Williams and Wilkins Co., Baltimore, 1933.
5. Clark, A. J., and Raventos, J.: The antagonism of acetylcholine and of quaternary ammonium salts. Quart. J. Exp. Physiol. *26*:375–392, 1937.
6. Cox, B. M., and Weinstock, M.: Quantitative studies of the antagonism by nalorphine of some of the actions of morphine-like analgesic drugs. Brit. J. Pharmacol. *22*:289–300, 1964.
7. D'Amour, F. E., and Smith, D. L.: A method for determining loss of pain sensation. J. Pharmacol. Exp. Ther. *72*:74–79, 1941.
8. Eddy, N. B., and Leimbach, D.: Synthetic analgesics. II. Dithienylbutenyl- and dithienylbutylamines. J. Pharmacol. Exp. Ther. *107*:385–393, 1953.
9. Finney, D. J.: *Statistical Methods in Biological Assay*, 2nd ed., Hafner Publishing Company, New York, 1964.
10. Green, R. D., III, and Fleming, W. W.: Agonist-antagonist interactions in the normal and supersensitive nictitating membrane of the spinal cat. J. Pharmacol. Exp. Ther. *156*:207–214, 1967.
11. Hayashi, G., and Takemori, A. E.: The type of analgesic-receptor interaction involved in certain analgesic assays. Europ. J. Pharmacol. *16*:63–66, 1971.
12. Hayashi, G., and Takemori, A. E.: *Unpublished observations*.

13. Mackay, D.: The mathematics of drug-receptor interactions. J. Pharm. Pharmacol. *18*:201–222, 1966.
14. Schild, H. O.: pA, a new scale for the measurement of drug antagonism. Brit. J. Pharmacol. *2*:189–206, 1947.
15. Schild, H. O.: The use of drug antagonists for the identification and classification of drugs. Brit. J. Pharmacol. *2*:251–258, 1947.
16. Schild, H. O.: pA$_x$ and competitive drug antagonism. Brit. J. Pharmacol. *4*:277–280, 1949.
17. Schild, H. O.: Drug antagonism and pA$_x$. Pharmacol. Rev. *9*:242–246, 1957.
18. Smits, S. E., and Takemori, A. E.: Quantitative studies on the antagonism by naloxone of some narcotic and narcotic-antagonist analgesics. Brit. J. Pharmacol. *39*:627–638, 1970.
19. Takemori, A. E., Hayashi, G., and Smits, S. E.: Studies on the quantitative antagonism of analgesics by naloxone and diprenorphine. Europ. J. Pharmacol. *20*:85–92, 1972.
20. Takemori, A. E., Kupferberg, H. J., and Miller, J. W.: Quantitative studies of the antagonism of morphine by nalorphine and naloxone. J. Pharmacol. Exp. Ther. *169*:39–45, 1969.
21. Takemori, A. E., Oka, T., and Nishiyama, N.: Alteration of analgesic receptor-antagonist interaction induced by morphine. J. Pharmacol. Exp. Ther. (*submitted*).

Narcotic Antagonists, edited by M. C. Braude, L. S. Harris, E. L. May, J. P. Smith, and J. E. Villarreal. *Advances in Biochemical Psychopharmacology, Vol. 8.* Raven Press, New York © 1974.

Effects of Narcotics and Narcotic Antagonists on Operant Behavior

D. E. McMillan

Department of Pharmacology, School of Medicine, University of North Carolina, Chapel Hill, North Carolina 27514

Operant behavior is a useful preclinical measure of the behavioral effects of narcotics and narcotic antagonists. Under multiple fixed-ratio fixed-interval schedules of food presentation, low doses of both narcotics and narcotic antagonists increase rates of responding during the fixed-interval component of the multiple schedule, whereas higher doses decrease rates under both components. In general, the potency of these drugs in affecting operant behavior in pigeons parallels their potency in man, except that naloxone, a relatively pure antagonist in man, has marked effects on operant behavior, while nalorphine, which has considerable potency in man, does not affect operant behavior until very large doses are given. At much lower doses than those that affect operant behavior, narcotic antagonists can block almost completely the effects of large doses of morphine and methadone on the operant behavior of pigeons. Operant behavior can also be used to study the development of tolerance and dependence phenomena in animals. When morphine or methadone is administered repeatedly to pigeons, the behavioral effects of these drugs disappear and the dose can be increased to many times the originally effective dose with little further effect on behavior. In contrast, only a slight tolerance can be shown to develop to pentazocine using these techniques. Finally, the operant behavior of pigeons tolerant to morphine is disrupted when small doses of naloxone are given, yet no signs of physical withdrawal can be observed, suggesting that operant behavior may also provide a sensitive reflection of drug dependence.

INTRODUCTION

It has long been recognized that the behavioral effects of narcotics and narcotic antagonists play an important role in determining the clinical usefulness of these drugs, as well as contributing to their abuse potential. Lasagna and Beecher (14) have suggested that the clinical assessment of analgesia may be influenced both by behavioral effects that contribute toward the analgesic effect of a drug and by the behavioral side effects that limit the usefulness of that drug. The importance of operant conditioning in maintaining drug-seeking behavior has been emphasized by Nichols (21), whereas Wikler (31) has suggested an important role for classical conditioning in contributing to relapse to opiates.

A useful approach for studying the behavioral variables influencing drug dependence is to regard these variables within an operant conditioning framework (23). Within this framework, future behavior is determined by the consequences of past behavior, and these consequences are referred to as reinforcers. In most operant conditioning experiments, food, water, and/or electric shock have been used as reinforcers to maintain or suppress behavior; however, drugs can also act as reinforcers of the behavioral responses that lead to their administration.

When drugs are used as reinforcers, they can affect behavior through mechanisms other than the process of reinforcement, since it has been demonstrated repeatedly that drugs interact with behavior maintained by conventional reinforcers such as food, water, and electric shock (3). Thus, it is important to study the interaction between narcotics, narcotic antagonists, and operant behavior in order to separate the effects of drugs as reinforcers from other effects that they have on behavior.

Although there have been many studies on the effects of morphine on operant behavior (5, 9, 12, 19, 26, 27), there are few studies on the effects of other narcotic analgesics on operant behavior, and perhaps even fewer studies on the effects of narcotic antagonists. This chapter emphasizes the effects of narcotic antagonists on operant behavior. Experiments on the effects of morphine and other narcotic analgesics on operant behavior are reviewed only when these effects can be compared with the effects of narcotic antagonists.

EFFECTS OF NARCOTICS AND NARCOTIC ANTAGONISTS ON OPERANT BEHAVIOR

The most extensive series of experiments on the effects of narcotics and narcotic antagonists on operant behavior have used the pigeon to study the effects of these drugs on performance maintained under a multiple fixed-ratio (30) fixed-interval (5 min) schedule of food presentation (mult FR 30 FI 5). In these experiments (18-20) food was presented after the pigeon pecked a response key 30 times (FR 30) in the presence of a blue stimulus light, or after the first response after 5 min had elapsed in the presence of a red stimulus light (FI 5). Each of the schedule components was available only for limited time periods, so that the components alternated either as a function of the passage of time when the bird did not peck the key, or as a function of the delivery of food when the bird met the schedule contingencies. During non-drug control sessions, responding under the FR component was characterized by steady, rapid rates of responding (usually two or three responses per second); responding under the FI component was characterized by a pause at the beginning of the 5-min FI, followed by a gradual acceleration of responding to a terminal high rate which occurred at the end of the interval. The mean rate of responding averaged across the inhomogeneous FI component was usually between 0.5 and 1.0 response per second. Representative cumulative response records of control performance are shown in Fig. 1.

In the first series of these experiments (19), morphine (1 mg/kg), nalor-

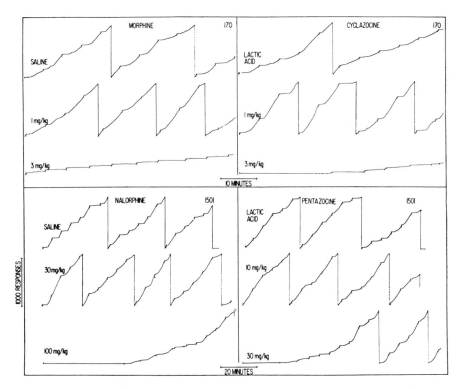

FIG. 1. Representative cumulative records of performances under the multiple FR 30 FI 5 schedule after control and drug injections. Abscissa: time. Ordinate: cumulative number of responses. The FR and FI components are alternated; the components change after the presentation of food (short diagonal lines on the cumulative record) or after an elapsed time of 4 min during the FR component or after the end of the FI component (not shown). Note that each drug increased the level of responding during the FI component at the lower dose shown and decreased responding in both FI and FR components at the higher dose. In many instances, responding was better sustained during FR components than during FI components. From reference (19).

phine (30 mg/kg), cyclazocine (1.0 mg/kg), and pentazocine (10 mg/kg) all increased the rate of responding under the FI component of the multiple schedule (Fig. 1). Most of the increase in the mean rate of responding occurred during the early part of the FI component where rates of responding were very low. At higher dose levels all four drugs decreased the rate of responding under both schedule components. None of these drugs increased the high rates of responding under the FR component at any of the doses studied, although drug-induced increases in the high rates of responding maintained by this schedule are possible with other classes of drugs (28).

In subsequent experiments, naloxone, EN 2265, and methadone (20), as well as both of the optical isomers of pentazocine and cyclazocine (18), were found to have effects on performance under the mult FR 30 FR 5 schedule of food presentation similar to those reported for morphine (19).

The effects of all of these narcotics and narcotic antagonists on schedule-controlled behavior can be summarized by comparing their effects on responding maintained by the FI component of the schedule. Figure 2 shows that all of the drugs studied increased the rates of responding under the FI component of the multiple schedule at low doses and decreased the rates of responding at higher doses. Because the lower ends of the dose-effect curves were not explored extensively, it is difficult to make any potency comparisons among these drugs for their rate-increasing effects; however, an arbitrary point can be picked on the descending leg of the dose-effect curve for potency comparison. If a dose is picked which decreased responding under the FI component by 50%, the order of potency can be determined as shown in Table 1, where the effects of narcotics and narcotic antagonists on pigeon behavior are compared with the effects of these drugs in some other measurement systems, including analgesia in man. In general, there is good agreement across these measures, although there are some differences. Perhaps the most striking of these differences is the low potency of nalorphine in affecting pigeon behavior. In the writing test and as an analgesic in man, nalorphine is only slightly less potent than morphine, whereas it is more potent on the guinea pig ileum. However, in decreasing FI responding in the pigeon, nalorphine is less than 1/10 as potent as morphine. Other investigators (30) have also found nalorphine to be rather inactive in tests of animal behavior, although there is at least one report of nalorphine activity on rat behavior at low doses (29).

Naloxone has been considered to be a relatively pure narcotic antagonist (2, 15) without agonist activity in most systems. Naloxone does suppress responding under both schedule components in the pigeon, and at even lower doses, FI responding is increased.

Holtzman and Jewett (10) have studied the effects of pentazocine on the

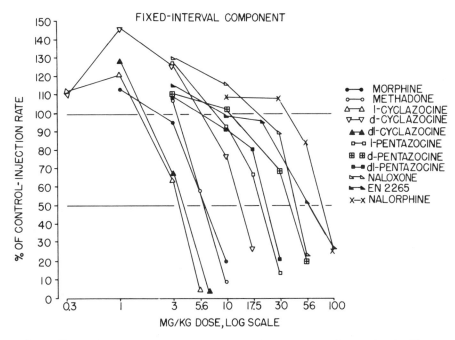

FIG. 2. Effects of narcotics and narcotic antagonists on responding under the FI component of the mult FI 5 FR 30 schedule. Abscissa: mg/kg. Ordinate: % of average control-injection rate of responding. Each point is the mean of single observations in each of four pigeons.

operant behavior of the rat. In these experiments, the rats were trained to press a lever under a continuous avoidance schedule (24). Each lever press postponed the delivery of electric shock to the feet of the rat. If no responding occurred, electric shocks were delivered to the feet of the rat every 15 sec. Under this schedule, rats pressed the lever at a rate of less than 0.1 response per second and avoided more than 90% of the shocks. Pentazocine, at dose levels from 2 to 16 mg/kg, increased the rate of avoidance responding. A higher dose of 32 mg/kg pentazocine decreased the rate of responding. The shape of this pentazocine dose-effect curve is very similar to that of pentazocine for responding maintained by the FI schedule of food presentation in the pigeon (Fig. 1), where low doses (3 mg/kg) of pentazocine increased the rate of responding, and higher doses (17.5 to 30 mg/kg) decreased the rate. Thus, the effects of pentazocine on food-reinforced responding in pigeons can be extended to shock-avoidance performance in rats, suggesting that the effects in pigeons are not species specific, nor do they depend on the type of reinforcer used to maintain behavior.

TABLE 1. Comparison of effects of narcotics and narcotic antagonists on the operant behavior of pigeons (dose to decrease by 50% the rate of responding under the FI component) with the effects of these drugs in other animal tests and in man.

Drug	Dose to decrease FI by 50% (mg/kg)	Writhing test (22) (mg/kg base)	Inhibition of coaxially stimulated guinea pig ileum (6) ($M \times 10^{-9}$)	Human analgesia potency ratio (22)
L-Cyclazocine	3.5	0.05	17	not tested
DL-Cyclazocine	3.8	0.10	11	30.0
Methadone	5.8	not tested	not tested	not tested
Morphine	6.0	0.44	460	1.0
D-Cyclazocine	17	inactive at 1.0	>36,800	not tested
L-Pentazocine	21	1.4	526	0.4
DL-Pentazocine	24	3.1	1368	0.2–0.4
D-Pentazocine	39	inactive at 32	24,912	inactive
Naloxone	44	inactive at 30	>27,800	inactive
EN 2265	58	not tested	not tested	not tested
Nalorphine	78	0.54	101	0.9

INTERACTIONS BETWEEN NARCOTICS AND NARCOTIC
ANTAGONISTS

The most extensive series of investigations of the interaction between narcotics and narcotic antagonists on operant behavior has also used the pigeon as an experimental animal (18, 20). In these experiments pigeons again were trained to respond with food as a reinforcer under a mult FR 30 FI 5 schedule of food presentation. Prior to the session, a narcotic antagonist was injected into one side of the breast muscle, followed immediately by a dose of morphine. Ten min later, an hour-long session under the multiple schedule began. Morphine dose-effect curves were determined before and after the interactions with narcotic antagonists to evaluate the role of any tolerance development following repeated administration of morphine.

Figure 3 shows a cumulative response record for the interaction between naloxone and morphine on the operant behavior of the pigeon. At 10 mg/kg, morphine severely disrupted responding under both schedule components. A dose of 10 mg/kg of naloxone completely blocked these rate-decreasing effects of morphine. In fact, naloxone even restored the complex curvature of the pattern of FI responding to its normal shape. Figure 4 shows more extensive data on the interaction between morphine and the optical isomers of cyclazocine. L-Cyclazocine (0.1 mg/kg) almost completely blocked the effects of morphine. D-Cyclazocine was less potent as a morphine antagonist, and at least part of the antagonism of the rate-decreasing effect of D-cyclazocine could be attributed to the rate-increasing effect of D-cyclazocine.

Table 2 uses several criteria to evaluate the potency of a number of narcotic antagonists against morphine. Although there is some variability from measure to measure, apparently based on the higher dose levels of antagonist required to reverse the rate decreases under the FR component than under the FI component, there is relatively good agreement among measures. In blocking the rate-decreasing effects of morphine, L-cyclazocine appears to be the most potent antagonist, followed by DL-cyclazocine and naloxone. D-Cyclazocine was less potent, and nalorphine was even less potent. Neither racemic pentazocine nor either of its optical isomers could block the rate-decreasing effects of morphine at doses up to 10 mg/kg. These 10 mg/kg dose levels of pentazocine approach the doses of pentazocine that decrease rates of responding in pigeons that have not received morphine (McMillan and Morse, 1967; McMillan and Harris, 1972), making it difficult to look for antagonist effects of higher doses of pentazocine. In some experiments it appears that pentazocine adds to the rate-decreasing effects of morphine on operant behavior (18, 20), rather than antagonizing these

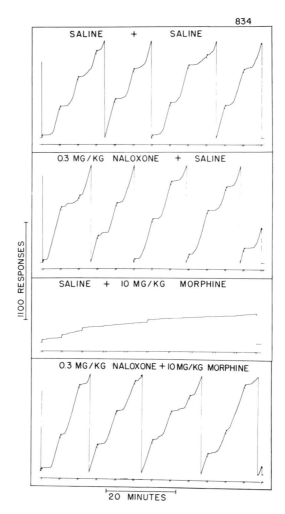

FIG. 3. Cumulative response records of bird 834 showing the effects of a control injection, naloxone, morphine, and a naloxone-morphine combination on patterns of responding. Abscissa: time. Ordinate: cumulative number of responses. The FI and the FR components are alternated. The components change after each presentation of food (short diagonal lines on the cumulative record and the horizontal line), or after an elapsed time of 40 sec after a response could produce food during the FI component (short diagonal lines on the horizontal line without diagonal lines on the cumulative record), or after 40 sec during the FR component (short diagonal lines on the horizontal line without diagonal lines on the cumulative record). From reference (20).

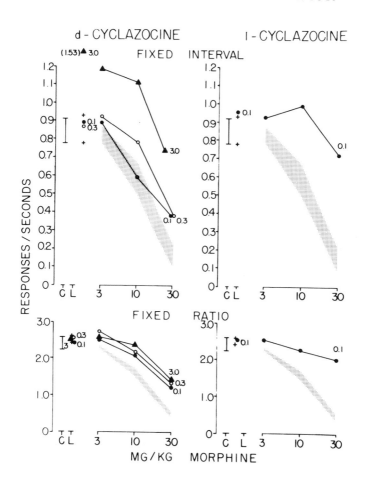

FIG. 4. Effects of morphine (with a lactic acid control injection) and morphine plus D- and L-cyclazocine on the average rate of responding under each component of the mult FR 30 FI 5 schedule of food presentation. Abscissa: dose, log scale. Ordinate: rate of responding during a complete session. The brackets at C show the range of values obtained on 14 noninjection days (Thursdays). The crosses at L show the values obtained after administration of the injection vehicles (lactic acid and distilled water). The other symbols at L show the effects of each dose of cyclazocine when it was given with the morphine injection vehicle (distilled water). The dose of cyclazocine is marked beside each point at L. The shaded area is the range of two determinations of the morphine dose-response curve, with one determination made before and one determination made after the study of antagonism. In the left column the filled circles represent the effects of morphine with 0.1 mg/kg of D-cyclazocine, the open circles represent the effects of morphine with 0.3 mg/kg of D-cyclazocine, and the filled triangles represent the effects of morphine with 3.0 mg/kg of D-cyclazocine. In the right column, the filled circles represent the effects of morphine with 0.1 mg/kg of L-cyclazocine. Each point is the mean of a single observation in each of four pigeons. From reference (18).

TABLE 2. *A comparison of the potency of narcotic antagonists in blocking the rate-decreasing effects of morphine.*

Antagonist	Dose (mg/kg) required to reverse 50% of the rate decreased produced by 30 mg/kg of morphine		Dose (mg/kg) required to reverse completely the rate decrease produced by 10 mg/kg of morphine		Average blocking dose (mg/kg)
	FI	FR	FI	FR	
L-Cyclazocine	0.1	0.1	0.1	0.1	0.1
DL-Cyclazocine	0.1	0.1	0.1	1.0	0.3
Naloxone	0.03	3.0	0.3	0.3	1.0
D-Cyclazocine	3.0	3.0	0.3	0.3–1.0	1.5
Nalorphine	1.0	1.0	10	1–10	4.6
L-Pentazocine*	>10	>10	>10	>10	>10
DL-Pentazocine*	>10	>10	>10	>10	>10
D-Pentazocine*	>10	>10	>10	>10	>10

* Inactive at 10 mg/kg; higher doses were not studied.

effects. With the exception of the inactivity of pentazocine as a narcotic antagonist, the potency order of these drugs as narcotic antagonists does not differ markedly from the potency order of these same drugs as antagonists in other systems (2, 22).

Although it is clear that powerful narcotic antagonists can block the rate-*decreasing* effects of morphine on operant behavior, the previous experiments do not indicate whether or not narcotic antagonists can block the rate-*increasing* effects of morphine. McMillan et al. (20) selected pigeons whose response rates were increased by approximately 50% during the FI component after small doses of morphine and pretreated these birds with naloxone. A dose of 0.1 mg/kg of naloxone blocked the rate-increasing effect of morphine almost completely. This, naloxone appears to be a powerful antagonist of both the rate-increasing and rate-decreasing effects of morphine on schedule-controlled behavior.

In all of the experiments discussed previously, the narcotic antagonists have been administered before the narcotic. However, a similar antagonism can be shown if the morphine is injected first. Kosersky and Harris (13) injected intravenous morphine (5.6 mg/kg) to suppress totally responding of pigeons whose behavior was maintained under an FR 60 schedule of food presentation. A dose of 0.3 mg/kg naloxone, through the same intravenous cannula, restored responding to normal rates within 10 sec.

Although naloxone has little agonist activity in many systems (2), many narcotic antagonists do have marked agonist activity (7). For example, the effects of cyclazocine in both animals (1) and man (11) can be blocked by naloxone. In this respect, the pigeon seems to differ from other species. McMillan et al. (20) attempted to block the rate-decreasing effects of cyclazocine on behavior under the multiple FR FI schedule. At doses up to 30 mg/kg of naloxone, there was no antagonism of the cyclazocine depression. In fact, high doses of naloxone seemed to potentiate the rate-decreasing effects of cyclazocine.

The interactions between naloxone and cyclazocine, when the operant behavior of the pigeon is studied, may be contrasted with interactions between naloxone and another benzomorphan narcotic antagonist, pentazocine, when the avoidance behavior of the rat is measured (10). In the rat experiments, naloxone blocked both the rate-increasing effects of low doses of pentazocine and the rate-decreasing effects of higher doses. It has not yet been determined whether these differences can be traced to the differences in species, to the different schedules maintaining responding, or to the different benzomorphan examined.

In summary, operant behavior appears to be a useful index of the potency of narcotic antagonists in blocking the effects of narcotics. Using the operant behavior of the pigeon, there is a fair degree of agreement between the human data and the pigeon with respect to the ordering of potency of the various narcotic antagonists. However, the situation is less clear when attempts are made to use powerful narcotic antagonists to antagonize the behavioral effects of other narcotic antagonists.

INTERACTIONS BETWEEN NARCOTIC ANTAGONISTS AND "DEPRESSANT DRUGS"

There have been few attempts to study the interaction between narcotic antagonists and drugs of classes other than the narcotic analgesics. The importance of such studies is obvious, since patients using narcotic antagonists might also be taking other drugs, either as prescribed by their physicians or for purposes of abuse.

In one study of this type (16), the interaction between naloxone and chlorpromazine on the operant behavior of the pigeon was studied. Inactive doses of naloxone enhanced chlorpromazine's rate-decreasing effect on operant behavior, while at doses where both drugs decreased the rate of responding, the combined effects of chlorpromazine and naloxone were greater than the sum of their individual rate-decreasing effects. It is not known to what extent these observations can be extended to other narcotic antagonists in addition to naloxone, to other CNS depressants in addition to chlorpromazine, and to other species.

OPERANT BEHAVIOR AS A BASELINE FOR STUDYING THE DEVELOPMENT OF DRUG TOLERANCE AND PHYSICAL DEPENDENCE

Operant behavior has been used to study the development of tolerance to morphine (4, 19, 25), methadone (8), and pentazocine (18). In these experiments, a stable baseline pattern of operant responding is established and then a drug is administered repeatedly. The initial injection produces a marked effect, but after repeated injections the effects of the drug are no longer observed. In some instances, the dose can then be increased to a large multiple of the original dose with little further effect on operant behavior.

Table 3 summarizes a typical experiment of this type. Pigeons, responding under a multiple FR FI schedule of food presentation were injected with 5.6 mg/kg of morphine, which almost completely eliminated responding under both schedule components. After nine injections of this dose of morphine (three times weekly), the rate of responding was almost at control levels. Subsequently, the dose of morphine was increased to 150 mg/kg, administered twice daily. Although each of these injections was more than 25 times the original dose, morphine no longer disrupted the rate or the pattern of responding. Since behavior was not affected at these doses, it seems likely that an even larger tolerance could have been demonstrated.

Heifetz and McMillan (8) showed that tolerance also develops to the effects of methadone on operant behavior. However, they could not demonstrate tolerance to the rate-increasing effect of methadone, even when

TABLE 3. *Operant responding as a measure of tolerance development to morphine-and naloxone-precipitated withdrawal from morphine.*

Treatment	Injection	FI rate	FR rate
Control range	—	0.60–1.01	2.02–2.55
5.6 mg/kg	1	0.01	0.87
5.6 mg/kg	6	0.54	1.94
56.0 mg/kg	7	0.10	0.50
56.0 mg/kg	20	0.38	1.07
56.0 mg/kg – 2/day	26	0.72	2.12
10.0 mg/kg naloxone	27	0.00	0.10
150.0 mg/kg – 2/day	41	0.79	2.03
24 hr without morphine		0.56	1.99
48 hr without morphine		0.72	2.11
10.0 mg/kg naloxone (72 hr without morphine)	42	0.42	1.48
96 hr without morphine		0.93	2.45
10.0 mg/kg naloxone (120 hr without morphine)	43	0.67	2.28

methadone was injected for 16 consecutive days after the rate-increasing effects were first observed.

A marked tolerance does not seem to develop to the repeated administration of pentazocine in pigeons (18). When a 17.5 mg/kg dose of pentazocine was administered, responding was greatly suppressed. This dose was administered three times weekly for 11 injections and then daily for six injections without tolerance development being observed. When the dose of pentazocine was increased to 35 mg/kg and the birds were injected twice daily, a limited tolerance development could be demonstrated.

Operant behavior also can be used to measure the effects of drug withdrawal on animal behavior. In one such experiment (17), pigeons were made tolerant to 56.0 mg/kg injections of morphine and then 10 mg/kg of naloxone was injected (Table 3). Although this dose of naloxone is far below that which depresses operant behavior in pigeons (20), naloxone almost entirely eliminated the responding of these pigeons that were tolerant to morphine. Despite the disruption of operant behavior, no overt signs of physical withdrawal could be observed. Subsequently, these pigeons were placed back on the morphine regimen. After a period of time the administration of morphine was discontinued in an attempt to observe signs of morphine abstinence. Again, no overt signs of abstinence could be observed; however, there was a very slight decrease in the rate of responding under both schedule components 24 hr after the last morphine injection (injection 42). Although behavior was normal 48 hr after the last morphine injection, 24 hr later a dose of 10 mg/kg naloxone again markedly decreased responding.

Operant behavior has been shown to be a useful measure of the behavioral effects of narcotic antagonists, as well as a measure of the efficacy and potency of narcotic antagonists in blocking the behavioral effects of narcotic analgesics. Although more experiments need to be done to illustrate the usefulness of operant behavior for studying drug tolerance and drug withdrawal syndromes, these experiments suggest that operant behavior may also be a sensitive measure of the behavioral state of the animal during tolerance development and during morphine abstinence.

CONCLUSIONS

Narcotics and narcotic antagonists have very similar effects on operant behavior in pigeons and rats. They differ from each other in potency.

With some exceptions, the potency order of narcotics and narcotic antagonists in affecting operant behavior in pigeons correlates positively with the analgesic potency of these drugs in man.

At doses much lower than those that affect operant behavior, powerful narcotic antagonists can block completely the effects of narcotic analgesics on operant behavior.

Operant behavior can be used to study drug tolerance and drug withdrawal phenomena in animals.

ACKNOWLEDGMENTS

Preparation of this manuscript was supported by U.S. Public Health Service Research Grant NB 06854 to Dr. Louis S. Harris. I wish to thank Mrs. Martha E. Byrd for preparation of the manuscript and the Williams and Wilkins Co. and my coauthors for permission to reproduce Figures 1, 3, and 4 from the original publications.

REFERENCES

1. Blumberg, H., Dayton, H. B., and Wolf, P. S.: Counteraction of narcotic antagonist analgesics by the narcotic antagonist naloxone. Proc. Soc. Exp. Biol. Med. *123*:755–758, 1966.
2. Blumberg, H., Wolf, P. S., and Dayton, H. B.: Use of the writhing test for evaluating analgesic activity of narcotic antagonists. Proc. Soc. Exp. Biol. Med. *118*:763–766, 1965.
3. Dews, P. B., and Morse, W. H.: Behavioral pharmacology. Ann. Rev. Pharmacol. *1*:145–174, 1961.
4. Djahanguiri, B., Richelle, M., Fontaine, O.: Behavioral effects of a prolonged treatment with small doses of morphine in cats. Psychopharmacologia *9*:363–372, 1966.
5. Geller, I., Bachman, E., and Seifter, G.: Effects of reserpine and morphine on behavior suppressed by punishment. Life Sci. *4*:226–231, 1963.
6. Harris, L. S., Dewey, W. L., Howes, J. F., Kennedy, J. S., and Pars, H.: Narcotic-antagonist analgesics: Interactions with cholinergic systems. J. Pharmacol. Exp. Ther. *169*:17–22, 1969.
7. Harris, L. S., and Pierson, A. K.: Some narcotic antagonists in the benzomorphan series. J. Pharmacol. Exp. Ther. *143*:141–148, 1964.
8. Heifetz, S. A., and McMillan, D. E.: Development of behavioral tolerance to morphine and methadone using the schedule-controlled behavior of the pigeon. Psychopharmacologia *19*:40–52, 1971.
9. Hill, H. E., Pescor, F. T., Belleville, R. E., and Wikler, A.: Use of differential bar-pressing rates of rats for screening analgesic drugs. I. Techniques and effects of morphine. J. Pharmacol. Exp. Ther. *120*:388–397, 1957.
10. Holtzman, S. G., and Jewett, R. E.: Some actions of pentazocine on behavior and brain monoamines in the rat. J. Pharmacol. Exp. Ther. *181*:346–356, 1972.
11. Jasinski, D. R., Martin, W. R., and Sapira, J. D.: Antagonism of the subjective, behavioral pupillary and respiratory depressant effects of cyclazocine by naloxone. Clin. Pharmacol. Ther. *9*:215–222, 1968.
12. Kelleher, R. T., and Morse, W. H.: Escape behavior and punished behavior. Fed. Proc. *23*:808–817, 1964.
13. Kosersky, D. S. and Harris, L. S.: Eur. J. Pharmacol. *21*:379–382, 1973.
14. Lasagna, L., and Beecher, H. K.: The analgesic effectiveness of nalorphine and nalorphine-morphine combinations in man. J. Pharmacol. Exp. Ther. *112*:356–363, 1954.
15. Martin, W. R.: Opoid antagonists. Pharmacol. Rev. *19*:463–522, 1967.
16. McMillan, D. E.: Interactions between naloxone and chlorpromazine on behavior under schedule control. Psychopharmacologia *19*:128–133, 1971.

17. McMillan, D. E., Dewey, W. L., and Harris, L. S.: Characteristics of tetrahydrocannabinol tolerance. Ann. N.Y. Acad. Sci. *191*:83–99, 1971.
18. McMillan, D. E., and Harris, L. S.: Behavioral and morphine-antagonist effects of the optical isomers of pentazocine and cyclazocine. J. Pharmacol. Exp. Ther. *180*:569–579, 1972.
19. McMillan, D. E., and Morse, W. H.: Some effects of morphine and morphine antagonists on schedule-controlled behavior. J. Pharmacol. Exp. Ther. *157*:175–184, 1967.
20. McMillan, D. E., Wolf, P. S., and Carchman, R. A.: Antagonism of the behavioral effects of morphine and methadone by narcotic antagonists in the pigeon. J. Pharmacol. Exp. Ther. *175*:443–458, 1970.
21. Nichols, J. R.: How opiates change behavior. Sci. Amer. *212*:80–88, 1965.
22. Pearl, J., and Harris, L. S.: Inhibition of writhing by narcotic antagonists. J. Pharmacol. Exp. Ther. *154*:310–323, 1966.
23. Schuster, C. R., and Thompson, T.: Self administration of and behavioral dependence on drugs. Ann. Rev. Pharmacol. 9:483–502, 1969.
24. Sidman, M.: Avoidance conditioning with brief shock and no exteroceptive warning signal. Science *118*:157–158, 1953.
25. Thompson, T., and Schuster, C. R.: Morphine self-administration, food reinforced and avoidance behaviors in rhesus monkeys. Psychopharmacologia 5:87–94, 1964.
26. Tsou, K.: Effects of morphine upon several types of operant conditionings in the rat. Acta Physiol. Sinica 26:143–150, 1963.
27. Verhave, T., Owen, J. E., and Robbins, E. B.: The effect of morphine sulfate on avoidance and escape behavior. J. Pharmacol. Exp. Ther. *125*:248–257, 1959.
28. Waller, M. B., and Morse, W. H.: Effects of pentobarbital on fixed-ratio reinforcement. J. Exp. Anal. Behav. 6:125–130, 1963.
29. Weiss, B.: The effects of various morphine-N-allyl-normorphine ratios on behavior. Arch. Int. Pharmacodyn. Ther. *105*:381–388, 1956.
30. Weiss, B., and Laties, V. G.: Analgesic effects in monkeys of morphine, nalorphine and a benzomorphan narcotic antagonist. J. Pharmacol. Exp. Ther. *143*:169–173, 1964.
31. Wikler, A.: On the nature of addiction and habituation. Brit. J. Addiction 57:73–79, 1961.

Narcotic Antagonists, edited by M. C. Braude, L. S. Harris, E. L. May, J. P. Smith, and J. E. Villarreal. *Advances in Biochemical Psychopharmacology, Vol. 8.* Raven Press, New York © 1974.

Self Administration: Positive and Negative Reinforcing Properties of Morphine Antagonists in Rhesus Monkeys

F. Hoffmeister and W. Wuttke

Institut für Pharmakologie der BAYER AG, Wuppertal-Elberfeld, West Germany

Three groups of rhesus monkeys restricted with harnesses were surgically prepared with indwelling jugular vein catheters which were connected to injection pumps. The pumps could be activated automatically or by lever-pressing responses of the monkeys. Monkeys of one group were trained to press a lever for codeine injections of 50 mg/kg. Every tenth response was followed by an injection (fixed ratio 10 schedule, FR 10). Codeine was available during daily 3-hr sessions. After responding was stabilized, codeine was replaced by different doses of heroin, codeine, pentazocine, propiramfumarate, nalorphine, and cyclazocine. The second group of monkeys performed under a schedule in which a response either terminated stimuli associated with intravenous injections (avoidance) or terminated the injections of nalorphine, cyclazocine, pentazocine, propiramfumarate, or codeine (escape). The third group performed under the same schedule with the difference that these monkeys were physically dependent on morphine. During the avoidance-escape experiment morphine dependence was maintained by automatic injections of morphine once every 4 hr. Under this schedule, nalorphine, pentazocine, and propiramfumarate were studied. In rhesus monkeys with a history of opiate self-administration who were not physically dependent, pentazocine and propiramfumarate have positive reinforcing properties qualitatively comparable to those of heroin and codeine since both maintain self-administration behavior. In contrast, nalorphine and cyclazocine appear to have punishing effects under these conditions, since the monkeys cease to press the lever when codeine was replaced by nalorphine and cyclazocine. In naive rhesus monkeys (i.e., subjects without any drug experience prior to the experiment) nalorphine and cyclazocine – in contrast to pentazocine, propiramfumarate, and codeine – have negative reinforcing properties; both have the capacity to initiate and maintain stable avoidance-escape behavior. In subjects physically dependent on morphine, nalorphine, pentazocine, and propiramfumarate act as negative reinforcers.

From clinical pharmacological studies it is known that analgesics possessing both morphine-agonistic and morphine-antagonistic actions can

361

show different psychic effects in man. Substances such as nalorphine or cyclazocine, which are more potent morphine antagonists than agonists, cause disphoric psychotomimetic effects in man at analgesic doses. Such aversive effects were found in individuals without opiate history as well as in individuals physically dependent on opiates (9, 13).

A second class of substances including, for example, pentazocine and propiram fumarate, which have relatively potent agonistic and weak antagonistic actions, mainly produce morphine-like euphoria at therapeutic doses in individuals not physically dependent on opiates. Nalorphine-like aversive effects only become evident at relatively high doses (4, 10, 12). However, in persons physically dependent on high doses of morphine, pentazocine and propiram fumarate only have aversive properties similar to those of nalorphine and cyclazocine. Therefore, at therapeutic doses, unlike nalorphine and cyclazocine, pentazocine and propiram fumarate are suitable for clinical use as analgesics (8, 11). Clinical trials have shown that substances with this type of action are potent analgesics which, owing to their relatively weak abuse potential, are superior to all other narcotic analgesics known at present. Therefore, we were interested in comparing the effects of pure morphine agonists with nalorphine-like as well as with pentazocine-like compounds on self-administration behavior in rhesus monkeys.

METHODS

Subjects were male and female rhesus monkeys (*Macaca mulatta*) weighing between 3 and 4 kg. Under pentobarbital anesthesia (30 mg/kg i.v.), silicone rubber catheters were passed through the internal jugular vein to the level of the right atrium. The surgically implanted catheter was led subcutaneously to the monkey's back where it exited through a stab wound in the skin. Each monkey was placed in a metal harness which was attached to a jointed metal restraining arm. The arm was fixed to the rear wall of the cubicle. The catheter passed through the restraining arm to the back of the cubicle where it was connected to an automatic injection pump. A lever and a stimulus light were mounted in the back wall of the cubicle. Intravenous injections could be automatically delivered or injections could be programmed to occur when monkeys pressed the lever (response). Injections consisted of 0.2 ml/kg of solution. Activation of the pump was clearly audible to the monkeys. Injection duration was regulated according to the monkey's body weight. The monkeys remained in their individual cubicles throughout the experiment with food and water freely available. Details of catheterization procedure and apparatus have been reported by Deneau et al. (2).

Experiment 1

Eight monkeys were used. A white stimulus light was presented for 8 hr a day, and each response during this time was followed by an injection of 50 mg/kg of codeine. Once responding was initiated, drug access was limited to a 3-hr daily session and the number of responses required to produce a codeine injection was increased to 10, that is, a 10-response fixed-ratio schedule of drug injection (FR 10).

When responding became stabilized, codeine was replaced by different doses of heroin, codeine, pentazocine, propiram fumarate, nalorphine, and cyclazocine. Each drug was tested on at least three monkeys. Decreasing doses of each drug were administered for each of six successive daily 3-hr sessions. Codeine was also replaced by saline for six daily sessions in each of the monkeys. For more extensive description of this procedure, see Hoffmeister and Schlichting (6).

Experiment 2

A total of seven rhesus monkeys were trained to press a lever to turn off a white light which was associated with annoying electric stimuli of 10-sec duration, scheduled to occur 30 sec after the onset of the light. Electric stimuli were administered by means of chronically implanted electrodes. Each response turned off the white light for a 1-min time-out period (1). After the subjects had learned to avoid or to escape most of the electric shocks during successive daily 2-hr sessions, the electric stimuli were replaced by a 10-sec infusion of saline solution. After lever pressing extinguished in the presence of the white stimulus light or decreased to a "saline-level" of low responding (when the monkeys "tolerated" a high number of saline injections), saline was replaced by different unit doses of nalorphine, cyclazocine, pentazocine, propiram fumarate, and codeine, each for six successive daily 2-hr sessions. The number of avoidance and escape responses was recorded. The degree of avoidance was calculated in individual monkeys as the number of infusions tolerated as a percent of the saline infusions tolerated during a 6-day control period. For further details concerning the procedure, see Hoffmeister and Wuttke (7).

Experiment 3

The subjects in this experiment were three rhesus monkeys with a history of morphine self-administration. Over a period of 2 months prior to the experiment, each monkey self-administered about 18 mg/kg/day, a dose sufficient to develop physical dependence on morphine, as assessed by intensity of precipitated abstinence signs (2, 14). During the experiment, morphine self-administration was discontinued and physical dependence was maintained by automatic injections of 3 mg/kg once every 4 hr. After 5 or more days, during which lever responses had no consequences, monkeys were tested under a discrete avoidance-escape schedule (1) on 2-hr daily sessions which started 1 hr after an automatic morphine injection. Under this schedule, a 10-sec nalorphine injection (10 mg/kg) was delivered every 30 sec in the presence of a green stimulus light. A response during the 30-sec green-light period terminated the light for a 60-sec time-out period and prevented the injection (avoidance). If the monkeys failed to respond, the green light remained on and a 10-sec injection began. A response during the injection terminated both the injection (escape) and the green light for the 60-sec time-out period. For further details of this procedure, see Goldberg et al. (5).

DRUGS

Codeine-phosphate, morphine-HCl-trihydrate, nalorphine-HCl, pentazocine-HCl, propiram fumarate, and cyclazocine-HCl were dissolved in saline solution. All doses refer to the bases of the drugs.

RESULTS AND DISCUSSION

Experiment 1

As indicated in Fig. 1, all compounds studied except nalorphine and cyclazocine were self-administered dose dependently. The peak rate of self-administration occurred at 0.5 mg/kg with heroin injections, 25 mg/kg with codeine injections, and 50 mg/kg with pentazocine and propiram fumarate injections. Neither nalorphine in injection doses from 5 to 500 mg/kg nor cyclazocine in injection doses from 0.1 to 10 mg/kg produced lever pressing below the saline self-administration level.

These cross self-administration experiments show that in rhesus monkeys with a history of opiate self-administration, but without current physical dependence on opiates, morphine antagonists of the nalorphine-cyclazocine type have no positive reinforcing properties. Since rates of self-administration are below those of saline for nalorphine and cyclazocine, these drugs appear to act as punishers. On the other hand, weak morphine antagonists such as pentazocine and propiram fumarate do maintain stable self-administration behavior although the doses necessary to engender maximum rates of self-administration are twice as high as for codeine and one hundred times as high as for heroin.

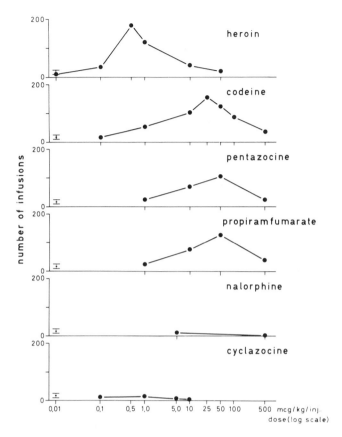

FIG. 1. Cross self-administration in rhesus monkeys trained for codeine self-administration. Symbols represent means of at least three monkeys per dose. Control: mean number (with confidence limits) of saline infusions per day of all eight monkeys involved in this experiment during a 6-day control period.

Experiment 2

Figure 2 shows the results for nalorphine and cyclazocine in the avoidance-escape procedure in naive subjects. Injection doses from 500 to 10 mg/kg of nalorphine and from 10 to 25 mg/kg of cyclazocine generate and maintain avoidance-escape behavior; injection doses of 1 mg/kg of nalorphine and 0.1 mg/kg of cyclazocine are tolerated by the subjects, as shown by the fact that lever-pressing behavior was extinguished. As indicated in Fig. 3, in injection doses of 50 mg/kg, propiram fumarate is tolerated like saline; pentazocine and codeine are tolerated even more than saline. The

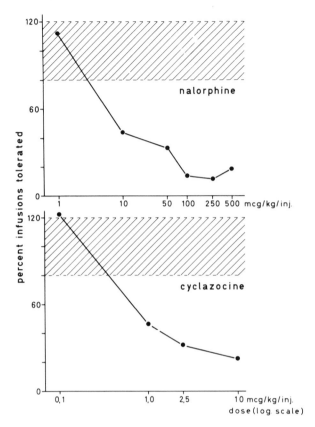

FIG. 2. Avoidance of and escape from nalorphine and cyclazocine infusions in naive rhesus monkeys. Abscissa: dose. Ordinate: number of drug infusions tolerated expressed as percent of the number of saline infusions tolerated during a 6-day control period. Symbols represent means of at least three monkeys per dose. Control: the mean number of saline infusions tolerated (with confidence limits) during a 6-day control period of all seven monkeys involved in the experiment was assigned the value of 100%.

results of this experiment show that nalorphine and cyclazocine have negative reinforcing properties.

Experiment 3

Only nalorphine, pentazocine and propiram fumarate were studied under the discrete avoidance schedule in morphine dependent monkeys. As indicated in Fig. 4, all three compounds initiate and maintain stable avoidance behavior in these subjects physically dependent on morphine. Injections

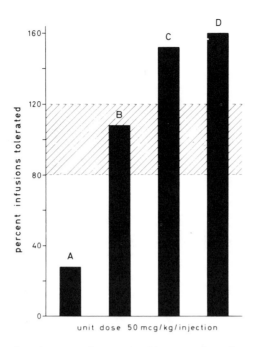

FIG. 3. Avoidance of and escape from nalorphine, propiram fumarate, codeine and pentazocine infusions in naive rhesus monkeys. Abscissa: dose. Ordinate: number of drug infusions tolerated expressed as percent of the number of saline infusions tolerated during a 6-day control period. Columns represent means of at least three monkeys per substance. Control: the mean number of saline infusions tolerated (with confidence limits) during a 6-day control period of all seven monkeys involved in the experiment was assigned the value of 100%.

neither of nalorphine at doses of 5 mg/kg nor of pentazocine and propiram fumarate at doses of 50 mg/kg are tolerated.

Summary of the Three Experiments

In rhesus monkeys with a history of opiate self-administration but without current physical dependence, pentazocine and propiram fumarate have positive reinforcing properties qualitatively comparable to those of heroin and codeine since both maintain self-administration behavior. In contrast, nalorphine and cyclazocine have punishing effects under these conditions, since the monkeys cease to press the lever when codeine is replaced by nalorphine and cyclazocine.

In naive rhesus monkeys, nalorphine and cyclazocine, but not pentazocine, propiram fumarate, or codeine, have negative reinforcing properties;

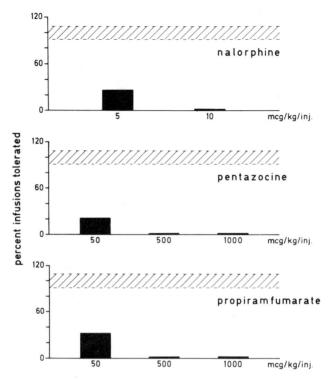

FIG. 4. Avoidance of and escape from nalorphine, pentazocine, and propiram fumarate infusions in rhesus monkeys physically dependent on morphine. Abscissa: dose. Ordinate: number of drug infusions tolerated expressed as percent of the number of saline infusions tolerated during a 6-day control period. Columns represent means of three monkeys. Control: the mean number of saline infusions tolerated (with confidence limits) during a 6-day control period of the three monkeys involved in the experiment was assigned the value of 100%.

only the former two drugs initiate and maintain stable avoidance-escape behavior.

In subjects physically dependent on morphine, nalorphine, pentazocine, and propiram fumarate act as negative reinforcers.

CONCLUSIONS

The results reported have shown that the different effects of agonists-antagonists of the nalorphine-cyclazocine type can be differentiated from those of pentazocine and propiram fumarate using self-administration procedures.

REFERENCES

1. Cook, L., and Catania, A. C.: Effects of drugs on avoidance and escape behavior. Fed. Proc. *23*:818–835, 1964.
2. Deneau, G. A., and Seevers, M. H.: Pharmacological aspects of drug dependence. Adv. Pharmacol. *3*:267–283, 1964.
3. Deneau, G. A., Yanagita, T., and Seevers, M. H.: Self-administration of psychoactive substances by the monkey. Psychopharmacologia *16*:30–48, 1969.
4. Fraser, H. F., and Rosenberg, D. E.: Studies on the human addiction liability of 2-hydroxy-5,9-dimethyl-2-(3,3-dimethyl-allyl)-6,7-benzomorphan (WIN 20.228): A weak narcotic antagonist. J. Pharmacol. Exp. Ther. *143*:149–156, 1964.
5. Goldberg, St. R., Hoffmeister, F., and Schlichting, U. U.: Morphine antagonists: Modification of behavioral effects by morphine dependence. In: Drug Addiction, Vol. I: Experimental Pharmacology, ed. by J. M. Singh, L. Miller, and H. Lal. Futura Publishing Co., Mount Kisco, New York, 1972.
6. Hoffmeister, F., and Schlichting, U. U.: Reinforcing properties of some opiates and opioids in rhesus monkeys with histories of cocaine and codeine self-administration. Psychopharmacologia *23*:55–74, 1972.
7. Hoffmeister, F., and Wuttke, W.: Negative reinforcing properties of morphine antagonists in naive rhesus monkeys. Psychopharmacologia (in press).
8. Jaffe, J. H.: Narcotic analgesics. In: The Pharmacological Basis of Therapeutics, 4th ed., ed. by L. S. Goodman and A. Gilman, pp. 237–275. Macmillan Company, New York, 1970.
9. Jasinski, D. R., Martin, W. R., and Sapira, J. D.: Antagonism of the subjective, behavioral, pupillary, and respiratory depressant effects of cyclazocine by naloxone. Clin. Pharm. Ther. *9*:215–222, 1968.
10. Jasinski, D. R., Martin, W. R., and Hoeldtke, R.: Studies of the dependence-producing properties of GPA-1657, profadol, and propiram in man. Clin. Pharm. Ther. *12*:613–649, 1971.
11. Lewis, J. W., Bentley, K. W., and Cowan, A.: Narcotic analgesics and antagonists. Ann. Rev. Pharmacol. *11*:241–270, 1971.
12. Martin, W. R.: Assessment of the dependence producing potentiality of narcotic analgesics. Int. Encyclopedia of Pharmacology and Therapeutics *1*:155–180, 1966.
13. Martin, W. R., and Gorodetzky, C. W.: Demonstration of tolerance to and physical dependence on N-allylnormorphine (nalorphine). J. Pharmacol. Exp. Ther. *150*:437–442, 1965.

Narcotic Antagonists, edited by M. C. Braude, L. S. Harris, E. L. May, J. P. Smith, and J. E. Villarreal. *Advances in Biochemical Psychopharmacology, Vol. 8.* Raven Press, New York © 1974.

Narcotic Antagonists as Stimulants of Behavior in the Rat: Specific and Nonspecific Effects*

Stephen G. Holtzman

Department of Pharmacology, Emory University, Atlanta, Georgia 30322

The actions of cyclazocine, pentazocine, and levallorphan were evaluated on two distinct types of behavior in adult male rats: operant behavior (lever pressing maintained under a continuous avoidance schedule) and locomotor activity. Drug effects on the total brain content of norepinephrine and dopamine were also examined. Dose-response curves were first determined for each drug administered alone, and then redetermined with concomitant administration of 8 or 16 mg/kg of naloxone. The three narcotic-antagonist analgesics increased avoidance responding and locomotor activity in a graded manner over a broad range of doses. The order of potency and peak activity in both procedures was cyclazocine > levallorphan > pentazocine. These drugs also produced dose-related decreases in brain catecholamine content ranging from 13 to 40%. Thus, the rat is a unique species in that its response to narcotic antagonists is characterized by graded behavioral stimulation. Naloxone, itself inactive in all procedures, blocked the effects of the narcotic-antagonist analgesics on operant behavior, but not their effects on locomotor activity and brain catecholamine levels. These results indicate that the agonistic component of action of narcotic antagonists in the rat is mediated by at least two mechanisms: one which is blocked by naloxone (i.e., specific), and one which is not (i.e., nonspecific).

Many narcotic antagonists can induce major changes in behavior when administered acutely to otherwise drug-free individuals (5, 15). However, in most infrahuman species narcotic antagonists have a relatively low order of behavioral activity, and there have been only a few studies which have attempted to evaluate systematically the effects of narcotic antagonists on animal behavior.

The present chapter describes the effects of the narcotic antagonists pentazocine, levallorphan, and cyclazocine on operant behavior and locomotor activity in the rat. Drug effects on brain levels of norepinephrine (NE) and dopamine (DA) were also determined since brain catecholamines have been implicated in the control of operant behavior and

---

* Publication no. 1085 of the Division of Basic Health Sciences of Emory University.

locomotor activity (23) as well as in some of the actions of morphine and related narcotic analgesics (22). Naloxone, a narcotic antagonist with little agonistic activity of its own (2, 11), blocks both the agonistic effects of narcotic antagonists and the effects of morphine-like drugs (15). Therefore, the three agonist-antagonists were tested alone and in the presence of naloxone. It will be demonstrated that narcotic antagonists can act as potent stimulants of behavior in the rat. Furthermore, evidence will be presented which indicates that the behavioral actions of the narcotic antagonists are mediated by at least two distinct mechanisms: one which is blocked by naloxone (i.e., "specific"), and one which is not (i.e., "nonspecific").

METHODS

Subjects

The subjects were adult male rats of the CFE strain (Carworth). The rats used in the operant behavior experiments were housed individually; all of the other rats were housed in group cages. The animal cages were maintained in a large colony room which was illuminated between 6:00 A.M. and 6:00 P.M. Food and water were continuously available to the animals.

Operant Behavior

Rats were trained to press a lever to a criterion of 90% avoidance under a continuous avoidance schedule (20) with an escape contingency (6). Every lever response by the rat postponed for 30 sec a scrambled 1.0 to 1.3 mA electric shock with a maximum duration of 3.0 sec which was delivered through the grid floor of the experimental chamber. In the continued absence of responses, shocks were delivered at 15-sec intervals. A response during the delivery of a shock immediately terminated the shock and initiated a 30-sec response-shock interval. More detailed descriptions of the apparatus and schedule parameters have previously been published (7–9).

Each rat was tested in two 4-hr experimental sessions per week held 3 to 4 days apart. Drugs were administered immediately before an experimental session, and were never tested in more than two sessions in succession. The appropriate drug vehicle was administered before all control (i.e., nondrug) sessions.

Locomotor Activity

Locomotor activity was measured in circular photoactivity cages, each 60 cm in diameter and 18 cm in height. Three visible light beams crossed at the center of a cage; the number of times that the rat interrupted a light beam was recorded on electromagnetic counters.

Rats were injected with either a drug or the drug vehicle and immediately placed in an activity cage, one rat per cage. After a 5-min adaptation period, locomotor activity was recorded for 1 hr.

Brain Catecholamines

Rats were killed by decapitation 60 to 75 min after receiving either a drug or the drug vehicle. The entire brain was rapidly removed, weighed, and homogenized by sonication (8). The brain homogenates were stored in a freezer until assay 1 to 3 days later. The amount of NE and DA in the homogenates was determined fluorometrically (1). Internal standards were included in every assay.

Drugs

The drugs used in these studies and the forms in which doses are expressed are levallorphan tartrate (generously supplied by Roche Laboratories, Nutley, N.J.), naloxone hydrochloride (generously supplied by Endo Laboratories, Inc., Garden City, N.Y.), and the free base of cyclazocine and pentazocine (both provided by Sterling Winthrop Research Institute, Rensselaer, N.Y.). Levallorphan and naloxone were dissolved in 0.9% saline. Cyclazocine and pentazocine were dissolved in three parts of 8.5% lactic acid; two parts of 1.0 N NaOH were added, raising the pH of the final solution to between 4 and 5. All drugs and drug vehicles were injected subcutaneously in a volume of 0.1 or 0.2 ml/100 g of body weight. Except where noted otherwise, when naloxone was given in combination with another drug, the two drugs were injected a few seconds apart into different subcutaneous sites.

RESULTS

Operant Behavior

The average rate of avoidance responding in the 4-hr experimental session was increased by 2.0 to 16 mg/kg of pentazocine (Fig. 1), by 0.5 to 64 mg/kg of levallorphan (Fig. 2), and by 0.125 to 2.0 mg/kg of cyclazocine (Fig. 3). The mean avoidance rate within a session often reached 200 to 300% of control values, especially during the first 1 to 2 hr following drug administration. Raising the dose of pentazocine to 32 mg/kg

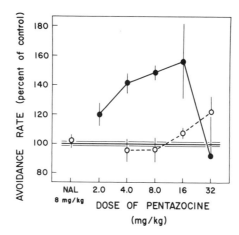

FIG. 1. Effects of pentazocine alone (solid circles, solid lines) and of pentazocine plus 8.0 mg/kg of naloxone (open circles, broken lines) on avoidance-response rate. The effect of 8.0 mg/kg of naloxone on avoidance rate is represented by the isolated point at the left. Data are expressed as a percent of the rate of responding in control sessions (control rate: 3.74 ± 0.05 responses per minute). Each point represents the mean of one observation in each of four rats in a 4-hr experimental session. Vertical lines and light horizontal lines represent ± 1 SEM. Data are modified from Holtzman and Jewett (8).

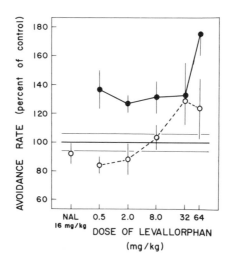

FIG. 2. Effects of levallorphan alone (solid circles, solid lines) and of levallorphan plus 16 mg/kg of naloxone (open circles, broken lines) on avoidance-response rate. The effect of 16 mg/kg of naloxone on avoidance rate is represented by the isolated point at the left. Data are expressed as a percent of the rate of responding in control sessions (control rate: 4.96 ± 0.30 responses per minute). Each point represents the mean of one observation in each of four rats in a 4-hr experimental session. Vertical lines and light horizontal lines represent ± 1 SEM. Data are from Steinert et al. (21).

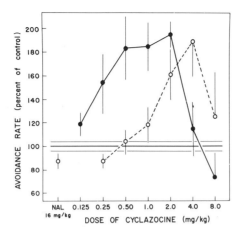

FIG. 3. Effects of cyclazocine alone (solid circles, solid lines) and of cyclazocine plus 16 mg/kg of naloxone (open circles, broken lines) on avoidance-response rate. The effect of 16 mg/kg of naloxone on avoidance rate is represented by the isolated point at the left. Data are expressed as a percent of the rate of responding in control sessions (control rate: 4.83 ± 0.21 responses per minute). Each point represents the mean of one observation in each of four rats in a 4-hr experimental session. Vertical lines and light horizontal lines represent ± 1 SEM. Data are from Holtzman and Jewett (10).

and the dose of cyclazocine to 4.0 and 8.0 mg/kg resulted in a disruption of operant behavior which was associated with prominent excitation of the animals. A higher dose of levallorphan (i.e., 128 mg/kg) also disrupted behavior but, at the same time, caused convulsions. Thus, the dose-response curve for levallorphan could not be extended further than 64 mg/kg.

The effects of pentazocine, levallorphan, and cyclazocine on avoidance response rate were antagonized by 8.0 or 16 mg/kg of naloxone. Analyses of variance showed that the dose-response curves generated by the three agonist-antagonists administered alone were significantly different from the curves generated in the presence of naloxone ($p < 0.01$ for all comparisons). The concomitant administration of 16 mg/kg of naloxone resulted in a shift to the right of the cyclazocine dose-response curve (Fig. 3). It was not possible to demonstrate similar total shifts of the pentazocine and levallorphan dose-response curves since higher doses of both drugs produced convulsions, even in the presence of naloxone. Naloxone alone had no significant effect on avoidance rate in any of the three series of experiments (Figs. 1–3).

Locomotor Activity

Pentazocine, levallorphan, and cyclazocine produced marked stimulation of locomotor activity which was graded over the dose ranges tested

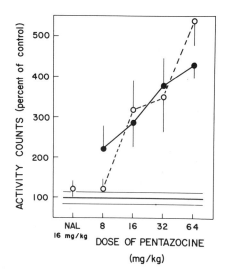

FIG. 4. Effects of pentazocine alone (solid circles, solid lines) and of pentazocine plus 16 mg/kg of naloxone (open circles, broken lines) on locomotor activity. The effect of 16 mg/kg of naloxone on locomotor activity is represented by the isolated point at the left. Data are expressed as a percent of locomotor activity in control sessions (control activity: 64 ± 10 counts per hour). Each point represents the mean of six observations in a 1-hr recording session. Vertical lines and light horizontal lines represent ± 1 SEM. Data are modified from Holtzman and Jewett (8).

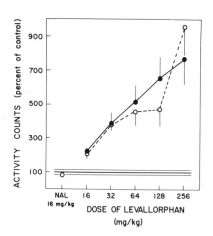

FIG. 5. Effects of levallorphan alone (solid circles, solid lines) and of levallorphan plus 16 mg/kg of naloxone (open circles, broken lines) on locomotor activity. The effect of 16 mg/kg of naloxone on locomotor activity is represented by the isolated point at the left. Data are expressed as a percent of locomotor activity in control sessions (control activity: 141 ± 24 counts per hour). Each point represents the mean of six observations in a 1-hr recording session. Vertical lines and light horizontal lines represent ± 1 SEM. Where vertical lines are absent, the SEM is less than the radius of the point. Data are from Steinert et al. (21).

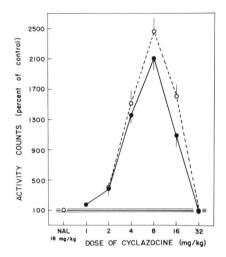

FIG. 6. Effects of cyclazocine alone (solid circles, solid lines) and of cyclazocine plus 16 mg/kg of naloxone (open circles, broken lines) on locomotor activity. The effect of 16 mg/kg of naloxone on locomotor activity is represented by the isolated point at the left. Data are expressed as a percent of locomotor activity in control sessions (control activity: 71 ± 6 counts per hour). Each point represents the mean of at least six observations in a 1-hr recording session. Vertical lines and light horizontal lines represent ± 1 SEM. Where vertical lines are absent, the SEM is less than the radius of the point. Data are from Holtzman and Jewett (10).

(Figs. 4–6). The dose-response curves generated by pentazocine and levallorphan were relatively shallow. An eightfold increase in the dose of pentazocine, from 8.0 to 64 mg/kg, resulted in an approximately twofold increase in locomotor activity. Similarly, a 16-fold increase in the dose of levallorphan, from 16 to 256 mg/kg, increased locomotor activity by about threefold. Both dose-response curves were monophasic up to doses which approached one-half of the LD_{50} of those drugs. Cyclazocine, in contrast, was clearly the most potent and active of the three drugs tested. Locomotor activity increased more than 20-fold as the dose of cyclazocine was raised from 1.0 to 8.0 mg/kg (Fig. 6). Furthermore, cyclazocine disrupted locomotor activity at higher doses, thus generating a biphasic dose-response curve.

Naloxone (16 mg/kg), administered 5 min before pentazocine and simultaneously with levallorphan and cyclazocine, failed to block the effects of those drugs on locomotor activity (Figs. 4–6). In fact, naloxone tended to enhance the increases in locomotor activity produced by cyclazocine (Fig. 6).

TABLE 1. *Effects of pentazocine and naloxone–pentazocine on brain catecholamine content[a]*

Dose of pentazocine (mg/kg)	Brain catecholamine concentration (μg/g of tissue)			
	NE		DA	
	Pentazocine	Naloxone[b]–Pentazocine	Pentazocine	Naloxone[b]–Pentazocine
0	100.0 ± 1.3[c]	102.6 ± 4.4	100.0 ± 1.5[c]	96.3 ± 1.8
8	101.1 ± 2.4	–	99.7 ± 3.6	–
16	94.1 ± 1.8[d]	88.6 ± 0.9[e]	92.0 ± 3.0[d]	81.3 ± 4.1[e]
32	81.6 ± 1.6[e]	74.6 ± 3.7[e]	77.7 ± 1.7[e]	66.7 ± 2.1[e]
64	71.6 ± 1.7[e]	61.7 ± 3.1[e]	59.9 ± 3.7[e]	57.7 ± 3.5[e]

[a] Data are modified from Holtzman and Jewett (8).
[b] Naloxone, 16 mg/kg, was administered 5 min before pentazocine.
[c] Data are expressed as a percent of the vehicle control. Each mean (± SEM) is based upon at least four observations. NE and DA levels after the administration of pentazocine vehicle were 0.457 ± 0.006 and 0.866 ± 0.013 μg/g of tissue, respectively.
[d] Significantly different from control, $p < 0.05$.
[e] Significantly different from control, $p < 0.01$.

Brain Catecholamines

Changes in brain catecholamine levels were found to be maximal approximately 1 hr after drug administration. Accordingly, dose-response curves were determined using this time interval. Tables 1–3 show that

TABLE 2. *Effects of levallorphan and naloxone–levallorphan on brain catecholamine content[a]*

Dose of levallorphan (mg/kg)	Brain catecholamine concentration (μg/g of tissue)			
	NE		DA	
	Levallorphan	Naloxone[b]–Levallorphan	Levallorphan	Naloxone[b]–Levallorphan
0	100.0 ± 1.4[c]	103.5 ± 3.9	100.0 ± 1.4[c]	103.9 ± 5.2
16	99.6 ± 2.8	98.8 ± 3.1	89.2 ± 1.4[d]	90.7 ± 2.0[d]
64	100.5 ± 5.6	80.3 ± 4.1[e]	85.0 ± 5.4[d]	85.1 ± 7.3[e]
256	69.4 ± 7.9[e]	76.3 ± 8.2[e]	72.0 ± 4.1[e]	81.1 ± 4.8[e]

[a] Data are from Steinert et al. (21).
[b] Naloxone, 16 mg/kg, was administered simultaneously with levallorphan.
[c] Data are expressed as a percent of the saline control. Each mean (± SEM) is based upon at least seven observations. NE and DA levels after the administration of saline were 0.461 ± 0.011 and 0.818 ± 0.029 μg/g of tissue, respectively.
[d] Significantly different from control, $p < 0.05$.
[e] Significantly different from control, $p < 0.01$.

TABLE 3. Effects of cyclazocine and naloxone–cyclazocine on brain catecholamine content[a]

| Dose of cyclazocine (mg/kg) | Brain catecholamine concentration (μg/g of tissue) | | | |
| | NE | | DA | |
	Cyclazocine	Naloxone[b]– Cyclazocine	Cyclazocine	Naloxone[b]– Cyclazocine
0	100.0 ± 1.3[c]	98.9 ± 3.7	100.0 ± 0.9[c]	99.3 ± 1.5
2	106.2 ± 3.7	104.4 ± 4.4	97.8 ± 3.6	97.0 ± 2.5
4	94.3 ± 2.0	101.3 ± 3.5	98.0 ± 1.9	98.1 ± 2.0
8	91.9 ± 2.4[d]	90.5 ± 3.5[d]	90.3 ± 2.6[c]	94.5 ± 2.6
16	90.3 ± 1.8[d]	87.7 ± 2.4[c]	84.8 ± 2.1[c]	89.4 ± 2.2[c]
32	86.8 ± 2.6[c]	80.7 ± 2.4[c]	83.8 ± 1.5[c]	81.5 ± 2.9[c]

[a] Data are from Holtzman and Jewett (10).

[b] Naloxone, 16 mg/kg, was administered simultaneously with cyclazocine.

[c] Data are expressed as a percent of the vehicle control. Each mean (± SEM) is based upon at least six observations. NE and DA levels after the administration of cyclazocine vehicle were 0.455 ± 0.006 and 0.853 ± 0.008 μg/g of tissue, respectively.

[d] Significantly different from control, $p < 0.05$.

[e] Significantly different from control, $p < 0.01$.

pentazocine, levallorphan, and cyclazocine all lowered the average brain content of NE and DA in a dose-related manner. The magnitude of drug effects ranged from a 13.2% reduction in brain NE content by 32 mg/kg of cyclazocine (Table 3) to a 40.1% reduction in the brain levels of DA by 64 mg/kg of pentazocine (Table 1). The depletion of brain catecholamines by the agonist-antagonists was not blocked by 16 mg/kg of naloxone (Tables 1–3).

DISCUSSION

Studies in our laboratory have shown that pentazocine, levallorphan, and cyclazocine, narcotic antagonists with agonistic properties, stimulate two types of behavior in the rat: operant behavior and locomotor activity. Naloxone, as previously reported (8), is inactive in these procedures. The general order of potency and peak activity of the drugs as behavioral stimulants is cyclazocine > levallorphan > pentazocine > naloxone. This is in accord with their analgesic activity in the rat as determined in the phenylquinone writhing test (4), except for levallorphan which is less active as an analgesic than as a behavioral stimulant.

Brain monoamines have been implicated in the stimulant effects of a number of drugs on behavior (23), and the depletion of brain catecholamines by pentazocine has been shown to correlate well with stimulation of locomotor activity (8). However, there does not appear to be any obvious relationship between the behavioral stimulation produced by levallorphan and cyclazocine and the catecholamine-depleting properties of these drugs.

Narcotic antagonists have a relatively low order of behavioral activity in most infrahuman species, a fact which has probably discouraged systematic investigations of these drugs. A few studies have determined dose-response relationships for the antagonists; for example, on the operant behavior of the pigeon (17, 18). While behavioral stimulation occurred under certain conditions, the predominant effect of the drugs was to disrupt ongoing behavior. Thus, the rat appears to be a unique species in that its response to narcotic antagonists is characterized by behavioral stimulation which is graded over a broad range of doses. This fact suggests that the rat may be a useful animal model for evaluating the stimulant effects of narcotic-antagonist analgesics on behavior.

Naloxone antagonized the effects of pentazocine, levallorphan, and cyclazocine on operant behavior but failed to block their effects on locomotor activity and brain catecholamines. This latter finding is unusual in view of naloxone's widely demonstrated ability to block the agonistic actions of the narcotic antagonists. Naloxone antagonizes the analgesic activity of pentazocine, levallorphan, and cyclazocine in the mouse and rat (3), the cyclazocine-induced depression of the flexor reflex in the chronic spinal dog (16), and in man the respiratory depressant effect of pentazocine (14) and the subjective, behavioral, pupillary and respiratory depressant effects of cyclazocine (13). Furthermore, naloxone can precipitate an abstinence syndrome in the pentazocine-dependent subject (12). On the other hand, naloxone does not block the rate-decreasing effects of cyclazocine on operant responding in the pigeon (19). Reports of a similar failure of naloxone to antagonize the disruption of operant behavior in the rat by levallorphan (25) and cyclazocine (24) are more difficult to evaluate since only single doses of the drugs were tested in those studies.

Martin (15) has advanced the concept of receptor dualism to explain the agonistic and morphine-antagonistic activity of the narcotic-antagonist analgesics. In this two-receptor model, morphine-like drugs interact with one receptor to produce an effect. The effect can be blocked by narcotic antagonists which combine with the morphine receptor but produce no effect of their own. It is through the second receptor that the agonistic actions of the narcotic antagonists are mediated. Since naloxone blocks the agonistic effects of narcotic antagonists as well as the effects of morphine, it was concluded that the two receptors are stereochemically similar or identical. However, the differential antagonism of the effects of pentazocine, levallorphan, and cyclazocine by naloxone described in this report indicates that at least some of the agonistic actions of narcotic antagonists are mediated by receptors which are quite distinct from those that mediate the actions of morphine-like drugs.

ACKNOWLEDGMENT

These studies were supported in part by U.S. Public Health Service Grants MH12870 and MH21699.

REFERENCES

1. Ansell, G. B., and Beeson, M. F.: A rapid and sensitive procedure for the combined assay of noradrenaline, dopamine and serotonin in a single brain sample. Anal. Biochem. *23*:196–206, 1968.
2. Blumberg, H., Dayton, H. B., George, M., and Rappaport, D. N.: N-Allynoroxymorphone: A potent narcotic antagonist. Fed. Proc. *20*:311, 1961.
3. Blumberg, H., Dayton, H. B., and Wolf, P. S.: Counteraction of narcotic antagonist analgesics by the narcotic antagonist naloxone. Proc. Soc. Exp. Biol. Med. *123*:755–758, 1966.
4. Blumberg, H., Wolf, P. S., and Dayton, H. B.: Use of writing test for evaluating analgesic activity of narcotic antagonists. Proc. Soc. Exp. Biol. Med. *118*:763–766, 1965.
5. Haertzen, C. A.: Subjective effects of narcotic antagonists cyclazocine and nalorphine on the Addiction Research Center Inventory (ARCI). Psychopharmacologia *18*:366–377, 1970.
6. Heise, G. A., and Boff, E.: Continuous avoidance as a base-line for measuring behavioral effects of drugs. Psychopharmacologia *3*:264–282, 1962.
7. Holtzman, S. G., and Jewett, R. E.: Interactions of morphine and nalorphine with physostigmine on operant behavior in the rat. Psychopharmacologia *22*:384–395, 1971.
8. Holtzman, S. G., and Jewett, R. E.: Some actions of pentazocine on behavior and brain monoamines in the rat. J. Pharmacol. Exp. Ther. *181*:346–356, 1972.
9. Holtzman, S. G., and Jewett, R. E.: Shock intensity as a determinant of the behavioral effects of morphine in the rat. Life Sci. *11* (Part I):1085–1091, 1972.
10. Holtzman, S. G., and Jewett, R. E.: *Unpublished observations.*
11. Jasinski, D. R., Martin, W. R., and Haertzen, C. A.: The human pharmacology and abuse potential of N-allylnoroxymorphone (naloxone). J. Pharmacol. Exp. Ther. *157*:420–426, 1967.
12. Jasinski, D. R., Martin, W. R., and Hoeldtke, R. D.: Effects of short- and long-term administration of pentazocine in man. Clin. Pharmacol. Ther. *11*:385–403, 1970.
13. Jasinski, D. R., Martin, W. R., and Sapira, J. D.: Antagonism of the subjective, behavioral, pupillary, and respiratory depressant effects of cyclazocine by naloxone. Clin. Pharmacol. Ther. *9*:215–222, 1968.
14. Kallos, T., and Smith, T. C.: Naloxone reversal of pentazocine-induced respiratory depression. J. Amer. Med. Ass. *204*:932, 1968.
15. Martin, W. R.: Opioid antagonists. Pharmacol. Rev. *19*:463–521, 1967.
16. McClane, T. K., and Martin, W. R.: Antagonism of the spinal cord effects of morphine and cyclazocine by naloxone and thebaine. Int. J. Neuropharmacol. *6*:325–327, 1967.
17. McMillan, D. E., and Harris, L. S.: Behavioral and morphine-antagonist effects of the optical isomers of pentazocine and cyclazocine. J. Pharmacol. Exp. Ther. *180*:269–279, 1972.
18. McMillan, D. E., and Morse, W. H.: Some effects of morphine and morphine antagonists on schedule-controlled behavior. J. Pharmacol. Exp. Ther. *157*:175–184, 1967.

19. McMillan, D. E., Wolf, P. S., and Carchman, R. A.: Antagonism of the behavioral effects of morphine and methadone by narcotic antagonists. J. Pharmacol. Exp. Ther. *175*:443–458, 1970.
20. Sidman, M.: Avoidance conditioning with a brief shock and no exteroceptive warning signal. Science *118*:157–158, 1953.
21. Steinert, H. R., Holtzman, S. G., and Jewett, R. E.: *Unpublished observations.*
22. Way, E. L. and Shen, F. H.: The effects of narcotic analgesics on specific systems. Catecholamines and 5-hydroxytryptamine. *In:* Narcotic Drugs, ed. by D. H. Clouet, pp. 229–253. Plenum Press, New York, 1971.
23. Weiss, B., and Laties, V. G.: Behavioral pharmacology. Ann. Rev. Pharmacol. *9*:297–326, 1969.
24. Wray, S. R.: A correlative evaluation of cyclazocine, LSD and naloxone on continuous discriminated avoidance in rats. Psychopharmacologia *26*:29–43, 1972.
25. Wray, S. R., and Cowan, A.: The effects of naloxone, chlorpromazine, and haloperidol pretreatment on levallorphan-induced disruption of rats' operant behavior. Psychopharmacologia *22*:261–270, 1971.

Narcotic Antagonists, edited by M. C. Braude, L. S. Harris, E. L. May, J. P. Smith, and J. E. Villarreal. *Advances in Biochemical Psychopharmacology, Vol. 8.* Raven Press, New York © 1974.

Subjective Effects of Narcotic Antagonists

Charles A. Haertzen

National Institute of Mental Health, Addiction Research Center, Lexington, Kentucky 40507

The two symptoms, tiredness and drunkenness, which are the most frequently reported acute effects of the narcotic antagonists nalorphine and cyclazocine are also typical actions of barbiturates and alcohol. Psychotomimetic effects also occur in the antagonists, but somewhat less frequently. The overall pattern is different from the psychotomimetic drug LSD, which produces more psychotomimetic symptoms, anxiety, and excitement, less drunkenness, and no sedation. In common with opiates, the two antagonists produce analgesia. Euphoria is a pronounced acute effect of opiates, but not of the antagonists. At low doses, opiate addicts express some liking for the antagonists, but this effect drops off with higher doses.

The similarity of a drug's subjective agonistic effects with those of nalorphine or morphine is associated with the drug's power to either precipitate or suppress abstinence symptoms in opiate addicts stabilized on morphine. Predictions of suppression or precipitation cannot be reliably made with drugs which have no agonistic effects.

The acute effects of cyclazocine are antagonized by naloxone according to Jasinski, Martin, and Sapira. Resnick, Fink, and Freedman found that naloxone lessened the occurrence of undesirable effects of cyclazocine. Tolerance develops to the agonistic subjective effects of the antagonists upon chronic administration, but not to the antagonistic action. The most frequently occurring abstinence symptoms following withdrawal of the antagonists in a study of opiate addicts by Martin et al. were restlessness, sleeplessness, nausea, headaches, bad dreams, chills, and shocks, but drug-seeking did not occur. Yawning, perspiration, rhinorrhea, gooseflesh, and diarrhea were also observable.

INTRODUCTION

According to Martin (24), the phrases "morphine-like agents" and "nalorphine-like antagonists" are unsatisfactory for classifying many of the newer drugs, as the "narcotic antagonists have both agonistic and antagonistic effects" and because the agonistic effects of some narcotic antagonists are qualitatively different from those produced by morphine. The *nalorphine syndrome* applies to the agonistic effects produced by nalorphine and nalorphine-like drugs, and the *opioid syndrome* refers to the pattern of pharmacological and agonistic effects that are similar to those induced by morphine. Martin has also suggested that the meaning of antagonists should be broadened to include partial agonists that may induce either the opioid or the nalorphine syndrome. Elsewhere, Martin (23) has reviewed the syndromes derived through the use of subjective and objective tests at the Addiction Research Center. The present chapter reviews the syndrome of acute subjective effects produced by nalorphine and morphine found in opiate addicts (6, 17–21, 23, 26–28), on the single-dose questionnaire (3, 23, 25), Addiction Research Center Inventory (12), and subjective drug-effect questionnaire (21). Attention is also given to the correlation between the syndrome of subjective effects produced by other opiates and antagonists with the syndromes for nalorphine and morphine and the significance of these correlations for predicting whether the drug precipitates or suppresses abstinence symptoms in subjects stabilized on morphine.

ACUTE SUBJECTIVE EFFECTS OF NARCOTIC ANTAGONISTS

The Single-Dose Questionnaire

The single-dose questionnaire (2, 3, 23, 25) has been used frequently in single-dose studies of opiates and narcotic antagonists (18–20, 26–28). Martin (23) extensively analyzed the utility and research findings on the test and presented the format and the system of scoring. Cochin (1) and Halbach and Eddy (11) also presented the test and reviewed ARC studies.

Opiate symptoms in the test are indexed by the occurrence of turning stomach, itchy skin, relaxed, coasting, soapboxing, pleasant sick, drive, sleepy, nervous, and drunken. Opiate signs rated by observers are indexed by scratching, red-eye, relaxed, coasting, soapboxing, vomiting, nodding, sleepy, nervous, and drunken. Dose equivalents have been found between the two antagonists and morphine using sums of both symptoms and signs. Most studies have used total scores on symptoms and signs. However, Martin et al. (26) found that itchy skin and coasting are dose-related specific symptoms for opiates, whereas drunken and sleepy are specific and dose-related items for the antagonists nalorphine and cyclazocine. Among the ratable signs, scratching, coasting, and soapboxing are specific for opiates, and sleepy and drunken are specific for antagonists.

To assess more fully the utility of the configuration of responses on symptoms and signs for judging similarity of drugs with morphine and nalorphine, data from all the single high doses of morphine (20 mg, i.v.; 30 mg s.c.; 30 mg i.m.; N = 90) and intermediate and high doses of nalorphine (16, 30, 32 mg s.c.; 14 mg i.v.; N = 44) were first pooled from the sources cited above. The number of subjects in various studies ranged from 8 to 12. The patterns or syndromes are operationally defined as the average percentage of responses on each item over 10 symptoms or 10 signs (Fig. 1). Then, these two drug patterns for symptoms and signs were separately correlated with the patterns for various low, medium, and high doses of other drugs given on a mg/70 kg basis. To represent these correlations in a dimensional framework, a diagonal factor analysis (4) was done by extracting the morphine pattern first and the nalorphine pattern second. Figure 2 shows the location of the average loadings for high doses of drugs only. An arbitrary line has been drawn to demarcate drugs whose acute effects are most similar to morphine (upper sector) or to nalorphine (lower sector). Cyclazocine (2.0 mg s.c.), levallorphan (12 mg s.c.), pentazocine (60 mg s.c.), and nalbuphine (72 mg s.c.) fall closer to nalorphine on the second, or nalorphine, dimension; codeine (90 mg i.v.), *d*-propoxyphene (180 mg i.v.), propiram (280 mg s.c.; 80 mg i.v.), GPA-1657 (7.0 mg i.v.; 20 mg s.c.), and

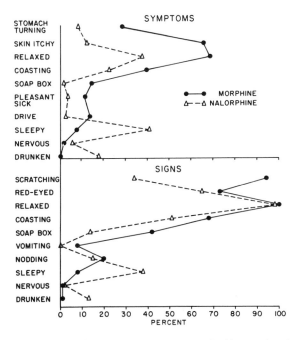

FIG. 1. Percentage of item endorsement on symptoms (subject ratings) and signs (observer ratings) for morphine and nalorphine. High doses of morphine (30 mg s.c. i.m.; 20 mg i.v., N = 90) and intermediate and high doses of nalorphine (16 mg s.c.; 30 and 32 mg s.c.; 14 mg i.v., N = 44) were pooled from several studies by Martin and Jasinski and coinvestigators (17–20, 26).

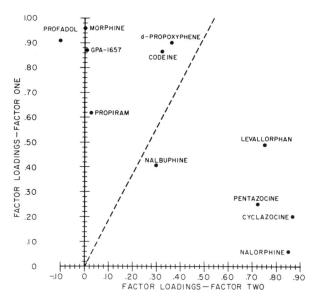

FIG. 2. Factors loadings of drugs on a morphine factor (one) and a nalorphine factor (two) for symptoms. The loadings refer to average loadings of the high doses of drugs cited in the reference to Fig. 1. Factors were extracted by the diagonal method of factor analysis (4) and morphine was extracted first.

profadol (100 mg s.c.) fall closer to morphine on the morphine dimension. The factor loadings of lower doses of the drugs tend to be similar to higher doses of the drugs reported in Fig. 2. However, the effect of a lower dose of pentazocine (40 mg) was closer to morphine, and the effect of the lowest dose of nalbuphine (8 mg) was too weak to be definitive. Naloxone (6, 12, or 24 mg s.c.) cannot be rated because of the lack of subjective effects (18).

The loadings on the morphine and nalorphine factors for each dose of the drugs cited were correlated with a suppression-precipitation index to obtain a multiple correlation with the index. The following weights were used to reflect roughly the level of suppression or precipitation of abstinence symptoms found upon challenge with a drug to subjects on either 60 or 240 mg of morphine per day: 4 = suppression of abstinence for those on 240 mg of morphine; 3 = suppression of abstinence for those on 60 mg of morphine and precipitation for those on 240 mg; 2 = failure to suppress for those on 60 mg of morphine and precipitation for those on 240 mg of morphine; and 1 = precipitation for those on 60 mg of morphine. A multiple correlation of 0.88 was obtained. This is considered a high level of predictability. Nalbuphine (8 mg and 24 mg) contributed the most error in prediction; this error is attributed to the very weak effect of the drug at these low doses. The morphine factor was most predictive of the index in the drugs used.

Results using signs are less certain as all drugs including nalorphine show a fairly substantial correlation with the morphine pattern. The product moment correlation between nalorphine and morphine was 0.79. Cyclazocine and levallorphan were most similar to nalorphine on signs.

Opiate addicts are asked to identify the drug given in the single dose questionnaire but narcotic antagonists are not provided as options. Opiates are uniformly identified as "dope" providing the dose is high enough. The narcotic antagonists cyclazocine and nalorphine are sometimes identified as dope especially at lower doses, but at higher doses they tend to be identified as barbiturates (26).

During chronic administration, opiate identifications occurred infrequently for antagonists such as cyclazocine (26). However, observers identified cyclazocine as dope. When addicts were simultaneously administered both cyclazocine (oral) and morphine chronically, some subjects identified it as dope (28). The investigators attributed the dope identification to some morphine-like effects of cyclazocine. Some dope identifications occurred also with antagonists such as nalbuphine (17).

In acute drug studies, opiate addicts showed some degree of liking for the antagonists: nalorphine (up to 16 mg/70 kg s.c.), cyclazocine [1.0 mg/70 kg s.c. (26)], pentazocine [40 mg s.c., (19)], levallorphan [12 mg, (18)], and nalbuphine [72 mg, (17)]. Liking for higher doses of nalorphine or cyclazocine tended to level off or decrease.

Liking for nalorphine or cyclazocine is not maintained during chronic administration. Thus, over a 10-week period, only one response of 420 was obtained for wanting the drug every day in six opiate addicts chronically given cyclazocine 13.2 mg/70 kg s.c. (26). Earlier, Isbell (15) had found that addicts disliked chronic nalorphine. When morphine and cyclazocine were simultaneously administered chronically, no addict wanted the drug every day (27).

Addiction Research Center Inventory (ARCI)

The ARCI has been used to assess the acute and simulated subjective effects of a large variety of drugs (5–7, 12), the chronic and withdrawal effects of opiates (9), associations to drugs (10), and differences between psychiatric clinical groups (7). Interest in extending the evaluation and quantification of the subjective effects of the antagonists cyclazocine and nalorphine with the ARCI was directly stimulated by the initial studies of

Martin et al. (6, 23, 26) on the single-dose questionnaire. The last test, as pointed out earlier, is a short test that contains several items that are sensitive to the effects of the antagonists.

The ARCI is a long test of 550 items and was designed by Hill et al. (12) with the intent of broadly sampling the content that would describe immediate subjective experiences (8). Mood, emotion, motivation, drive, appetite, sensation and perception, cognition, bodily symptoms, etc. were regarded as relevant. The test also samples items that differentiate clinical groups such as psychopaths and the mentally ill.

Typically, more than one drug scale for a given drug has been constructed. An empirical scale is made by selecting items which differentiate a drug in question from placebo, the universal standard, to provide a summary of a drug's effects (13). Other scales reflect the pattern of effects which a drug has in common with other drugs and are referred to as group variability scales (5). Development of a new group variability scale is contingent on the uniqueness of the effect of the drug. For instance, in the first analysis of drug patterns, a general drug effect pattern was found and was characterized by the greater incidence of some symptoms in all drugs tested relative to placebo. Feeling different, weird, and floating fall in this category. Morphine and amphetamine, as contrasted with LSD, pentobarbital, chlorpromazine, pyrahexyl, and alcohol produced relatively greater effects on items that appear to signify euphoria; this pattern is referred to as the morphine-benzedrine group variability (MBG) pattern. Pentobarbital, chlorpromazine, and alcohol (PCAG pattern), in contrast, produced relatively greater effects on items suggesting low motivation, sedation, and physical weakness. LSD produced effects of anxiety, depersonalization, and other psychotomimetic effects that appeared relatively specific for it (LSD pattern). Some items contribute to more than one pattern. For instance, feeling weird is a general drug item, but it is also an LSD item in the sense that LSD produces a much greater weirdness effect than the other drugs tested.

The narcotic antagonists such as nalorphine or cyclazocine were not included as part of the names of the above patterns as these drugs had not been tried. If the effects of these antagonists had been incorporated in the pattern analysis, they would have been included as a part of the definition of some patterns. These drugs would have contributed positively to the definition of the pattern for a general drug effect (GDE), low motivation (PCAG), psychotomimetic effects (LSD), and to inefficiency, an effect opposite that exemplified by amphetamine.

As new drugs or conditions have been tested, the question has always arisen as to whether the effects of the drug on items can be accounted for by its differential pattern on existing scales. The most impressive indication that a high dose of a drug defines a new pattern on items is a higher or lower percentage of true responses on an item than any other drug. As more drugs or conditions have been tested, the satisfaction of this criterion has been met infrequently. The criterion which can be met more frequently is a pattern of differences between a drug and other drugs over many items or scales.

The criteria referred to above have been applied to cyclazocine and nalorphine. The effects of these drugs were compared with placebo given in the same experiment as well as with drugs from other experiments. Subsequently, the empirical and group variability scales derived from the analysis of these drugs were included among others in a discriminant function analysis to determine if these scales contributed independent sources of variation for differentiating drugs including antagonist drugs that have been tested (7).

Methods

ARCI tests were obtained from post addicts in two single blind studies in 1965 (6). In one study (see Fig. 3 for the N values listed as "a") about half of 32 subjects were randomly given no drug, placebo, two intramuscular doses of morphine (15 or 30 mg/70 kg), pentobarbital (125 or 250 mg/70 kg), cyclazocine (.6 mg or 1.2 mg/70 kg), or nalorphine (16 or 32 mg/70 kg). In the second study, low doses of cyclazocine (0.3 mg/70 kg) and nalorphine (8 mg/70 kg) were substituted for morphine and pentobarbital in an attempt to evaluate the occurrence of euphoria in the antagonists.

Subjects were given their drug at 8:00 A.M. and tested an hour later with the ARCI. Differences between the two highest doses of cyclazocine and nalorphine were determined on each of the 550 ARCI items and between placebo and the average effect of these two drugs with chi square. A scale was developed to show differences between 20 mg of morphine (i.m.) from a prior study by Hill et al. (13) and the average of the two highest doses of cyclazocine and nalorphine.

Analyses of variance (drugs × doses × subjects) were run on ARCI scales to show the effects of doses and the difference between cyclazocine and nalorphine mentioned above. A discriminant function method was also applied to the drugs shown in Fig. 3 (7) on 23 ARCI scales.

Results

The subjective effects of cyclazocine and nalorphine were similar as only five out of 550 items differentiated these drugs at the highest dose at the

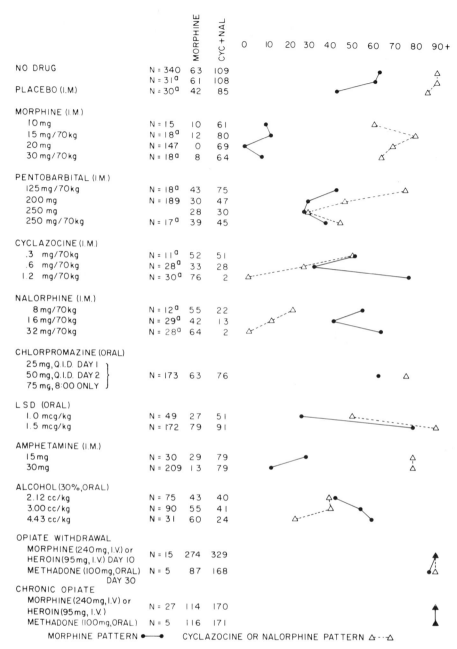

		MORPHINE	CYC+NAL	0 10 20 30 40 50 60 70 80 90+
NO DRUG	N = 340	63	109	
	N = 31[a]	61	108	
PLACEBO (I.M.)	N = 30[a]	42	85	
MORPHINE (I.M.)				
10 mg	N = 15	10	61	
15 mg/70kg	N = 18[a]	12	80	
20 mg	N = 147	0	69	
30 mg/70kg	N = 18[a]	8	64	
PENTOBARBITAL (I.M.)				
125mg/70kg	N = 18[a]	43	75	
200 mg	N = 189	30	47	
250 mg		28	30	
250 mg/70kg	N = 17[a]	39	45	
CYCLAZOCINE (I.M.)				
.3 mg/70kg	N = 11[a]	52	51	
.6 mg/70kg	N = 28[a]	33	28	
1.2 mg/70kg	N = 30[a]	76	2	
NALORPHINE (I.M.)				
8 mg/70kg	N = 12[a]	55	22	
16mg/70kg	N = 29[a]	42	13	
32mg/70kg	N = 28[a]	64	2	
CHLORPROMAZINE (ORAL)				
25mg, Q.I.D. DAY 1				
50mg, Q.I.D. DAY 2	N = 173	63	76	
75 mg, 8:00 ONLY				
LSD (ORAL)				
1.0 mcg/kg	N = 49	27	51	
1.5 mcg/kg	N = 172	79	91	
AMPHETAMINE (I.M.)				
15mg	N = 30	29	79	
30mg	N = 209	13	79	
ALCOHOL (30%, ORAL)				
2.12 cc/kg	N = 75	43	40	
3.00 cc/kg	N = 90	55	41	
4.43 cc/kg	N = 31	60	24	
OPIATE WITHDRAWAL				
MORPHINE (240mg, I.V.) or HEROIN (95mg, I.V.) DAY 10	N = 15	274	329	
METHADONE (100mg, ORAL) DAY 30	N = 5	87	168	
CHRONIC OPIATE				
MORPHINE (240mg, I.V.) or HEROIN (95mg, I.V.)	N = 27	114	170	
METHADONE (100mg, ORAL)	N = 5	116	171	

MORPHINE PATTERN ●—●   CYCLAZOCINE OR NALORPHINE PATTERN △--△

FIG. 3. Sum of t^2 for differences between various drug conditions and two standards for morphine and cyclazocine plus nalorphine on 23 ARCI scales. t-Tests on each scale were calculated for a theoretical N of 10 for each subsample after scores had been corrected for four scales by a discriminant function method (7). Conditions designated by "a" were drawn from a study of antagonists (6). Other drug effects were obtained from the study by Hill et al. (13). Chronic and withdrawal opiate effects for morphine and heroin were obtained from Haertzen and Hooks (9), and chronic and withdrawal methadone effects were described by Martin et al. (31).

0.05 level and these five questions failed to distinguish the drugs at the lower doses. Cyclazocine was much more potent than nalorphine (range of 15 to 26) on five drug-oriented scales: General Drug Effect, Morphine Empirical, Efficiency, Pentobarbital-Chlorpromazine-Alcohol Group Variability (PCAG) scale, and LSD. The dose effect for the two highest doses of both drugs was greatest for PCAG ($F = 30.04$, 1/28 d.f.) and next highest on LSD ($F = 17.14$). No effect was found on the Morphine Benzedrine Group scale (MBG, $F = 0.04$), and a negative effect was found on Efficiency ($F = 7.36$) which measures amphetamine effects.

One hundred and thirty-six items differentiated the high doses of the antagonists from placebo (ARCI scale #152). Table 1 illustrates some of the item content on which differences were found and the direction of scoring. Three major classes of effects were prominent. The first class includes sedation, physical weakness, and loss of interest and motivation for intellectual and physical activities. These effects are also common for the PCAG scale in the ARCI. Drunkenness increased on relevant speech, gait, and orientation items; a Drunk scale summarizes such effects. Psychotomimetic effects increased and included anxiety, depersonalization, and various weird experiences associated with LSD. Social and cognitive efficiency was impaired. In addition subjects reported an impairment of vision.

The effects of the highest doses of cyclazocine and nalorphine were greater than those for 20 mg of morphine on items referring to tiredness, cognitive difficulty, distortions in sensation and perception, discouragement, incoordination, anxiety, misery, hangover, and social inadequacy. On the other hand, euphoria, sense of humor, sentimentality, self-control, patience, fewer worries, greater appetite for ice cream or cigarettes, and more itching sensations were more common under morphine. A Narcotic Antagonist scale (NAnt, ARCI #153) measures these differences (6) and is included in the set of 23 drug-sensitive scales (7).

Figure 3 indicates the degree of similarity or difference of many different drug conditions with the combined pattern of the highest doses of cyclazocine and nalorphine and the pattern for morphine as determined from a modified discriminant function analysis. The numbers refer to the sum of t^2 (t-test for a constant theoretical N of 10; the sum of t^2 is a general distance function) over 23 ARCI drug-sensitive scales between the standards, that is, morphine and the antagonists, and each of the other conditions listed in the figure. In this system of analysis, the smaller the sum of t^2, the greater the similarity. As can be seen from the figure, the various doses of morphine are most similar to the morphine standard as indicated by the low sum of t^2. The effects of the intermediate doses of both nalorphine and cyclazo-

TABLE 1. *Items which differentiate cyclazocine and nalorphine from placebo*

1. *INTERESTS* (8 ITEMS)
   39F I FEEL LIKE CATCHING UP ON ALL MY WORK.
   225T I DON'T FEEL LIKE READING ANYTHING RIGHT NOW.

2. *ENERGY* (13 ITEMS)
   9T I FEEL WEAK. 384F I AM FULL OF ENERGY.

3. *HEARING* (4 ITEMS)
   480T I HEAR EVERY LITTLE SOUND AROUND ME EVEN WHEN I TRY NOT TO.

4. *INTERNAL SENSATIONS* (14 ITEMS)
   76T MY HEAD FEELS HEAVY.
   458T SOME PARTS OF MY BODY FEEL NUMB.
   452T I FEEL DIZZY.

5. *PAIN* (2 ITEMS)
   285T MY HEAD ACHES. 300T MY NECK ACHES.

6. *TASTE* (8 ITEMS)
   413T I HAVE A BITTER TASTE IN MY MOUTH.
   227T I FEEL AS IF I HAVE A LUMP IN MY THROAT.

7. *TIME* (3 ITEMS)
   503T I AM HAVING SOME DIFFICULTY KEEPING TRACK OF TIME.
   537T TIME IS PASSING MORE SLOWLY THAN USUAL.

8. *TOUCH* (3 ITEMS)
   461T MY SKIN FEELS ROUGH.
   495T MY CLOTHES FEEL DIFFERENT TO THE TOUCH.

9. *VISION* (10 ITEMS)
   534T MY SIGHT SEEMS TO COME AND GO.
   494T THIS ROOM SEEMS TO BE CHANGING SIZE.

10. *TEMPERATURE* (12 ITEMS)
    79T MY FACE FEELS HOT.

11. *COORDINATION* (10 ITEMS)
    257F I WOULD HAVE NO TROUBLE WALKING A CHALK LINE.
    475T MY SPEECH IS SLURRED.

12. *ABILITY* (22 ITEMS)
    529T MY THOUGHTS SEEM TO COME AND GO.

112T THESE QUESTIONS SEEM VERY UNCLEAR AND CONFUSING.
280T I HAVE DIFFICULTY REMEMBERING.

13. *WEIRD EXPERIENCES* (6 ITEMS)
    267T I HAVE A WEIRD FEELING.
    125T I HAVE FELT MY BODY DRIFT AWAY FROM ME.
    147T IT SEEMS AS IF SOMEONE ELSE IS ANSWERING THESE QUESTIONS FOR ME.

14. *EUPHORIA* (7 ITEMS)
    319F I WOULD BE HAPPY ALL THE TIME IF I FELT AS I DO NOW.
    398T THIS IS ONE DAY I'LL PUT MY TROUBLES ON THE SHELF.

15. *HOSTILITY AND CONTROL* (8 ITEMS)
    189F I HAVE BETTER CONTROL OVER MYSELF THAN USUAL.
    331T I WOULD DESCRIBE MYSELF AS FEELING MEAN.

16. *INTERPERSONAL RELATIONS* (7 ITEMS)
    54T I FEEL LIKE AVOIDING PEOPLE, ALTHOUGH I USUALLY DO NOT FEEL THIS WAY.
    469T MY FAMILY WOULD REALLY BE DISGUSTED IF THEY SAW ME NOW.
    62F I THINK I WOULD ACT LIKE MY USUAL SELF AT A PARTY.

17. *ANXIETY* (7 ITEMS)
    201T I FEEL ANXIOUS AND UPSET.
    487T IT WOULD MAKE ME NERVOUS IF SOMEONE PUT HIS HAND ON ME.
    179T IF I WERE TO TALK I MIGHT SAY THE WRONG THING.
    182T I FEEL SO MISERABLE THAT OTHER PEOPLE MUST BE AWARE OF IT.
    528T MY HEAD FEELS AS IT DOES DURING A HANGOVER.

cine appear more similar to the pattern for morphine than do the highest doses. As the doses of the antagonists were increased, the pattern became more similar to the pattern for the highest doses of these drugs. Opiate withdrawal and chronic opiate effects appear most distant from both the acute effects of morphine and the antagonists. The scores for the no-drug condition are also highly different from those for morphine and the antagonists. The effects of alcohol and the barbiturates appear most similar to the antagonists because the sum of t^2 is least for these. In view of the fact that the antagonists produce some psychotomimetic effects, it is of interest that the effects of LSD become increasingly different from those for the antagonists with dose elevation of LSD. Psychotomimetic symptoms on the whole are more marked under LSD; in addition, low motivation and drunkenness increase more with the antagonists and excitement increases more with LSD.

The Subjective Drug-Effect Questionnaire

Following the ARCI study reported above, portions of the PCAG, MBG, and LSD scales were used as a supplement to the single-dose questionnaire to quantify the agonistic actions of opioids and nalorphine-like agonists (12, 18–20, 23). The three scales represent a large proportion of the drug-differentiating power that is obtainable with the total ARCI. Elevations on the PCAG and LSD scales and no change on the MBG scale characterize the nalorphine syndrome; an elevation on MBG and no change on PCAG and LSD characterize the opioid syndrome (6, 20, 23). The nalorphine syndrome has been found in single dose studies of nalorphine (30 mg s.c.), cyclazocine (1.0 mg), levallorphan (12 mg s.c.), nalbuphine (72 mg s.c.), and pentazocine (60 mg s.c.). Naloxone has no acute subjective effects. Appropriate challenging doses of the first four drugs precipitate abstinence symptoms in opiate addicts stabilized on 60 mg of morphine. Pentazocine precipitates abstinence symptoms in those stabilized on 240 mg of morphine.

On the other hand, the acute effects of high doses of GPA-1657 (7.0 mg i.v.), codeine (90 mg i.v.), and *d*-propoxyphene (180 mg i.v.) were most similar to those of morphine. These drugs at appropriate doses suppressed abstinence in those addicts stabilized on 240 mg of morphine. In a study of GPA-1657 (20 mg s.c.), positive effects were found on both MBG and PCAG.

Elevations on MBG, PCAG, and LSD were seen following an acute dose of propiram (280 mg s.c.). Profadol (100 mg i.m.) had significant positive effects on PCAG and MBG, but the changes were not significantly different from morphine (30 mg i.m.). Both of these drugs suppressed abstinence in opiate addicts stabilized on 60 mg of morphine but precipitated abstinence in those on 240 mg of morphine.

CHRONIC EFFECTS

Martin et al. (26) have found tolerance to both opiate symptoms and signs in subjects chronically given cyclazocine (13.2 mg/70 kg s.c.) as tested by a challenge of either 3.3 mg/70 kg of cyclazocine or 16 mg/70 kg of nalorphine. There is no tolerance to the opiate antagonistic effects of cyclazocine (29). The acute effects of cyclazocine are antagonized by naloxone according to Jasinski et al. (21). Subsequently, other investigators have found that the disturbing symptoms which arise during cyclazocine induction can be allayed by administration of naloxone (32). Complaints occurring during oral cyclazocine induction (up to 4 mg/day, oral) include sedation, sleeplessness, headache, and constipation. One subject required 33 days to reach stabilization and encountered difficulty in sleeping, irritability, and uncontrolled thoughts; he also had hallucinations of a girl. Such symptoms disappeared on stabilization (29). In the case of nalbuphine, Jasinski and Mansky (17) found some tolerance to its effects. However, when the dose was increased disturbing symptoms emerged starting at the chronic level of 142 mg on the 10th day. These consisted of "headache, difficulty in concentration, strange thoughts, irritability, nervousness, blurring vision, depression, and strange dreams." Such symptoms lingered to a certain extent and two subjects would not tolerate doses above 147 mg. Three subjects got up to 240 mg by the 51st day. Earlier, Isbell (15) found difficulty in increasing the dose of nalorphine in a chronic study. Martin et al. (26) circumvented this problem by starting with a very small dose (1 mg).

ABSTINENCE

As rated by the Himmelsbach system of scoring (14), abstinence signs have been found after withdrawal of all the antagonists except naloxone. Martin et al. (26) found subjective abstinence symptoms after withdrawal of 13.2 mg/70 kg s.c. of cyclazocine. The symptoms in decreasing order of frequency in six opiate addicts were restlessness or sleeplessness, nausea, headache, bad dreams, chills, shocks, and back pain. Observable signs in order of frequency of occurrence included lacrimation, yawning, perspiration, rhinorrhea, gooseflesh, and diarrhea. The occurrence of shock-like sensations was especially notable and has also been found following withdrawal of oral cyclazocine and to nalorphine (27). These shocks appeared to be precipitated by hot or cold drinks. Itching is also a distinctive sign compared with opiates.

DISCUSSION

Martin (24) elaborated on the theoretical basis for the agonistic and antagonistic effects of the drugs. The theory has been applied by Martin and Jasinski (30) and Jasinski (16) to newer drugs reviewed here. The pharmacology of the newer drugs has been reviewed by Lewis et al. (23). Some similarity of acute subjective effects of morphine and nalorphine has been found; however, the differences are great enough to make the overall patterns distinctive. The degree of correlation between a drug's actions and the syndromes for morphine and nalorphine is prognostic of whether the drug will suppress or precipitate abstinence symptoms in opiate addicts stabilized on morphine. The agonistic subjective effects of high doses of levallorphan, cyclazocine, and nalbuphine were similar to the nalorphine syndrome. These drugs precipitated abstinence when appropriate doses were administered to subjects stabilized on 60 mg of morphine per day. The acute effects of a high dose of pentazocine (60 mg) were also similar to the nalorphine syndrome; it precipitated abstinence in subjects stabilized on 240 mg of morphine but not for those stabilized on 60 mg. The five drugs (codeine, *d*-propoxyphene, GPA-1657, profadol, and propiram), whose acute effects were more similar to those of morphine as rated by the single-dose questionnaire, suppressed abstinence when the morphine stabilization dose was 60 mg, but the partial agonists profadol and propiram precipitated abstinence in those on 240 mg of morphine. The multiple correlation of 0.88 between the suppression-precipitation index and the morphine and nalorphine factor loadings shows a high level of predictability.

Whether a distinctive morphine or nalorphine pattern occurs is generally dependent on the magnitude of the dose. Distinctiveness is indexed in part by the variability in the differences between scores on items or scales for a drug. The agonistic effects of nalorphine (32 mg) and cyclazocine (1.2 mg) are quite distinctive on ARCI scales for the total inventory at these high doses, and their effects can be distinguished from other drugs. While the effects of these drugs bear some similarity to those for pentobarbital and alcohol at the high doses, the similarity is even greater at the lower doses (7). Using the total ARCI, the correct prediction of which drug a person is taking is dose dependent. The effect of dose on the correlation of patterns applies also to samples from various studies on morphine and nalorphine on the single-dose questionnaire.

In assessing the similarity of drugs by correlating patterns of responses, the N in the sample is a significant variable in determining the size of the correlations especially in tests in which only a true-false option is given, as the standard error for a true-false option is extremely large. The N can partially compensate for the lack of distinctiveness of patterns typically associated with low doses of drugs. Thus, the average r of the patterns for 10 samples of low doses of morphine with the high-dose morphine pattern was 0.78 ($z = 1.045$) on the single-dose questionnaire; the r obtained after pooling the 10 samples was 0.91 ($z = 1.528$). This difference is equivalent to an r of .45. The effect of N was less on the intermediate dose (r of 0.85 vs. 0.93 for an effective difference equivalent to an r of 0.41). The average r increased to 0.95 on the highest dose. Because of the problems of sample size, particularly with low doses, the r values with the morphine and nalorphine patterns cited in Fig. 2 may be more accurate than those obtained in a particular sample in which the Ns ranged from 8 to 12. The problems associated with sample size can be obviated partly by having subjects make ratings on a five-point rather than a two-point scale.

With respect to suggestions for measurement and evaluation of psychoactive drugs in a general sense, a measure of a general drug effect is highly useful as a means for matching different drugs for potency. A rating of "feeling the medicine" or the rating of the strength of the drug's effect are useful single items and have been used in the single-dose questionnaire. A rating of the degree of physical sickness may be a good general indicator of withdrawal symptoms. To obtain a comprehensive evaluation of the effects of a drug, the same measures need to be given during each phase of drug administration. If psychotomimetic effects, for instance, occur when an antagonist is given as a single dose or as a challenge to subjects stabilized on morphine, the effect can be described formally in relative terms if the LSD scale is used in every phase. It is suggested that subjective measures of euphoria, sedation, drunkenness, excitement, psychotomimetic symptoms, chronic opiate or nalorphine effects, and opiate or nalorphine withdrawal be obtained during acute, day-after acute dose, chronic, substitution, and withdrawal phases of studies.

CONCLUSIONS

The overall pattern of subjective effects for the narcotic antagonists nalorphine and cyclazocine is highly similar. These effects are similar to those of morphine in some respects, but the overall pattern is quite different. The correlation between the pattern of subjective effects produced by a drug with those for morphine or nalorphine is predictive of the drug's power to precipitate or suppress abstinence symptoms in subjects stabilized on morphine. In the predictive equation, similarity with the morphine pattern appears most important.

ACKNOWLEDGMENT

Drs. W. R. Martin, D. R. Jasinski, and D. C. Kay reviewed the manuscript and gave valuable suggestions. Dr. D. R. Jasinski provided some single-dose questionnaire data for naloxone and levallorphan which had not been presented (18).

REFERENCES

1. Cochin, J.: Methods for the appraisal of analgetic drugs for addiction liability. In: Selected Pharmacological Testing Methods, Vol. 3, Ed. by A. Burger, pp. 121–167. Marcel Dekker, Inc., New York, 1968.
2. Fraser, H. F.: Methods for testing for narcotic addiction in animals and man and their efficacy for predicting human abuse. In: Methods in Drug Evaluation, ed. by P. Mantegazza and F. Piccinini, pp. 297–311. North-Holland Publishing Co., Amsterdam, 1966.
3. Fraser, H. F., Van Horn, G. D., Martin, W. R., Wolbach, A. B., and Isbell, H.: Methods for evaluating addiction liability. (A) "Attitude" of opiate addicts toward opiate-like drugs, (B) A short-term "direct" addiction test. J. Pharmacol. Exp. Ther. *133*:371–387, 1961.
4. Fruchter, B.: Introduction to Factor Analysis. Van Nostrand, New York, 1954.
5. Haertzen, C. A.: Development of scales based on patterns of drug effects, using the Addiction Research Center Inventory (ARCI). Psychol. Rep. *18*:163–194, 1966.
6. Haertzen, C. A.: Subjective effects of narcotic antagonists cyclazocine and nalorphine on the Addiction Research Center Inventory (ARCI). Psychopharmacologia *18*:366–377, 1970.
7. Haertzen, C. A.: Manual and Appendix of Addiction Research Center Inventory Scales (ARCI). In preparation.
8. Haertzen, C. A., Hill, H. E., and Belleville, R. E.: Development of the Addiction Research Center Inventory (ARCI): Selection of items that are sensitive to the effects of various drugs. Psychopharmacologia *4*:155–166, 1963.
9. Haertzen, C. A., and Hooks, N. T., Jr.: Changes in personality and subjective experience associated with the chronic administration and withdrawal of opiates. J. Nerv. Ment. Dis. *148*:606–614, 1969.
10. Haertzen, C. A., and Hooks, N. T., Jr.: Dictionary of drug associations to heroin, benzedrine, alcohol, barbiturates and marijuana. J. Clin. Psychol. *29*:115–164, 1973.
11. Halbach, H., and Eddy, N. B.: Tests for addiction (chronic intoxication) of morphine type. Bull. Wld. Hlth. Org. *28*:139–173, 1963.
12. Hill, H. E., Haertzen, C. A., and Belleville, R. E.: The ARC Inventory. National Institute of Mental Health, Addiction Research Center, Lexington, Ky., 1958.
13. Hill, H. E., Haertzen, C. A., Wolbach, A. B., Jr., and Miner, E. J.: The Addiction Research Center Inventory: Standardization of scales which evaluate subjective effects of morphine, amphetamine, pentobarbital, alcohol, LSD-25, pyrahexyl and chlorpromazine. Psychopharmacologia *4*:167–183, 1963.
14. Himmelsbach, C. K.: The morphine abstinence syndrome, its nature and treatment. Ann. Intern. Med. *15*:829–839, 1941.
15. Isbell, H.: Attempted addiction to nalorphine. Fed. Proc. *15*:442, 1956.
16. Jasinski, D. R.: Effects in man of partial morphine agonists. Presented at Symposium on Agonist and Antagonist Actions of Narcotic Analgesic Drugs, Aberdeen, Scotland, July 12–15, 1971.
17. Jasinski, D. R., and Mansky, P. A.: Evaluation of nalbuphine for abuse potential. Clin. Pharmacol. Ther. *13*:78–90, 1972.

18. Jasinski, D. R., Martin, W. R., and Haertzen, C. A.: The human pharmacology and abuse potential of N-allylnoroxymorphone (naloxone). J. Pharmacol. Exp. Ther. *157*:420–426, 1967.
19. Jasinski, D. R., Martin, W. R., and Hoeldtke, R. D.: Effects of short- and long-term administration of pentazocine in man. Clin. Pharmacol. Ther. *11*:385–403, 1970.
20. Jasinski, D. R., Martin, W. R., and Hoeldtke, R.: Studies of the dependence producing properties of GPA-1657, profadol, and propiram in man. Clin. Pharmacol. Ther. *12*:613–649, 1971.
21. Jasinski, D. R., Martin, W. R., and Sapira, J. D.: Antagonism of the subjective, behavioral, pupillary, and respiratory depressant effects of cyclazocine by naloxone. Clin. Pharmacol. Ther. *9*:215–222, 1968.
22. Lewis, J. W., Bentley, K. W., and Cowan, A.: Narcotic analgesics and antagonists. A. Rev. Pharmacol. *11*:241–270, 1971.
23. Martin, W. R.: Clinical evaluation for narcotic dependence. In: New Concepts in Pain and Its Clinical Management. F. A. Davis Co., Philadelphia, 1967.
24. Martin, W. R.: Opioid antagonists. Pharmacol. Rev. *19*:463–521, 1967.
25. Martin, W. R., and Fraser, H. F.: A comparative study of physiological and subjective effects of heroin and morphine administered intravenously in post addicts. J. Pharmacol. Exp. Ther. *133*:388–399, 1961.
26. Martin, W. R., Fraser, H. F., Gorodetzky, C. W., and Rosenberg, D. E.: Studies of the dependence producing potential of the narcotic antagonist 2-cyclopropylmethyl-2'-hydroxy-5, 9-dimethyl-6, 7-benzomorphan (cyclazocine, Win 20, 740, ARC II-C-3). J. Pharmacol. Exp. Ther. *150*:426–436, 1965.
27. Martin, W. R., and Gorodetzky, C. W.: Demonstration of tolerance to and physical dependence on N-allylnormorphine (nalorphine). J. Pharmacol. Exp. Ther. *150*:437–442, 1965.
28. Martin, W. R., and Gorodetzky, C. W.: Cyclazocine an adjunct in the treatment of narcotic addiction. Int. J. Addict. *2*:85–93, 1967.
29. Martin, W. R., Gorodetzky, C. W., and McClane, T. K.: An experimental study in the treatment of narcotic addicts with cyclazocine. J. Clin. Pharmacol. Ther. *7*:455–465, 1966.
30. Martin, W. R., and Jasinski, D. R.: The mode of action and abuse potentiality of narcotic antagonists. In: Pain: Basic Principles – Pharmacology – Therapy, Ed. by R. Janzen, W. D. Keidel, A. Herz, and C. Steichele and ed. by J. P. Payne and R. A. P. Burt (English edition), pp. 225–234. Georg Thieme Publishers, Stuttgart, 1972.
31. Martin, W. R., Jasinski, D. R., Haertzen, C. A., Kay, D. C., Jones, B. E., Mansky, P. A., and Carpenter, R. W.: Methadone – A reevaluation. Arch. Gen. Psychiat. *28*:286–295, 1973.
32. Resnick, R. B., Fink, M., and Freedman, A. M.: Cyclazocine treatment of opiate dependence: A progress report. Compr. Psychiat. *12*:491–502, 1971.

Narcotic Antagonists, edited by M. C. Braude, L. S. Harris, E. L. May, J. P. Smith, and J. E. Villarreal. *Advances in Biochemical Psychopharmacology, Vol. 8.* Raven Press, New York © 1974.

Requirements for Extinction of Relapse-Facilitating Variables and for Rehabilitation in a Narcotic-Antagonist Treatment Program

Abraham Wikler

Department of Psychiatry, College of Medicine, University of Kentucky, University of Kentucky Medical Center, Lexington, Kentucky 40506

Clinical and experimental data strongly suggest that two sets of variables generated during chronic opioid intoxication provide sources of reinforcement for renewed self-administration of opioids long after "detoxification" (DTX): (1) the secondary "protracted" opioid-abstinence syndrome (14) and (2) classically conditioned facilitation of the primary "early" opioid-abstinence syndrome coupled with operantly conditioned opioid-seeking behavior (OSB) (32). Therefore, maintenance on a narcotic antagonist after DTX (15), preferably one without agonistic actions, should be continued beyond the duration of "protracted abstinence." However, DTX alone (with or without conventional psychotherapy) does not accomplish extinction (EXT) of the conditioned responses, classical or operant. Such EXT may occur during narcotic-antagonist maintenance if the patient attempts, often enough, to achieve "euphoria" (UPH) or to suppress "conditioned abstinence" (CA) by injection of opioids after discharge from the hospital, but unless he "misbehaves" in this manner, relapse is as likely to occur after the antagonist is withdrawn as after previous "cures." Hence, active EXT procedures, e.g., supervised self-injections of opioids under antagonist blockade, should be initiated after DTX and continued until the patient desists, while still in the hospital. After discharge, the patient should be returned to his home environment in the expectation that, in response to CA, he will self-inject opioids but without the possibility of reinforcing CA through reestablishment of "unconditioned" physical dependence or reinforcing OSB through achievement of UPH or suppression of CA. Concomitantly, socially acceptable behaviors should be reinforced by appropriate therapies.

The basic rationale for the use of narcotic antagonists in the postdetoxification treatment of opioid-dependent persons has been stated succinctly by Martin et al. (15) in their report on the potential usefulness of cyclazocine for this purpose: "On the basis of our studies, 4 mg per day of cyclazocine will provide protection against the euphorogenic actions of large doses of narcotics, prevent the development of physical dependence, and will thereby control the pharmacological actions which are held responsible for narcotic addiction. . . . There may be other benefits. Wikler (30) stated that two of the important reasons for relapse of the abstinent narcotic addict are conditioned abstinence which may be evoked by stimuli that have been associated with the addict's hustling activity to acquire drugs, and reinforcement of drug-seeking behavior through repeated reductions of abstinence by drug. It is possible that in subjects who attempt to readdict themselves while receiving a narcotic antagonist such as cyclazocine, there may be extinction of physical dependence and drug-seeking behavior."

The purposes of this chapter are to consider how a narcotic-antagonist treatment program should be designed to maximize the chances for true extinction of known and putative relapse-facilitating variables, in the light of certain experimental data on such variables and on the pharmacological properties of narcotic antagonists; and to consider also the problems that may arise in consequence of success in depriving a former opioid-dependent individual of some major "reinforcers," generated during previous episodes of opioid dependence.

RELAPSE-FACILITATING VARIABLES

A. "Euphorigenic" Actions of Opioids

That in some "normal" persons, and without exception in former opioid-dependent ones, opioids can produce a subjective state of "unusual well being" that is incommensurate with the objective reality of the situation (euphoria) is so well known as to require no documentation. To infer, however, that the "quest for euphoria" is sufficient to account for relapse is to strain the credulity even of those who accept the "pain-pleasure principle" (an empty tautology) as a scientific explanation of behavior, inasmuch as such a view ignores the facts that on continued self-administration of opioids, tolerance to most of the "euphorigenic" effects develops rapidly, "dysphoria" prevails, enforced "cold turkey" withdrawals are apt to occur, and none of these "painful" experiences are forgotten or repressed (8, 27, 30, 32). To be sure, monkeys will initiate and continue to self-administer morphine intravenously at unit doses that are too low to generate peripheral effector signs of physical dependence (38) but this observation should stimulate investigation of the biochemical-neurophysiological mechanisms of drug reinforcement, rather than speculation about whether or not such a monkey experiences "euphoria."

B. Physical Dependence on Opioids

It is universally conceded that once physical dependence on opioids develops, self-administration of opioids is continued "in order to" avoid or suppress opioid-abstinence phenomena. Clinicians generally assume that physical dependence disappears within 2 or 3 weeks after withdrawal of opioids, and, therefore, can play no significant role in the genesis of relapse. However, as early as 1942, Himmelsbach (10) demonstrated that disturbances in physiological homeostasis can persist for up to 6 months after withdrawal of morphine from tolerant and physically dependent subjects. Similarly, Martin et al. (17) demonstrated that with the subsidence of the early ("primary," "acute") morphine-abstinence syndrome in the rat, a protracted ("secondary," "chronic") abstinence syndrome develops which lasts at least 6 months. Also, more recent studies by Martin and Jasinski (16) have revealed that in man, a protracted morphine-abstinence syndrome consisting of decreased blood pressure, pulse rate, body temperature, and pupil diameter can persist for up to 30 weeks after abrupt withdrawal of morphine in tolerant and physically dependent subjects. Martin (14) suggests that in consequence of such changes, the "postaddict" is physiologically (as well as psychologically) more vulnerable to stress than normal individuals.

C. Conditioning Factors

An intensive psychodynamic study of a patient during self-regulated readdiction to morphine, conducted in 1947 (27), yielded anamnestic and on-going behavioral evidence that: (a) the cycle of very early abstinence changes developing within a few hours after a dose of morphine in the tolerant state, and their suppression by the next dose, is appetitively, not aversively, reinforcing (analogous to "appetite," in contrast to "hunger"); and (b) relapse after "cure" (detoxification) may be based in part upon previous classical conditioning of opioid-abstinence changes to the physical and/or social environment in which the user becomes physically dependent, coupled with previous operant conditioning of drug-seeking behavior (hustling). As formulated in terms of a Pavlovian conditioning paradigm (26), stimuli that are temporally contiguous with administration of morphine on repeated occasions come to evoke conditioned responses that are quite different in the nontolerant and in the tolerant, physically dependent subject, in consequence of successively changing "adaptive" responses to the initial effects of the drug. As tolerance increases, such initial effects decline in intensity and duration, and what become classically conditioned are the central "adaptive" (and "counteradaptive") changes that succeed the initial (agonistic) effects of the opioid which, if not suppressed by renewed administration of the drug, emerge as "abstinence phenomena." Also included in this formulation are the assumptions that unconditioned opioid-abstinence phenomena, although of low intensity, persist for many months after withdrawal of the drug (10, 16) and that the central "counter-adaptations" responsible for these serve to reinforce "conditioned abstinence," thus delaying spontaneous extinction; and that "anxiety due to abstinence changes and its relief by morphine is of great importance in establishing a habit pattern of relieving anxiety due to other factors (e.g., neurotic conflicts) by the use of morphine and similar drugs" (26). According to these concepts, physical dependence can play a powerful role in altering the "personality" of the opioid-dependent individual. Given the temporal contiguities appropriate for conditioning (automatically provided by the "street environment" with its "bad associates," variable interval schedule of drug reinforcement, "hustling," and innumerable sources of "neurotic conflict"), the detoxified patient is by no means "cured," inasmuch as drug withdrawal alone, while reducing his "unconditioned drive" does not extinguish the "conditioned drive" generated by such temporal contiguities, at least as long as some residua of physical dependence persist, or physical dependence is reestablished by renewed self-administration of opioids.

In the course of the original studies on precipitation of opioid-abstinences syndromes in man (34), some evidence was obtained that such abstinence syndromes can be conditioned (33). Five "postaddicts" who volunteered for the experiments were made tolerant to morphine or methadone by multiple daily subcutaneous injections of these drugs (40 to 400 mg/day). At irregular intervals on different days, these subjects received single subcutaneous injections of either nalorphine (5 or 15 mg) or normal saline in lieu of one of the regularly scheduled doses of morphine or methadone. The nalorphine injections always evoked typical opioid-abstinence phenomena of varying degrees of severity. During the first 2 to 3 weeks of interspersing saline injections, the latter evoked, within 30 min after administration, complaints of "hot and cold all over," "cramps," "nausea" and/or "gagging," and, frequently, yawning, lacrimation, rhinorrhea, and mydriasis. The saline injections rapidly ceased to evoke any response, and inquiry revealed that the subjects had been watching each other and if the first one to receive an injection did not get "sick" within 2 to 3 minutes, they all concluded (correctly) that the "shot was a blank," and reacted accordingly.*

More success in conditioning the nalorphine-precipitated abstinence syndrome was achieved by Goldberg and Schuster (5, 6) in the monkey. In their earlier study (5) repeated pairing of a tone with intravenous injection of nalorphine in three monkeys physically dependent on morphine eventually resulted in the appearance of conditioned abstinence changes either on presentation of the tone and intravenous injection of normal saline, or presentation of the tone alone. These conditioned abstinence changes, consisting of transitory suppression of food-reinforced lever pressing, emesis, excessive salivation, and bradycardia, were similar to those evoked by nalorphine except that the latter produced tachycardia. Extinction of the conditioned abstinence changes was accomplished by presenting the tone plus saline injection repeatedly over 40 to 45 sessions, but they could be reinstated by a few pairings of the tone with nalorphine injection. Similar results were obtained in their later study (6), using a red light instead of a tone as the conditional stimulus, and it was also found that conditioned suppression of food-reinforced lever pressing and bradycardia could be evoked by presentation of the red light plus intravenous saline injection once monthly over periods of 60 to 120 days after permanent withdrawal of morphine. These conditioned responses extinguished rapidly when red light plus saline injection was presented daily, but they could be reinstated rapidly by a few red light plus nalorphine injections. Complementing these studies, Goldberg et al. (7) found that morphine-dependent monkeys increased the rate of intravenous self-injection of saline in response to a red light which previously had been paired repeatedly with intravenous injection of nalorphine. Schuster and Woods (22) reported that, in monkeys, a red light stimulus that had been paired repeatedly with intravenous self-injection of morphine during self-maintained dependence on morphine acquired secondary (conditioned) reinforcing properties that persisted up to 19 days after complete withdrawal of morphine, i.e., transitory increases in lever-pressing rates occurred when, during the morphine-abstinent period, such lever presses resulted in presentation of the red light plus intravenous injection of saline. "Thus, stimuli associated with either the nalorphine-induced withdrawal syndrome or with morphine reinforcement can acquire conditioned rein-

---

*The finding that "decoding" of the experimental design by the subjects altered the properties of the conditioned stimulus (saline injections) calls attention to the power of "cognitive labeling" in man, and suggests that verbal psychotherapy may be more effective in treatment than it has been if "craving" is recognized as "conditioned abstinence," and verbal psychotherapy is directed toward assisting in the extinction of the latter by the behavioral procedures discussed below.

forcing properties which result in their playing an important role in the control of self-administration of drugs" (7).

More analogous to the "natural" situation in man, however, are studies on conditioning of abstinence phenomena provoked by abrupt withdrawal of morphine, instead of by administration of nalorphine or other narcotic antagonists. Thus, my co-workers and I (30, 35) demonstrated that, in the rat, at least one abstinence sign that follows abrupt withdrawal of morphine, namely, increase in "wet dog" shake frequency, can be conditioned to an environment that had been temporally contiguous with early morphine abstinence on repeated occasions during previously maintained physical dependence. Such evidence of "conditioned abstinence" persisted for up to 155 days after morphine withdrawal. In these experiments, all physically dependent rats were subjected to the classical conditioning procedure. In addition, half of the experimental rats also received operant training in suppressing morphine-abstinence phenomena by no-choice drinking of etonitazene (10 mcg/ml aqueous solution) (34a) over 12-hr periods in the presence of discriminatory cues, while the other half received "pseudotraining," i.e., only water was available for the same periods of time in the presence of the same discriminatory cues under the same conditions of morphine abstinence. Two groups of control rats which received saline injections i.p. on the same schedule as the morphine injections for the experimental rats were operantly "trained" and "pseudotrained" in the same manner, except that the etonitazene concentration was 5 mcg/ml for the operantly "trained" control group. Surprisingly, on "relapse" choice drinking tests conducted at intervals of 1 to 3 weeks over a period of 155 days after withdrawal of morphine (or saline), both the operantly "trained" and "pseudotrained" experimental ("postaddict") rats consumed more etonitazene than their respective control groups in terms of percentage of total fluids (etonitazene solution, 5 mcg/ml, plus water) ingested, up to the 58th withdrawal day. Similar results (both as regards conditioned increases in "wet dog" shake frequencies and "relapse") were obtained in a supplementary study (35, Study 2) on operantly "trained" and "untrained" experimental and control rats; in this study, both "trained" and "untrained," formerly physically dependent rats consumed significantly more etonitazene in choice tests following morphine withdrawal than their respective control groups through the 142nd day of morphine abstinence. In another study (36) completely "untrained" rats previously made physically dependent on morphine (final "maintenance" level, 200 mg/kg, i.p., once daily) consumed significantly greater mean volumes of etonitazene solution (5 mcg/ml) than rats that had received saline i.p. on the same schedule in choice tests after withdrawal of morphine (or saline) for a period of approximately 1 year, whereas mean volumes of water consumed in these choice tests did not differ significantly.

These results raise the question of whether or not previous physical dependence alone is sufficient to generate relapse long after opioid withdrawal. The data of Nichols et al. (20) would seem to demonstrate the importance of operant conditioning as well as of physical dependence, inasmuch as those physically dependent rats that had been forced (by prior fluid deprivation) to drink morphine solutions (0.5 mg/ml) during morphine withdrawal ingested more of the morphine solution in choice tests (morphine versus water) up to 7 weeks of morphine abstinence than rats with previous physical dependence that had not been so forced, or had been forced to drink quinine or alum solutions, "equiaversive" to the morphine solution. Using a modified form of water deprivation and forced drinking of morphine solutions (23), Kumar and Stolerman (12) reported that even 110 days of enforced abstinence from morphine solutions did not prevent previously morphine-dependent rats from resuming oral self-administration of the originally aversive morphine solution. The importance of conditioning factors in relapse is also suggested by the report of Thompson and Ostlund (25) who found that rats made physically dependent on morphine by forced oral self-administration of the drug and retained in the "addiction" environment for 30 days after morphine was withdrawn ingested more morphine solution in choice tests conducted in the "addiction" environment than in a completely different environment. Likewise, physically dependent rats that were removed to the different environment for 30 days after morphine withdrawal ingested more morphine solution in choice tests conducted in the original "addiction" environment than in the different environment.

However, interpretation of such data is rendered difficult because of the possibility that the originally aversive morphine solutions may have acquired their reinforcing properties, not because of the pharmacological actions of morphine, but through association with thirst relief during forced-drinking training periods. This possibility is not ruled out with certainty by control with "equiaversive" solutions of quinine, etc., since changes in thresholds for aversiveness after repeated ingestion of the solutions may be different for quinine and morphine.

Such problems may be avoided by use of the intravenous self-injection technique for animal experimentation, but since lever pressing is not in the "natural" behavioral repertoire of animals, and must be learned by them, other difficulties in interpretation may arise. With this technique, which they had originally developed, Weeks and Collins (25a) prepared five groups of rats: "postaddict" (morphine by self-injection, then abstinence from morphine for 4 weeks); "morphine pretreated" (morphine by passive injection, then 4 weeks of abstinence); "water conditioned" (training on lever pressing for water, then no lever presentations for 4 weeks); "combined morphine pretreated plus training on lever pressing for water"; and "normal" (naive, untreated, untrained). Upon replacement in the operant cages where lever pressing produced intravenous morphine injections, the "postaddict" and the "combined morphine pretreated plus training on lever pressing for water" groups promptly resumed lever pressing at relatively high and equal rates, while the "water conditioned," "normal," and "morphine pretreated" groups responded at lower rates, in that descending order. In all groups except the "morphine pretreated," the average number of daily self-injections of morphine increased over the 7 days of "relapse" testing. These investigators conclude that "Prior exposure to morphine is only a minor factor in etiology of relapse; a more important factor seems to be conditioning, established during active addiction by repeated incipient abstinence and its relief by lever pressing for morphine. Then, when returned to the experimental cage with access to morphine, a powerful drive to press the lever is activated and this is reduced by morphine."

However, since in the experiments of Weeks and Collins (25a) the "normal" rats, even without training on lever pressing, initiated and over a 7-day period increased the frequency of morphine self-injections, the difficulty remains in separating those reinforcing properties of opioids that (presumably) are not consequences of abstinence suppression ("psychic dependence") from those that are ("physical dependence") in relation to the genesis of relapse. Monkeys, too, will initiate and maintain self-injection of morphine (4) even when the unit doses delivered are very small (38). In contrast, Jones and Prada (11) found that most naive dogs will not initiate self-injection of morphine, although they will readily initiate and maintain self-injection of amphetamine. However, after inducing physical dependence by passive intravenous injection of morphine, all six dogs so treated learned to maintain their "addiction" by intravenous self-injections of the drug. Moreover, these animals resumed morphine self-injection within minutes or hours after being replaced in the operant chamber 1 to 6 months following removal to their home cages and withdrawal of morphine. As stated by these investigators, "It thus appears that in post-addict dogs that had self-administered morphine during their addiction effects other than those experienced during the initial exposure to morphine are responsible for relapse."

That previously "neutral" or even slightly aversive stimuli can acquire secondary (conditioned) reinforcing properties through temporal contiguity with suppression of opioid-abstinence on repeated occasions, and that such acquired reinforcing properties can persist long after morphine withdrawal, was demonstrated by my colleagues and me (37). Two groups of morphine-tolerant rats maintained on 200 mg/kg of morphine, i.p., in a single dose each morning (hence, in early abstinence each night) had access (from 8:00 P.M. to 8:00 A.M.) to single drinking tubes containing anise-flavored etonitazene (5 mcg/ml) for one-half of the rats and anise-flavored water for the other half. Two groups of naive rats receiving normal saline i.p. on the same schedule were treated likewise. None of the four groups was ever fluid-deprived and food was always abundantly available. Such conditioning sessions were conducted on 9 irregularly spaced nights over a period of 25 days, after which morphine (or saline) injections were terminated abruptly. Twenty-four hours after termination of injections, the two physically dependent groups showed significantly lower colonic temperatures and significantly higher "wet dog" shake frequencies (reliable morphine-abstinence signs) than the two control groups. In subsequent choice-drinking tests (anise-flavored water versus plain water), the previously physically dependent group that had ingested anise-flavored etonitazene solution during the conditioning sessions drank significantly greater mean volumes of anise-flavored *water* than any other group for at least 137 days after withdrawal of morphine or saline, whereas choice consumption of plain water was not significantly different among the four groups. These investigators suggest that as in the case of anise-flavor, an "exteroceptive" (gustatory-olfactory) cue, "interoceptive" stimuli, such as certain of the pharmacological actions of opioids (including etonitazene), can acquire long-persisting secondary (conditioned) reinforcing properties by virtue of their close temporal contiguity with morphine-abstinence suppression, and thus account for relapse even in the absence of any observer-manipulated operant "training" procedures. Translated into "real life" terms, this hypothesis implies that the behavior of "postaddicts" is, in part, under the control of a variety of secondary reinforcers generated during previous episodes of physical dependence, including "bad associates," opioid drugs, and "internal stimuli" of nondrug origin which are mediated by central neural pathways that are also involved in the mediation of the morphine-abstinence syndrome (31).

EXPERIMENTAL EXTINCTION

If it is accepted that conditioning factors generated during previous episodes of physical dependence play an important role in the genesis of relapse, then the notoriously high relapse rate of patients "detoxified" with or without conventional psychotherapy can be readily understood. Mere withdrawal of opioids and prolonged retention of the patient in a drug-free environment does not extinguish the conditioned responses, any more than satiating a rat with food (i.e., reducing its "hunger drive") and keeping it away from the Skinner box for a period of time will "cure" it of its lever pressing "habit," previously reinforced by food rewards under conditions of food deprivation (30). Nor can one expect verbal psychotherapy to extinguish the conditioned responses, if only because neither the patient nor his therapist is likely to be aware of such on-going conditioning processes (31). By analogy with extinction procedures known to be effective in the laboratory, postdetoxification treatment programs should include procedures for *active* extinction of both "conditioned abstinence" and pharmacologically reinforced opioid-seeking behavior, namely: (a) repeated elicitation of "conditioned abstinence" without the possibility of reinforcing this conditioned response by reestablishment of unconditioned physical dependence; and (b) frequent repetition of the addict heroin self-injection "ritual" under conditions that preclude suppression of opioid-abstinence phenomena, conditioned or unconditioned.

Before the potential utility of cyclazocine for extinction became known through the work of Martin et al. (15), I (30) suggested that this end might be accomplished by the development of two new drugs, namely, one which if substituted for heroin or morphine would produce, on abrupt withdrawal, a prolonged, though not necessarily severe abstinence syndrome, and another which, though ineffective in suppressing such abstinence phenomena, would be sufficiently reinforcing on other grounds, so that initially, the addict would "work" for it on some schedule of reinforcement, to be determined empirically. Inasmuch as the second drug would not suppress the abstinence phenomena generated by withdrawal of the first drug, it was surmised that eventually, the patient would cease to self-inject the second drug, i.e., the "ritual" of self-injection *under conditions of opioid-withdrawal distress* would be extinguished. The present availability of orally effective narcotic antagonists affords a simpler method for achieving extinction provided that these drugs are used in combination with behavioral extinction procedures that are appropriate to the mode of interaction between specific narcotic antagonists and opioid agonists. Of particular importance for use in extinction therapy is the capacity of opioid antagonists for preventing the development of physical dependence on potent opioid agonists. In the case of nalorphine, this was demonstrated in a study (33) carried out in 1954, which was designed to test the hypothesis of Tatum, Seevers, and Collins (24) concerning the roles of "depressant" and "stimulant" actions of morphine in the genesis of physical dependence. It was found that no morphine effects and no hind limb morphine-abstinence phenomena developed in three chronic spinal dogs that had received morphine, 2.5 mg/kg, s.c., every

6 hr and nalorphine, 5 mg/kg, s.c., every 3 hr for 28 days before simultaneous abrupt withdrawal of both drugs. In contrast, the typical cycle of morphine effect, tolerance and the hind limb abstinence syndrome (flexor and crossed extensor hyperreflexia, running movements, etc.), appeared in one of the three chronic spinal dogs when it was readdicted to morphine, 2.5 mg/kg, s.c., every 6 hr alone, and then abruptly withdrawn. Inasmuch as the hypothesis of Tatum, Seevers, and Collins attributed the development of physical dependence to cumulative "stimulant" actions of morphine, and in the 1950's it was widely held that nalorphine did not antagonize such "stimulant" actions, the demonstration that concomitant administration of nalorphine with morphine in suitable dose ratios and time schedules prevents the development of physical dependence on morphine was considered to refute that hypothesis. Although, because of its short duration of opioid-antagonistic action and its psychotomimetic effects (28), nalorphine would be impractical for use in a therapeutic extinction program, these early experiments illustrate one important property of narcotic antagonists, of which use should be made in therapeutic extinction programs. Even after prolonged maintenance on cyclazocine (or, hopefully, an orally effective long-acting narcotic antagonist without agonistic effects of any sort), extinction of conditioned responses, both physiological and behavioral, will not take place unless "conditioned abstinence" is elicited repeatedly by presentation of appropriate conditioned stimuli, and the subject tries repeatedly, but without success, to suppress such abstinence phenomena by self-injection of what he knows to be heroin or morphine. Unless these requirements are "programmed" while the patient is still in the hospital (after detoxification and stabilization on the narcotic antagonist), reliance will have to be made on the patient's "misbehaving" after discharge (still maintained on the antagonist), i.e., returning to his "bad associates," "hustling" for and self-injecting himself with heroin. To be sure, the evidence for "conditioned abstinence" in man under "street" conditions is still inferential (from histories of relapse because of "the flu" or some such vague complaints that are reminiscent of opioid-abstinence phenomena) and devising appropriate conditioned stimuli for eliciting "conditioned abstinence" in a hospital setting would be no easy task, but it should be attempted. Likewise, self-injection of heroin (under narcotic-antagonist maintenance), guaranteed "pure" by the therapist, may not have the same symbolic significance as self-injecting a "bag" on the street, but one could hope that "laboratory" extinction of the operant will generalize to some extent. Furthermore, briefer additional extinction sessions could be carried out under more "natural" conditions in an out-patient facility in the patient's home environment after discharge from the hospital, using "bags" and other

features of the "ritual" and perhaps in the presence of "bad associates" who have seen the error of their ways.

Another problem that will have to be resolved is how long a patient should be maintained on the antagonist to ensure extinction of conditioned responses. The animal data reviewed in this chapter indicate that conditioned autonomic, somatic, and behavioral responses take a long time to extinguish and that "protracted abstinence" can persist for 10 months in man. Therefore, approximately 1 year of narcotic-antagonist maintenance would seem to be a reasonable estimate, provided that urinary detection tests for opioids and other drugs of abuse remain negative for several months.

REHABILITATION

It is generally accepted that any treatment program for drug-dependent persons should include job-counseling, psychotherapy, and other rehabilitative efforts. What is rarely considered, however, are the special needs of persons who have become dependent on opioids and have undergone the "personality" changes consequent to "protracted abstinence" and the conditioning processes discussed above. Writing in 1955, I (29) suggested that the state of physical dependence ". . . fulfills a need which has been generally overlooked, but appears to be of prime importance for human beings — the need for continuous activity directed toward attainable, but recurring goals. The consequence of failure to satisfy this need is an intolerable state of boredom. This may be achieved temporarily by the use of any of a large number of drugs which alter affective behavior, but only those that produce pharmacological dependence can furnish a continually recurring 'synthetic' need that can be satisfied. The activity necessary for assuring a continuous supply of drugs (termed 'hustling' in the addict's jargon) provides a sense of accomplishment, much as the acquisition of money by law-abiding citizens, and serves to enhance the prestige of the 'hustler' in the eyes of himself and his fellow addicts. Under favorable conditions, particularly if different goals for sustained activity are acquired by re-education, relapses to drug use may not occur. But since the manifestations of 'natural' needs can become 'conditioned,' those of 'synthetic' needs may also be activated in response to specific stimuli, and hence pharmacological dependence can become an important factor in the genesis of subsequent relapse."

It may be remarked that the self-reinforcing function of "hustling" postulated above for "human beings," has its counterpart in animals. Neuringer (19) reported that pigeons and rats perform learned behaviors to get food even in the presence of free food in abundant supply, regardless of whether they are food-deprived or not: "The act of producing food can serve as its own motivation and therefore as its own reward." Similar observations have been reported by Carder and Berkowitz (3). Furthermore, it appears that the greater the "effort" expended in "hustling," the greater is its reward, inasmuch as it has been shown that in rats, greater "effort" during acquisition of an instrumental response results in greater resistance to extinction and that, other factors being equal, partial reward increases resistance to extinction more than continuous reward (1, 13). Perhaps in the case of the addict, occasionally unsuccessful "hustling" for drugs constitutes "partial reward" (variable interval reinforcement schedule, with variable magnitudes of reinforcer).

Having successfully extinguished "hustling" for drugs by appropriate extinction procedures under narcotic-antagonist maintenance, a new problem presents itself: how to entrain the patient to "hustle" for socially acceptable reinforcers? Vocational training, job counseling, and the like are certainly required, but two variables complicate the problem, namely, the convincing evidence that the great majority of "detoxified," formerly opioid-dependent persons suffer from some type of psychopathology, and the as-yet-to-be assessed influence of "state-dependent learning" on the capacities of such persons to function in the drug-free state. Thus, in the most recently published study on the personalities of "postaddicts," Monroe et al. (18) administered the Lexington Personality Inventory (LPI) to a total of 837 "detoxified" subjects at the Clinical Research Centers at Lexington, Kentucky, and Fort Worth, Texas, between the years 1965 and 1968. For the population as a whole (including "NARA" patients who were admitted under the Narcotic Addict Rehabilitation Act of 1966, voluntary patients, probationers, and prisoners), characterological disorder ("psychopathy" or "sociopathy") was indicated by the LPI data in 42%, emotional disturbance in 29%, and thinking disorder in 22%, whereas only 7% were asymptomatic. In the subcategories of patients, the NARA group could be differentiated from all the others in terms of heterogeneity of psychopathology (characterological disorder, 31%; emotional disturbance, 31%; thinking disorder, 29%). One finding that is consistent with the results of earlier studies (9) is the high incidence of "psychopathy" (31% to 52%) within all groups, despite the title of the report by Monroe et al. (loc. cit.). Among the behavioral characteristics displayed by the "psychopath" is the inability to emit sustained goal-directed activity under the control of long-delayed reinforcement (operant language for the psychiatric phrase, "inability to delay gratification"). Theoretically, vocational training and job counseling should be directed toward occupations that "pay off" on a piece-work basis by the hour or day, rather than by the week or month (if there are any such in our society). "Emotional disturbances" and "thinking disorder," with or without "psychopathy," may also require special treatment, possibly pharmacological ("nonaddicting"). As for the possible influence of "state-dependent learning," the only study on opioids that appears to have been published (21) is that of Belleville (2) in the rat. This investigator found that rats trained to press a lever for food rewards under morphine, amphetamine, or saline conditions showed less resistance to extinction when the extinction procedure was carried out under a drug condition different from that obtaining during acquisition, than when drug-produced "internal states" were the same during acquisition and extinction. If it should be demonstrated that opioids produce "state-dependent learning" in man, then it may be necessary to retrain "detoxified" and "extinguished" former opioid users in such socially and personally useful behaviors as he may have acquired during years of living and coping in the opioid-altered "internal state."

ACKNOWLEDGMENTS

The research reported in this chapter was supported in part by the U.S. Public Health Service, National Institute of Mental Health grant nos. 13194 and 17748.

REFERENCES

1. Aiken, E. G.: The effort variable in the acquisition, extinction and spontaneous recovery of an instrumental response. J. Exp. Psychol. *53*:47–51, 1957.
2. Belleville, R. E.: Control of behavior by drug-produced internal stimuli. Psychopharmacologia *5*:95–105, 1964.
3. Carder, B., and Berkowitz, K.: Rats' preference for earned in comparison with free food. Science *167*:1273–1274, 1970.
4. Deneau, G., Yanagita, T., and Seevers, M. H.: Self-administration of psychoactive substances by the monkey. Psychopharmacologia *16*:30–48, 1969.
5. Goldberg, S., and Schuster, C. R.: Conditioned suppression by a stimulus associated with nalorphine in morphine-dependent monkeys. J. Exp. Anal. Behav. *10*:235–242, 1967.
6. Goldberg, S. R., and Schuster, C. R.: Conditioned nalorphine-induced abstinence changes: Persistence in post-dependent monkeys. J. Exp. Anal. Behav. *14*:33–46, 1970.
7. Goldberg, S. R., Woods, J. H., and Schuster, C. R.: Morphine: Conditioned increases in self-administration in rhesus monkeys. Science *166*:1306–1307, 1969.
8. Haertzen, C. A., and Hooks, N. T.: Changes in personality and subjective experience associated with the chronic administration and withdrawal of opiates. J. Nerv. Ment. Dis. *148*:606–614, 1969.
9. Hill, H. E., Haertzen, C. A., and Glaser, R.: Personality characteristics of narcotic addicts as indicated by the MMPI. J. Gen. Psychol. *62*:127–139, 1960.
10. Himmelsbach, C. K.: Clinical studies of drug addiction: Physical dependence, withdrawal and recovery. Arch. Intern. Med. *69*:766–772, 1942.
11. Jones, B. E., and Prada, J. A.: Relapse to morphine use in dog. Psychopharmacologia *30*:1–12, 1973.
12. Kumar, R., and Stolerman, I. P.: Resumption of morphine self-administration by ex-

addict rats: An attempt to modify tendencies to relapse. J. Comp. Physiol. Psychol. *78*:457–465, 1972.

13. Lawrence, D. H., and Festinger, L.: Deterrents and Reinforcements. The Psychology of Insufficient Reward. Chapter 7: Effort, expectation and amount of reward. Stanford University Press, Stanford, 1962.

14. Martin, W. R.: Pathophysiology of narcotic addiction: Possible roles of protracted abstinence in relapse. *In:* Drug Abuse – Proceedings of the International Conference, edited by C. J. D. Zarafonetis, pp. 153–159. Lea and Febiger, Philadelphia, 1972.

15. Martin, W. R., Gorodetzky, C. W., and McClane, T. K.: An experimental study in the treatment of narcotic addicts with cyclazocine. Clin. Pharmacol. Ther. *7*:455–465, 1966.

16. Martin, W. R., and Jasinski, D. R.: Physiological parameters of morphine dependence in man – Tolerance, early abstinence, protracted abstinence. J. Psychiat. Res. *7*:9–17, 1969.

17. Martin, W. R., Wikler, A., Eades, C. G., and Pescor, F. T.: Tolerance to and physical dependence on morphine in the rat. Psychopharmacologia *4*:247–260, 1963.

18. Monroe, J. J., Ross, W. F., and Berzins, J. I.: The decline of the addict as "psychopath": Implications for community care. Int. J. Addictions, *6*:601–608, 1971.

19. Neuringer, A. J.: Animals respond for food in the presence of free food. Science *166*:399–401, 1969.

20. Nichols, J. R., Headlee, C., and Coppock, W.: Drug addiction. I. Addiction by escape training. J. Amer. Pharmaceut. Assoc. *(Sci. ed.)* *45*:788–791, 1956.

21. Overton, D. A.: Discriminative control of behavior by drug states. *In:* Stimulus Properties of Drugs, edited by T. Thompson and R. Pickens, pp. 87–110. Appleton-Century-Crofts, New York, 1971.

22. Schuster, C. R., and Woods, J. H.: The conditioned reinforcing effects of stimuli associated with morphine reinforcement. Int. J. Addictions *3*:223–230, 1968.

23. Stolerman, I. P., and Kumar, R.: Preferences for morphine in rats: Validation of an experimental model of dependence. Psychopharmacologia *17*:137–150, 1970.

24. Tatum, A. L., Seevers, M. H., and Collins, K. H.: Morphine addiction and its physiological interpretation based on experimental evidences. J. Pharmacol. Exp. Ther. *36*:447–475, 1929.

25. Thompson, T., and Ostlund, W.: Susceptibility to readdiction as a function of the addiction and withdrawal environment. J. Comp. Physiol. Psychol. *59*:388–392, 1965.

25a. Weeks, J. R., and Collins, R. J.: Patterns of intravenous self-injection by morphine-addicted rats. *In:* The Addictive States, edited by A. Wikler, Res. Publ. Assoc. Nerv. Ment. Dis., Vol. 46, pp. 288–298. Williams and Wilkins, Baltimore, 1968.

26. Wikler, A.: Recent progress in research on the neurophysiological basis of morphine addiction. Amer. J. Psychiat. *105*:329–338, 1948.

27. Wikler, A.: A psychodynamic study of a patient during self-regulated re-addiction to morphine. Psychiat. Quart. *26*:270–293, 1952.

28. Wikler, A.: Clinical and electroencephalographic studies on the effects of mescaline, N-allylnormorphine and morphine in man. J. Nerv. Ment. Dis. *120*:157–175, 1954.

29. Wikler, A.: Rationale of the diagnosis and treatment of addictions. Connecticut State Med. J. *19*:560–569, 1955.

30. Wikler, A.: Conditioning factors in opiate addiction and relapse. *In:* Narcotics, edited by D. I. Wilner and G. G. Kassebaum, pp. 85–100. McGraw-Hill, New York, 1965.

31. Wikler, A.: Some implications of conditioning theory for problems of drug abuse. *In:* Drug Abuse. Data and Debate, edited by P. Blachly, pp. 104–113. Charles C. Thomas, Springfield, 1970. Republished with permission in Behav. Sci. *16*:92–97, 1971.

32. Wikler, A.: Sources of reinforcement for drug-using behavior. A theoretical formulation. *In:* Pharmacology and the Future of Man, pp. 18–30, 1973.

33. Wikler, A.: *Unpublished observations.*

34. Wikler, A., Fraser, H. F., and Isbell, H.: N-allylnormorphine: effects of single doses and precipitation of acute "abstinence syndromes" during addiction to morphine, methadone or heroin in man (postaddicts). J. Pharmacol. Exp. Ther. *109*:8–20, 1953.

34a. Wikler, A., Martin, W. R., Pescor, F. T., and Eades, C. G.: Factors regulating oral consumption of an opioid (etonitazene) by morphine-addicted rats. Psychopharmacologia 5:55–76, 1963.

35. Wikler, A., and Pescor, F. T.: Classical conditioning of a morphine abstinence phenomenon, reinforcement of opioid-drinking behavior and "relapse" in morphine-addicted rats. Psychopharmacologia 10:255–284, 1967.

36. Wikler, A., and Pescor, F. T.: Persistence of "relapse-tendencies" of rats previously made physically dependent on morphine. Psychopharmacologia 16:375–384, 1970.

37. Wikler, A., Pescor, F. T., Miller, D., and Norrell, H.: Persistent potency of a secondary (conditioned) reinforcer following withdrawal of morphine from physically dependent rats. Psychopharmacologia 20:103–117, 1971.

38. Woods, J. H., and Schuster, C. R.: Reinforcement properties of morphine, cocaine and SPA as a function of unit dose. Int. J. Addictions, 3:231–237, 1968.

Narcotic Antagonists, edited by M. C. Braude, L. S. Harris, E. L.
May, J. P. Smith, and J. E. Villarreal. *Advances in Biochemical
Psychopharmacology, Vol. 8*. Raven Press, New York © 1974.

Behavioral Procedures: An Overview

William L. Dewey

The data presented in this section of the volume show that by using
operant techniques one can obtain potency estimates, duration of action,
and the ability to produce tolerance and/or physical dependence of narcotic
agonists or antagonists. The agonists and antagonists have similar effects
on operant behavior but significantly different potencies. The drug sensitivity of these procedures is such that operant behavioral changes are
observed at doses below those which alter the physical appearance of the
animal. Although the pigeon is an excellent species to use to obtain analgesic agonist or antagonist ratios, pigeons do not give clear-cut withdrawal
symptoms and they are of limited use in opiate dependency studies.

It has been demonstrated that operant behavior techniques can be used
to differentiate between those narcotic antagonists which produce positive
reinforcing properties and those which produce negative reinforcing properties. Hoffmeister and his colleagues presented data which showed that
pentazocine, propiram fumarate, and codeine had positive reinforcement
properties whereas nalorphine and cyclazocine were negatively reinforcing.

Data were presented which showed a clear distinction in the potency of
narcotic antagonists to produce adverse effects in drug-free as opposed to
post-dependent monke/s. It took much less naloxone or nalorphine to produce these apparently adverse effects in post-dependent monkeys than in
previously drug-naive animals. Concern was expressed that the adverse
effects of the narcotic antagonists could be a problem in their use in treating post-opiate addicts. This problem may be minimized in light of the fact
that tolerance appears to develop to many of the subjective effects of
cyclazocine but not to its antagonistic property. This tolerance has been
shown to develop in man during very slow administration of relatively high
doses of cyclazocine. The dysphoric effects are not always observed following acute low doses of this drug.

It was pointed out that the subjective effects of cyclazocine and nalorphine are quite similar. Although in some ways these effects are similar to
those produced by morphine, by and large the overall pattern is quite different from that of morphine. It was proposed that the pattern of subjective

effects produced by a drug can be used to predict that drug's ability to suppress or precipitate withdrawal in patients dependent on morphine.

A theoretical model presented by Wikler suggested that the use of narcotic antagonists in the treatment of the post-opioid addict would be facilitated by the development of extinction. He further suggested that post-addicts, while hospitalized and on an antagonist, might be required to inject themselves repeatedly with an opioid. They will not experience the usual euphoria and this will initiate the development of extinction.

The narcotic antagonist analgesics cyclazocine, levallorphan, and pentazocine increased the rates of responding in an avoidance schedule and increased spontaneous activity while producing a decrease in rat whole brain norepinephrine levels. Naloxone did not block the effect of these drugs on locomotor activity or on the decrease in whole brain norepinephrine but did antagonize their stimulatory effect on the operant behavior. These data were interpreted to suggest that, of the three effects of these drugs, only the stimulatory effect on the operant behavior was specific, and that these agonistic effects were produced by at least two different mechanisms.

Narcotic Antagonists, edited by M. C. Braude, L. S. Harris, E. L.
May, J. P. Smith, and J. E. Villarreal. Advances in Biochemical
Psychopharmacology, Vol. 8. Raven Press, New York © 1974.

Chronic Effects of Select Narcotic Antagonists in Mice

Jo Ann Nuite and Louis S. Harris

Department of Pharmacology, University of North Carolina, Chapel Hill, North
Carolina 27514

Recently, chronic administration of narcotic antagonists has become a
clinical reality. As early as the 1960's, a pellet implantation method, developed by Huidobro and later modified by Way, made it possible to study
the chronic effects of morphine in mice. We have further modified this technique to study the general effects of prototype narcotic antagonists in this
experimental paradigm. Nalorphine, naloxone, and cyclazocine were formulated into pellets similar to the morphine pellets of Way et al. and implanted
s.c. into C.R. species mice. The effects of these compounds were then
compared to those of morphine. Parameters studied included: body weight,
motor activity, analgesic activity (as measured by the tail-flick test), and
naloxone-precipitated abstinence. Moreover, the ability of these compounds to antagonize morphine was studied over time. As expected, morphine exhibited its previously reported characteristic effects. The mice
became noticeably tolerant to the acute effects of morphine, and naloxone
precipitated jumping behavior in morphine-dependent mice. In contrast, the
antagonists exhibited a dissimilar pharmacological profile. In addition, the
antagonistic activity of the antagonists was evident and varied over time.
Tolerance did not appear to develop to the antagonistic effect.

Chronic administration of narcotic antagonists is now a clinical reality.
The narcotic antagonists presently in use demonstrate a wide spectrum of
activity, varying from the "pure" antagonist naloxone to the mixed agonist-
antagonists pentazocine and cyclazocine. There has been a good deal of
interest in developing techniques which characterize both antagonistic and
agonistic activity acutely in rodents (2, 7, 8, 11). No attempt will be made
to summarize all of the available literature. As an overview, however, it
should be mentioned that these acute procedures rely on the measurement
of opiate effects, such as increased threshold to pain in classical procedures,
increased locomotor activity, the Straub-tail effect, and depression of respiration (1, 2, 10). Notably, narcotic antagonists are conspicuous for their
lack of activity in these types of procedures, whereas they are unique in
their ability to reverse the characteristic effects of opiates (10).

The chronic effects of narcotic antagonists have only begun to be studied in rodents. Recently, a pellet implantation technique developed by Huidobro (9), and later modified by Way et al. (13, 14), has provided a convenient means to study the chronic effects of morphine in mice. Mice, implanted subcutaneously with morphine pellets over a 3-day period, exhibit a characteristic syndrome. Changes in body weight, motor activity, and analgesic activity are evident. Also, analogous to the clinical situation, tolerance develops to these agonistic effects. Moreover, the narcotic antagonists reverse morphine's analgesic activity and precipitate prominent behavioral changes in morphine-dependent mice. Specifically, Way et al. have reported that naloxone administration to morphine-dependent mice produces a characteristic jumping behavior which they have used as one index of the "abstinence syndrome."

Both their chemical similarity to morphine and recent clinical developments with the narcotic antagonists prompted the study of the chronic effects of select antagonists in mice. The pellet implantation technique made it possible: (1) to compare the chronic effects of morphine with those of the narcotic antagonists in mice, and (2) to study the ability of the antagonists to block the acute effects of morphine at various times after implantation. It is this data which will be presented.

METHODS

Pellet Composition and Method of Implantation

Pellets of morphine and the antagonists were formulated according to the method of Way et al. (4, 13, 14). Morphine pellets contained 75 mg base; cyclazocine pellets contained 4.0 mg base. Nalorphine and naloxone pellets were made with two amounts of drug, either 4.0 or 40.0 mg base. Placebo pellets contained all other components of the drug pellets (cellulose, calcium stearate, and silicon dioxide) except drug.

Pellets were implanted subcutaneously in male Swiss Webster mice weighing from 25 to 30 g under light ether anesthesia. Animals recovered as soon as the anesthesia wore off, usually within 1 or 2 min. Incisions were well healed within a day or two permitting subcutaneous injections without difficulty.

Parameters Measured

The following parameters were measured: body weight, motor activity, analgesic activity (as measured in the tail flick) (3, 5), and naloxone "precipitated abstinence." In addition, the ability of pellets of antagonists to reverse morphine's analgesia at various times after implantation was studied. Mice were used once only.

Body weight was measured daily and immediately after implantation using a standard mouse laboratory scale. Values for control, test, and placebo animals were averaged and at least six animals per group were used. Change in body weight was expressed as follows:

$$\% \text{ Change} = \frac{\text{Weight on Day 1} - \text{Weight on Day 3}}{\text{Weight on Day 1}} \times 100$$

Thus, increases or decreases in body weight were expressable as percent of change from premedication weight.

Motor activity of implanted animals was similarly measured over a 3-day period using a photocell activity cage (Actophotometer, Woodard Laboratories). Animals were divided into groups of three. Values from two groups were averaged. Groups of placebo and test animals were run simultaneously in randomized cages. After an initial acclimatization period of 5 min, motor activity was determined over the next 15 min each day. Animals were tested on day 1, 2 hr after implantation and for the next 3 days. All activity is compared with placebo animals run at the same time. Thus, changes in activity were expressed as:

$$\frac{\text{Test value} - \text{Placebo value}}{\text{Placebo value}} \times 100 = \% \text{ Change}$$

Analgesic activity over a 3-day period was measured in the tail-flick procedure (6). Placebo animals served as controls. To prevent tissue damage due to repeated prolonged exposure to the noxious stimulus, a 5-sec cut-off time was used in the morphine-implanted animals. Therefore, to observe the development of tolerance in the morphine-implanted animals, a separate experiment was performed. Two sets of mice (n = six per group) were implanted with either morphine or placebo pellets. Three days after implantation, the pellets were removed under light ether anesthesia. After 8 hr, a dose-response curve was run for morphine in both sets of animals using the tail-flick procedure. Both morphine and placebo animals served as their own controls. Percent maximal possible effect (% MPE) versus log-dose of morphine was plotted and the ED_{50} dose determined (6). ED_{50} values for morphine in animals previously implanted with either morphine or placebo pellets were then compared.

Naloxone-precipitated jumping behavior was measured using the method of Way et al. (13). Three days after pellet implantation of either morphine, cyclazocine, or nalorphine, the antagonist naloxone (10 mg/kg) was injected subcutaneously and jumping behavior observed for 15 min. Results were expressed as:

$$\frac{\text{No. of animals jumping}}{\text{Total No. of animals}} \times 100 = \% \text{ Jumping}$$

Antagonistic activity was measured at various times after implantation of pellets of cyclazocine, nalorphine, and naloxone using the tail-flick procedure and subcutaneous administration of 10 mg/kg of morphine sulfate. Two procedures were used: (a) groups of mice were implanted with either antagonist or placebo pellets. At various times after implantation, control tail-flick readings were taken. Then, morphine sulfate (10 mg/kg, s.c.) was injected and analgesia measured at 20 min. Each group received no prior injection of morphine. Percent MPE was calculated using a 10-sec cut-off time. (b) At a time when antagonism seemed to disappear due to the pellets alone, morphine and a low dose of the particular antagonist were injected simultaneously. Test groups included animals previously implanted with antagonist or placebo pellets as well as untreated controls. Percent MPE was calculated. This allows an estimation of the degree of tolerance to the antagonistic effects of these compounds.

RESULTS

Effects of Pellets Over a 3-Day Period

Mice implanted with morphine pellets over a 3-day period exhibited the previously described characteristic syndrome (Table 1). On the first day, the morphine animals were hyperactive, demonstrating a marked increase in motor activity (approximately 500% increase on day 1) over placebo animals run at the same time. However, by the third day, there was a marked decrease in activity compared to the activity on day 1. This is in comparison to placebo animals run at the same time. Morphine-implanted animals showed a characteristic weight loss (13%) over the 3-day period. Moreover, marked tolerance to morphine analgesia developed. A 9- to 10-fold increase in the ED_{50} for morphine in the tail flick was observed after 3 days of implantation with morphine pellets. Placebo animals showed no change in sensitivity to morphine after 3 days of implantation.

In contrast to morphine, animals implanted with pellets of a low dose (4.0 mg) of nalorphine, naloxone, and cyclazocine showed no measurable effects in any of these parameters. They looked remarkably like placebo animals.

TABLE 1. *Effects of pellets of morphine, nalorphine, and naloxone on body weight, analgesic activity, and motor activity over a 3-day period in S.W. mice*

Group[1]	Body weight[2]	Analgesic activity[2]	Motor Activity[2]
Placebo	4 (↑)	No activity	
Morphine[3]	13 (↓)	Nine- to 10-fold ↑[4]	128 (↓)
Nalorphine[3]	6 (↑)	No activity	No change
Naloxone[3]	0.0	No activity	No change

[1] n = five at least

[2] Values expressed as $= \dfrac{\text{Day 3 value} - \text{Day 1 value}}{\text{Day 1 value}} \times 100 = \%$ Change.

[3] Morphine pellet contained 75.0 mg base, nalorphine and naloxone 4.0 mg base.

[4] Expressed as the increase in the ED_{50} for morphine in animals implanted for 3 days.

A higher dose of nalorphine and naloxone (40 mg/pellet) still showed no measurable effect in the tail flick or on body weight over the 3-day period (Table 2). Yet motor activity increased over the 3-day period. In contrast to morphine, both nalorphine and naloxone caused an initial decrease in motor activity, which returned to slightly above control values on day 3.

In this study, all animals implanted with morphine for 3 days exhibited the characteristic jumping behavior within 15 min after injection of naloxone. Animals implanted with either nalorphine, at two dose levels, or cyclazocine did not exhibit this behavior. Even when additional injections of nalorphine and cyclazocine (50 mg/kg and 10 mg/kg respectively, s.c.) were given on

TABLE 2. *Effects of pellets of nalorphine and naloxone containing 40.0 mg base each on body weight, analgesic activity, and motor activity over a 3-day period*

Group[1]	Body weight[2]	Analgesic activity	Motor Activity[2]
Placebo	0.0	No activity	
Nalorphine	3 (↑)	No activity	108 (↑)
Naloxone	3 (↑)	No activity	158 (↑)

[1] n = five at least

[2] Values expressed as $= \dfrac{\text{Day 3 value} - \text{Day 1 value}}{\text{Day 1 value}} \times 100 =$ % Change.

days 2 and 3, a challenge with naloxone did not cause this characteristic jumping behavior. Control animals were similarly unaffected.

Antagonism of Morphine Analgesia

A time-related and lasting antagonism of morphine analgesia was found in mice implanted with pellets of the antagonists. Cyclazocine's effect is apparent in Fig. 1. The ability of cyclazocine to reverse morphine analgesia varied over time but was still significant 48 hr after implantation.

Nalorphine (Fig. 2) demonstrated a more rapid decrease over time. At 24 hr, antagonistic activity was virtually gone. At this time, in order to ascertain if tolerance had developed to the antagonistic effect, an acute dose of nalorphine was administered. The effect of morphine injected at the same time was measured. As is evident in Fig. 2, there was no apparent difference between animals previously implanted with placebo or nalorphine pellets. In both sets of animals a low acute dose of nalorphine completely antagonized 10 mg/kg of morphine.

Naloxone-implanted animals (Fig. 3) demonstrated an analogous effect. Antagonistic activity decreased with time. However, it was still present at 24 hr in contrast to the effect of nalorphine. Again, when naloxone was administered acutely to animals previously implanted, there was no dif-

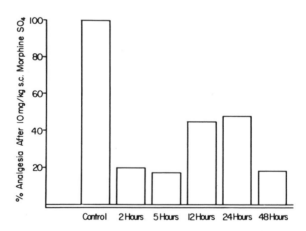

FIG. 1. Effect of cyclazocine pellet (4.0 mg base) on morphine analgesia in C.R. mice over a 48-hr period (n = six). All animals were tested 30 min after an injection of morphine and after the various time intervals following implantation with pellets of antagonists. Control animals were implanted with placebo pellets. Percent analgesia is measured $\frac{\text{Test} - \text{Control}}{10 \text{ s.c.} - \text{Control}} \times 100$.

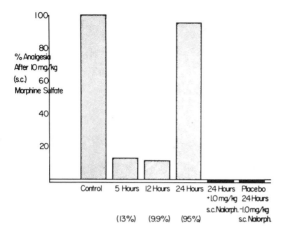

FIG. 2. Effect of nalorphine pellet (4.0 mg nalorphine HCl) on morphine analgesia in C.R. mice over a 24-hr period (n = six).

ference in antagonism between animals previously implanted with either naloxone or placebo pellets. Moreover, a dose-response curve for naloxone antagonism of morphine in naloxone- and placebo-implanted animals was similar, reiterating the initial result.

At a higher dose of both nalorphine and naloxone (40 mg/pellet) antagonistic activity was still evident 72 hr after implantation.

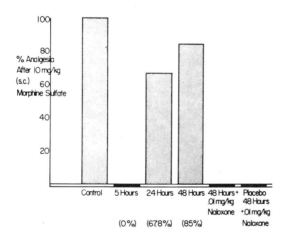

FIG. 3. Effect of naloxone pellet (4.0 mg naloxone HCl) on morphine analgesia in C.R. mice over a 48-hr period (n = six).

CONCLUSION

Pellets of select narcotic antagonists implanted in Swiss Webster mice exhibit a profile of activity dissimilar from that of morphine. A time-related and lasting antagonism was seen with pellets of nalorphine, naloxone, and cyclazocine in doses which did not cause significant behavioral or opiate-like effects. In equal amounts, cyclazocine lasted longer than naloxone which lasted longer than nalorphine. No tolerance to the antagonistic effect was evident.

Techniques similar to the implantation technique described may be useful in analyzing and predicting the chronic effects of narcotic antagonists. Combined with acute techniques for assessing antagonistic and agonistic effects of this type of compounds, the pellet implantation technique (or adaptions of it) may serve as a useful vehicle for delineating the effects of narcotic antagonists in mice and for predicting activity in man.

ACKNOWLEDGMENTS

Particular acknowledgments are extended to Drs. Louis S. Harris and William L. Dewey for their attention and guidance throughout this work; in addition, to Drs. James Olsen and J. Stephen Kennedy who assisted in the formulation of the pellets and in the spirit of encouragement throughout the study. In addition, a word of thanks is extended to all those working in Dr. Harris' laboratory for creating and maintaining an atmosphere which made the work not only rewarding but enjoyable. These studies were supported in part by grants from the NIMH (MH 19759) and the NAS-NRC Committee on Problems of Drug Dependence (D-71-6).

SOURCE OF COMPOUNDS

Cyclazocine (Sterling Winthrop Research Institute, Rensselaer, N.Y.); Morphine alkaloid and sulfate (S.B. Penick and Company, Chemical Division, New York, N.Y.); Nalorphine (Merck and Company, Inc., Rahway, N.J.); Naloxone (Endo Laboratories Inc., Garden City, N.Y.).

REFERENCES

1. Blane, G. F., and Dugdall, D.: Interactions of narcotic antagonists and antagonist-analgesics. J. Pharm. Pharmacol. *20*:547–552, 1968.
2. Collier, H. O. J., and Schneider, D.: Profiles of activity in rodents of some narcotic and narcotic antagonist drugs. Nature *224*:610–612, 1969.
3. D'Amour, F. E., and Smith, D. L.: A method for determining loss of pain sensation. J. Pharmacol. Exp. Ther. *72*:74–79, 1941.

4. Gibson, R. D., and Tingstad, J. E.: Formulation of a morphine implantation pellet suitable for tolerance and physical dependence studies in mice. J. Pharm. Sci. *59*:426–427, 1964.
5. Harris, L. S., Dewey, W. L., Howes, J. F., Kennedy, J. S., and Pars, H.: Narcotic antagonist analgesics, possible cholinergic mechanisms. J. Pharmacol. Exp. Ther. *169*:17–22, 1969.
6. Harris, L. S., and Pierson, A. K.: Some narcotic antagonists in the benzomorphan series. J. Pharmacol. Exp. Ther. *143*:141–148, 1964.
7. Hayashi, C., and Takemori, A. E.: The type of analgesic-receptor interaction involved in certain analgesic assays. Europ. J. Pharmacol. *16*:63–66, 1971.
8. Hendershot, L. C., and Forsaith, S.: Antagonism of the frequency of phenylquinone-induced writhing in the mouse by weak analgesics and non-analgesics. J. Pharmacol. Exp. Ther. *125*:237–240, 1959.
9. Hiudobro, F., Hiudobro, J. P., and Lorrain, G: Tolerance to morphine in white mice. Acta Physiol. Lat. Amer. *18*:59–75, 1968.
10. Martin, W. R.: Opioid antagonists. Pharmacol. Rev. *19*:463–521, 1967.
11. Perrine, T. D., Atwell, L., Tice, J. B., Jacobson, A. E., and May, E. L.: Analgesic activity as determined by the Nilson method. J. Pharm. Sci. *61*:86–88, 1972.
12. Smits, S. E., and Takemori, A. E.: Quantitative studies on the antagonism by naloxone of some narcotic and narcotic antagonist analgesics. Br. J. Pharmacol. *39*:627–638, 1970.
13. Way, E. L., Loh, H. H., and Shen, F. H.: Morphine tolerance, physical dependence and synthesis of brain 5-hydroxytryptamine. Science *162*:1290–1292, 1968.
14. Way, E. L., Loh, H. H., and Shen, F. H.: Simultaneous quantitative assessment of morphine tolerance and physical dependence. J. Pharmacol. Exp. Ther. *167*:1–8, 1969.

Narcotic Antagonists, edited by M. C. Braude, L. S. Harris, E. L. May, J. P. Smith, and J. E. Villarreal. *Advances in Biochemical Psychopharmacology, Vol. 8.* Raven Press, New York © 1974.

Evaluation in Nonhuman Primates: Evaluation of the Physical Dependence Capacities of Oripavine-Thebaine Partial Agonists in Patas Monkeys

Alan Cowan

Department of Pharmacology, Pharmaceutical Division, Reckitt and Colman Limited, Hull, England

The physiological and behavioral changes observed in patas monkeys after abrupt withdrawal of high doses of cyclazocine, nalorphine, or pentazocine and after naloxone challenge have been compared with those seen after the chronic administration of narcotic antagonist analgesics of the oripavine-thebaine series. Continual yawning, shaking, stereotyped self-scratching, and an apparent lack of distress characterized the abstinence syndromes of cyclazocine, nalorphine, and oripavine-thebaine derivatives such as cyprenorphine and RX 281-M. Primary dependence studies using mice did not differentiate between those oripavine-thebaine partial agonists possessing mild to medium and those possessing negligible physical dependence capacities in monkeys. The most promising oripavine, buprenorphine [N-cyclopropylmethyl-7-α (1-[S]-hydroxy-1,2,2-trimethylpropyl)-6,14-*endo*-ethano-6,7,8,14-tetrahydronororipavine], precipitated signs of abstinence in monkeys receiving cyclazocine chronically. In contrast to the reference partial agonists, there were no physiological or behavioral changes on abrupt withdrawal of buprenorphine, or again after naloxone challenge. It is predicted that the physical dependence liability of this narcotic antagonist analgesic will be of a low order in man.

INTRODUCTION

Recent single-dose suppression studies in monkeys at Hull and the University of Michigan have given equivocal results for several pharmacologically interesting oripavine-thebaine derivatives. A number of these narcotic antagonist analgesics have been reinvestigated in primary dependence tests with a view to predicting more precisely their physical dependence liabilities in man. Since cyclazocine, cyprenorphine (M-285), nalorphine, and pentazocine were used as reference partial agonists, it is now possible to present a general impression of the naloxone-induced

427

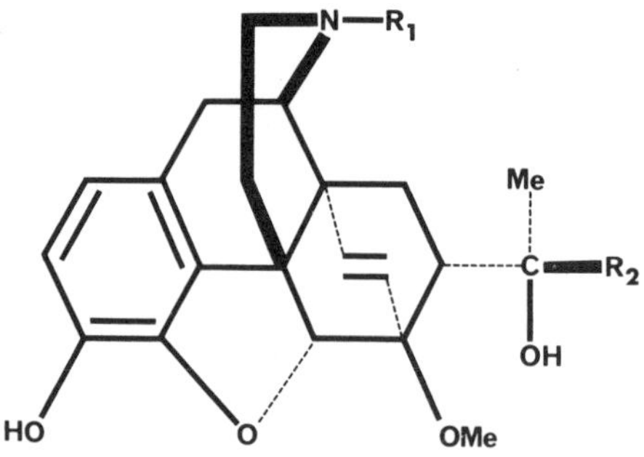

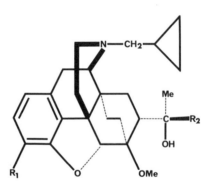

FIG. 1. Etheno compounds of the oripavine-thebaine series.

Compound	R$_1$	R$_2$
Alletorphine (RX 218-M)	allyl	n-Pr
Cyprenorphine (RX 285-M)	cpm	Me
RX 5217-M	"	Et
RX 289-M	"	n-Pr
RX 5205-M (3-Me ether of RX 5217-M)	"	Et
RX 281-M (3-Me ether of RX 289-M)	"	n-Pr

FIG. 2. Ethano compounds of the oripavine-thebaine series.

Compound	R$_1$	R$_2$
Diprenorphine (RX 5050-M)	OH	Me
RX 6007-M	"	n-Pr
Buprenorphine (RX 6029-M)	"	t-Bu
RX 6021-M	CH$_3$O	"
RX 6057-M	"	s-Bu

abstinence syndrome obtained with this class of analgesic, as opposed to the well-recognized signs of abstinence of the morphine type.

An additional feature of these studies has been a comparison of the monkey data with corresponding profiles obtained from primary dependence tests in mice. Although reasonably confident predictions can be advanced for strong agonist analgesics using mice (12, 16, 19), the value of these procedures for analgesics with mixed agonist-antagonist properties has yet to be firmly established.

On the basis of the rodent and primate results, the most promising of the partial agonists investigated (Figs. 1 and 2) was buprenorphine [N-cyclo-propylmethyl-7-α(1-[S]-hydroxy-1,2,2-trimethylpropyl)-6,14,-*endo*-ethano-6,7,8,14-tetrahydronororipavine] (M-6029).

METHODS

The mouse antiwrithing test and the rat tail-pressure procedures for assessing agonistic and antagonistic activities have previously been described (2). In the mouse tail-flick test for morphine (45 mg/kg, s.c.) antagonism, the nociceptive stimulus was hot water set at 55°C; those animals failing to withdraw their tails within 5 sec were termed pain killed.

In the mouse primary dependence test (19) two groups of 10 to 12 male mice (TO strain, 22 to 25 g) were injected s.c. with seven doses of test drug at 9 A.M., 4 P.M., and 10:30 or 11:30 P.M., respectively. The dose was doubled at each evening injection if toxic effects were absent. Three hr after the seventh injection, group 1 was challenged with nalorphine (10 mg/kg, s.c.) and group 2 received naloxone (10 mg/kg, s.c.). The number of jumps during successive 15-min periods was recorded automatically (3) and the number of mice jumping at least once during the 60-min session provided a means of ranking the physical dependence capacities of the compounds.

For the primate-dependence studies, groups of three drug-naïve patas monkeys (*Erythrocebus patas*) of both sexes weighing 3 to 4 kg were housed together in large cages (2.5 × 3.5 × 5 ft, see Fig. 3) and allowed food (Spratts Laboratory Diet No. 1) and water *ad libitum*. As a prophylactic against tuberculosis, isoniazid was injected into fruit to provide approximately 10 mg/kg/day for each animal.

Monkeys were injected once with naloxone (2 mg/kg, s.c.) and several times with physiological saline before each study began, to test for signs which might later be attributable to an abstinence syndrome. Drugs were administered s.c. at 9 A.M., 4 P.M., and 10:30 or 11:30 P.M. for 30 to 32 consecutive days. The development of physical dependence was monitored on days 14 and 28 by challenging each primate with naloxone (2 mg/kg, s.c.)

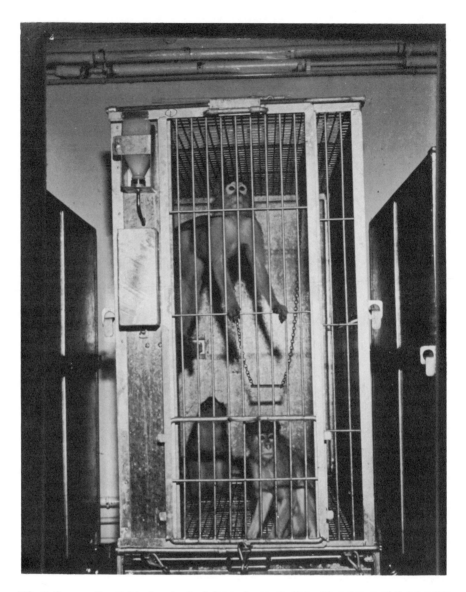

FIG. 3. Cage unit suitable for physical dependence studies with a group of three patas monkeys.

3 to 4 hr after the last dose of drug and noting signs of abstinence over 1 hr. The syndrome was classified as mild, moderate, or severe according to the protocol described by Deneau and Seevers (7). Physiological saline was injected during the week following abrupt withdrawal and the colony was observed for long periods through a oneway mirror at this time.

Drugs and their sources are nalorphine hydrobromide (Burroughs Wellcome and Co.), naloxone hydrochloride (Endo Laboratories Inc.), cyclazocine and pentazocine lactate (Fortral, Sterling Winthrop), and morphine sulfate (Macfarlan Smith). All doses refer to the soluble salt (usually hydrochloride) except buprenorphine, pentazocine, and RX 6007-M which are expressed in terms of the base.

RESULTS

The relative agonist-antagonist properties of the etheno (Fig. 1) and ethano (Fig. 2) series of compounds under investigation for dependence potential are presented in Tables 1 and 2. Thus, contrasting profiles are in evidence with RX 289-M, RX 6007-M, and alletorphine (high potency in both agonist tests with only moderate activity in the tail-flick procedure); with RX 281-M, RX 5205-M, RX 6021-M, and RX 6057-M (lower potency as both agonists and antagonists) and with diprenorphine (negligible agonistic but impressive antagonistic activity). Reference has previously been

TABLE 1. *Antinociceptive activities of oripavine-thebaine derivatives and reference compounds in rodents*

Compound	Antinociceptive ED_{50} (mg/kg, s.c. or i.p.)	
	Mouse writing	Rat tail pressure
RX 289-M	0.002 (0.001–0.005)	0.005 (0.003–0.011)
Alletorphine	0.005 (0.003–0.007)	0.033 (0.026–0.041)
Cyprenorphine	0.028 (0.008–0.078)	>100
RX 5217-M	0.037 (0.016–0.082)	>100
RX 281-M	0.39 (0.18–0.78)	1.3 (0.66–2.4)
RX 5205-M	1.6 (1.0–2.3)	10 (3.1–29)
RX 6007-M	0.003 (0.001–0.009)	0.008 (0.004–0.016)
Buprenorphine	0.033 (0.013–0.065)	0.024 (0.012–0.049)
RX 6057-M	0.52 (0.32–0.86)	0.61 (0.41–0.92)
RX 6021-M	2.8 (1.4–5.6)	4.3 (1.9–10)
Diprenorphine	>100	>100
Morphine	0.64 (0.10–3.2)	1.8 (1.2–2.4)
Cyclazocine	0.77 (0.40–1.5)	1.8 (0.73–4.2)
Pentazocine	3.0 (1.2–8.2)	18 (12–37)

Confidence limits (95%) are in parentheses.

TABLE 2. *Morphine antagonistic activities of oripavine-thebaine derivatives and reference compounds in rodents*

Compound	Morphine antagonistic AD_{50} (mg/kg, s.c. or i.p.)	
	Mouse tail flick	Rat tail pressure
RX 289-M	3.6 (1.2–12)	>10
Alletorphine	5.5 (1.1–24)	>10
Cyprenorphine	0.005 (0.002–0.015)	0.013 (0.006–0.028)
RX 5217-M	0.006 (0.003–0.013)	0.007 (0.004–0.012)
RX 281-M	31 (17–56)	>100
RX 5205-M	14 (6.9–26)	>100
RX 6007-M	5.6(2.0–16)	>10
Buprenorphine	0.22 (0.091–0.55)	>100
RX 6057-M	>100	>10
RX 6021-M	36 (15–86)	>100
Diprenorphine	0.003 (0.001–0.009)	0.008 (0.004–0.014)
Cyclazocine	0.70 (0.26–1.9)	>50
Pentazocine	28 (13–61)	>60
Naloxone	0.058 (0.023–0.145)	0.165 (0.060–0.454)

made to the inability of oripavine-thebaine partial agonists to show both antinociceptive and morphine antagonistic activities in the tail-pressure test (14).

Data obtained with these compounds from primary dependence studies in mice are shown in Table 3. It should be noted that, with the exception of

TABLE 3. *Direct dependence tests in mice*

Compound	Dose (mg/kg s.c.)	Factor × mouse A/W ED_{50}	No. mice jumping on day 3		No. mice jumping on day 5	
			Nalorphine	Naloxone	Nalorphine	Naloxone
Alletorphine	2.5–40	500	3/11	9/12	10/11	12/12
Cyprenorphine	15–240	500	0/11	0/11	1/12	1/12
RX 5217-M	10–160	270	0/10	1/12	1/12	0/12
RX 289-M	1–16	500	1/11	0/11	1/12	1/12
RX 5205-M	20–100	10	1/12	2/11	0/11	2/23
RX 281-M	4–64	10	1/12	0/12	1/12	3/12
RX 6007-M	1.5–25	500	0/11	0/11	0/12	1/12
Buprenorphine	15–50	450	1/11	2/12	1/12	2/11
RX 6021-M	3–48	10	3/12	1/12	4/12	4/12
RX 6057-M	5–40	10	0/11	0/11	1/12	0/12
Morphine	5–80	10	4/12	6/12	9/12	11/12
Nalorphine	20–320	10	—	0/12	—	0/12
Pentazocine	3–48	10	0/12	1/12	1/12	0/12

Jumping was recorded during 1 hr after nalorphine or naloxone challenge (both 10 mg/kg, s.c.) in mice having received seven or 13 injections of test drug. A/W = antiwrithing test.

alletorphine, initial doses as high as 500 times the antiwrithing ED_{50} failed to show antagonist-precipitated jumping to the extent seen with those mice receiving relatively lower agonistic doses of morphine. In fact, with the majority of these narcotic antagonist analgesics, the mice that actually jumped did so fewer than five times during 1 hr whereas the morphine group averaged 44 jumps on nalorphine challenge on day 5.

It is now well established that morphine antagonistic activity *per se* in a molecule does not preclude the possibility of inherent physical dependence potential (20). Consequently, an appreciation of the effects of standard partial agonists in patas monkeys seemed desirable as a preliminary to tests with the oripavine-thebaine compounds. These experiments are summarized in Table 4. The most striking feature of the abstinence syndromes with cyclazocine, nalorphine, and pentazocine was the absence of the distress (e.g., loud and persistent vocalization, extreme irritability and restlessness, continual fighting) so characteristic of morphine abstinence in this species. Despite the high frequency of yawning (Fig. 4), shaking, and stretching,

TABLE 4. *A comparison of naloxone-induced abstinence syndromes in groups of three patas monkeys receiving reference compounds over 1 month*

Compound	Dose (mg/kg, s.c.)	Naloxone challenge (2 mg/kg, s.c.) days 14 and 28
Diprenorphine	10	No signs of abstinence No signs on abrupt withdrawal
Pentazocine	2.0–9.0 10	No signs of abstinence Yawning; stretching. Low incidence of yawning and shaking 20 to 74 hours after abrupt withdrawal
Cyclazocine Nalorphine	0.5–1.0 10	(a) Morphine-like signs: yawning; shaking; stretching and restlessness (both nalorphine only); (b) other signs: stereotyped scratching; normal activity patterns; alert; normal defensive attitudes to human approach; duration of syndrome, 40 to 50 min; (c) abrupt withdrawal: significant yawning, shaking and scratching over 3 days; no obvious discomfort.
Morphine	3.0	Yawning; shaking; stretching; cries of apparent distress; emesis; irritability; fighting; restlessness then "on the nod"; lying on back and side; no playful interaction; piloerection; either disinterest or unusual aggression on human approach; peak effects, 2 to 20 min. A similar, but attenuated syndrome which included anorexia, was evident for 3 to 4 days after abrupt withdrawal.

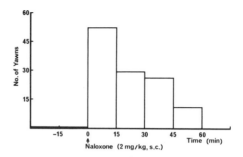

FIG. 4. Naloxone-induced yawning in monkeys (79 and 82) having received nalorphine for 14 days.

normal behavioral interactions were evident between the primates and between the primates and the observer on his approach.

Since the stereotyped scratching of either the cheeks, ears, chest, thighs, or buttocks (and occasionally the cage floor) was another marked feature of the cyclazocine and nalorphine syndromes, there does seem to be a case for considering these syndromes as being qualitatively different in some respects to that of morphine (rather than merely a mild manifestation). Such signs as yawning, shaking, and stretching are, of course, common to both syndromes. These observations parallel those seen in man where the

TABLE 5. *The effect of naloxone challenge or abrupt withdrawal of drug in groups of three monkeys receiving oripavine-thebaine derivatives chronically*

Compound	Dose (mg/kg, s.c.)	Naloxone challenge (2 mg/kg, s.c.) Day 14	Naloxone challenge (2 mg/kg, s.c.) Day 28	Abrupt withdrawal
Etheno series				
Alletorphine	0.25–0.50	++(moderate)	++(moderate)	−
Cyprenorphine	10	+	+	+
RX 5217-M	0.10	++(moderate)	++(moderate)	++(mild)
RX 289-M	0.01–0.02	+	.	.
RX 5205-M	7.5	++(moderate)	++(moderate)	++(mild)
RX 281-M	2.0–4.0	+	.	.
Ethano series				
RX 6007-M	0.20–0.90	−	+	+
	0.25–2.0	−	+	+
Buprenorphine	1.5–3.0	−	−	−
	3.0–12.5	−	−	−
RX 6021-M	5.0	++(mild)	++(moderate)	++(mild)
RX 6057-M	3.0	++(mild)	++(moderate)	−

− no abstinence syndrome; + cyclazocine-like syndrome; ++ morphine-like syndrome.

cyclazocine and nalorphine withdrawal syndromes have elements in common with that of morphine but are considered qualitatively different and cause only minimal discomfort (17, 18).

Diprenorphine and buprenorphine were the only compounds of those investigated (Tables 4 and 5) that failed to produce behavioral or physiological changes in the primates on both naloxone challenges. It must be stated, however, that one monkey receiving the low-dose regimen of buprenorphine displayed a few stretching responses on day 14. The interesting findings for both etheno and ethano series were (a) the recognition in some cases of syndromes resembling that of cyclazocine rather than that of morphine and (b) the mildness (or absence) of the morphine-like syndrome on abrupt withdrawal, in contrast to the quite moderate intensities recorded in the same animals on naloxone challenge.

DISCUSSION

In the search for an analgesic with low abuse potential, interest has focused recently on the wide spectrum of mixed agonist and antagonist actions seen in monkeys and man with compounds such as cyclazocine, GPA 1657, nalbuphine, pentazocine, profadol, and propiram (9–20). The present work has revealed a further intriguing profile in that of buprenorphine, where the high agonistic and antagonistic activities observed in the rodent tests represent a unique balance which may well be manifested in the biphasic dose-response curve (4, 13) and the low physical dependence capacity in animals.

In retrospect, it seems unreasonable to read too much into the optimistic data for buprenorphine and the other oripavine-thebaine partial agonists in the mouse direct dependence tests. With this procedure, the physical dependence capacities of strong agonists possessing weak or negligible antagonistic activities may be predicted (e.g., alletorphine, morphine); however, on the basis of the primate data, the jumping test is of little value in differentiating between partial agonists with low dependence potential (e.g., diprenorphine) and those displaying syndromes resembling that of cyclazocine (e.g., cyprenorphine, RX 281-M) or again, from those showing mild or even moderate abstinence of the morphine type (e.g., RX 5205-M, RX 5217-M). Perhaps the precision of the test would be improved by dosing over longer periods of time and measuring several components of the mouse abstinence syndrome rather than just one.

Difficulties are also encountered in the evaluation of these partial agonists using traditional single-dose suppression tests in monkeys (6, 20). For example, alletorphine suppresses some signs of morphine abstinence in this species but exacerbates others (21). In view of these findings, the oripavine-thebaine derivatives described in the present work have been compared with reference partial agonists in the more definitive primary dependence procedure in patas monkeys. The choice of the patas rather than the rhesus monkey was based purely on historical grounds. Extensive use of both types of monkey in this laboratory for several years has given the impression of similar signs of abstinence after chronic dosing with reference agonists and partial agonists.

Signs of abstinence were only observed in those primates receiving *large* doses of pentazocine. The abstinence syndrome to this compound was not characterized by the stereotyped scratching as seen after cyclazocine and nalorphine administration. Parenthetically, it is of interest that the latter two drugs also contrast with pentazocine in not being associated with drug-seeking behavior in man (17, 18).

Additional studies with cyclazocine-dependent monkeys have shown that smaller doses of naloxone (0.5 mg/kg, s.c.) will precipitate immediate scratching episodes only in those animals that have not received the maintenance dose of cyclazocine for at least 2 hr. In these cases the prior injection of mepyramine (0.5 mg/kg, s.c.) did not reduce the frequency of scratching or, indeed, modify the abstinence syndrome. Scratching was also a feature of the syndrome seen with the strong etheno antagonist, cyprenorphine (1, 22). It is of interest that the injection of a conventional dose of nalorphine (2 mg/kg, s.c.) on day 30 failed to precipitate signs of abstinence in those animals on cyprenorphine despite the presence of yawning and scratching produced by naloxone challenge on day 28 and on abrupt withdrawal (day 32). Pertinent to this observation are the reports by Fraser and Rosenberg (8) and Jasinski, Martin, and Hoeldtke (10) that nalorphine failed to precipitate an acute abstinence syndrome in humans receiving cyclazocine or pentazocine, whereas naloxone produced signs of abstinence in the pentazocine subjects. Naloxone has not yet been tested in cyclazocine-dependent individuals.

In the etheno series (15) the abstinence syndromes of RX 289-M and the 3-methyl ether RX 281-M resembled that of cyclazocine rather than morphine whereas the reverse applied with RX 5217-M and the 3-methyl ether RX 5205-M. The monkeys receiving RX 5205-M differed from those on RX 5217-M, however, when challenged with naloxone (2 mg/kg, s.c.) 2 weeks after abrupt withdrawal. Mild signs of abstinence were only noted with the former animals.

The profiles of alletorphine and RX 6057-M were unusual in that a moderate naloxone precipitated-abstinence syndrome on day 28 was followed by normal behavioral and physiological patterns on abrupt withdrawal of drug on day 32.

Morphine-like signs of abstinence were recorded for compounds of both the etheno (e.g., RX 5205-M) and ethano (e.g., RX 6021-M) series despite the presence of the N-cyclopropylmethyl grouping in the molecule. Nevertheless, two ethano oripavines with this grouping, RX 6007-M and buprenorphine, are of especial interest, in view of their profiles in the dependence tests. RX 6007-M, a strong agonist and CNS depressant, did not suppress signs of withdrawal in withdrawn morphine-dependent monkeys (21). Moreover, no signs of abstinence were apparent on the first naloxone challenge in primary dependence tests (Table 5). After the second naloxone challenge, an unusually long period (25 to 30 min) elapsed before the onset of yawning, shaking, and scratching. These signs also appeared on abrupt withdrawal.

The interesting agonist-antagonist properties of buprenorphine in rodents (5) are replicated in the monkey. A dose as low as 0.03 mg/kg, s.c., precipitated a mild abstinence syndrome in nonwithdrawn morphine-dependent monkeys. Moreover, buprenorphine (0.5 mg/kg, s.c.) precipitated scratching, yawning, and shaking in monkeys that had received cyclazocine chronically for 30 days.

Buprenorphine has undoubtedly the lowest physical dependence capacity of the oripavine-thebaine partial agonists examined in the present study. It is predicted that the physical dependence liability of this compound will be of a low order in man.

CONCLUSIONS

The naloxone-induced abstinence syndrome in patas monkeys receiving partial agonists such as cyclazocine, nalorphine, cyprenorphine, or RX 281-M has elements in common with the morphine syndrome but is characterized by stereotyped self-scratching and the absence of distress. Primary dependence studies using mice do not differentiate between those oripavine-thebaine partial agonists possessing mild to medium and those possessing negligible physical dependence capacities in monkeys. Since buprenorphine is a narcotic antagonist analgesic with low dependence potential and an interesting profile in animals, it is recommended that the preliminary studies in humans be extended in a variety of pain situations.

ACKNOWLEDGMENTS

It is a pleasure to thank Dr. John Lewis and Mr. Ian Macfarlane for numerous helpful discussions. Samples of cyclazocine from Dr. R. A. P. Burt and naloxone from Dr. H. Blumberg are gratefully acknowledged.

REFERENCES

1. Bentley, K. W., Boura, A. L. A., Fitzgerald, A. E., Hardy, D. G., McCoubrey, A., Aikman, M. L., and Lister, R. E.: Compounds possessing morphine-antagonizing or powerful analgesic properties. Nature 206:102–103, 1965.
2. Blane, G. F.: Blockade of bradykinin-induced nociception in the rat as a test for analgesic drugs with particular reference to morphine antagonists. J. Pharm. Pharmacol. 19:367–373, 1967.
3. Cowan, A., and Cowan, P.: Automatic recording of the abstinence syndrome in opioid-dependent mice. Experientia 28:1126–1127, 1972.
4. Cowan, A., Lewis, J. W., and Macfarlane, I. R.: Analgesic and dependence studies with oripavine partial agonists. Br. J. Pharmacol. 43:461P–462P, 1971.
5. Cowan, A., Harry, E. J. R., Lewis, J. W., and Macfarlane, I. R.: *In preparation.*
6. Cowan, A.: *Unpublished observations.*
7. Deneau, G. A., and Seevers, M. H.: Drug dependence. *In:* Evaluation of Drug Activities: Pharmacometrics, Vol. 1, edited by D. R. Laurence and A. L. Bacharach, pp. 167–179, Academic Press, London, 1964.
8. Fraser, H. F., and Rosenberg, D. E.: Comparative effects of (1). chronic administration of cyclazocine (ARC II-C-3) (2). substitution of nalorphine for cyclazocine (3). chronic administration of morphine pilot crossover study. International Journal of the Addictions, 1:86–98, 1966.
9. Jasinski, D. R., and Mansky, P. A.: Evaluation of nalbuphine for abuse potential. Clin. Pharmacol. Ther. 13:78–90, 1972.
10. Jasinski, D. R., Martin, W. R., and Hoeldtke, R. D.: Effects of short- and long-term administration of pentazocine in man. Clin. Pharmacol. Ther. 11:385–403, 1970.
11. Jasinski, D. R., Martin, W. R., and Hoeldtke, R.: Studies of the dependence-producing properties of GPA-1657, profadol, and propiram in man. Clin. Pharmacol. Ther. 12:613–649, 1971.
12. Kaneto, H., and Nakanishi, H.: A simple quantitative method for the evaluation of physical dependence liability of morphine in mice. Jap. J. Pharmacol. 21:411–413, 1971.
13. Lewis, J. W.: Ring C-bridged derivatives of thebaine and oripavine. *This volume.*
14. Lewis, J. W., and Cowan, A.: R&S 6029-M. Presented at the 34th Annual Scientific Meeting of the Committee on Problems of Drug Dependence, Ann Arbor, U.S.A., 1972.
15. Lewis, J. W., Bentley, K. W., and Cowan, A.: Narcotic analgesics and antagonists. Ann. Rev. Pharmacol. 11:241–270, 1971.
16. Marshall, I., and Weinstock, M.: Quantitative method for assessing one symptom of the withdrawal syndrome in mice after chronic morphine administration. Nature 234:223–224, 1971.
17. Martin, W. R., and Gorodetzky, C. W.: Demonstration of tolerance to and physical dependence on N-allylnormorphine (nalorphine). J. Pharmacol. Exp. Ther. 150:437–442, 1965.
18. Martin, W. R., Fraser, H. F., Gorodetzky, C. W., and Rosenberg, D. E.: Studies of the dependence-producing potential of the narcotic antagonist 2-cyclopropylmethyl-2'-hydroxy-5, 9-dimethyl-6, 7-benzomorphan (cyclazocine, WIN-20, 740, ARC II-C-3). J. Pharmacol. Exp. Ther. 150:426–436, 1965.
19. Saelens, J. K., Granat, F. R., and Sawyer, W. K.: The mouse jumping test—a simple screening method to estimate the physical dependence capacity of analgesics. Arch. Int. Pharmacodyn. Thérap. 190:213–218, 1971.
20. Villarreal, J. E.: Recent advances in the pharmacology of morphine-like drugs. *In:* Advances in Mental Science, Vol. 2, edited by R. T. Harris, C. R. Schuster, and W. McIsaac, pp. 83–116, University of Texas Press, Houston, 1970.
21. Villarreal, J. E.: *Personal communication.*
22. Wray, S. R., and Cowan, A.: The behavioural effects of levallorphan, cyprenorphine (M 285) and amphetamine on repeated Y-maze performance in rats. Psychopharmacologia 21:257–267, 1971.

Narcotic Antagonists, edited by M. C. Braude, L. S. Harris, E. L. May, J. P. Smith, and J. E. Villarreal. *Advances in Biochemical Psychopharmacology, Vol. 8*. Raven Press, New York © 1974.

Certain Theoretical and Practical Considerations Involved in Evaluating the Overall Abuse Potential of Opiate Agonists and Antagonists

H. Frank Fraser

1131 Merrick Drive, Lexington, Kentucky 40502

It has been pointed out that in evaluating a new drug, be it morphine agonist or antagonist, one must consider not only its capacity for inducing physical and psychic dependence but also its capacity for provoking harm to the individual and/or society. Taking into consideration all of these parameters, one arrives at an overall abuse potential of a given agent and this should determine the extent to which it would be controlled. It should be realized, however, that we have "socially acceptable" forms of addiction or abuse, such as alcohol and tobacco, versus "socially taboo" forms such as heroin abuse.

Evidence has been reviewed to support the thesis of Martin that there is a separate and distinct receptor site for morphine-like and for nalorphine-like drugs; that both types of drugs may act as agonists; and that both types may have distinct intrinsic activity as well as affinity for both receptor sites. This hypothesis forms the basis for new studies to evaluate the capacity of certain morphine-like drugs to substitute for morphine.

In evaluating the overall abuse of a new agent, one encounters difficulties in extrapolating to man in three areas: (a) extrapolation from animal studies, for example, analgesia evaluation in mice and abuse potential in monkeys; (b) extrapolation from one type of abuse test or one route of drug administration; and (c) extrapolations from multiple tests if each parameter evaluated is not qualitatively and quantitatively considered.

The therapeutic value and reduced diversion characteristics of certain combinations of agonists and antagonists are discussed (for example, methadone and naloxone).

Studies of abuse suggest certain characteristics for treating narcotic addiction. There are essentially three types of antagonists that might be selected for therapeutic use: (a) those that induce dysphoria, e.g., nalorphine; (b) those that are neutral, e.g., naloxone; and (c) those that have euphoric properties.

Our experience with addicts indicate that they would best accept a euphoric antagonist. Such an agent might be developed from a partial agonist or, most probably, from a combination of drugs.

439

INTRODUCTION

Definition of Terms and Scope of This Review

In 1964 the World Health Organization (WHO) Expert Committee on Addiction-Producing Drugs recommended using the term "drug dependence" instead of "drug addiction" or "drug habituation." Drug dependence was defined as a state arising from the repeated administration of a drug on a periodic or continuous basis and connoted "psychic" as well as "physical" dependence. Its characteristics vary with the agent involved, but drug dependence was a general term selected for its applicability to all types of drug abuse. It carried no connotation regarding the degree of risk to the public or need for a particular type of control.

In order to consider the concept of drug dependence in terms of its degree of risk to the public, the term "abuse" has been added to the WHO definition. We define abuse for the purposes of this review as follows: abuse of a drug exists if its use so harmfully affects the individual and/or society as to require its control. The degree of risk to the public is usually reflected in the type and extent of the controls promulgated. It should be realized, however, that we have socially acceptable forms of addiction or abuse such as addiction to alcohol and tobacco versus socially taboo forms such as heroin abuse.

In studies of abuse potential one must consider not only the subjective effects induced by a given drug but also its capacity to produce physical dependence. For example, the amphetamines and cocaine induce psychogenic dependence of a high degree, but do not produce significant physical dependence. On the other hand, nalorphine (18) produces physical dependence: a well-documented abstinence syndrome is demonstrated after chronic administration in high dosage. Nevertheless, it has no recognized abuse capacity because it is a dysphoric agent and no drug-seeking behavior is exhibited when nalorphine is abruptly withdrawn. There are drugs which induce both psychic and physical dependence, such as alcohol, barbiturates, and morphine. It will be emphasized throughout this chapter that a comprehensive pharmacological profile of a drug is essential in animals and man and that a battery of tests for dependence and administration of the drug by several routes may be necessary before an unknown drug can be appropriately classified as to relative abuse (25). In addition, the chief sources for possible error in projecting the abuse potential of an unknown drug will be pointed out.

This presentation will cover the proposals of Martin (15) regarding the nature of the opiate agonist and antagonist receptor sites, and outline how these concepts have formed the basis for experiments that have been useful in assessing the abuse potential of the antagonists in animals and in man (11, 15, 19, 21). Although evidence will be developed that antagonists may act as agonists, for convenience, the term *agonists* will refer to morphine-like agents, and the term *antagonists* will refer to nalorphine-like drugs.

The therapeutic value of certain combinations of opiate agonists and antagonists will be discussed as well as suggestions derived from studies of abuse as to the ideal type of antagonist that should be sought for treating narcotic addiction.

THE EVIDENCE FOR TWO RECEPTOR SITES AND THE IMPLICATIONS OF THIS IN THE ASSESSMENT OF ABUSE POTENTIAL OF OPIATE ANTAGONISTS

Houde's Studies

Houde (7) investigated the capacity of graded doses of nalorphine to antagonize the analgesic effect of 5 and 10 mg of morphine and observed that partial antagonism was effected in a ratio of 1:8 (nalorphine to morphine). When the ratio was 1:4, complete antagonism was attained, but at a ratio of 1:2 partial antagonism was again observed. When the ratio was 1:1, analgesia was further increased, but the appearance of undesirable subjective effects precluded the completion of the study. Yim et al. (24) observed a similar diphasic curve for mixtures of levallorphan and levorphan. It is not possible to explain such experiments on the basis of competitive antagonism for one receptor site. It is possible to explain the phenomenon, according to Martin (15), by assuming that both morphine and nalorphine have (a) distinct and different agonistic sites (e.g., for their analgesic action), (b) an intrinsic activity for either compound on a given receptor site, and (c) a specific affinity of either morphine-like or nalorphine-like agents for each receptor site. For example, nalorphine may have a relatively high affinity for the morphine receptor site with limited intrinsic activity at this receptor site.

Difference in Subjective Effects Induced by Single Doses of Morphine-like Agents as Compared with Nalorphine-like Drugs

There are differences in the type of subjective effects induced by nalorphine and cyclazocine as compared to morphine, employing the single-dose opiate questionnaire (5). Signs and symptoms of sleepiness and drunkenness increase in a dose-related fashion for cyclazocine and nalorphine (17, 18), whereas symptoms such as drive, "coasting," relaxation, and itchy skin are dose related for morphine-like agents (16). Haertzen (5, 6) and Jasinski et al. (9) compared the effects of cyclazocine and nalorphine with those of morphine, utilizing the PCAG (pentobarbital-chlorpromazine-alcohol), LSD, and MBG scales. The PCAG scale refers to a group of items prominent after administering pentobarbital, chlorpromazine, and alcohol; LSD concerns items related to psychotomimetic effects; and the MBG scale refers to items classified as "euphoria" after administering morphine or benzedrine.

They found that scores on the PCAG scale and the LSD scale were positively related to the doses of cyclazocine and nalorphine that were administered, whereas the dose of morphine was positively dose related only on the MBG scale. The subjective effects of the antagonists differed. For example, pentazocine (10) in low doses resembled the effects of morphine, but, in doses of 60 to 70 mg/kg, pentazocine developed attributes related to the PCAG and LSD scores. These results indicate that pentazocine had characteristics of both morphine and nalorphine.

Qualitative Differences in the Abstinence Syndrome for Agonists of the Morphine Type as Compared with Nalorphine-type Agonists

Martin and his collaborators (18) demonstrated that the abstinence syndrome following abrupt withdrawal of nalorphine differed qualitatively from that which followed the abrupt withdrawal of morphine (Table 1). By this we mean that the proportion of points from the Himmelsbach score differs for nalorphine and morphine. For example, in the case of morphine, 31.1% of the total points were derived from hyperpnea and 25.5% of these points were derived from an increase in systolic blood pressure. On the other hand, only 10.8% of the points from nalorphine abstinence resulted from hyperpnea and 9.5% resulted from an increase in blood pressure. The most important source for abstinence points in the case of nalorphine was an increase in body temperature, which accounts for 35.8% of the nalorphine abstinence score. Again, in the case of morphine, only 4.4% of the points were plus signs, whereas with nalorphine withdrawal, 11% of the points were plus signs (Table 1). The proportion of points for pentazocine, profadol, propiram, and (−)-β-2'-hydroxy-2,9-dimethyl-5-phenyl-6,7-benzomorphan (GPA-1657) are also illustrated in Table 1. The spectrum of absti-

TABLE 1. Relative percentages and ranks of Himmelsbach points for the 10 days following abrupt withdrawal in subjects dependent on morphine, nalorphine, profadol, propiram, or GPA-1657

Source of points	Morphine (M) % of total points	Rank	Nalorphine (N) % of total points	Rank	Pentazocine (P) % of total points	Rank	Profadol (C) % of total points	Rank	Propiram (B) % of total points	Rank	GPA-1657 % of total points	Rank
+ Signs	4.4	6	11.0	3	9.4	4	12.6	5	17.7	4	12.5	5
++ Signs	9.3	5	3.8	7	29.2	1	17.4	2	21.4	3	18.1	2
Caloric intake	1.9	8	6.7	6	3.2	8	2.3	9	2.2	7	1.9	8
Restlessness	0.8	9	1.1	8	0.0	9	5.2	7	1.2	8	5.4	6
Emesis	2.8	7	0.0	9	4.6	6	2.6	8	0.0	9	0.0	9
Fever	12.3	3	35.8	1	15.5	3	17.5	1	26.8	1	15.5	3
Hyperpnea	31.1	1	10.8	4	26.2	2	13.5	4	23.6	2	28.8	1
Systolic blood pressure	25.5	2	9.5	5	3.5	7	16.4	3	3.4	6	14.4	4
Weight loss	11.5	4	20.9	2	8.4	5	12.5	6	4.4	5	3.4	7

M × N = .60; M × P = .60; M × C = .72; M × B = .70; M × G = .70; N × P = .40; N × C = .50; N × B = .73; N × G = .63.
Comparisons were made with the Spearman rank correlation coefficients (R_s). (From Jasinski, Martin, and Hoeldtke, Progress report on the abuse potential of weak narcotic antagonists. Reported to the Committee on Problems of Drug Dependence, N.A.S./N.R.C., 1969.)

443

nence points varies with the antagonist tested, and the deviation from the morphine pattern depends largely on the extent to which the drug is related to morphine or to nalorphine in its overall pattern.

The Importance of the Two-Receptor Theory in Designing Experiments for Assessing the Physical Dependence of Opiate Antagonists

The two-receptor thesis as postulated by Martin, that is, one receptor for the agonist property of morphine-like drugs and the other for the nalorphine type, takes into consideration not only the concept of dual receptors but the concept of agonists of weak, moderate, and high intrinsic potency, as well as the affinity of both types of agonists for their receptor sites. The application of these concepts is illustrated below in substitution studies with the drug profadol, which is a weak morphine antagonist, but nevertheless has properties of a weak morphine agonist (11).

In customary substitution studies, patients are rendered dependent on a high daily dose of morphine, e.g., 240 mg. Under these conditions it is assumed that most of the receptor sites for morphine would be occupied. If in this substitution situation a drug such as profadol, with equal affinity for the morphine receptor site, is substituted for morphine, one would anticipate that fewer morphine effects would occur, and hence abstinence might well develop when profadol was substituted for 240 mg of morphine daily. On the other hand, if the daily dose of morphine were only 60 mg, not all of the morphine receptor sites would be occupied. In this case, when profadol, a partial morphine agonist, was substituted, more morphine receptor sites would be occupied and substitution would be effected. These postulates of Martin and his collaborators have been confirmed in the case of profadol; when a stabilization dose of 240 mg of morphine was used, substitution of profadol precipitated abstinence, but, when the daily dose of morphine was 60 mg, substitution of profadol suppressed abstinence. Not all the antagonists fall into the category ascribed for profadol. For example, pentazocine, although a morphine antagonist, precipitated abstinence whether the daily dose of morphine was 240 or 60 mg (10).

Insofar as the two-receptor theory is concerned, naloxone is an astounding compound since it exhibits no agonist activity at either the morphine or nalorphine receptor sites (9). It is potent in precipitating abstinence in the case of both morphine and nalorphine, indicating that it has a high affinity for both of these sites, yet it is quite inert from any other pharmacological point of view (9).

THE IMPORTANCE OF SPECIES DIFFERENCES WHEN ATTEMPTS ARE MADE TO EXTRAPOLATE TO MAN FROM ANIMALS FOR BOTH AGONISTS AND ANTAGONISTS

Difference Between Species

An important point to realize in extrapolating from animal to man is the qualitative differences in the action of morphine in the various species. The potent stimulating effects of morphine in the cat are well knowns, whereas in man, although exhibiting some stimulating properties, it has overall sedative or depressant effects. In the monkey morphine dilates the pupil, and during withdrawal causes an excessive drop in body temperature, effects which are contrary to those observed in man. In the rat chronically administered morphine has a definite stimulative effect immediately after each dose, whereas the effects of morphine on body temperature are dissimilar for the rat and man.

Evidence for Differences Between the Monkey and Man in Respect to Abuse Potential

In the United States for the past 15 years the accepted protocol for screening morphine-like drugs in animals for abuse potential is to utilize the mouse for determining analgesic potency and to determine abuse liability in the monkey.[1] At that point the abuse potential observed in the monkey is extrapolated to man. Overall, this procedure has been very effective since qualitatively the monkey and man have exhibited similarities, although in a few instances quantitative differences have been observed. It would not be surprising, however, to find significant differences between man and monkey, in view of the above qualitative differences among the species. As a matter of fact, such differences have been well documented, particularly in the benzomorphan series. For example, phenazocine has exhibited only minimal capacity to substitute for morphine in the monkey, but in man the potency of phenazocine was 45 times that found in the monkey (2). In the case of GPA-1657, profadol, and propiram, there was also discrepancy between man and monkey. All of these agents were judged to be narcotic antagonists in the monkey, since in nonwithdrawn morphine-

---

[1] For a more complete description of the methods employed the reader is referred to The Bulletin on Narcotics (United Nations), Vol. 22, No. 1, Page 11, 1969. (This program has been sponsored by the Committee on Problems of Drug Dependence, National Research Council.)

dependent monkeys they precipitated abstinence and they did not substitute for morphine in morphine-dependent monkeys (20). In subsequent studies in the monkey utilizing the direct addiction technique, Villarreal (21) demonstrated physical dependence in the monkey on GPA-1657, since large doses of nalorphine would precipitate mild signs of abstinence, and abrupt withdrawal of GPA-1657 showed mild signs of abstinence also. Observations in man demonstrated a different pattern of effects (11). In man GPA-1657 was three times as potent as morphine in the induction of morphine-like effects in single doses and it did not produce significant elevations in the PCAG or LSD scale scores. When GPA-1657 was substituted for morphine in patients dependent on 240 mg of morphine daily, it suppressed and did precipitate abstinence. In this respect, GPA-1657 was equipotent with morphine. In direct addiction tests, GPA-1657 behaved as a morphine-like drug (11).

In man profadol was one-third as potent as morphine in single doses and, like GPA-1657, it did not elevate scores of the PCAG and the LSD scales (a nalorphine characteristic) (11). When profadol was substituted for morphine in patients dependent on 240 mg of morphine, it precipitated abstinence, but, in patients dependent on 60 mg of morphine sulfate daily, profadol suppressed abstinence. In direct addiction tests, following abrupt withdrawal, the abstinence syndrome observed more closely resembled that of morphine than that of nalorphine (11).

In man, propiram was one-tenth as potent as morphine in inducing morphine-like effects in single doses. However, scores on the PCAG and LSD scales were higher for propiram than for morphine, which indicates that propiram had some nalorphine-like characteristics (11). When propiram was substituted for morphine in patients dependent on 240 mg of morphine daily, propiram precipitated abstinence. In patients dependent on 60 mg of morphine daily, propiram suppressed abstinence. In direct addiction tests with propiram, following abrupt withdrawal there was drug-seeking behavior, but the abstinence syndrome had characteristics of both morphine and nalorphine abstinence (11).

These observations suggest that, for certain compounds at least, it may be hazardous to extrapolate from mice and monkeys to men. This difficulty may in part be circumvented by assessing the potency of each compound as an analgesic and as a morphine-like drug of abuse in the same species. In the monkey, evaluation for analgesia might utilize the method of Malis and Gluckman (14). To complement the studies of physical dependence in the monkey, observations for self administration, such as those conducted by Woods (22), could be added. Yanagita et al. (23) found this procedure valuable in assessing the abuse potential of sedative hypnotics. An alternative would be to employ another species, such as the rat or mouse, to assess analgesia and dependence in the same species. It should be pointed out, however, that extrapolation to man of dependence observations for the mouse and the rat have not as yet been validated to the same extent as extrapolations from the monkey.

THE LIMITATIONS OF ANY SINGLE TEST FOR EVALUATING THE ABUSE POTENTIAL OF AGONISTS AND ANTAGONISTS

In certain instances there probably has been a tendency to evaluate the abuse potential of a new drug using only one procedure (e.g., evaluating the ability of a drug with morphine attributes to substitute for morphine in morphine-dependent monkeys or in man). Single-test procedures are hazardous for predicating overall abuse potential, particularly if the pharmacological pattern of the compound deviates in any significant way from that of morphine. An example of a possibility for misinterpretation of data is afforded by the study of Kay, Gorodetzky, and Martin (13) in which the comparative effects of codeine and morphine were evaluated by administering single intramuscular doses of these agents to postaddicts and interpreting the relative potency of these drugs for several parameters contained in the single-dose opiate questionnaire, which provides for responses by subjects and observers. (Note: The author does not wish to imply that these authors extrapolated from their study as to the overall relative abuse potential of codeine and morphine, since the objective of their measurements was to determine the relative potency of these agents for these parameters when the drugs were administered by one route, namely, intramuscular.) The relative potency and the parameters for codeine and morphine signs and symptoms are illustrated in Table 2. Assuming that this was the only available evidence as to the relative abuse potential of codeine and morphine, one would conclude that these drugs had equivalent abuse potential, except for relative potency, and that one only needed to administer codeine in approximately 10 times the dose of morphine in order to attain equivalent subjective and objective effects, since the authors demonstrated very few significant differences in codeine and morphine when equally effective doses were compared. Furthermore, the authors observed no evidence that the dose of codeine was limited by toxic effects; i.e., there was no ceiling for codeine (Table 2).

One knows, however, from vast clinical experience with both codeine and morphine and from other experimental studies on postaddicts that codeine and morphine are not equivalent in overall abuse potential. A good illustra-

TABLE 2. *Potency of codeine relative to morphine*[a]

Measure	Total[b]	Peak[c]
Miosis	14.2 (11.0, 18.8)	9.9 (5.9, 15.4)
Opiate signs	8.2 (6.5, 10.4)[d]	9.0 (7.2, 11.4)[d]
Opiate symptoms	10.8 (8.4, 13.7)	9.3 (7.8, 11.2)
Liking (observers)	9.9 (7.9, 12.1)	6.6 (4.7, 8.8)[d]
Liking (subjects)	10.4 (8.2, 13.1)	7.1 (5.4, 9.2)[d]

[a] Relative potency expressed as milligrams of codeine phosphate equivalent in effect to 1.0 mg of morphine sulfate (95% confidence limits for valid assays).

[b] Sum of five hourly observations; 20 subjects.

[c] Sum of effects ($N = 20$) at hour of maximal effect for each dose, corrected by placebo at that hour.

[d] Six-point assay showed significantly greater ($p < 0.05$) codeine effect with differing preparations. A valid five-point assay was obtained by omitting the lowest dose of morphine. [From Kay et al. (13).]

tion of this point is the study of Fraser et al. (4) which may be described as follows.

These workers demonstrated that veteran narcotic addicts in an experimental setting were able to differentiate subjectively between a placebo and an active drug, as well as between active drugs of varying potencies. These investigators reported, however, that in several instances there was considerable discrepancy between responses recorded by narcotic addicts (subjective evaluation) and responses of observers (behavioral evaluation). In this study of eight subjects, the drugs used and the initial and final daily doses attained during an intoxicating interval of 18 to 20 days were as follows: morphine subcutaneously, 32 and 240 mg; morphine orally, 32 and 240 mg; codeine orally, 200 and 1,500 mg; phenazocine, 4.8 and 12 to 36 mg; L-phenacylmorphan, 4 to 4.8 and 24 to 36 mg; diphenoxylate, 40 to 64 and 160 to 480 mg; D-3-methoxy-N-phenethyl-morphinan, 180 to 1,200 mg; oral placebo. The chronic dosage questionnaire was completed daily by patients and observers. The extent to which patients and observers identified the various agents as "dope," the potency, and the extent to which these doses were classified in the categories "would you like to take this drug daily?" "don't care," and "no" were recorded for both the patient (P) and the observers (A), as tabulated in Fig. 1. This experiment brings out the fact that the degree of acceptance of a drug may be evaluated one way from single-dose tests (4), but that a different interpretation results when the drug is chronically administered. It is obvious that codeine administered by the oral route in a chronic test had a very minimal degree of acceptance by

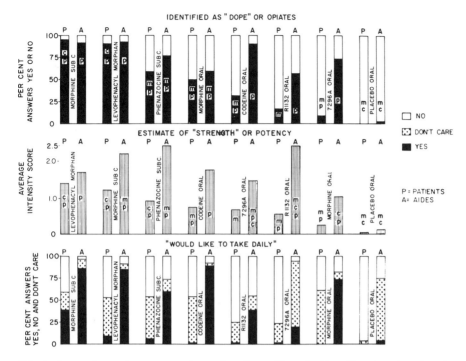

FIG. 1. Comparison of average ratings of patients (P) and aides (A) using the chronic dosage questionnaire for opiates in a "short" addiction test of 18 to 20 days involving seven drugs and a placebo.

Statistical comparisons by the paired *t* test among drugs tested for identification as "dope" or opiate and "strength" or potency are summarized separately for patients and aides. A significant difference (*p*<0.05) between morphine subcutaneously and other drugs, including a placebo, is shown by the symbol m; between codeine orally and other drugs by the symbol c; and between a placebo orally and other drugs by the symbol p.

[Reprinted from Fraser et al. (4).]

the patients, as evidenced by their replies to the question "Would you like to take this drug daily?" On the other hand, observers did not differentiate the effects of codeine from those of morphine administered subcutaneously. In fact, codeine was rated somewhat higher by the observers.

Additional studies with codeine by the intravenous route have demonstrated that the release of histamine is excessive in the case of codeine as compared with morphine, and the intense tingling and flush effect which is provoked is disturbing to the addict. Furthermore, codeine on rapid intravenous injection causes severe hypotension and even fainting, an effect which is upsetting to the addict. These experiments illustrate that codeine has potent and acceptable morphine-like effects when administered in single doses intramuscularly, but has disturbing effects when administered intravenously and minimally acceptable effects when given orally in chronic tests. Fraser et al. (4) indicate the need for conducting different modalities of tests on an unknown agent if one is to evaluate satisfactorily its overall abuse potential. All the experiments cited point up the inadequacy of the single-dose opiate questionnaire of Fraser et al. (4) as a sole predictor for overall abuse potential.

EVEN WHEN MULTIPLE TESTS FOR ABUSE POTENTIAL ARE EMPLOYED, IT IS NECESSARY TO EVALUATE QUALITATIVELY AND QUANTITATIVELY EACH TEST IN ARRIVING AT AN OVERALL EVALUATION OF THE ABUSE POTENTIAL OF A NEW DRUG

Table 3 presents the results observed when several different parameters were evaluated for the abuse potential of morphine-like drugs (morphine,

TABLE 3. *Results observed for several parameters used in evaluating the human abuse potential of certain opiate agonists and antagonists*

	Morphine	Codeine	Propoxyphene	Pentazocine	Nalorphine
Subjective effects Intramuscular (single doses)	morphine euphoria	morphine euphoria	morphine euphoria	morphine euphoria in smaller doses; nalorphine-like in larger doses	dysphoria
Subjective effects Intravenous (single doses)	morphine euphoria	morphine euphoria (partial)	morphine euphoria	same as intramuscular	dysphoria
Substitution for morphine (240 mg/day)	+	+	+	precipitates abstinence	precipitates abstinence
Direct addiction:					
1. Abstinence syndrome	+	+	+	+	+
2. Drug-seeking behavior	+	+	+	+	0
3. Precipitation of abstinence by naloxone	+			+	?
4. Precipitation of abstinence by nalorphine	+	+	+	+	0

codeine, and propoxyphene), and two antagonists (pentazocine and nalorphine). When such a tabular presentation is employed in a comparison of codeine and morphine by intramuscular injection, identical results are described for every parameter. However, as we have described above, there are qualitative as well as quantitative differences between morphine and codeine with regard to their abuse potential.

In a similar manner, the abuse potential of propoxyphene as construed from this table is identical to that of morphine. This is obviously incorrect, since Fraser and Isbell (1) demonstrated that the abuse potential of propoxyphene was not only less than that of morphine, but substantially less than that of codeine. Table 3, for example, does not bring out the fact that in substitution studies in patients dependent on morphine, propoxyphene significantly, yet only partially, suppressed morphine abstinence (1). When an attempt was made to suppress abstinence completely by augmenting the dose of propoxyphene, a grand mal convulsion developed and the study was terminated (1). Furthermore, propoxyphene is a potent tissue irritant; when it is given intravenously, veins are progressively occluded (3). When an attempt was made to increase the oral dose of propoxyphene in single doses and during chronic administration to attain equivalent morphine-like euphoria, the patients complained of anxiety and nervousness, and in certain instances psychotic effects developed (1).

Both pentazocine and nalorphine exhibit an identical abstinence pattern in Table 3, but a very important point is missed by considering only this aspect. The abstinence syndrome is qualitatively different during withdrawal of morphine from that observed when pentazocine and nalorphine are withdrawn, especially since drug-seeking behavior is not seen during withdrawal from nalorphine; the same is true for the parameter *precipitation of abstinence with naloxone and nalorphine.* Not only do the antagonists resemble each other in the table, but they are also similar to morphine, codeine, and propoxyphene in many respects.

The point is made that when one evaluates compounds for their relative abuse potential, one must consider all the parameters involved in a qualitative and a quantitative manner. Attempts to simplify may be misleading.

ABUSE POTENTIAL OF COMBINATIONS OF AGONISTS AND ANTAGONISTS

A combination of agonist and antagonist has been advocated for drugs to be taken orally. For example, with a combination of methadone and naloxone, the premise is that when given orally the analgesic, euphoric, and "blocking action for heroin" of methadone would not be impaired, whereas intravenous injection of such a combination would precipitate abstinence by the naloxone and thus preclude the abuse of methadone intravenously. This concept has been practically demonstrated at the Addiction Research Center (12). However, a word of caution is necessary. The combination should not have too high a concentration of naloxone, because in a morphine type of dependency a very violent abstinence syndrome may be precipitated. In addition, there is no evidence that a "spree" abuse of methadone might not occur in a person nondependent on opiates. For example, Isbell and Fraser (8) administered various combinations of morphine and nalorphine chronically to initially nondependent addicts. Dependency on morphine developed during the test, as demonstrated by the appearance of an abstinence syndrome with each injection of the combination. However, undesirable symptoms subsided in approximately 2 hr (the length of action of nalorphine), and the effects of morphine took over. The subjects did not particularly like the test, but all persisted in taking the combination for 30 days.

The same logic might be applied to a combination of propoxyphene and naloxone designed for oral administration. If such combinations are to be employed, it would be preferable to have the agonist (methadone or propoxyphene) combined with an antagonist of longer action than naloxone.

INFORMATION OBTAINED FROM EVALUATION OF THE ABUSE POTENTIAL OF ANTAGONISTS AND THEIR SELECTION AS PROPHYLACTIC AGENTS

Theoretically there are three types of antagonists that might be selected for therapeutic use: (a) those that induce dysphoria, e.g., nalorphine, (b) those that are neutral, e.g., naloxone, or (c) those that have euphoric properties. The long history of disulfiram (Antabuse®) suggests that an aphoric agent is not sufficient. We might well look for a euphoric type of antagonist that has restricted toxicity and limited physical dependence capacity. Partial agonists capable of precipitating abstinence could be satisfactory (the partial agonists so far explored, however, have shown too much drug-seeking behavior to be satisfactory), or it might require a combination of drugs, i.e., a partial agonist and an antagonist.

REFERENCES

1. Fraser, H. F., and Isbell, H.: Pharmacology and addiction liability of *dl*- and *d*-propoxyphene. Bull. Narcot. *12*:9–14, 1960.
2. Fraser, H. F., and Isbell, H.: Human pharmacology and addiction liabilities of phenazocine and levophenacylmorphan. Bull. Narcot. *12*:15–23, 1960.
3. Fraser, H. F., Martin, W. R., Wolbach, A. B., and Isbell, H.: Addiction liability of an

isoquinoline analgesic, 1-(p-chlorophenethyl)-2-methyl-6,7-dimethoxy-1,2,3,4-tetrahy-droisoquindline. Clin. Pharmacol. Ther. *2*:287–299, 1961.

4. Fraser, H. F., Van Horn, G. D., Martin, W. R., Wolbach, A. B., and Isbell, H.: Methods for evaluating addiction liability. (A) "Attitude" of opiate addicts toward opiate-like drugs; (B) A short-term "direct" addiction test. J. Pharmacol. Exp. Ther. *133*:371–387, 1961.
5. Haertzen, C. A.: Subjective effects of narcotic antagonists cyclazocine and nalorphine on the Addiction Research Center Inventory (ARCI). Psychopharmacology *18*:366–377, 1970.
6. Haertzen, C. A.: Subjective effects of narcotic antagonists. *This Volume.*
7. Houde, R. W., and Wallenstein, S. L.: Clinical studies of morphine-nalorphine combinations. Fed. Proc. *15*:440–441, 1956.
8. Isbell, H., and Fraser, H. F.: *Unpublished data.*
9. Jasinski, D. R., Martin, W. R., and Haertzen, C. A.: The human pharmacology and abuse potential of N-allylnoroxymorphone (naloxone). J. Pharmacol. Exp. Ther. *157*:420–426, 1967.
10. Jasinski, D. R., Martin, W. R., and Hoeldtke, R. D.: Effects of short- and long-term administration of pentazocine in man. Clin. Pharmacol. Ther. *11*:385–403, 1970.
11. Jasinski, D. R., Martin, W. R., and Hoeldtke, R. D.: Studies of the dependence producing properties of GPA-1657, profadol, and propiram in man. Clin. Pharmacol. Ther. *12*:613–649, 1971.
12. Jasinski, D. R., and Nutt, J. G.: Studies of methadone-naloxone mixtures in man (abstract). Fifth International Congress on Pharmacology, Abstracts of Volunteer Papers, p. 115, July 23–28, 1972.
13. Kay, D. C., Gorodetzky, C. W., and Martin, W. R.: Comparative effects of codeine and morphine in man. J. Pharmacol. Exp. Ther. *156*:101–106, 1967.
14. Malis, J. L., and Gluckman, M. L.: Assaying narcotic antagonist drugs for analgesic activity in rhesus monkeys. *This Volume.*
15. Martin, W. R.: Opioid antagonists. Pharmacol. Rev. *19*:463–521, 1967.
16. Martin, W. R., and Fraser, H. F.: A comparative study of physiological and subjective effects of heroin and morphine administered intravenously in postaddicts. J. Pharmacol. Exp. Ther. *133*:388–399, 1961.
17. Martin, W. R., Fraser, H. F., Gorodetzky, C. W., and Rosenberg, D. R.: Studies of the dependence producing potential of the narcotic antagonist 2-cyclopropylmethyl-2′-hydroxy-5,9-dimethyl-6,7-benzomorphan (cyclazocine, Win-20,740, ARC II-C-3), J. Pharmacol. Exp. Ther. *150*:426–436, 1965.
18. Martin, W. R., and Gorodetzky, C. W.: Demonstration of tolerance to and physical dependence on N-allylnormorphine (nalorphine), J. Pharmacol. Exp. Ther. *150*:437–442, 1965.
19. Martin, W. R., and Jasinski, D. R.: The mode of action and abuse potentiality of narcotic antagonists. *In:* Pain: Basic Principles – Pharmacology – Therapy, edited by R. Janzen, W. D. Keidel, A. Herz, and C. Steichle, pp. 225–234. Georg Thieme Pub. Stuttgart, 1972.
20. Villarreal, J. E.: Recent advances in the pharmacology of morphine like drugs. *In:* Advances in Mental Science, Vol. 2, edited by R. T. Harris, W. M. McIsaac, and C. R. Schuster, University of Texas Press, Houston, 1970.
21. Villarreal, J. E., and Dummer, G. E.: Evaluation of the physical dependence capacity of narcotic antagonists on Rhesus monkeys. *This Volume.*
22. Woods, J. H.: Blockade of self administration of narcotics. *This Volume.*
23. Yanagita, T., and Takahashi, S.: Dependence liability of several sedative-hypnotic agents evaluated in monkeys. J. Pharmacol. Exp. Ther. *185*:307–316, 1973.
24. Yim, G. K. W., Keasling, H. H., and Gross, E. G.: Simultaneous minute volume and tooth pulp threshold changes following chronic administration of levorphan and a levorphan-levallorphan mixture in rabbits. J. Pharmacol. Exp. Ther. *118*:193–197, 1956.
25. Zarafonetis, C. J. D.: Preference of addicts for certain narcotic drugs and routes of administration. *In:* Drug Abuse. Proceedings of the International Conference, p. 143. Lea & Febiger, Philadelphia, 1972.

Narcotic Antagonists, edited by M. C. Braude, L. S. Harris, E. L. May, J. P. Smith, and J. E. Villarreal. *Advances in Biochemical Psychopharmacology, Vol. 8.* Raven Press, New York © 1974.

Neuroanatomical and Chemical Correlates of Naloxone-Precipitated Withdrawal

E. Leong Way, H. H. Loh, I. K. Ho, E. T. Iwamoto, and Eddie Wei

Department of Pharmacology, University of California School of Medicine, San Francisco, California 94143, Langley Porter Neuropsychiatric Institute, San Francisco, California 94143, and Division of Environmental Health Sciences, School of Public Health, University of California, Berkeley, California 94720

Physical dependence on morphine is manifested by a highly characteristic behavior when morphine intake is abruptly terminated or when a morphine antagonist is administered. In the rodent rendered dependent on morphine by subcutaneous morphine pellet implantation, one of the most characteristic signs of withdrawal precipitated by naloxone administration is stereotyped jumping behavior. In experiments utilizing the application of crystalline naloxone to discrete brain areas of the morphine-dependent rat, the thalamus was found to be one of the, if not the, most sensitive regions responding to precipitated withdrawal. Severe withdrawal signs were elicited after administration of naloxone in the thalamus but not in the neocortical, hippocampal, hypothalamic, or tegmental areas of the brain. A study of the biochemical changes occurring during naloxone-precipitated withdrawal in the mouse revealed that the jumping response was accompanied by a sudden elevation of dopamine in the caudate nucleus while norepinephrine and serotonin remained unchanged. Pharmacologic manipulations designed to block the sudden dopamine increase effected an inhibition of the jumping response. That the dopamine increase was not the consequence of the jumping action was evidenced by the fact that dopamine increased even though jumping was prevented by D-tubocurarine. Increase in cholinergic activity by cholinesterase inhibition reduced the dopamine increase as well as the jumping response.

INTRODUCTION

One of the most dramatic responses elicited by narcotic antagonists is the phenomenon of precipitated abstinence. In the subject highly dependent on narcotics, the administration of an antagonist provokes an explosive syndrome. The signs and symptoms that ensue are highly characteristic and similar to those obtained during abrupt withdrawal. However, unlike the latter state, the signs of precipitated withdrawal are rapid in onset, very intense, and of brief duration, lasting generally less than 1 to 2 hr. Precipitated abstinence was first described in 1953 by Wikler, Isbell, and Fraser who studied the effects of nalorphine in subjects physically dependent on morphine, methadone, or heroin (40). It is now well established that the response can be evoked by other antagonists not only in humans but in the narcotic-dependent animal as well, particularly the monkey, dog, and rodent. Moreover, the withdrawal response precipitated by an antagonist is used as a rapid diagnostic test for narcotic dependence (20, 40) since the evidence can be obtained within minutes instead of hours as required in abrupt withdrawal.

The withdrawal syndrome occurring in the narcotic addict is believed to be a counter adaptive response to the effects resulting from frequent repeated administrations of high doses of a narcotic. As a consequence of bodily adjustments to maintain homeostasis, a state of rebound latent hyperexcitability occurs when a prolonged drug-induced depression is suddenly terminated by abrupt discontinuance of the drug (12, 28, 39). The precise anatomic sites and biochemical mechanisms involved have not been elucidated, but the topic has been the subject of several reviews (4, 5, 12, 16, 21, 34, 39). In recent years, studies in this area have been greatly facilitated by procedures for rapid induction of physical dependence on morphine and by the narcotic antagonists, which have reduced the observation period of the withdrawal state and magnified certain abstinence signs to an intensity that allows for their quantitative measurement. Although it is recognized that the mechanisms involved in abrupt abstinence and precipitated abstinence are not identical in many details, the resemblance is such that most workers have used antagonist-precipitated abstinence for studying physical dependence mechanisms. In order that proper perspective and meaning be gleaned from such studies, therefore, it is important to study the many facets of antagonist-precipitated withdrawal responses. The studies to be described summarize much of the work that is being carried out in our laboratories along these lines.

INDUCTION OF DEPENDENCE IN RODENTS

Many investigators have used the mouse or rat for assessing physical dependence on morphine because the procedures are simple and inexpensive. The animal model appears to have validity since the classic effects of morphine such as analgesia (antinociception), tolerance, and physical dependence can easily be demonstrated in both species. In the past, quantitative studies of the abstinence syndrome have been limited because frequent repeated injections of high doses of morphine over a prolonged period were required to render the animals sufficiently dependent. In recent years the subcutaneous pellet implantation procedure described by Huidobro and Maggiolo has been widely used to produce physical dependence (15). Using a modified pellet, we have been able to accelerate markedly the development of dependence and obtain a high degree of physical dependence (32, 33).

The pellet consists of morphine base, 75 mg; microcrystalline cellulose, 75 mg; fumed silicon dioxide, 0.75 mg; and calcium stearate, 1.5 mg. The size of the tablet is 3 mm and the hardness 15 Strong Cobb units (10).

Implantation of the pellet results in detectable dependence within a few hours but the effect is not maximal until 3 days after implantation. Physical dependence on morphine can be noted after removal of the pellet by characteristic signs of withdrawal or by the loss in body weight (1, 13, 14). However, more dramatic signs are manifested by precipitating withdrawal with the narcotic antagonist naloxone (13, 33, 36). The withdrawal signs after abrupt precipitated withdrawal in both the mouse and rat are similar, but, like in man, after precipitated withdrawal, the signs are more rapid in onset, of greater intensity, and of much shorter duration.

NALOXONE-PRECIPITATED WITHDRAWAL

Precipitated abstinence in the morphine-dependent mouse is characterized by defecation, urination, sniffing, increased motor activity with exploratory behavior, tremors, sometimes convulsions (32, 33), and most characteristically by stereotyped jumping (32, 33).

Precipitated abstinence in the rat has been studied in several laboratories. The reports have been previously cited (37). The syndrome is characterized by hyperactivity within the first minute consisting of rearing on the hind legs, sniffing, and exploratory behavior. This is soon followed by hypernea, ear blanching, teeth chattering, and wet shakes. The animal will immediately leap out when placed in a jar (escape attempts) and may exhibit stereotyped jumping similar to the mouse when placed on a platform. After approximately 5 min, rhinorrea, abnormal posturing, salivation, swallowing movements, vocalization upon touching, and ptosis are usually observable. Diarrhea generally occurs after 10 min. Less frequent signs are exopthalmos, chromodacryorrhea, penile erection, and seminal emission (37).

ASSESSMENT OF PHYSICAL DEPENDENCE BY NALOXONE-PRECIPITATED WITHDRAWAL

A point scoring system may be used to measure the degree of dependence, but dependence can also be quantified on an all or none basis by estimating the naloxone ED_{50} to produce a given withdrawal sign (13, 33, 36). In selecting only one sign of withdrawal for assessing dependence intensity, consideration must always be given to the possibility that any experimental manipulation of the dependent state might selectively affect only the withdrawal sign and not the total syndrome. This criticism can be met by using several withdrawal signs for quantal assay of dependence with naloxone. If the total dependent state is altered by some experimental maneuver, parallel changes in the naloxone ED_{50} should be effected in all the behavioral parameters that are assessed provided, of course, that a particular withdrawal sign is not selectively altered by the maneuver. In the rat, the more reliable indexes of precipitated abstinence are diarrhea, abnormal posturing, ear blanching, swallowing movements, teeth chattering, escape attempts, and wet shakes. The latter two signs, while highly characteristic, require higher doses of naloxone to elicit (37). In the mouse, by far the most striking response of precipitated withdrawal is the stereotyped jumping behavior (32, 33).

STEREOTYPED JUMPING AND NALOXONE ED_{50} AS INDEXES FOR DEPENDENCE ASSESSMENT

The degree of physical dependence on morphine can be assessed without removal of the pellet by estimating the amount of naloxone needed to precipitate jumping. Using jumping from a circular platform as a quantal response to varying doses of naloxone, the median effective dose of naloxone (ED_{50}) can easily be determined. An inverse relationship exists between the two parameters; the higher the degree of dependence, the lower the naloxone ED_{50}. Jumping does not occur in mice not dependent on morphine even after toxic doses of naloxone. Although the jumping response was not elicited by 12 mg/kg of naloxone in animals challenged immediately after implantation, the dose of naloxone required to elicit the effect became progressively less with increasing implantation time, as shown in Fig. 1. It was possible to precipitate jumping with naloxone after only 3 hr of implantation but the dose required was 70 times that after 72 hr. At 3 hr after pellet implantation, the naloxone ED_{50} was 3.2 mg/kg and after 72 hr it decreased to 0.045 mg/kg (33).

It was possible to decrease or increase the amount of naloxone for precipitating the abstinence syndrome by removing the morphine pellet and selecting the time for naloxone challenge. Less naloxone was required to elicit withdrawal jumping when the animals were tested at a time (8 to 12 hr after pellet removal) when abstinence was maximal after abrupt withdrawal. Conversely, more naloxone was required if the animals were challenged

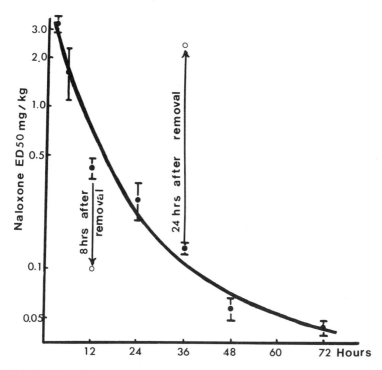

FIG. 1. Relationship of the degree of physical dependence to the duration of implant of a morphine pellet as measured by the amount of naloxone required to precipitate withdrawal jumping in the mouse (32). Filled circles indicate experiments on implanted mice without removal of the morphine pellet. Open circle on the same group after removal of the pellet.

24 hr after pellet removal when dependence to morphine had largely subsided. For example, in the 12-hr implanted group which exhibited a naloxone ED_{50} of 0.42 (0.36 to 0.48) mg/kg, removal of the pellet and retesting 8 hr later resulted in a fourfold decrease in the ED_{50} to 0.10 (0.079 to 0.127) mg/kg. On the other hand, in a group of mice implanted for 36 hr, the naloxone ED_{50} was 0.135 (.123 to .148) mg/kg; removal of the pellet and retesting with naloxone after 24 hr yielded nearly a 20-fold increase in the ED_{50} to 2.4 (1.85 to 3.2) mg/kg (33).

ANATOMICAL CORRELATES OF NALOXONE-PRECIPITATED WITHDRAWAL

The neuroanatomical areas related to the abstinence syndrome have not been clearly defined. It can be concluded from studies by various investigators (8, 11, 18, 22, 31, 41) that dependence on morphine can develop in many loci within the central nervous system, although the degrees of sensitivity to morphine effects may vary. Kerr and Pozuelo reported that withdrawal signs, precipitated by opioid antagonists in the morphine-dependent rat, were suppressed or markedly reduced when a major part of the ventromedial nucleus of the hypothalamus had been lesioned. Herz and his associates (11) postulated that structures in the caudal brainstem, most probably in the floor of the fourth ventricle, are important substrates for the development of dependence on morphine. In experiments utilizing the application of crystalline naloxone hydrochloride to discrete brain areas of the morphine-dependent rat, we find the thalamus to be one of the, if not the, most sensitive regions for precipitating withdrawal (35, 37).

A 20 gauge stainless steel guide cannula, filed to a predetermined length, was stereotaxically implanted into the left hemisphere of the rat brain under ether anesthesia. One to 5 days later, dependence on morphine was induced by the subcutaneous implantation of a morphine pellet. To precipitate withdrawal, naloxone hydrochloride was applied to the brain 70 to 76 hr after pellet implantation. An inner cannula, 0.5 mm longer than the guide cannula, was tamped in crystalline naloxone hydrochloride and inserted into the guide cannula. Although the precise amount of naloxone delivered to brain tissue in this manner cannot be ascertained, the treatment was uniformly administered to all animals and the procedure successfully discriminated between brain areas of relative sensitivity.

The abstinence syndrome precipitated by application of naloxone to the brain is very similar to that described earlier after systemic administration of naloxone in morphine-dependent rats. Abstinence signs which are dose dependent on naloxone, such as diarrhea, ear blanching, abnormal posturing, ptosis, teeth chattering, escape attempts, and wet shakes, appear within 10 min after cerebral application of naloxone in sensitive areas. Since leaping attempts to escape from the jar and wet shakes represent distinctive abstinence behavior and a high degree of physical dependence, their neuroanatomical correlates were investigated. The naloxone ED_{50} for precipitating wet shakes and escape attempts is five to 10 times greater than for the other abstinence signs. If a rat made two or more escape attempts or had three or more wet shakes within 10 min after cerebral application of naloxone, it was considered to have undergone precipitated withdrawal. Under identical experimental conditions, cerebral application of naloxone hydrochloride to the thalamus of six nondependent rats did not induce the abstinence syndrome. At the termination of these experiments, the animals were sacrificed and the site of the cannula tip was determined by gross microscopic dissection, and the stereotaxic atlas by Konig and Klippel (19) was used as the reference guide to locate the anatomical sites.

The areas in the brain that were studied are illustrated in Fig. 2. The abstinence syndrome was most frequently evoked in and around the medial thalamic nuclei (area 3a and Table 1). The region surrounding the parafascicularis nucleus, in particular, was sensitive to naloxone-precipitated withdrawal. Application of naloxone to lateral thalamic nuclei did not precipitate withdrawal (area 3b and Table 1), but positive responses were obtained in area 4 which is 1 to 1.5 mm caudal to the parafascicularis nucleus. Neocortical (area 1) and hippocampal (area 2) areas above the thalamus, as well as medial mesencephalic (area 5) and hypothalamic (area 6) regions, were not responsive to naloxone-precipitated withdrawal.

It should be noted that only selected acute abstinence signs were systematically investigated. Although we chose to observe escape attempts and wet shakes, other abstinence signs such as teeth chattering, diarrhea, and ear blanching appeared to increase, both in frequency and intensity, in the proximity of the sensitive thalamic structures. However, other abstinence signs may develop in neural elements which are not exclusively located in the forebrain. For example, the spinal cord may be involved in the persistence of some withdrawal signs described by Martin et al. as the chronic abstinence syndrome (22).

Recent histochemical (25, 29) and physiological (23) studies of the medial thalamic nuclei provide a basis which indicates that these nuclei may be the site for some of the action of morphine. The medial thalamic nuclei may be

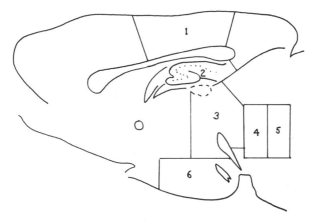

FIG. 2. Areas of precipitated abstinence in morphine-dependent rats. The figure represents a sagittal section of the rat brain, 0.4 mm lateral to the midline (35).

TABLE 1. *Areas of precipitated abstinence in morphine-dependent rats*

Anatomical areas	No. in Fig. 1	Medial-lateral extension of area (mm)	No. of rats	No. exhibiting severe abstinence
Neocortex	1	0–2.0	9	1
Hippocampus	2	0–3.0	12	0
Thalamus	3	0–2.0	21	20
Medial thalamus	4	0–1.4	20	9

Diencephalic-
  mesencephalic
  junctures
	5	0–1.5	20	13

Mesencephalon	6	0–2.5	16	0
Hypothalamus	7	0–2.0	7	0

From Wei et al. (35)

part of the neural circuitry which mediates the effect component of pain perception (17). Olds (24) and Stein (30) have shown that electrical or cholinergic stimulation of medial diencephalic structures has negative reinforcing properties on behavior. The centrum medianum-parafascicularis nucleus in the medial thalamus receives cholinergic innervation from the tegmentum (27) and also has a relatively high cholinesterase activity (25). It has been known for some time that morphine inhibits the release of acetylcholine in nervous tissue and that opioid antagonists reverse this inhibition (26). If morphine should act by inhibiting the release of acetylcholine in medial thalamic nuclei, depending upon the circuitry, the pharmacologic consequences could be excitatory or inhibitory. Since naloxone-precipitated withdrawal jumping is suppressed by cholinesterase inhibition, elevation of acetylcholine appears to have an inhibitory effect on this response.

BIOCHEMICAL CORRELATES OF NALOXONE-PRECIPITATED WITHDRAWAL JUMPING

Many studies have been made trying to implicate the pharmacologic effects of morphine and its surrogates on the bioamines in the central nervous system. The approach has been based on the premise that the amines have transmitter functions in the brain and on the knowledge that the disposition of the amines in the brain can be influenced by narcotics. Particular interest in dopamine in the tolerant and dependent state has been stimulated by the findings of Clouet and Ratner who observed that its turnover is increased after morphine but tolerance develops to this effect after repeated morphine administration (3).

In order to assess the roles of the biogenic amines in stereotyped jumping behavior precipitated by naloxone in morphine-dependent mice, dopamine (DM), norepinephrine (NE), and serotonin (5HT) were estimated in mice 0, 2, 5, and 10 min after administering naloxone. Brain DM levels suddenly increased after naloxone administration while NE and 5HT were not affected. Figure 3 shows the brain levels of 5HT, DM, and NE in mice injected with naloxone, 5 mg/kg, s.c. Brain levels of DM were increased almost 30% above control values after naloxone injection; the increased levels were evident at 2 min and remained elevated at 10 min after naloxone injection. Placebo-implanted control mice did not exhibit the increase in brain DM after naloxone injection. A 0.5 mg/kg dose of naloxone caused less increase in DM (+ 15%) whereas 10 mg/kg of naloxone was no more effective than 5 mg/kg.

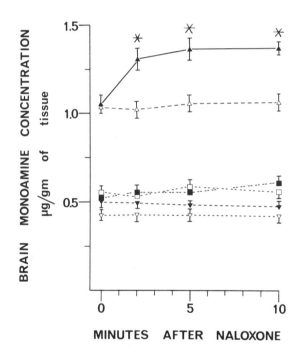

MINUTES AFTER NALOXONE

FIG. 3. Levels of brain monoamines in morphine-dependent mice at various intervals after the injection of naloxone. Naloxone (5 mg/kg, s.c.) was given 6 hr after pellet removal in 72-hr morphine- and placebo-implanted mice which were sacrificed at various times after injection. ▲———▲, DM levels in morphine-implanted mice. △— — —△, DM levels in placebo-implanted mice. ■— — — ■, 5-HT levels in morphine-implanted mice. □— — —□, 5-HT levels in placebo-implanted mice. ▼— — —▼, NE levels in morphine-implanted mice. ▽— — —▽, NE levels in placebo-implanted mice. Each point represents the mean monoamine level in three experiments using four mice each. The vertical lines represent ± S.E.M. *, significantly different from placebo-implanted control, $p < .01$.

A study of distribution of biogenic amines during naloxone-precipitated withdrawal in tissue from four brain areas indicated that a sudden increase occurred in the mouse cortex striatum. Figure 4 shows the disposition of 5HT, NE, and DM in mouse cortex striatum, brainstem, cerebellum, and hypothalamus at 0, 5, 10, and 20 min after naloxone, 5 mg/kg, s.c. The cortex striatum, which had the highest concentration of DM, 2.1 μg/gm, also showed the greatest relative change in DM concentration following naloxone. A 25% increase in DM levels was observed 10 min after naloxone

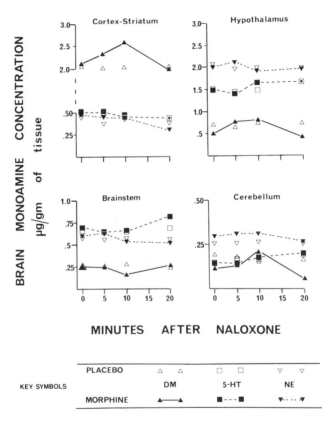

FIG. 4. Monoamine levels in various brain regions of morphine-dependent mice after naloxone challenge. Naloxone (5 mg/kg, s.c.) was administered 6 hr after pellet removal in 72-hr morphine- or placebo-implanted mice. Each point represents a single determination from two pooled cortical hemispheres and striata, three pooled brainstems, seven pooled cerebella, or 10 pooled hypothalami. The average weights in mg ± S.D. of each of the pooled brain areas were cortex striatum (including the hippocampus), 396 ± 43; brainstem (thalamus, corpora quadragemini, medulla, and pons), 352 ± 46; hypothalamic area, 226 ± 38; and cerebellum, 420 ± 51 (N equals eight for each pooled area).

injection and the response subsided 10 min later. Placebo-implanted control mice did not exhibit the increase in brain DM after naloxone. 5HT and NE concentrations did not change appreciably in any of the brain regions investigated in either morphine or placebo-implanted animals.

In the rat a similar response was noted. A large increase in brain DM occurred in the corpus striatum after the administration of naloxone in morphine-implanted, but not in placebo-implanted, rats. Levels of DM in morphine-implanted rats rose to almost 50% above control values 20 min after the naloxone challenge whereas the levels in placebo-implanted animals remained unaltered. Again, 5HT and NE were not altered appreciably in either placebo- or morphine-implanted animals.

Biogenic amine levels were compared in jumping and nonjumping dependent mice after naloxone-precipitated withdrawal. Eleven out of 15 mice jumped after receiving naloxone, 1 mg/kg, during the 10-min observation period. Brain DM was determined in the four nonjumpers and four out of 11 jumpers selected at random. Additionally, four mice were selected from a group of 10 dependent mice which did not jump when given saline instead of naloxone. DM levels were found to increase in dependent mice that jumped after administration of naloxone but not in nonjumpers. Table 2 summarizes the levels of biogenic amines in morphine-implanted mice receiving saline or naloxone 6 hr after pellet removal. The level of brain DM in the mice that jumped was almost 20% greater than either the saline control or the group that did not jump. Brain levels of 5HT and NE remained the same.

To rule out the possibility that the DM increase caused by naloxone in

TABLE 2. *Brain monoamine levels in morphine-dependent nonjumping and jumping mice[a] following a naloxone challenge*

Treatment	Group designation	DM	NE	5-HT
		μg/gm $\pm$ S.E.M.[b] (N = 4)		
Saline	Nonjumpers	1.04 ± 0.07	0.42 ± 0.01	0.55 ± 0.01
Naloxone	Nonjumpers	1.03 ± 0.05	0.41 ± 0.01	0.58 ± 0.01
	Jumpers	1.22 ± 0.07[c]	0.43 ± 0.01	0.58 ± 0.01

[a] Mice were implanted with a pellet of morphine, s.c., for 72 hr. Six hr after pellet removal, the animals were given an s.c. injection of either saline or naloxone, 1 mg/kg, and the mice that jumped within 10 min were separated from the nonjumpers.

[b] Mice were sacrificed 10 min after saline or naloxone injection.

[c] Significantly different from the nonjumpers receiving either naloxone or saline, $p < .05$.

dependent animals was caused by the act of jumping, D-tubocurarine was administered to effect paralysis by neuromuscular blockade. It was found that although the jumping response was blocked by D-tubocurarine, it did not prevent the increase in brain DM. Comparisons were made in morphine-implanted mice pretreated with either saline or D-tubocurarine (0.25 mg/kg, i.p.) 15 min before a challenge of either saline or naloxone, 5 mg/kg, s.c., and sacrificed 5 min later. D-Tubocurarine *per se* did not alter the steady-state concentrations of any of the biogenic amines, and, after naloxone, the increase in DM which resulted (20%) was nearly identical with that of the noncurarized group which exhibited a 100% incidence of jumping after naloxone. Brain 5HT and NE levels remained unaltered in all groups of mice. Thus, although jumping may be associated with an increase in DM, the response itself did not affect the increase in DM that occurred during naloxone-precipitated jumping.

Participation of cholinergic pathways in the naloxone-precipitated jumping response was demonstrated in a previous study in this laboratory. Inhibition of cholinesterase by physostigmine or diisopropylfluorophosphate greatly attenuated the jumping response (2). This was confirmed by a repeat of these experiments and, in addition, brain amine levels were determined (2). It was found that physostigmine not only inhibited the jumping response but also that the sudden increase in brain DM did not occur.

Recent reports (9, 27) have supported the view that stereotyped behavior is caused by an increase in neostriatal (caudate nucleus and putamen) dopamine neuronal activity. Systemic injection of L-DOPA in combination with a peripheral DOPA decarboxylase inhibitor produces stereotyped sniffing behavior; repeated doses of L-DOPA produce vigorous biting behavior in rats (9). The stereotyped behavior after amphetamine (sniffing, licking, and biting) was attributed to cerebral dopamine (27). Dopamine receptor stimulation via intraneostriatal injection of apomorphine in the rat was found to produce stereotyped forward walking, sniffing, licking, or biting (6, 9). Very high doses of L-DOPA have been found to produce fighting and jumping behavior in mice (7). When apomorphine was given to rats intravenously, stereotyped behavior, described as "cliff jumping," was observed (38). Thus, the stereotyped jumping behavior observed after a naloxone challenge in morphine-dependent mice and rats appears to have behavioral and biochemical characteristics in common with the stereotyped jumping produced by various other pharmacological agents.

The possibility that a cholinergic-dopaminergic interaction may be involved in the jumping syndrome is suggested not only by our observation that inhibition of naloxone-induced withdrawal jumping by physostigmine also resulted in blockade of the sudden increase in brain dopamine but by other work in the literature. Shute and Lewis (29) have reported a dense cholinergic innervation of the neostriatum, and, as pointed out by Randrup and Munkvad (27), dopamine and cholinergic paths to the neostriatum are probably antagonistic in function. The efficacy of anticholinergic drugs for treating parkinsonism, in which there is a dopamine deficiency, is well known. Hence, it appears conceivable that an elevation of acetylcholine levels acts to antagonize dopamine-induced stereotyped jumping in morphine-dependent mice.

The present study defines only one sign of antagonist-precipitated withdrawal in narcotic dependence and does not provide the mechanism of abstinence. The withdrawal syndrome consists of a constellation of signs and symptoms which involve many sites and pathways in the central nervous system, as well as several neurotransmitters. A particular abstinence sign represents merely the end response of a very complicated manifestation, but knowledge of its basis contributes in a small way to the ultimate understanding of physical dependence processes.

ACKNOWLEDGMENTS

The studies described were supported largely by U.S. Public Health Service grants RG-01839, MH-17017, DA-00564, and MH-19944.

REFERENCES

1. Akera, T., and Brody, T. M.: The addiction cycle to narcotics in the rat and its relation to catecholamines. Biochem. Pharmacol. *17*:675–688, 1968.
2. Bhargava, H. N., and Way, E. Leong: Acetylcholinesterase inhibition and morphine effects in morphine tolerant and dependent mice. J. Pharmacol. Exp. Ther. *183*:31–40, 1972.
3. Clouet, D. H., and Ratner, M.: Catecholamine biosynthesis in brains of rats treated with morphine. Science *168*:854–856, 1970.
4. Clouet, D. H.: Theoretical biochemical mechanisms for drug dependence. *In:* Chemical and Biological Aspects of Drug Dependence, edited by S. J. Mule and H. Brill, pp. 545–561. CRC Press, Cleveland, 1972.
5. Cochin, J.: Possible mechanisms in development of tolerance. Fed. Proc. *29*:19–32, 1970.
6. Ernst, A. M., and Smelik, P. G.: Site of action of dopamine and apomorphine in compulsive gnawing behavior in rats. Experientia *12*:837–838, 1966.
7. Everett, G. M., and Borcherding, J. W.: L-Dopa: Effect on concentrations of dopamine, norepinephrine, and serotonin in brains of mice. Science *168*:849–850, 1970.
8. Foltz, E. L., and White, L. E.: Modification of morphine withdrawal by frontal lobe cingulum lesions. *In:* First International Congress of Neurological Sciences, edited by L. Von Bogaert and Z. Radermeker, pp. 163–168. Pergamon Press, London, 1959.
9. Fuxe, K., and Ungerstedt, U.: Interaction of amphetamines with biogenic amines: Histochemical, biochemical and functional studies on central monoamine neurons after acute and chronic amphetamine administration. *In:* Amphetamines and Related Compounds, edited by E. Costa and S. Garattini, pp. 257–288. Raven Press, New York, 1970.

10. Gibson, R. D., and Tingstad, J. E.: Formulation of morphine implantation pellet suitable for tolerance-physical studies in mice. J. Pharm. Sci. *59*: 426–427, 1970.
11. Herz, A.: Central nervous sites of action of morphine in dependent and non-dependent rabbits. Fifth International Congress on Pharmacology, San Francisco, 1972.
12. Himmelsbach, C. K.: With reference to physical dependence. Fed. Proc. *2*:201–203, 1943.
13. Ho, I. K., Lu, S. E., Stolman, S., Loh, H. H., and Way, E. Leong: Influence of p-chlorophenylalanine on morphine tolerance and physical dependence and regional serotonin turnover studies in morphine tolerant-dependent mice. J. Pharmacol. Exp. Ther. *182*:155–165, 1972.
14. Hosoya, E.: Some withdrawal symptoms of rats to morphine. Pharmacologist *1*:77, 1959.
15. Huidobro, F., and Maggiolo, C.: Some features of the abstinence syndrome to morphine in mice. Acta Physiol. Latinoamer. *18*:201–209, 1961.
16. Jaffe, J. H., and Sharpless, S. K.: Pharmacologic denervation supersensitivity in the central nervous system: A theory of physical dependence. *In:* The Addictive States, edited by A. Wikler, pp. 226–246. Williams and Wilkins, Baltimore, 1968.
17. Jasper, H.: *In:* Brain Mechanisms and Consciousness, edited by E. Adrian, H. Bremer, and H. Jasper, p. 374. Blackwell Scientific Publication, Oxford, 1954; Papez, J. W.: Electroencephalogr. Clin. Neurophysiol. *8*:117, 1956.
18. Kerr, F. L., and Pozuelo, J.: Suppression of physical dependence and induction of hyperthalamic lesions in addicted rats. Proc. Mayo Clinic *46*:653–665, 1971.
19. Konig, J. F. R., and Klippel, R. A.: The Rat Brain: A Stereotaxic Atlas of the Forebrain and Lower Parts of the Brain Stem. Williams and Wilkins, Baltimore, 1963.
20. Martin, W. R.: Opioid antagonists. Pharmacol. Rev. *19*:464–521, 1967.
21. Martin, W. R.: Pharmacological redundancy as an adaptive mechanism in the central nervous system. Fed. Proc. *29*:13–27, 1970.
22. Martin, W. R., and Eades, C. G.: A comparison between acute and chronic physical dependence in the chronic spinal dog. J. Pharmacol. Exp. Ther. *146*:385–394, 1964.
23. Mizoguchi, K., and Mitchell, C. L.: An evaluation of the effects of morphine on electrocortical recruitment in the cat and dog. J. Pharmacol. Exp. Ther. *166*:134–145, 1969.
24. Olds, M. E., and Olds, J.: Approach-avoidance analysis of rat diencephalon. J. Comp. Neurol. *120*:259–295, 1963.
25. Olivier, A., Parent, A., and Poirier, L. J.: Identification of the thalamic nuclei on the basis of their cholinesterase content in the monkey. J. Anat. *106*:37–50, 1970.
26. Jhamandas, K., Phillis, J. W., and Pinsky, C.: Effects of narcotic analgesics and antagonists on the *in vivo* release of acetylcholine from the cerebral cortex of the cat. Brit. J. Pharmacol. *43*:53–66, 1971.
27. Randrup, A., and Munkvad, I.: Behavioural stereotypes induced by pharmacological agents. Pharmakopsychiatrie Neuro-Psychopharmakologie *1*:18–26, 1968.
28. Seevers, M. H.: Characteristics of dependence on and abuse of psychoactive drugs. *In:* Chemical and Biological Aspects of Drug Dependence, edited by S. J. Mule and H. Brill, pp. 13–21. CRC Press, Cleveland, 1972.
29. Shute, C. C. D., and Lewis, P. R.: The ascending cholinergic reticular systems: Neocortical, olfactory and subcortical projections. Brain *90*:497–519, 1967.
30. Stein, L.: *In:* Psychopharmacology, A Review of Progress, 1957–1967, edited by D. H. Efron, pp. 105–124. Public Health Service Publication No. 1836, 1968.
31. Trafton, C. L., and Marques, P. R.: Effects of septal area and cingulate cortex lesions on opiate addiction behavior in rats. J. Comp. Physiol. Psychol. *75*:277–285, 1971.
32. Way, E. Leong, Loh, H. H., and Shen, F. H.: Morphine tolerance, physical dependence and synthesis of brain 5-hydroxytryptamine. Science *162*:1290–1292, 1968.
33. Way, E. Leong, Loh, H. H., and Shen, F. H.: Simultaneous quantitative assessment of morphine tolerance and physical dependence. J. Pharmacol. Exp. Ther. *167*:1–8, 1969.
34. Way, E. Leong, and Shen, Fu-Hsiung: The effect of narcotic analgesic drugs on specific systems: Catecholamines and 5-hydroxytryptamine. *In:* Narcotic Drugs: Biochemical Pharmacology, edited by D. H. Clouet, pp. 229–253. Plenum Press, New York, 1971.

35. Wei, Eddie, Loh, Horace H., and Way, E. Leong: Neuroanatomical correlation of morphine dependence. Science *177*:616–617, 1972.
36. Wei, Eddie, Loh, Horace H., and Way, E. Leong: Brain sites of precipitated abstinence in morphine-dependent rats. J. Pharmacol. Exp. Ther. *185*:108–115, 1973.
37. Wei, Eddie, Loh, Horace H., and Way, E. Leong: Quantitative aspects of precipitated abstinence in morphine-dependent rats. J. Pharmacol. Exp. Ther. *184*:398–403, 1973.
38. Weissman, A.: Cliff jumping in rats after intravenous treatment with apomorphine. Psychopharmacologia *21*:60–65, 1971.
39. Wikler, A.: Theories related to physical dependence. *In:* Chemical and Biological Aspects of Drug Dependence, edited by S. J. Mule and H. Brill, pp. 359–377. CRC Press, Cleveland, 1972.
40. Wikler, A., Fraser, H. F., and Isbell, H.: N-Allylnormorphine: Effects of single doses and precipitation of "abstinence syndromes" during addiction to morphine, methadone or heroin in man (post-addicts). J. Pharmacol. Exp. Ther. *109*:8–20, 1953.
41. Wikler, A., Rescor, M. J., Kalbaugh, E. P., and Angelucci, R. J.: Effects of frontal lobotomy on the morphine abstinence syndrome in man. Arch. Neurol. *67*:510–521, 1952.

Narcotic Antagonists, edited by M. C. Braude, L. S. Harris, E. L. May, J. P. Smith, and J. E. Villarreal. *Advances in Biochemical Psychopharmacology, Vol. 8.* Raven Press, New York © 1974.

Interactions of Narcotic Antagonists with Receptor Sites

Avram Goldstein

Addiction Research Laboratory, Department of Pharmacology, Stanford University, Stanford, California 94305

Evidence is summarized, from the work of others, indicating that narcotic antagonists occupy receptor sites passively and reversibly, whereas agonists occupy the same sites actively, promoting conformation change in the receptor. A derivative conclusion is that narcotic receptor sites do not ordinarily interact with any essential endogenous substrate such as a neurotransmitter. The receptor, however, could have two sites — one for an endogenous substrate, the other an allosteric site interacting with narcotic agonists and antagonists. A method is described whereby the interaction of naloxone with brain proteolipid can be followed and compared with the similar interactions of levorphanol. The system may be conducive to obtaining direct evidence about induced conformational change. The guinea pig ileum longitudinal muscle-myenteric plexus preparation from tolerant-dependent guinea pigs is tolerant to morphine and also to catecholamines, is supersensitive to serotonin, and has unchanged sensitivity to acetylcholine. An interpretation of these findings is offered, explaining the basis of tolerance and dependence. Some receptors in the central nervous system, which are responsible for precipitated withdrawal caused by naloxone, have different kinetic properties from those that mediate various acute effects of the narcotics. The interaction between naloxone and these receptors is noncompetitive with respect to narcotic agonists. A well-known discrepancy between the duration of action of methadone as an agonist and as a suppressor of withdrawal points in the same direction.

I. INTRODUCTION

Narcotic antagonists have two main effects — blockade or reversal of the actions of narcotic agonists, and precipitation of acute withdrawal phenomena in dependent animals or man. I shall consider in this chapter the relationship between these two effects, and what they imply about narcotic receptor sites. The availability of naloxone, a pure antagonist devoid of the mixed agonist-antagonist effects displayed by such compounds as nalorphine and levallorphan, has made possible a more unambiguous interpretation than before.

II. BLOCKING EFFECTS OF THE ANTAGONISTS

In order to discuss the interactions between agonists or antagonists and the narcotic receptors, I will first introduce and define two terms: *passive interaction* and *active interaction*. A *passive interaction* between a receptor and a ligand is typified by the class of enzyme inhibitors that act by merely occupying the enzyme active center. If the interaction is reversible, they are likely to be competitive inhibitors; if irreversible, they will be noncompetitive. In either case, occupancy of the active center is a sufficient condition for the drug action. Moreover, a significant fraction of the total active centers must be occupied; otherwise no significant change in the substrate flux can result. An *active interaction* is one in which the ligand brings about a conformational change in the receptor, as with allosteric enzyme inhibitors or activators. Here site occupancy is a necessary but not sufficient condition for manifesting the drug action. In the case of allosteric effects upon enzymes, significant fractional occupancy is again necessary, since stoichiometry dictates a low ratio (often 1:1) of substrate sites to allosteric sites.

Allosteric effects on other kinds of receptor can be manifested, in principle, at low fractional occupancy. One can imagine a conformational change in only one out of many thousand receptors in a membrane, which would be sufficient to depolarize that membrane. At a nerve terminal this could directly cause the release of neurotransmitter; at a dendritic process or neuronal cell body it could initiate a propagated impulse. Pharmacologic action due to an effect upon a small fraction of a receptor pool has been postulated in theory (26, 29, 36) and is supported by recent evidence on the acetylcholine receptor (2, 25).

The opiate antagonists provide us with important evidence concerning the interactions with narcotic receptors (24, 30, 31). The antagonists have exactly the same structures as the agonists, except for an allyl, cyclopropylmethyl, or other small substituent instead of methyl on the nitrogen atom. Moreover, the same high degree of stereospecificity is observed among the antagonists as among the agonists. In both cases only the D(−) isomers are active. Thus, dextrallorphan, the N-allyl analogue of dextrorphan [L(+)], is neither an agonist nor an antagonist (10), just as dextrorphan is devoid of agonistic properties. But levallorphan, the N-allyl analogue of levorphanol [D(−)], is an effective antagonist. Naloxone is the N-allyl analogue of the effective agonist, D(−)-oxymorphone. Furthermore, antagonists in the oripavine series, in which the agonists (such as etorphine) have very high potency, are also very potent (1, 12). Although alternatives have been advanced (24), it seems more likely, on the basis of the structure-activity relationships, that the antagonists and agonists can occupy the same receptor sites. This conclusion is strongly supported by the abundance of direct evidence showing that blocking actions of antagonists against a variety of narcotic agonist effects follow strictly competitive kinetics (23, 37).

These arguments lead to the logical conclusion that site occupancy is not a sufficient condition for producing narcotic effects, since naloxone occupies the site yet produces no effect. Clearly, site occupancy is the necessary and sufficient condition for antagonist effect, but something more is required for agonist effect. Consonant with modern biochemical concepts, we have to suppose that "something more" is the production of a conformational change. Thus, agonists interact *actively,* antagonists interact *passively* with the receptors.

A derivative conclusion may be drawn: the narcotic receptor sites have no dynamic ongoing function in the nervous system. By "sites" I mean the specialized topographic regions on the receptor macromolecules, which accommodate the ligand molecules. The distinction between a receptor and a receptor site is analogous to that between an enzyme and its active site. By "dynamic ongoing function" I mean a function upon which the normal status of the nervous system depends, and which requires the flux of some endogenous molecule through the site. If the site accepted a normal substrate (i.e., if it were an enzyme active center), or if it accepted a neurotransmitter (i.e., if it were a postsynaptic receptor site), site occupancy alone (e.g., by naloxone) would obviously disturb normal function. This is not the same as saying the receptor as a whole has no function. The receptor macromolecule could have two sites — one for interacting with an endogenous substrate or neurotransmitter, and a different (allosteric) site for interacting with narcotic agonists and antagonists. Then only the active interaction with an agonist would induce allosteric modification of the endogenous substrate or neurotransmitter site. Alternatively, the receptor could be a membrane protein with an essential role, but not ordinarily interacting with any endogenous compound. The essential point about all this is that the normal state of the receptor does not appear to be altered by its combination with naloxone, and that the altered state resulting from its combination with an agonist reverts to normal in the presence of naloxone.

Some experimental findings are not easily explained by simple mutual displacement of agonists and antagonists at the same sites; such difficulties led to the formulation of a "dual receptor" hypothesis (24). Let me cite a particularly striking example first noted in Kosterlitz's laboratory (8, 23) and repeatedly observed in our own work. In the guinea pig ileum longitudinal muscle-myenteric plexus preparation, some narcotic agonists depress the twitch amplitude for a long time (e.g., 1 hr or longer) despite repeated thorough washes. Addition of naloxone at any time during this period of prolonged inhibition restores the full twitch amplitude immediately. Washout of the naloxone results in a return to the inhibited state. Eventually, whether or not naloxone has been used, the twitch amplitude and sensitivity to agonists both return to normal. This finding is obviously not consistent with simple competitive displacement. Nevertheless, in the same tissue under the same conditions, classical competitive kinetics are observed, i.e., a constant ratio of antagonist to agonist concentration for a given degree of twitch inhibition.

The phenomenon described above resembles the classical atropine-acetylcholine antagonism, which is characterized by apparently competitive kinetics despite the well known very long duration of action of atropine. Acetylcholine seems to displace atropine from receptor sites, yet when the acetylcholine is removed, the atropine is clearly still present. This "atropine anomaly" (16) has been attributed to spare receptors, it being supposed that in addition to the receptors blocked by atropine, many more remain free and capable of being activated by combination with acetylcholine. Although this explanation may be tenable for a persistent antagonist, it clearly will not work for a persistent agonist. If the prolonged occupancy of sites by an opiate agonist produces a prolonged functional derangement, how could the occupancy of other (spare) receptors by an antagonist abolish the agonist effect, especially when the antagonist has no discernible action of its own?

There is a way out of the dilemma. If agonist molecules are not actually displaced from the receptor sites, it follows that the occupancy of free receptor sites by an antagonist must somehow alter the properties of the receptor, so as to nullify the functional impairment caused by agonist occupancy. This suggests a set of allosterically related sites, such as the four oxygen-binding sites of hemoglobin. The simplest model would be a dimer, with two identical sites capable of accommodating either agonist or antagonist molecules. This may be represented schematically, with M symbolizing an agonist (e.g., morphine), N an antagonist (e.g., naloxone), and R a receptor site:

$$R.R \quad + M = R.R\text{-}M$$
$$R.R\text{-}M + M = M\text{-}R.R\text{-}M \quad \Big\} - \text{agonist effect, receptor conformation altered}$$

$$R.R \quad + N = R.R\text{-}N$$
$$R.R\text{-}N + N = N\text{-}R.R\text{-}N \quad \Big\} - \text{no effect, receptor conformation normal}$$

$$\left.\begin{array}{l} R.R\text{-}M + N = N\text{-}R.R\text{-}M \\ R.R\text{-}N + M = M\text{-}R.R\text{-}N \end{array}\right\} \begin{array}{l} -\text{no effect (antagonism),} \\ \text{receptor conformation normal} \end{array}$$

I propose, in other words, that the reversible binding of antagonist to either site stabilizes the conformation of the dimeric receptor in its fully functional state. Prior binding of antagonist would prevent the conformational change otherwise induced by agonist binding to free receptor; and binding of antagonist to the agonist-receptor complex would return the receptor to its normal functional conformation. Such a model provides a chemical basis for the logical necessity outlined earlier. An appealing feature is that different kinds of receptor sites need not be postulated for the agonists and antagonists. Mixed agonist-antagonist properties (e.g., nalorphine) can also be rationalized within this conceptual framework.

I can now present some preliminary evidence about the binding of naloxone to brain extracts. We have been studying the binding of radioactive levorphanol to brain proteolipids, as described in previous publications (14, 15, 19, 28). Mouse brain is homogenized in chloroform-methanol (2:1). The extract is washed with one-fifth vol of water, reduced in volume under N_2, then incubated at room temperature with radioactive levorphanol or naloxone at concentrations in the pharmacologically effective range (0.1 to 1.0 μM). The material is placed on a Sephadex LH-20 column, on which separation occurs both by molecular size and by polarity (35). Elution is with increasing concentrations of methanol in the mixture with chloroform. Typical elution diagrams are shown in Fig. 1. In the upper diagram it can be seen that the bulk of the levorphanol emerges at approximately fraction 40, corresponding to the behavior of free levorphanol in control experiments. There is a distinct peak of radioactivity at fraction 20, toward the end of the pure chloroform elution. We have found, in other experiments, that levorphanol is bound stereospecifically in this peak. Moreover, the material responsible for the binding is ether precipitable, in this respect having the character of proteolipid protein rather than of many lipids.

Free naloxone emerges at fraction 14. There are at least three peaks representing bound naloxone, one of which is nearly coincidental with the peak of bound levorphanol.

When the chloroform-methanol extract was first incubated with a high concentration (10^{-3} M) of nonradioactive levorphanol, a precipitate formed, as described in an earlier publication (14). This was removed by centrifugation, and the supernatant solution was incubated with radioactive naloxone (10^{-6} M), as before, and then fractionated on a Sephadex LH-20 column

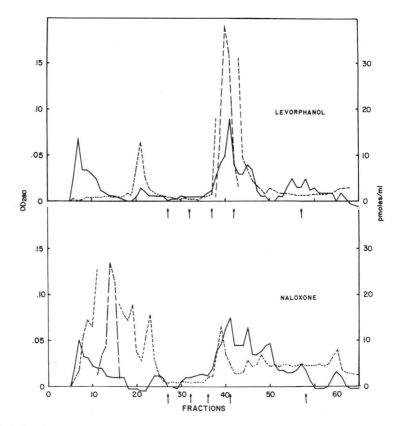

FIG. 1. Binding of levorphanol and naloxone to mouse brain proteolipids. Chloroform-methanol (2:1) extracts of mouse brain were washed with one-fifth vol of water, reduced in volume, incubated with radioactive levorphanol or naloxone, and fractionated on Sephadex LH-20 columns. Each 4-ml fraction was assayed for protein (optical density at 280 nm) and radioactivity. Initial elution was with chloroform, then at successive arrows with chloroform-methanol 15:1, 10:1, 6:1, 4:1, and 1:1. Solid lines = optical density 280. Broken lines = radioactivity; scale changed by a factor of 10 to accommodate the major peaks, as shown.

equilibrated with 10^{-3} M levorphanol. All eluting solutions contained the same concentration of levorphanol. Under these conditions, the peak of bound naloxone at fraction 23, which most nearly approximated the position of the bound levorphanol (cf. Fig. 1), was completely absent. Other naloxone peaks were virtually unaffected. It is likely, therefore, that naloxone competes for the same binding sites as levorphanol, although possible alternative interpretations have not yet been ruled out.

It is of interest that the behavior of the levorphanol-proteolipid complex on these columns is entirely different from that of the ligand-free proteolipid. When the brain extract was first fractionated on Sephadex LH-20, and the capacity of each fraction to bind levorphanol was studied separately by a phase-distribution procedure (40) two major binding peaks were found. One peak emerged very early in the elution pattern (at about fraction 7), the other quite late (at about fraction 37). There was no binding capacity in the region where the peak of bound levorphanol is seen in Fig. 1. On the other hand, as Fig. 1 shows, when the levorphanol and the extract were allowed to interact first, and then fractionated, no binding was seen near fraction 7, but bound complex emerged at fraction 20. This means that the complex has very different physical properties than the proteolipid alone, perhaps suggesting a conformation change induced by the ligand. Experiments are in progress to ascertain if naloxone alters the properties of the proteolipid in a similar way. Our hypothesis, that an agonist induces conformation change whereas an antagonist does not, could possibly be tested directly in this system.

III. ANTAGONIST EFFECTS IN THE TOLERANT-DEPENDENT STATE

A major question is whether or not precipitated withdrawal in dependent animals and man results from interaction of antagonists with the same receptors as in the blockade of acute agonist effects. Unitary theories have been proposed (5–7, 17, 18, 34) according to which changes in the number or properties of the narcotic receptors would account for both tolerance and dependence. These theories are supported by the findings that tolerance and dependence seem to develop and subside concurrently (3, 20, 39), and that both can be prevented by chronic treatment with antagonists (27) or inhibitors of protein synthesis (9, 38). An attractive and parsimonious feature of these theories is that they explain precipitated withdrawal as the natural consequence of an antagonist competitively reversing agonist effects at quantitatively or qualitatively altered receptor sites.

Direct evidence for altered receptor function in the tolerant-dependent state has been obtained recently by Schulz in my laboratory (32, 33). The electrically stimulated longitudinal muscle-myenteric plexus preparation from the guinea pig ileum is inhibited by very low concentrations of narcotics (22). Catecholamines act in the same way as morphine. Acetylcholine and serotonin are excitatory, causing contraction of the unstimulated strip. Naloxone blocks the morphine action competitively, has no effect of its own, and does not block the catecholamines, acetylcholine, or serotonin.

Preparations from guinea pigs made tolerant and dependent with morphine pellet implants were tolerant (six- to 10-fold) to morphine. In these tolerant strips, although there was no change in the sensitivity to exogenous acetylcholine, supersensitivity (10-fold) to exogenous serotonin was observed. At the same time, the strips were tolerant to exogenous catecholamines. Since extensive washing had removed morphine from these strips, we were not surprised to find that naloxone had no action of its own, although it effectively blocked the higher concentrations of morphine needed to inhibit the twitch.

We propose that the electrically stimulated twitch is mediated by the release of serotonin at a synapse, the postsynaptic element of which is the cholinergic neuron that innervates the muscle. We suggest that morphine acts by preventing the release of serotonin or its action upon the postsynaptic receptors, or both, and that the adaptive supersensitivity to serotonin may be responsible for both tolerance and dependence, as proposed by Collier (6). The demonstrated inhibition of tryptophan hydroxylase by morphine, and the adaptive increase of enzyme activity after chronic morphine administration (21) may also play a role here. *In vivo*, with normal parasympathetic stimulation, naloxone would evoke hyperexcitability by abolishing the morphine inhibition. In the morphine-free isolated preparation, this result would not be obtained, but the supersensitivity itself would be revealed by application of exogenous serotonin.

Withdrawal effects precipitated by naloxone *in vivo* are evidently mediated, at least in part, by a central mechanism, as shown by Eidelberg and Barstow (13) in monkeys, and more recently by Wei et al. (41) in rats. The central receptors for this action may have different kinetic properties from those (both central and peripheral) mediating the usual agonist effects. One such indication is found in the experiments of Cheney (4), showing that, in contrast to the well-established competitive antagonism of opiate effects by naloxone, the precipitation of withdrawal in dependent mice was noncompetitive. Dependence was measured quantitatively by determining the ED_{50} for naloxone-precipitated jumping activity. When levorphanol was injected every 8 hr, a steady state of dependence was eventually established. Each levorphanol injection was followed by a decrease in the naloxone ED_{50} (i.e., increase in dependence). This effect developed fully in a few hours, then wore off again, to return to the initial level at the end of the 8-hr interval, when the next levorphanol injection was due. If naloxone displaced levorphanol competitively from receptor sites involved in the precipitated withdrawal, it should have required a great deal more naloxone to elicit jumping activity after a levorphanol injection (when the brain was flooded with levorphanol) than before. No such effect was observed. The naloxone ED_{50} was virtually the same (actually somewhat lower) after a levorphanol injection as it was just before a levorphanol injection, even though the measured brain concentration of levorphanol was 12 times higher after levorphanol than before. In man, too, it had been observed that a withdrawal syndrome precipitated by an antagonist could not be terminated by administering large doses of a narcotic (42).

Finally, there is an old paradox concerning the duration of action of methadone, which may also bear upon this question. The early studies with this narcotic in man (11) showed clearly that its duration of action after systemic administration was almost identical to that of morphine, at equi-effective doses. Analgesia, pupillary constriction, and sedation were the effects measured. On the other hand, the duration of action of this drug in suppressing withdrawal symptoms is clearly very much longer than that of morphine; indeed, this is the main reason for its use in narcotic detoxi-fication. These discrepancies between the time courses of agonistic and dependence-sustaining effects suggest again that the receptors primarily involved in the centrally mediated withdrawal effects may have unique properties.

ACKNOWLEDGMENTS

I am grateful to Louise I. Lowney and Karin Schulz for expertly carrying out several experiments described here. Naloxone and levorphanol were gifts from Endo Laboratories and Hoffmann-LaRoche, respectively. This investigation was supported by grants 18963 and 22230 from the National Institute of Mental Health.

REFERENCES

1. Blaine, G. F., Boura, A. L. A., Fitzgerald, A. E., and Lister, R. E.: Actions of etorphine hydrochloride (M99): A potent morphine-like agent. Br. J. Pharmacol. *30*:11–22, 1967.
2. Burgen, A. S. V., and Spero, L.: The action of acetylcholine and other drugs on the efflux of potassium and rubidium from smooth muscle of the guinea-pig intestine. Br. J. Pharmacol. *34*:99–115, 1968.
3. Cheney, D. L., and Goldstein, A.: Tolerance to opioid narcotics, III. Time course and reversibility of physical dependence in mice. Nature *232*:477–478, 1971.
4. Cheney, D. L., Judson, B. A., and Goldstein, A.: Failure of an opiate to protect mice against naloxone-precipitated withdrawal. J. Pharmacol. Exp. Ther. *182*:189–194, 1972.
5. Collier, H. O. J.: A general theory of the genesis of drug dependence by induction of receptors. Nature *205*:181–182, 1965.
6. Collier, H. O. J.: Tolerance, physical dependence and receptors. A theory of the genesis of tolerance and physical dependence through drug-induced changes in the number of receptors. Adv. in Drug Res. *3*:171–188, 1966.
7. Collier, H. O. J.: Humoral transmitters, supersensitivity, receptors and dependence. *In:* Scientific Basis of Drug Dependence, edited by H. Steinberg, pp. 49–66. Churchill, London, 1969.

8. Cowie, A. L., Kosterlitz, H. W., and Watt, A. J.: Mode of action of morphine-like drugs on autonomic neuro-effectors. Nature *220*:1040–1042, 1968.
9. Cox, B. M., Ginsburg, M., and Osman, O. H.: Acute tolerance to narcotic analgesic drugs in rats. Br. J. Pharmacol. *33*:245–256, 1968.
10. Cox, B. M., and Weinstock, M.: The effect of analgesic drugs on the release of acetylcholine from electrically stimulated guinea-pig ileum. Br. J. Pharmacol. *27*:81–92, 1966.
11. Denton, J. E., and Beecher, H. K.: New analgesics, II. A clinical appraisal of the narcotic power of methadone and its isomers. JAMA *141*:1146–1153, 1949.
12. Dobbs, H. E.: Effect of cyprenorphine (M285), a morphine antagonist, on the distribution and excretion of etorphine (M99), a potent morphine-like drug. J. Pharmacol. Exp. Ther. *160*:407–414, 1968.
13. Eidelberg, E., and Barstow, C. A.: Morphine tolerance and dependence induced by intraventricular injection. Science *174*:74–76, 1971.
14. Goldstein, A.: The search for the opiate receptor. Pharmacology and the Future of Man. Proc. 5th Int. Congr. Pharmacol., San Francisco 1972, *1*:140–150, Karger, Basel, 1973.
15. Goldstein, A.: Recent studies on the binding of opiate narcotics to possible receptor sites. In: New Concepts in Neurotransmitter Regulation, edited by A. J. Mandell, pp. 297–309. Plenum Press, New York, 1973.
16. Goldstein, A., Aronow, L., and Kalman, S. M.: Principles of Drug Action. Harper and Row, New York, 1968.
17. Goldstein, A., and Goldstein, D. B.: Possible role of enzyme inhibition and repression in drug tolerance and addiction. Biochem. Pharmacol. *8*:48, 1961.
18. Goldstein, D. B., and Goldstein, A.: Enzyme expansion theory of drug tolerance and physical dependence. Proc. Assoc. Res. Nerv. Ment. Dis. *46*:265–267, 1968.
19. Goldstein, A., Lowney, L. I., and Pal, B. K.: Stereospecific and nonspecific interactions of the morphine congener levorphanol in subcellular fractions of mouse brain. Proc. Nat. Acad. Sci. *68*:1742–1747, 1971.
20. Goldstein, A., and Sheehan, P.: Tolerance to opioid narcotics. I. Tolerance to the "running fit" caused by levorphanol in the mouse. J. Pharmacol. Exp. Ther. *169*:175–184, 1969.
21. Knapp, S., and Mandell, A. J.: Some drug effects on the functions of the two physical forms of tryptophan-5-hydroxylase; influence on hydroxylation and uptake of substrate. *In:* Serotonin and Behavior, edited by J. Barchas and E. Usdin. Academic Press, New York, 1973.
22. Kosterlitz, H. W., Lydon, R. J., and Watt, A. J.: The effect of adrenaline, noradrenaline and isoprenaline on inhibitory α- and β-adrenoceptors in the longitudinal muscle of the guinea-pig ileum. Br. J. Pharmacol. *39*:398–413, 1970.
23. Kosterlitz, H. W., and Watt, A. J.: Kinetic parameters of narcotic agonists and antagonists with particular reference to N-allylnoroxymorphine (naloxone). Br. J. Pharmacol. *33*:266–276, 1968.
24. Martin, W. R.: Opioid antagonists. Pharmacol Rev. *19*:463–521, 1967.
25. Miledi, R., and Potter, L. T.: Acetylcholine receptors in muscle fibres. Nature *233*:599–603, 1971.
26. Nickerson, M.: Receptor occupancy and tissue response. Nature *178*:697–698, 1956.
27. Orahovats, P. D., Winter, C. A., and Lehman, E. G.: The effect of N-allylnormorphine upon the development of tolerance to morphine in the albino rat. J. Pharmacol. Exp. Ther. *109*:413–416, 1953.
28. Pal, B. K., Lowney, L. I., and Goldstein, A.: Further studies on the stereospecific binding of levorphanol by a membrane fraction from mouse brain. In: Agonist and Antagonist Actions of Narcotic Analgesic Drugs. Proc. Symp. Brit. Pharmacol. Soc., Aberdeen, July 1971, edited by H. W. Kosterlitz, H. O. J. Collier, and J. E. Villarreal, pp. 62–69. Macmillan, London, 1973.
29. Paton, W. D. M.: A theory of drug action based on the rate of drug-receptor combination. Proc. Roy. Soc. Ser. B, *154*:21–69, 1961.
30. Portoghese, P. S.: A new concept on the mode of interaction of narcotic analgesics with receptors. J. Med. Chem. *8*:609–616, 1965.

31. Portoghese, P. S.: Stereochemical factors and receptor interactions associated with narcotic analgesics. J. Pharm. Sci. *55*:865–887, 1966.
32. Schulz, R., and Goldstein, A.: Morphine tolerant longitudinal muscle strip from guinea pig ileum. Brit. J. Pharmacol., in press.
33. Schulz, R., and Goldstein, A.: Supersensitivity to serotonin in myenteric plexus of morphine tolerant guinea pig. Nature *244*:868–870, 1973.
34. Shuster, L.: Repression and de-repression of enzyme synthesis as a possible explanation of some aspects of drug action. Nature *189*:314–315, 1961.
35. Soto, E. F., Pasquini, J. M., Placido, R., and LaTorre, J. L.: Fractionation of lipids and proteolipids from cat grey and white matter by chromatography on an organophilic dextran gel. J. Chromatog. *41*:400–409, 1969.
36. Stephenson, R. P.: A modification of receptor theory. Br. J. Pharmacol. *11*:379–393, 1956.
37. Takemori, A. E., Kupferberg, H. J., and Miller, J. W.: Quantitative studies of the antagonism of morphine by nalorphine and naloxone. J. Pharmacol. Exp. Ther. *169*:39–45, 1969.
38. Way, E. L., Loh, H. H., and Shen, F. H.: Morphine tolerance, physical dependence, and synthesis of brain 5-hydroxytryptamine. Science *162*:1290–1292, 1968.
39. Way, E. L., Loh, H. H., and Shen, F. H.: Simultaneous quantitative assessment of morphine tolerance and physical dependence. J. Pharmacol. Exp. Ther. *167*:1–8, 1969.
40. Weber, G., Borris, D. P., De Robertis, E., Barrantes, F. J., La Torre, J. L., and De Carlin, M.: The use of a cholinergic fluorescent probe for the study of the receptor proteolipid. Molec. Pharmacol. *7*:530–537, 1971.
41. Wei, E., Loh, H. H., and Way, E. L.: Neuroanatomical correlates of morphine dependence. Science *177*:616–617, 1972.
42. Wikler, A., Fraser, H. F., and Isbell, H.: N-allylnormorphine: Effects of single doses and precipitation of acute "abstinence syndrome" during addiction to morphine, methadone or heroin in man (post-addicts). J. Pharmacol. Exp. Ther. *109*:8–20, 1953.

Narcotic Antagonists, edited by M. C. Braude, L. S. Harris, E. L.
May, J. P. Smith, and J. E. Villarreal. Advances in Biochemical
Psychopharmacology, Vol. 8. Raven Press, New York © 1974.

Stereoisomers of Viminol: Catalepsy and Brain Monoamine Turnover Rate

E. Costa, D. Cheney, and A. Revuelta

Laboratory of Preclinical Pharmacology, National Institute of Mental Health, Saint Eliza-
beths Hospital, Washington, D.C. 20032

Viminol R_2 (10 mg/kg i.p.) causes analgesia and catalepsy and increases
the concentration and turnover rate of striatal dopamine. Cerebellar
norepinephrine content is not increased by R_2 but its turnover is accelerated.
Doses of R_2 (2.5 mg/kg i.p.) which cause analgesia can still increase brain
catecholamine turnover rate. S_2 does not antagonize the catalepsy elicited
by R_2 (molar ratio 2:1) and does not antagonize the accumulation of striatal
dopamine elicited by R_2. S_2 (20 mg/kg i.p.) changes neither steady state
concentrations nor turnover rate of brain catecholamines. Neither S_2 nor
R_2 affects steady state or turnover rate of brain serotonin.

Viminol, or 1-[α(N-O-chlorobenzyl)-pyrryl] 2-di-sec butylamine ethanol,
is a central analgesic (7) which exhibits cross-tolerance to morphine. This
report concerns two of the stereoisomers of viminol (S_2 and R_2).

R_2 is $C_{①}R$; $C_{②}R$ and $C_{③}$ — ([α]_D 20° Δ 19.46). S_2 is $C_{①}S$;
$C_{②}S$ and $C_{③}$ — ([α]_D 20° + 1.10°).

The compound R_2 is a slightly more active analgesic than morphine (9),
whereas the compound S_2 is not analgesic but antagonizes analgesia elicited
by R_2 and morphine (8). Although S_2 antagonizes R_2 analgesia at a molar
ratio (S_2/R_2) smaller than that required to antagonize the analgesia elicited
by morphine, S_2 can antagonize physical dependence caused by morphine

and elicit withdrawal symptoms when injected into morphine-dependent mice (8).

The present report shows that S_2 (10 mg/kg i.p.) antagonizes neither the running activity elicited by morphine (100 mg/kg i.p.) in mice nor, at doses of 20 mg/kg i.p., the catalepsy elicited by R_2 (10 mg/kg i.p.) in rats. R_2 increases striatal dopamine (DM) concentrations and accelerates the turnover rate of striatal DM and cerebellar norepinephrine (NE). S_2 changes neither striatal DM nor cerebellar NE steady state concentrations or turnover rate. The acceleration of DM and NE turnover rates occurs after analgesic doses of R_2 and cannot be related to the catalepsy elicited by this drug.

EFFECT OF VIMINOL STEREOISOMERS AND MORPHINE ON MOTOR ACTIVITY OF MICE AND RATS

We injected intraperitoneally 100 mg/kg of morphine to two groups of 10 mice each (male, 20 to 25 g). One group received S_2[1] (10 mg/kg s.c.), the other group received saline. The motor activity of each group was monitored continually for 9 hr at intervals of 15 min using a photocell activity meter (Metron, Sweden) (5). The data reported in Fig. 1 show that S_2 fails to increase motor activity and to antagonize the running activity elicited by morphine. In these experiments, the molar ratio of S_2 to morphine was 1:10. Since the antagonism of morphine analgesia requires a molar ratio of 1:1, we cannot conclude that the running activity elicited by morphine fails to be antagonized by S_2. Due to the toxicity of viminol S_2, we could not reach a molar ratio of 1:1 in the experiments reported in Fig. 1.

Male Sprague-Dawley rats (180 to 200 g) were injected intraperitoneally with various doses of viminol R_2 and S_2. Their exploratory activity, muscle tone, and posture were monitored by inspection at fixed time intervals after the injection. Every dose tested elicited tail rigidity and a dose-dependent decrease of motor activity, which appeared after a latency of about 10 min. Rats receiving 5 mg/kg i.p. or more of R_2 exhibited catalepsy, and the severity of this symptom appeared to be dose dependent. We estimated the intensity of catalepsy by a conventional three-point score system described in Table 1. The data reported in this table show that R_2 in doses of 10 and 5 mg/kg i.p. causes catalepsy which is dose related in its intensity. Moreover, S_2 in a molar ratio 2:1 does not antagonize the catalepsy elicited by R_2.

---

[1] The two stereoisomers of viminol (S_2 and R_2) are dissolved in a small volume of glacial acetic acid and diluted to desired volume with saline. The solution is injected at a pH between 4.5 and 5. We are indebted to Dr. D. Della Bella for the gift of hydroxybenzoate salts of the two viminol stereoisomers used in this study.

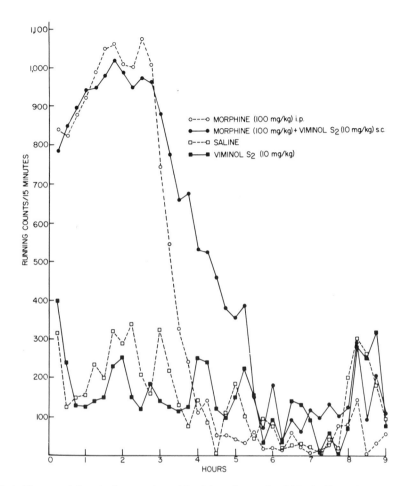

FIG. 1. Motor activity of mice monitored for 9 hr at intervals of 15 min. Ten mice were used per treatment.

ACTION OF VIMINOL ISOMERS ON MONOAMINE CONCENTRATIONS OF VARIOUS PARTS OF RAT BRAIN

We measured brain concentrations of serotonin (5-HT), NE, and DM according to a published procedure (11) and dissected the brain as described earlier (4). The data reported in Table 2 show that R_2 (15 mg/kg i.p.) increases the striatal DM concentrations but fails to change the concentration of 5-HT and NE in telencephalon. This dose causes death in about 30% of the rats, the death occurring between 2 and 4 hr after the

TABLE 1. *Catalepsy in rats receiving various doses of viminol (R₂ or S₂)*

Viminol (mg/kg i.p.)	Cataleptic score[a] after minutes			
	10	20	40	80
R_2 (10)	5	12	12	12
R_2 (5)	0	5	6	6
R_2 (2.5)	0	0	0	0
S_2 (20)	0	0	0	0
S_2 (20) + R_2 (10)	6	12	12	12

[a] The intensity of catalepsy was scored in groups of four rats each injected with various doses of the two stereoisomers of viminol. Reduced exploratory behavior = 1; absolute immobility and rigidity = 2; imposed abnormal postures persisting longer than 1 min = 3. Figures express the total score in each group. A 10-min time interval elapsed between two successive injections of viminol stereoisomers.

injection. In contrast, a dose of 20 mg/kg i.p. of the less toxic S_2 fails to change the concentrations of the three amines (Table 3).

In Table 4 we have reported the time course for the onset of catalepsy and of the increase of striatal dopamine concentrations in rats receiving various doses of viminol R_2. Only the doses of R_2 that elicit catalepsy increase the concentration of striatal DM. Noncataleptic doses of the compound fail to change striatal DM concentrations. When S_2 is given 10 min before R_2 (molar ratio 2:1), it fails to change the increase of striatal DM concentrations elicited by R_2, nor does this treatment affect either the intensity or the time course of the cataleptic effects of R_2.

TABLE 2. *Monoamine concentrations (nmoles/g $\pm$ SE) in brain parts of rats receiving 15 mg/kg i.p. of viminol R_2*

Minutes after injection	Telencephalon		Striatal dopamine
	NE	5-HT	
0	2.7 ± 0.084	2.2 ± 0.11	41 ± 3.2
30	2.6 ± 0.041	1.9 ± 0.02	55 ± 4.6[a]
60	2.6 ± 0.19	2.1 ± 0.18	61 ± 10[a]
90	3.3 ± 0.58	2.3 ± 0.43	55 ± 8.6[a]

Each value is the average of four assays
[a] $p < 0.05$

TABLE 3. *Monoamine concentrations (nmoles/g) in brain parts of rats receiving 20 mg/kg i.p. of viminol S_2*

Minutes after injection	Telencephalon		Striatal dopamine
	NE	5-HT	
0	3.1 ± 0.13	3.2 ± 0.19	43 ± 6.2
30	3.3 ± 0.10	3.4 ± 0.24	48 ± 2.8
60	2.9 ± 0.16	3.1 ± 0.22	42 ± 4.0
90	3.2 ± 0.11	3.1 ± 0.15	44 ± 2.6

Each value is the mean of four assays

ACTION OF VIMINOL STEREOISOMERS ON BRAIN MONOAMINE TURNOVER RATE

Drugs may affect the function of monoaminergic neurons without changing the steady state concentrations of the putative transmitter they store (10). Drugs that interact with processes regulating intraneuronal metabolism (6) and storage of transmitters can change the concentration of the putative transmitter, but drugs that increase or decrease the rates of neuronal pulse flow do not necessarily change the transmitter steady state concentrations. These considerations suggest that the measurement of brain monoamine concentrations is not conclusive to exclude drug interactions with monoaminergic neurons.

The data reported in Table 5 show that neither S_2 nor R_2 affects brain

TABLE 4. *Time course of catalepsy and of increase of striatal DM concentrations (nmoles/g $\pm$ SE) in rats receiving various doses of viminol (R_2 or S_2)*

Viminol[a] (mg/kg i.p.)	Minutes after viminol (R_2 or S_2)					
	15		30		60	
	DM	Catalepsy	DM	Catalepsy	DM	Catalepsy
R_2 (10)	48 ± 1.8	8	53 ± 2.2^b	12	56 ± 2.4^b	12
S_2 (20)	45 ± 2.4	0	—	0	—	0
S_2 (20) + R_2 (10)	54 ± 4.0^b	7	59 ± 5.8^b	12	67 ± 7.6^b	12
R_2 (5)	51 ± 6.3	6	—	7	—	7
R_2 (2.5)	45 ± 3.3	0	42 ± 4.1	0	41 ± 3.7	0

[a] The second viminol isomer was injected after a time interval of 10 min. Catalepsy was scored with the three-point system reported in Table 1.

[b] $p < 0.05$ when compared to saline-treated rats. Values referring to DM are the average of four rats; figures referring to catalepsy are the total score in four rats. The DM concentration in striatum of rats receiving saline 43 ± 2.3 nmoles/g.

TABLE 5. *Turnover rate of 5-HT in brain of rats receiving viminol (R_2 or S_2)*

Viminol	Turnover rate (nmoles/g/hr)	
(mg/kg i.p.)	Accumulation of serotonin	Decline of 5-hydroxyindoleacetic acid
Saline	1.8	1.6
R_2 (10)	1.7	1.6
S_2 (20)	1.6	1.4

Groups of four rats each were killed at 10, 20, and 40 min after injection of pargyline (75 mg/kg i.p.) which was given 10 min after R_2 or S_2. 5-HT and 5-hydroxyindoleacetic acid concentrations were measured at various times. Turnover rates were estimated according to the method of Neff and Tozer (12).

5-HT turnover rate when estimated by two different methods: accumulation of 5-HT and decrease of 5-hydroxyindoleacetic acid at various times after pargyline (12).

It is generally assumed that formation of 3,4-dihydroxyphenylalanine (DOPA), the first enzymatic reaction involved in catecholamine biosynthesis, is rate limiting (17); however, only indirect techniques are available to estimate tyrosine hydroxylation *in vivo*. During the last year, we have been working on more direct techniques to measure specific activity of DM and DOPA in tissues that contain a uniform population of catecholamine neurons (only dopaminergic or only noradrenergic) (2, 3). This investigation has been made possible by recent developments of analytical techniques which allow analysis of tissue concentrations of amines and amino acids

TABLE 6. *Turnover rate of striatal DM in rats receiving viminol (R_2 or S_2) 10 min before 3,5-³H-tyrosine (1 mC/kg i.v.)*

Viminol (mg/kg i.p.)	nmoles/g ± SE	k/hr	nmoles/g/hr[a]
Saline	46 ± 3.4	0.46	21
R_2 (10)	47 ± 3.2	0.95	47
S_2 (20)	48 ± 4.8	0.45	22

Groups of four rats each were killed at 5, 10, and 15 min after injection of ³H-tyrosine. Viminol did not change the concentration (nmole/g) of tyrosine (37 ± 0.29), DOPA (0.23 ± 0.034), or DM (46 ± 3.4).

[a] Estimated from the change of DOPA (D)- and dopamine (DM)-specific activities at 2.5-min intervals (Δ_t) from 5 to 20 min after injection of ³H-tyrosine (30 C/mmole)

$$\frac{(DM_{t_2} - DM_{t_1})2}{[(D_{t_2} - DM_{t_2}) + (D_{t_1} - DM_{t_1})]\Delta_t}$$

TABLE 7. *Turnover rate of cerebellar NE in rats receiving viminol R_2 or S_2 10 min before 3,5-^{3}H-tyrosine (1 mC/kg i.v.)*

Viminol (mg/kg i.p.)	nmole/g ± SE	k/hr	nmole/g/hr[a]
Saline	0.81 ± 0.067	0.22	0.18
R_2 (10)	0.84 ± 0.082	0.52	0.43
S_2 (20)	0.86 ± 0.096	0.29	0.20

Groups of four rats each were killed at 5, 10, and 15 min after injection of ^{3}H-tyrosine. Viminol stereoisomers did not change the concentrations of tyrosine, DOPA, or dopamine.

[a] Estimated from the change with time of DOPA- and NE-specific activity at 2.5-min intervals (for details see Table 6)

with a single ion-exchange column. Moreover, the identification and assay of small concentrations of amines is possible by multiple ion detection (2). The data reported in Tables 6 and 7 were obtained with such techniques. Specifically, the data in Table 6 show that R_2 doubles DM turnover rate in striatum, as measured from the change with time of DOPA- and dopamine-specific radioactivity in rats receiving a tracer dose of ^{3}H-tyrosine. In contrast, S_2 does not increase striatal DM turnover rate. In order to ascertain if the action of R_2 is selective for brain dopaminergic tracts, we studied the turnover rate of cerebellar NE in rats receiving R_2 and S_2. We selected this brain area because it contains only brain noradrenergic tracts; therefore, in cerebellum the DOPA formed from tyrosine functions exclusively as the precursor of NE. The data reported in Table 7 show that R_2 increases the turnover rate of cerebellar NE without changing the steady state concentration of this amine. In contrast, S_2 changes neither the steady state concentration nor the turnover rate of cerebellar NE.

CATALEPSY AND BRAIN CATECHOLAMINE TURNOVER RATE

To determine if the increase of catecholamine turnover rate elicited by R_2 could be linked to the catalepsy in a causal relationship, we investigated the time-course relationships of the catalepsy and of the increase of catecholamine turnover rate. The data reported in Table 1 show that catalepsy occurs within 10 min after the injection of 10 mg/kg of R_2. We have therefore studied whether, during 10 min immediately following the injection of R_2, there is an increase in the amount of radioactive tyrosine incorporated into striatal DM or cerebellar NE. The data reported in Table 8 show that neither R_2 (10 mg/kg i.p.) nor S_2 (20 mg/kg i.p.) changes the incorporation of radioactive tyrosine into striatal DM or cerebellar NE during the 10

TABLE 8. *Incorporation of 3,5-³H-tyrosine into striatal DM or cerebellar NE before the onset of catalepsy elicited by viminol (S_2 or R_2)*

Viminol (mg/kg i.p.)	Tyrosine				DM or NE			
	dpm/nmole × 10⁻³ ± SE		nmoles/g ± SE		dpm/nmole × 10⁻³ ± SE		nmole/g ± SE	
	Striatum	Cerebellum	Striatum	Cerebellum	Striatum DM	Cerebellum NE	Striatum DM	Cerebellum NE
Saline	5.9 ± 0.60	6.0 ± 0.26	37 ± 0.29	52 ± 11	0.75 ± 0.14	0.88 ± 0.085	46 ± 2.1	0.86 ± 0.062
R_2 (10)	5.2 ± 0.53	6.6 ± 0.36	41 ± 0.35	58 ± 15	0.76 ± 0.077	0.87 ± 0.032	39 ± 4.9	0.88 ± 0.040
S_2 (20)	5.5 ± 0.66	6.1 ± 0.18	42 ± 0.52	59 ± 3.5	0.77 ± 0.15	0.72 ± 0.092	42 ± 4.6	0.92 ± 0.056

3,5-³H-tyrosine (1 mC/kg i.v.; S.A. 30 C/mmole) was injected intravenously. Five min later rats received viminol (S_2 or R_2) or saline and were killed 15 min after injection of the radioactive label. Each value is the average of at least three assays.

TABLE 9. *Incorporation of 3,5-³H-tyrosine into striatal DM or cerebellar NE after the onset of the pharmacological effects elicited by viminol (S₂ or R₂)*

Viminol (mg/kg i.p.)	Tyrosine				DM or NE			
	dpm/nmole × 10⁻³ ± SE		nmoles/g ± SE		dpm/nmole × 10⁻³ ± SE		nmoles/g ± SE	
	Striatum	Cerebellum	Striatum	Cerebellum	Striatum DM	Cerebellum NE	Striatum DM	Cerebellum NE
Saline	6.0 ± 0.60	7.7 ± 0.95	40 ± 5.3	48 ± 5.4	0.35 ± 0.076	0.46 ± 0.026	54 ± 6.2	1.1 ± 0.15
R₂ (10)	6.9 ± 0.41	10 ± 1.2	41 ± 2.4	39 ± 6.2	1.2 ± 0.15[a]	1.1 + 0.10[a]	46 ± 5.5	0.86 ± 0.16
R₂ (5)	5.4 ± 0.57	10 ± 2.9	40 ± 6.0	56 ± 11	0.77 ± 0.21[a]	0.64 ± 0.097[a]	64 ± 4.0	1.2 ± 0.098
R₂ (2.5)	5.7 ± 1.3	12 ± 1.9	33 ± 4.6	49 ± 11	1.0 ± 0.18[a]	0.91 ± 0.21[a]	55 ± 3.2	1.2 ± 0.12
S₂ (20)	7.4 ± 1.4	8.5 ± 1.1	37 ± 3.2	38 ± 6.8	0.51 ± 0.077	0.59 ± 0.12	60 ± 5.9	1.2 ± 0.092

3,5-³H-tyrosine (1 mC/kg i.v.; S.A. 3 C/mmole) was injected intravenously 10 min after various doses of viminol S₂ and R₂. The doses of 10 and 5 mg/kg of R₂ elicited catalepsy; R₂ (2.5 mg/kg) and S₂ (20 mg/kg) did not cause catalepsy. The animals were killed 10 min after the label and 20 min after viminol. Each value refers to the mean of three assays.

[a] $p < 0.05$

491

min immediately following the injection of the two drugs. In contrast, R_2 but not S_2 increases the rate of incorporation of ^{3}H-tyrosine into cerebellar NE and striatal DM when tested between 10 and 35 min after the drug injection (Tables 6 and 7). It appears from our data that R_2-induced catalepsy precedes the increase in brain catecholamine turnover rate, suggesting that this increase is the consequence rather than the cause of some mechanism triggered specifically by R_2 which is directly involved in eliciting the catalepsy.

To ascertain if the catalepsy occurs every time there is an increase of brain catecholamine turnover rate, we studied the effect of various doses of R_2 on the incorporation of ^{3}H-tyrosine into DM and NE in striatum and cerebellum. The results of these experiments are reported in Table 9. These data show that a dose of 2.5 mg/kg of R_2 which fails to elicit catalepsy (Table 1) increases the incorporation rate of ^{3}H-tyrosine into the catecholamine stored in cerebellum and striatum. It is interesting to note that this dose of R_2 can cause analgesia by a central mechanism (8).

DISCUSSION

Drugs interacting with catecholaminergic neurons can increase turnover rate by changing one of several mechanisms involved in adrenergic neuronal function. Drugs can: (a) inhibit uptake mechanisms; (b) increase the afferent stimulatory synaptic input impinging onto catecholaminergic neurons; (c) block the postsynaptic receptors. The mechanism outlined in (a) was tested by measuring the uptake of tracer doses of L-^{3}H-NE *in vivo* by heart of rats receiving either saline or R_2 (10 mg/kg i.p.). These experiments indicated that viminol R_2 does not interfere with the uptake of radioactive NE by rat heart. The mechanism outlined in (c) might be linked with that outlined in (b) because it is known (10) that a blockade of dopaminergic postsynaptic receptors can activate excitatory neuronal loops that bring about an increase of afferent stimulation into the cell bodies of the catecholaminergic neurons whose postsynaptic receptors are blocked. Assuming that blockade of postsynaptic receptors in striatum accounts for the catalepsy, we have tested whether stimulation of these receptors could overcome this catalepsy. In preliminary experiments we have found that catalepsy elicited by R_2 (10 mg/kg i.p.) could be reversed with 5 mg/kg i.p. of apomorphine, which is thought to stimulate DM receptors in brain (1).

A blockade of postsynaptic receptors by R_2 as a cause of the catalepsy is consistent with the reversal of the catalepsy by apomorphine; moreover, the time course of the onset of the increase of DM turnover is greater than the time interval required for the appearance of R_2-induced catalepsy, as would have been expected if the DM receptor blockade were the mechanism involved. An increase of DM and NE turnover rate in brain was reported to occur after high doses of methadone (14) and morphine (15, 16).

Tolerance and cross-tolerance can develop to the morphine effects on brain catecholamine turnover rate (18). Moreover, continued administration of morphine may cause physical dependence in catecholamine synthesis; in fact, mice receiving a dose schedule of morphine causing dependence cannot synthesize normal amounts of catecholamines unless they receive the dose of morphine required to maintain their drug dependence (13).

We are continuing our investigation on the effects of R_2 on catecholamine synthesis to determine if analgesia occurs only when catecholamine synthesis is increased. We have only established that S_2 given in a molar ratio that antagonizes the analgesic effects of R_2 fails to curtail the accumulation of striatal DM and the catalepsy elicited by viminol R_2. It remains to be established whether S_2 can antagonize the increase of catecholamine turnover rate elicited by analgesic doses of viminol R_2 since S_2 can counteract the analgesic effect of R_2. In view of the speculation made on the involvement of brain 5-HT in morphine action (18), it is of interest that neither R_2 nor S_2 increases the concentration or the turnover rate of brain 5-HT.

REFERENCES

1. Andén, N. E., Rubenson, A., Fuxe, K., and Hockfelt, T.: Evidence for dopamine receptor stimulation by apomorphine. J. Pharm. Pharmacol. *19*:627–631, 1967.
2. Costa, E.: The fundamental role of immediate precursors to estimate turnover rate of catecholamines by isotopic labeling. Proc. International Congress of Pharmacology, July, 1972, in press.
3. Costa, E., Green, A. R., Koslow, S. H., LeFevre, H. F., Revuelta, A., and Wang, C.: Dopamine and norepinephrine in noradrenergic axons: A study in vivo of their precursor product relationship by mass fragmentography and radiochemistry. Pharmacol. Rev. *24*:167–190, 1972.
4. Costa, E., Groppetti, A., and Revuelta, A.: Action of fenfluramine on the monoamine stores of rat tissues. Brit. J. Pharmacol. *41*:57–64, 1971.
5. Costa, E., Naimzada, K. M., and Revuelta, A.: Phenmetrazine, aminorex and (±) *p*-chloramphetamine: Their effect on motor activity and turnover rate of brain catecholamines. Brit. J. Pharmacol. *43*:570–579, 1971.
6. Costa, E., and Neff, N. H.: The physiological role of monoamine oxidase (MAO) in monoamine storage as revealed by monoamine oxidase inhibitors (MAOI). In: Cheymol, J. and Boissier, J. R. (eds.): Proceedings of the 3rd International Pharmacological Meeting, Oxford, Pergamon Press, Vol. 10, pp. 15–32, 1968.
7. Della Bella, D.: Identificazione e sviluppo di Una Nuova classe di analgesici centrali. Boll. Chim. Farm. *111*:5–9, 1972.
8. Della Bella, D.: Stereoisomers of viminol: Preliminary pharmacological profile. *This symposium*.
9. Della Bella, D., Ferrari, V., Frigeni, V., and Lualdi, P.: Agonistic and antagonistic properties of diesteresisomers in a new central analgesic. Nature, in press, 1973.
10. Neff, N. H., and Costa, E.: Effect of tricyclic antidepressants and chlorpromazine on brain

catecholamine synthesis. In: Garattini, S. and Dukes, M. N. G. (eds.): Proceedings of the International Symposium on Antidepressant drugs, New York, Excerpta Medica Foundation, pp. 28–34, 1967.

11. Neff, N. H., Spano, P. F., Groppetti, A., Wang, C., and Costa, E.: A simple procedure for calculating the synthesis rate of brain norepinephrine, dopamine and serotonin after a pulse injection of radioactive tyrosine and tryptophan. J. Pharmacol. Exp. Ther. *176*:701–710, 1971.

12. Neff, N. H., and Tozer, T. N.: In vivo measurement of brain serotonin turnover. Advances in Pharmacology, Vol. 6A, 97–109. 1967.

13. Rosenman, S. J., and Smith, C. B.: ^{14}C-Catecholamine synthesis in mouse brain during morphine withdrawal. Nature *240*:153–155, 1972.

14. Sesame, H. A., Perez-Cruet, J., DiChiara, G., Tagliamonte, A., Tagliamonte, P., and Gessa, G. L.: Evidence that methadone blocks dopamine receptors in brain. J. Neurochem. *19*:1953–1957, 1972.

15. Smith, C. B., Sheldon, M. I., Bednarczyk, J. H., and Villareal, J. E.: Morphine induced increase in the incorporation of ^{14}C tyrosine into ^{14}C dopamine and ^{14}C norepinephrine in the mouse brain: antagonism by naloxone and tolerance. J. Pharmacol. Exp. Ther. *180*: 547–557, 1972.

16. Smith, C. B., Villarreal, J. E., Bednarczyk, J. H., and Sheldon, M. I. Tolerance to morphine induced increases in ^{14}C catecholamine synthesis in mouse brain. Science *170*:1106–1108, 1970.

17. Udenfriend, S.: Tyrosine hydroxylase. Pharmacol. Rev. *18*:43–51, 1966.

18. Way, L. E. and Shen, F. H.: Catecholamines and 5-hydroxytryptamine. In: Clouet, D. H. (ed.): Narcotic Drugs, Plenum Press, New York, pp. 229–250, 1971.

Narcotic Antagonists, edited by M. C. Braude, L. S. Harris, E. L. May, J. P. Smith, and J. E. Villarreal. *Advances in Biochemical Psychopharmacology, Vol. 8.* Raven Press, New York © 1974.

Pharmacokinetics and Neurochemical Effects of Pentazocine and Its Optical Isomers

Barry Berkowitz

Pharmacology Section, Department of Physiologic Chemistry, Roche Institute of Molecular Biology, Nutley, New Jersey 07110

Using fluorometric and gas chromatographic methods, the pharmacokinetics of pentazocine have been extensively studied. The absorption of pentazocine is rapid following parenteral administration to man with peak plasma levels occurring within 1 hr. Slower absorption and greater metabolism result in a delay in achieving maximal plasma levels after oral administration with the highest levels occurring between the first and third hours. Metabolism of pentazocine is extensive and involves oxidation of the N-dimethylallyl side chain and glucuronide conjugation on the phenolic moiety. Individual differences in the metabolism of pentazocine can account for differences in its pharmacologic effect as those individuals who metabolized pentazocine the least are most strongly affected. The analgesic activity of pentazocine resides in the parent compound, specifically the L-isomer. However, the D- and L-isomers are equipotent in lowering the levels of rat brain norepinephrine and probably do so by increasing neuronal release. Brain dopamine concentration is reduced to a much greater extent by the analgetically active L-isomer. Thus, dopamine may play an important role in mediating the effects of pentazocine and possibly other narcotic antagonists.

Pentazocine, the first narcotic antagonist analgesic to achieve widespread therapeutic use in man, has been extensively studied. The development of sensitive and specific assays for pentazocine and its metabolites in body tissues and fluids has allowed detailed analyses of its absorption, distribution, metabolism, and excretion (6, 19, 25). This review will illustrate the findings and interpretations of these pharmacokinetic studies as well as the methods employed. Recent studies on the effects of pentazocine on biogenic amines will also be summarized.

METHODS

Radioisotopic (13, 14), gas chromatographic (3, 4, 18, 25, 26), and fluorometric analyses (6, 9, 13) have been utilized in the studies of pentazocine. As with all methods, each has advantages and limitations. Early studies with radioisotopically labeled pentazocine lacked specificity for most tissues as only total radioactivity was measured, and metabolites could not be differentiated from the parent compound (13, 14). Radioisotopic pentazocine was also found to be fairly unstable. Moreover, studies in man are always limited with radioisotopic procedures.

Fluorometric procedures were therefore developed and expanded by Berkowitz and Way (6, 9) and El-Mazati and Way (12) which, when coupled with extraction procedures, were found to have adequate sensitivity and specificity for pentazocine for both clinical and animal studies. The limit of sensitivity of this procedure allowed levels in human plasma to be followed for several hours after analgesic doses. Urinary drug levels were followed by utilizing a buffer wash in the extraction procedure to remove interfering metabolites. However, these metabolites were not able to be quantitatively or qualitatively examined by this procedure. Gas chromatographic analysis of pentazocine recovered from body fluids yielded data in good agreement with the fluorometric methods (3, 4, 11, 18, 19). Pittman (25) and collaborators (26) were also able to quantitate and identify pentazocine metabolites in the urine. The fluorometric and gas chromatographic procedures are limited by the need to extract the drug from tissues and by a limit of sensitivity of about 50 ng. These limitations may be overcome by the use of radioimmunoassays. Spector and Parker (28, 29) have developed a radioimmunoassay for morphine which not only does not require solvent extraction but is 100 times more sensitive than fluorometric or gas chromatographic procedures, easily detecting picogram quantities of the narcotic. All of the protein-coupling procedures employed to make morphine antigenic and elicit antibody formation are applicable to the narcotic antagonists pentazocine, naloxone, cyclazocine, nallorphine, and structural congeners.

ABSORPTION

Pentazocine is absorbed rapidly following intramuscular or subcutaneous administration. Maximal plasma levels averaging 0.14 μg/ml were obtained between 15 and 45 min after intramuscular administration of 45 mg/70 kg (7) as shown in Fig. 1. Moreover, maximal analgesia and respiratory depression were observed within 60 min following injection (1, 2, 5, 7, 8).

When given orally, pentazocine was more slowly absorbed than after administration by injection. Peak plasma levels occurred between 1 and 3 hr after drug ingestion (4, 8) as did peak analgesia (2). It is clear that less pentazocine reached the blood after oral administration than intramuscular

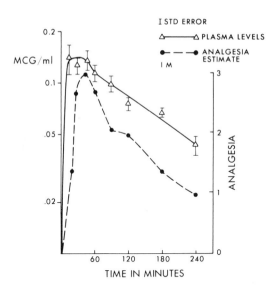

FIG. 1. Plasma levels of pentazocine and pain relief after intramuscular administration of 45 mg/70 kg. Pain evaluation or analgesia: 0 = no pain relief; 1 = slight relief; 2 = moderate relief; 3 = good relief; complete relief. The results represent the average of eight subjects for each determination.

administration. Twice the intramuscular dose given orally produced similar peak plasma levels (7). Additionally, four times the intravenous dose administered intramuscularly resulted in only one to two times higher blood levels (4). Thus relatively slower absorption necessitates about a twofold higher oral than intramuscular dose. A probable contributing factor requiring higher oral than injected doses is that more pentazocine is metabolized following oral administration (7, 11).

DISTRIBUTION

Pentazocine is widely distributed throughout the body as determined from animal studies (12, 13). In the rat, pentazocine was found in the highest concentrations in the lung, spleen, and kidney following intravenous administration. Lower than expected levels were present in tissues after oral administration apparently because of rapid metabolism by the liver (13).

Pentazocine rapidly enters the brain (9, 18, 22) of rats and mice. Peak levels are achieved within 30 min after subcutaneous or intraperitoneal injection. In comparison to morphine, pentazocine enters the brain more rapidly and achieves a much higher brain-to-plasma ratio and also leaves the brain more rapidly (9, 18). The brain-to-plasma ratio for pentazocine is about four (9, 18) whereas that for morphine is less than one (17). This means that at equivalent plasma concentrations there is at least four times more pentazocine than morphine in the brain. Thus, although pentazocine is estimated to be one-third less potent as an analgesic in man than morphine, at the molecular level it is probably a far less potent agonist.

METABOLISM AND EXCRETION

Metabolism of pentazocine limits its action since less than 5% of the administered dose is excreted unchanged (7, 25). Intersubject differences in metabolism appear to play a major role in determining the effects of pentazocine. In man those subjects with the greatest incidence of side effects excreted the least amount of pentazocine metabolites, but three times as much pentazocine as subjects without side effects (8). Supporting evi-

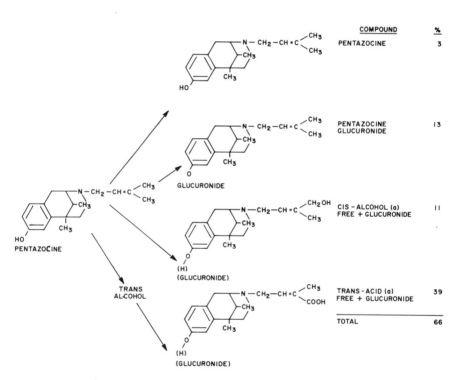

FIG. 2. Metabolic pathway of pentazocine. The structures and percent excretion indicated by (a) are from the studies of Pittman and co-workers (25, 26).

dence for variable effects of pentazocine resulting from differences in metabolism has been reported by Paalzow and Arbin (22). They found those mice which had the least analgesic effect after pentazocine had lower serum pentazocine levels and higher metabolite levels than mice which exhibited greater analgesia.

The pathway of metabolism in man is primarily by oxidation of the N-dimethylallyl side chain (25) with lesser amounts being conjugated with glucuronic acid (8, 25). In man the half-life of pentazocine in plasma is 2 hr (7). Excretion is primarily in the urine and occurs mainly during the first 24 hr. However, as much as 30% of the administered dose remains in the body or is in the form of unidentified metabolites (6, 14) (Fig. 2).

MECHANISM OF PENTAZOCINE ACTION

It is probable that pentazocine and not a metabolite is responsible for the analgesic activity of this compound. In man there is a good correlation between maximal plasma pentazocine levels and peak analgesia following intramuscular administration (7). There is additional evidence in rats and mice suggesting a correlation between analgesia and central nervous system concentration of pentazocine (9, 22). Perhaps the most direct evidence for analgesia residing in the parent molecule is that the known metabolites are practically devoid of analgesic activity (9), and in mice receiving pentazocine those having the highest serum content of pentazocine metabolite exhibited the least analgesia (22).

The L-optical isomer of pentazocine is responsible for the bulk of analgesia, respiratory depression, and narcotic antagonism (5, 15, 23, 24). This does not mean that the D-isomer is devoid of pharmacologic activity. In man an appreciable incidence of side effects including sedation, sweating, and subjective effects is caused by the D-isomer (5, 15). McMillan and Harris (20) recently reported significant behavioral activity of D-pentazocine in the pigeon. However, although differential pharmacologic effects can be attributed to specific isomers, the molecular mechanisms subserving the pharmacologic action of pentazocine, or for that matter any strong analgesic, are not understood.

The quest for an explanation for the differences in effects between the D- and L-isomers has primarily involved the brain, since studies in the rat have established that differences in absorption, distribution, metabolism, or excretion cannot account for the differences in pharmacologic activity of the isomers (9). There were no differences in the regional central nervous system distribution of D- or L-pentazocine although the L-isomer was about 15 times more potent as an analgesic (9). If differences in pharmacokinetics

TABLE 1. *Effect of* D- *or* L-*pentazocine on norepinephrine and dopamine in the rat cortex*

Drug	Dose	Norepinephrine (μg/g)	Dopamine (μg/g)
Control	—	0.27 ± 0.02	1.56 ± 0.08
D-isomer	15	0.24 ± 0.02	1.34 ± 0.10
	30	0.18 ± 0.02*	1.10 ± 0.11*
	60	0.16 ± 0.02*	1.16 ± 0.25*
L-isomer	15	0.18 ± 0.02*	0.97 ± 0.04*
	30	0.14 ± 0.05*	0.62 ± 0.12*
	60	0.19 ± 0.04*	0.66 ± 0.10*

Pentazocine was administered subcutaneously and rats killed 1 hr later. Tissues from five rats were analyzed for each dose of each isomer. Results are ± standard error of the mean.
* Statistically significant $p < 0.05$.

do not explain the actions of pentazocine, a more promising approach has been to study the effects of pentazocine on biogenic amines.

Pentazocine toxicity (27), behavioral effects (16), and analgesia (21) may be modulated by an action of norepinephrine, serotonin, or dopamine in the brain. Since these studies were all done using D- and L-pentazocine it was important to examine the effect of the optical isomers of pentazocine on these amines. As shown in Table 1 D-,L-pentazocine reduced the concentration of norepinephrine in the cortex to the same extent, whereas the L-isomer produced a greater decrease than the D-isomer in the concentration of dopamine.

The mechanism of amine alteration appears to be the result of an increased neuronal release (10). The effect of the D-isomer on brain catecholamines may provide a biochemical basis for some of its behavioral activity (5, 20), whereas the marked effect of the L-isomer on brain dopamine suggests this amine might be more important in mediating analgesic activity.

REFERENCES

1. Beaver, W. T., Wallenstein, S. L., Houde, R. W., and Rogers, A.: A comparison of the analgesic effects of pentazocine and morphine in patients with cancer. Clin. Pharmacol. Ther. 7:740–751, 1966.
2. Beaver, W. T., Wallenstein, S. L., Houde, R. W., and Rogers, A.: A clinical comparison of the effects of oral and intramuscular administration of analgesics: Pentazocine and phenazocine. Clin. Pharmacol. Ther. 9:582–597, 1968.
3. Beckett, A. H., and Taylor, J. F.: Blood concentrations of pethidine and pentazocine in mother and infant at time of birth. J. Pharm. Pharmacol. 19 (suppl.):50, 1967.
4. Beckett, A. H., Taylor, J. F., and Kourounakis, P.: The absorption, distribution and excretion of pentazocine in man after oral and intravenous administration. J. Pharm. Pharmacol. 22:123–128, 1970.

5. Bellville, J. W., and Forrest, W. H.: Respiratory and subjective effects of D- and L-pentazocine. Clin. Pharmacol. Ther. *9*:142–151, 1968.
6. Berkowitz, B.: Influence of plasma levels and metabolism on pharmacological activity: Pentazocine. Ann. NY Acad. Sci. *179*:269–281, 1971.
7. Berkowitz, B. A., Asling, J. H., Shnider, S. M., and Way, E. L.: Relationship of pentazocine plasma levels to pharmacological activity in man. Clin. Pharmacol. Ther. *10*:320–328, 1969.
8. Berkowitz, B., and Way, E. L.: Metabolism and excretion of pentazocine in man. Clin. Pharmacol. Ther. *10*:681–689, 1969.
9. Berkowitz, B. A., and Way, E. L.: Analgesic activity and central nervous system distribution of the optical isomers of pentazocine in the rat. J. Pharmacol. Exp. Ther. *177*:500–508, 1971.
10. Berkowitz, B. A.: *To be published.*
11. Burt, R. A. P., and Beckett, A. H.: The absorption and excretion of pentazocine after administration by different routes. Br. J. Anaesth. *43*:427–437, 1971.
12. El-Mazati, U., and Way, E. L.: The biologic disposition of pentazocine in the rat. J. Pharmacol. Exp. Ther. *177*:332–341, 1971.
13. Ferrari, R. A.: Differential distribution of pentazocine-³H and cis-3-chloroallylnorpentazocine-³H in the cat.[1] Toxicol. Appl. Pharmacol. *12*:404–416, 1968.
14. Flavell Matts, S. G., McCready, V. R., James, K. W., Gwyther, Myfanwy, M., and Hammersley, P. A. G.: Radio-isotopic studies of the urinary excretion of pentazocine as an aid to pharmacotherapeutic application. Clin. Trials J. *4*:842, 1967.
15. Forrest, W. H., Beer, E. G., Bellville, J. W., Ciliberti, B. J., Miller, E. V., and Paddock, R.: Analgesic and other effects of the D- and L-isomers of pentazocine. Clin. Pharmacol. Ther. *10*:468–476, 1969.
16. Holtzman, S. G., and Jewett, R. E.: Some actions of pentazocine on behavior and brain monoamines in the rat. J. Pharmacol. Exp. Ther. *181*:346–356, 1972.
17. Kupferberg, H. J., and Way, E. L.: Pharmacologic basis for the increased sensitivity of the newborn rat to heroin. J. Pharmacol. Exp. Ther. *141*:105, 1963.
18. Medzihradsky, F., and Ahmad, K.: The uptake of pentazocine into brain. Life Sci. *10*:711–720, 1971.
19. Mitchard, M.: Pharmacokinetic studies on pentazocine. Acta Pharmacol. Toxicol. *3*:172–180, 1971.
20. McMillan, D. E., and Harris, L. S.: Behavioral and morphine-antagonist effects of the optical isomers of pentazocine and cyclazocine. J. Pharmacol. Exp. Ther. *180*:569–579, 1972.
21. Paalzow, L.: Studies on the mechanism of analgesic action of pentazocine. Proceedings of the Fifth International Congress on Pharmacology 174, 1972.
22. Paalzow, L., and Arbin, A.: Serum and brain concentrations of pentazocine in relation to analgesic activity in mice. J. Pharm. Pharmacol. *24*:552–557, 1972.
23. Pearl, J., and Harris, L. S.: Inhibition of writhing by narcotic antagonists. J. Pharmacol. Exp. Ther. *154*:319–323, 1966.
24. Pearl, J., Stander, H., and McKean, D.: Effects of analgesics and other drugs on mice in phenylquinone and rotarod tests. J. Pharmacol. Exp. Ther. *167*:9–13, 1969.
25. Pittman, K. A.: Human metabolism of orally administered pentazocine. Biochem. Pharmacol. *19*:1833–1835, 1970.
26. Pittman, K. A., Rosi, D., Cherniak, R., Merola, A. J., and Conway, W. D.: Metabolism *in vitro* and *in vivo* of pentazocine. Biochem. Pharmacol. *18*:1673–1678, 1969.
27. Rogers, K., and Thornton, J.: The interaction between monoamine oxidase inhibitors and narcotic analgesics in mice. Br. J. Pharmacol. *36*:470–480, 1969.
28. Spector, S.: Quantitative determination of morphine in serum by radioimmunoassay. J. Pharmacol. Exp. Ther. *178*:253–263, 1971.
29. Spector, S., and Parker, C.: Morphine: Radioimmunoassay. Science *168*:1347–1349, 1970.

Narcotic Antagonists, edited by M. C. Braude, L. S. Harris, E. L. May, J. P. Smith, and J. E. Villarreal. *Advances in Biochemical Psychopharmacology, Vol. 8.* Raven Press, New York © 1974.

Disposition and Metabolism of ³H-Cyclazocine in Dogs

S. J. Mulé, C. W. Gorodetzky,* and T. H. Clements*

New York State Narcotic Addiction Control Commission, Testing and Research Laboratory, Brooklyn, New York 11217

The metabolism of ³H-cyclazocine was studied in nontolerant, tolerant, and abstinent dogs after a 1.25 mg/kg (free base) s.c. injection of the drug. Norcyclazocine and cyclazocine were identified in the urine of these dogs after extraction and direct application of hydrolyzed and unhydrolyzed urine samples to chromatographic paper buffered with 0.1 M phosphate or impregnated with silicic acid. The chromatograms were developed with tertiary amyl alcohol-*n*-butyl ether-water (80:7:13, v/v) or ethyl acetate-methanol-NH₄OH (85:10:5, v/v). Methods were developed for the estimation of ³H-cyclazocine and ³H-norcyclazocine in biologic material with a minimal sensitivity of 3 ng/ml. The mean percentage recovery of the administered dose of ³H-cyclazocine obtained from urine and feces for both free and conjugated drug over a period of 120 hr was 43.7% from nontolerant dogs, 58.5% from tolerant dogs, and 40.7% from abstinent dogs. In the urine of nontolerant, tolerant, and abstinent dogs, 2.3 to 2.7% of the ³H-cyclazocine was recovered as free norcyclazocine and an equal amount as conjugated norcyclazocine. In the feces of these dogs, from 1.5 to 2.4% of the free and 0.02 to 0.7% of the conjugated norcyclazocine was obtained. Norcyclazocine was not found in the brain of the dogs at various time intervals, but the metabolite was obtained in peripheral tissues. No drug was found in the CNS of a 24-hr abstinent dog. Urine samples were subjected to acid and enzymatic hydrolysis, using β-glucuronidase and phenol sulfatase. The data indicated that the conjugate of both cyclazocine and norcyclazocine was a glucuronide. The results indicated that potency of cyclazocine but not latency of abstinence was correlated with distribution. Norcyclazocine (1.0 mg/kg) did not significantly depress the flexor reflex of the chronic spinal dog. It is concluded that norcyclazocine is not an active metabolite of cyclazocine and that 47 to 66% of the administered ³H-cyclazocine was accounted for as free and conjugated cyclazocine and norcyclazocine, as determined over a 5-day period.

---

* Present address: National Institute of Mental Health, Addiction Research Center, Lexington, Kentucky 40507

503

INTRODUCTION

It has been shown (1–3) that patients chronically receiving cyclazocine develop tolerance to this drug and cross tolerance to nalorphine. An abstinence syndrome developed when cyclazocine was abruptly withdrawn and it reached a maximum only on the 7th day of abstinence. The signs of abstinence persisted for a period of 6 weeks and were quantitatively different from that observed with morphine (4, 5).

The observations on abstinence, the potent analgesic activity (6), and the use of cyclazocine in the treatment of narcotic drug dependence (7, 8) were of such interest to warrant a thorough distribution and metabolic study of cyclazocine. The results of this study are reported in this chapter.

METHODS

The preparation of ³H-cyclazocine, its radiochemical purity, the estimation of ³H-cyclazocine and ³H-norcyclazocine, specificity, biological procedures, and chromatographic techniques were all as described previously (9, 10).

RESULTS

1. Cyclazocine

The data on the urinary and fecal excretion of ³H-cyclazocine appear in Table 1. The percentage recovery of ³H-cyclazocine from urine and feces in nontolerant, tolerant, and abstinent dogs appears in Table 1. The mean percentage recovery of ³H-cyclazocine from urine was quite similar in the nontolerant, tolerant, and abstinent dogs for free (4.3 to 4.7%) and conjugated (29.8 to 36.2%) cyclazocine. However, a distinct increase in the mean excretion of free cyclazocine was observed in the feces of the tolerant dogs (16%) in comparison to the nontolerant (4.3%) and abstinent dogs (5.6%). The percentage recovery of the conjugated drug from the feces was similar in the nontolerant, tolerant, and abstinent dogs. Thus, the total percentage recovery (urine plus feces) of the injected dose of ³H-cyclazocine accounted for over a period of 120 hr ranged from 40.7 to 58.5%. The largest percentage recovery accounted for was obtained with the tolerant dogs and was due to the increased excretion of free cyclazocine in the feces.

At 120 hr, both free and conjugated cyclazocine were found in the urine of nontolerant and tolerant dogs at levels of 0.01 to 0.02% of the injected

TABLE 1. Percentage of ^{3}H-cyclazocine recovered from urine and feces of nontolerant, tolerant, and abstinent dogs after a 1.25 mg/kg (free base) s.c. injection of ^{3}H-cyclazocine

	Percentage recovery from urine[a]								
	Free			Conjugated			Total		
Dog No.[b]	Non-tolerant	Tolerant	Abstinent	Non-tolerant	Tolerant	Abstinent	Non-tolerant	Tolerant	Abstinent
30	5.8	2.4	6.5	29.4	29.1	24.3	35.2	31.5	30.8
31	4.0	1.5	4.3	35.2	40.1	29.8	39.2	41.6	34.1
33	3.5	10.2	2.2	35.2	39.6	35.3	38.7	49.8	37.5
	Percentage recovery from feces[c]								
30	2.7	29.5	4.0	0.8	3.4	1.0	3.5	32.9	5.0
31	6.6	12.9	7.5	1.5	0.3	1.2	8.1	13.2	8.7
33	3.7	5.8	5.3	2.6	0.7	0.7	6.3	6.5	6.0
	Mean percentage recovery from urine and feces[d]								
Biologic material									
Urine	4.4	4.7	4.3	33.3	36.3	29.8	37.7	41.0	34.1
Feces	4.3	16.0	5.6	1.6	1.5	1.0	6.0	17.5	6.6
Total	8.7	20.7	9.9	34.9	37.8	30.8	43.7	58.5	40.7

[a] Figures represent the percentage of the administered dose of ^{3}H-cyclazocine recovered from urine collected over a period of 120 hr (5 days).
[b] Dogs 30, 31, and 33 were studied in the nontolerant, tolerant, and abstinent physiologic states.
[c] Figures represent the percentage of the administered dose of ^{3}H-cyclazocine recovered from feces collected over a period of 120 hr.
[d] Figures represent the mean values obtained from the urine and feces, from dogs 30, 31, and 33, over a collection period of 120 hr.

drug. In the abstinent dogs, 0.06 to 0.13% of the injected cyclazocine was obtained in the 120-hr urine sample as free and conjugated drug. From 0.01 to 0.07% of the injected ³H-cyclazocine was obtained as free and conjugated drug in the nontolerant, tolerant, and abstinent dog feces during the 96- to 120-hr period. During the first 8 hr, the nontolerant, tolerant, and abstinent dogs excreted in the urine 60 to 84% of the free cyclazocine and 56 to 69% of the conjugated drug. The values decreased rapidly after 8 hr, but ranged between 1 and 15% at the 48- to 120-hr time interval for both free and conjugated drug.

During the first 48 hr, 62 to 74% of the free drug and 59 to 85% of the conjugated drug were found in the feces of the nontolerant and tolerant dogs. Seven to 15% of the free and conjugated drug was obtained at this time in the feces of the abstinent dogs. A significantly high percentage of drug was excreted during the 48- to 96-hr period by the nontolerant and tolerant dogs. In the feces of the abstinent dogs, 83 to 90% of the free and conjugated drug was obtained in the 48- to 96-hr sample. The percentage of drug (free and conjugated) found in the 96- to 120-hr period ranged from 0.6 to 3% in the nontolerant, tolerant, and abstinent dogs.

The total radioactivity found in the urine and feces of the nontolerant, tolerant, and abstinent dogs (30, 31, and 33) appears in Table 2. The largest percentage of radioactivity appeared in the urine (42.9 to 58.5%) of these dogs over a 5-day period. The mean percentage radioactivity was higher in the feces of the tolerant dogs (28.3%) in comparison to the nontolerant (13.9%) and abstinent dogs (16.0%). The total radioactivity accounted for ranged from 58.8% in the abstinent dogs to 86.9% in the tolerant dogs.

Maximal levels of free drug in plasma were observed 30 min after cyclazocine administration in both nontolerant and tolerant dogs (100 to 150 ng/ml). The concentration of free drug fell to one-half the maximal level at about 2 hr (biologic half-life) in both the nontolerant and tolerant dog. The mean levels of free cyclazocine in the nontolerant and tolerant dogs were almost identical through 12 hr. At this time, the concentration was 3 ng/ml in both the nontolerant and tolerant dogs.

Maximal levels of conjugated cyclazocine were observed at 90 min in both the nontolerant and tolerant dogs. The mean concentration of conjugated drug fell to one-half the maximal level at about 3 hr in the nontolerant dogs and at 4 hr in the tolerant dogs (biologic half-life). The mean levels of conjugated cyclazocine were lower in the nontolerant as compared to the tolerant animals at each time interval through 8 hr. At 8, 12, and 24 hr, the mean levels were 60, 52, and 9 ng/ml, respectively, in the nontolerant dogs, and 80, 43, and 18 ng/ml, respectively, in the tolerant dogs.

Levels of free and conjugated cyclazocine were obtained in the abstinent

TABLE 2. Total radioactivity found in the urine and feces of nontolerant, tolerant, and abstinent dogs after a 1.25 mg/kg (free base) s.c. injection of ³H-cyclazocine

| | Percent of administered ³H-cyclazocine[a] | | | | | | | | |
| | Urine | | | Feces | | | Total | | |
Dog	Non-tolerant	Tolerant	Abstinent	Non-tolerant	Tolerant	Abstinent	Non-tolerant	Tolerant	Abstinent
30	65.8	46.2	53.5	6.1	48.1	21.1	72.0	94.3	74.6
31	58.6	60.7	33.9	16.8	24.3	16.4	75.3	85.1	50.2
33	43.3	68.7	41.4	18.9	12.6	10.4	62.2	81.3	51.8
Mean	55.9	58.5	42.9	13.9	28.3	16.0	69.8	86.9	58.8

[a] Duplicate determinations were performed as described under Methods on each urine and fecal sample obtained over a period of 120 hr. The results were averaged and totaled, and the percentage of ³H-cyclazocine administered calculated.

507

dogs at 8, 12, and 24 hr after the last 1.25 mg/kg (free base) subcutaneous injection of ³H-cyclazocine. At these time intervals, the mean levels for free drug were 6, 3, and 0 ng/ml and 81, 32, and 13 ng/ml for conjugated drug. Blood samples were not obtained during the first 8 hr because the cyclazocine levels were considered to be the same as that described for the tolerant dogs.

Distribution of ³H-Cyclazocine in the Central Nervous System of Nontolerant and Tolerant Dogs

The levels of ³H-cyclazocine were quite similar in gray or white matter of the individual anatomical areas at the various time intervals for both nontolerant and tolerant dogs (Table 3). Maximal mean levels of drug were observed at 1 hr in gray and white matter for both nontolerant and tolerant dogs. The rate at which cyclazocine appeared to leave the cerebrum was faster for the nontolerant animals in comparison to the tolerant, so that levels of 36 to 56 ng/g and 100 to 117 ng/g were obtained 6 hr after drug administration. Free cyclazocine was not detected in the cerebral cortex or subcortical areas of an abruptly withdrawn dog 24 hr after the last injection. The biologic half-life of free cyclazocine in gray and white matter for both nontolerant and tolerant dogs ranged between 2 and 3 hr.

The data concerning the distribution of free ³H-cyclazocine in selected areas of the CNS, in the cerebrospinal fluid (CSF), and in plasma at the time of sacrifice appear in Table 4. Maximal levels of free cyclazocine were obtained 1 hr following drug in both nontolerant and tolerant dogs. The highest concentrations appeared to be in the hypothalamus and dorsal thalamus at this time. The levels of cyclazocine were similar to the cerebral cortex at each time interval. As in the cerebral cortex, the concentration of cyclazocine appeared to be higher at 4 and 6 hr in the tolerant dogs in comparison to the nontolerant values.

The CSF levels of free drug were similar to plasma values in the nontolerant and tolerant dogs, but considerably less than the values observed for CNS tissue.

Distribution of ³H-Cyclazocine in Various Tissues of Nontolerant and Tolerant Dogs

Presented in Table 5 are the data concerning the levels of ³H-cyclazocine in various tissues and bile of nontolerant and tolerant dogs. The levels of free cyclazocine in the heart, duodenum, and colon were quite similar to those found in the CNS 1 hr after drug, whereas the levels in the spleen,

TABLE 3. Distribution of free ^{3}H-cyclazocine in the cerebral cortex of nontolerant and tolerant dogs after a 1.25 mg/kg (free base) s.c. injection

	Mean concentration[a]							
	Nontolerant dogs				Tolerant dogs			
Area of Cerebrum	1 hr	2 hr	4 hr	6 hr	1 hr	2 hr	4 hr	6 hr
				(ng/g)				
Temporal								
Gray	1216	690	117	34	1165	706	188	125
White	759	632	132	60	1021	687	211	104
Sensorimotor								
Gray	1227	727	129	25	1332	761	207	116
White	931	650	140	61	1154	720	216	111
Prefrontal								
Gray	1207	704	127	50	1220	662	207	111
White	1040	674	131	55	1157	628	211	105
Occipital								
Gray	1218	704	113	35	1299	621	208	101
White	908	651	126	53	1159	622	197	100
Parietal								
Gray	1206	705	125	38	1280	649	225	133
White	836	630	131	52	1048	592	225	81
Cortical mean[b]								
Gray	1215 ± 24	706 ± 13	122 ± 7	36 ± 4	1259 ± 56	680 ± 94	207 ± 19[c]	117 ± 5
White	895 ± 35	647 ± 13	132 ± 5	56 ± 2	1108 ± 47[c]	650 ± 91	212 ± 18[c]	100 ± 5
Gray/white ratio	1.36	1.09	0.92	0.65	1.14	1.05	0.97	1.17

[a] Duplicate determinations were performed on the individual tissues of each animal and the results averaged. Three nontolerant and tolerant dogs were sacrificed at 1 and 4 hr, two at 2 hr, and one at 6 hr. A single tolerant dog was sacrificed 24 hr after receiving a 1.25 mg/kg (free base) s.c. injection of ^{3}H-cyclazocine and abruptly withdrawn from drug. No ^{3}H-cyclazocine was detected in the cerebral cortex or selected subcortical areas of the CNS of this dog.

[b] Mean ± standard error of the mean.

[c] $p < .01$ as compared to the corresponding nontolerant value.

509

TABLE 4. *Distribution of free ³H-cyclazocine in the central nervous system of non-tolerant and tolerant dogs after a 1.25 mg/kg (free base) s.c. injection*

CNS tissue or fluid	Mean concentration[a]							
	Nontolerant dogs[b]				Tolerant dogs[b]			
	1 hr	2 hr	4 hr	6 hr	1 hr	2 hr	4 hr	6 hr
	(ng/g or ml)							
Cerebellum gray	1001	588	93	36	1121	687	157	107
Cerebellum white	843	556	113	25	976	526	158	83
Midbrain	971	571	98	30	1105	546	169	92
Corpus callosum	747	586	104	25	859	585	265	89
Olfactory tracts	1035	612	105	N.S.[c]	1077	572	194	83
Olfactory bulbs	909	481	85	6	912	586	135	85
Fornix	1087	709	132	N.S.	1241	628	236	111
Optic tr. N. chiasma	814	602	132	N.S.	952	626	207	49
Pyriform area	975	750	138	45	982	728	235	105
Hypothalamus	1060	671	102	55	1443	697	207	90
Dorsal thalamus	1233	785	123	37	1755	739	234	111
Cerebral peduncle	894	585	108	58	940	609	191	92
Medulla	947	610	114	33	943	560	212	97
Pons	897	601	114	44	920	598	206	182
Caudate nucleus	969	688	126	44	1217	694	220	102
Cervical spinal cord	840	603	179	64	638	544	263	138
Cerebrospinal fluid	107	96	25	9	142	85	40	24
Plasma (sacrifice)	118	76	12	8	134	62	49	21

[a] Duplicate determinations were performed on the individual tissues of each animal and the results were averaged. The values of individual animals seldom deviated by more than ± 16% from the mean.

[b] Three dogs were sacrificed at 1 and 4 hr, two at 2 hr, and one at 6 hr.

[c] N.S., not significant.

kidney, adrenals, pancreas, and lung were two- to fourfold higher. The values found in the liver were similar to the CNS at 1 and 2 hr in the non-tolerant dogs, but considerably higher in the tolerant dogs. Although the data appeared to be similar for the nontolerant and tolerant dogs, distinctly higher levels of drug were present in the tolerant tissues at 6 hr in comparison to nontolerant values. Free cyclazocine were still detectable in the liver, colon, kidney, and pancreas 24 hr after the last dose of cyclazocine.

The bile contained the highest nanograms per milliliter levels of ³H-cyclazocine found in either nontolerant or tolerant dogs. Peak concentrations of free and conjugated drug occurred at 2 hr for the nontolerant dogs, at 1 hr for free and at 6 hr for conjugated drug in the tolerant dogs. Free and conjugated cyclazocine represented 1.1 and 12.8%, respectively, of the administered drug in the 24-hr sample of bile.

TABLE 5. Distribution of free ³H-cyclazocine in various tissues of nontolerant and tolerant dogs after a 1.25 mg/kg (free base) s.c. injection

| | Mean concentration[a] | | | | | | | | |
| | Nontolerant dogs[b] | | | | Tolerant dogs[b] | | | | |
Tissue or fluid	1 hr	2 hr	4 hr	6 hr	1 hr	2 hr	4 hr	6 hr	24 hr[c]
					(ng/g or ml)				
Heart	972	566	79	20	1,004	585	167	86	N.S.[d]
Liver	973	1,040	227	102	3,474	3,313	938	2,668	187
Duodenum	1,028	1,019	709	139	1,256	1,295	314	662	N.S.
Colon	184	539	103	43	750	1,347	183	183	2,571
Spleen	2,701	1,813	249	71	2,752	1,976	380	262	N.S.
Kidney	3,825	1,608	335	86	3,467	2,919	422	840	55
Adrenal	2,233	1,224	194	52	2,269	1,416	312	264	N.S.
Pancreas	3,943	2,377	518	141	4,377	2,180	744	382	33
Lung	4,255	1,171	348	90	2,289	1,133	309	154	N.S.
Bile	1,370	14,572	5,947	11,518	11,185	3,845	3,452	7,639	10,804
Bile conjugated	19,889	182,318	174,472	145,421	96,970	120,736	42,980	208,540	126,692

[a] Duplicate determinations were performed on the individual tissues of each animal and the results were averaged. The values of the individual animals seldom deviated by more than ±22% from the mean.

[b] Three dogs were sacrificed at 1 and 4 hr, two at 2 hr, and one at 6 hr.

[c] A single tolerant dog received a 1.25 mg/kg (free base) s.c. injection of ³H-cyclazocine, was abruptly withdrawn, and sacrificed 24 hr later.

[d] N.S., not significant.

2. Norcyclazocine

Urinary and Fecal Excretion of ^{3}H-Norcyclazocine in Nontolerant, Tolerant, and Abstinent Dogs

The mean percentage excretion of ^{3}H-norcyclazocine from ^{3}H-cyclazocine (Table 6) in the urine of nontolerant, tolerant, and abstinent dogs was quite similar for free (2.3 to 2.7%) and for conjugated norcyclazocine (2.4 to 2.8%). However, there was a slightly higher excretion of free norcyclazocine (2.4%) in the feces of the tolerant dog in comparison with that of the nontolerant and abstinent dogs (1.5 to 1.6%). Less than 1% of the administered ^{3}H-cyclazocine appeared as conjugated norcyclazocine in the feces of these dogs. Thus, the total percentage recovery of norcyclazocine from cyclazocine ranged from 6.3% in the abstinent dogs to 7.5% in the nontolerant and tolerant animals.

At the 96- to 120-hr period, both free and conjugated norcyclazocine were found in the urine of nontolerant and tolerant dogs at levels of 0.002 to 0.015% of injected cyclazocine. In the abstinent dogs, 0.095% was obtained as free norcyclazocine and 0.027% as conjugated norcyclazocine during this time period. From 0.69 to 0.78% of injected cyclazocine was obtained as free norcyclazocine in the feces of the nontolerant and abstinent dogs in the 96- to 120-hr sample. In the conjugated form, from 0.004 to 0.063% of norcyclazocine was obtained in these dogs. Neither free nor conjugated cyclazocine was found in the 96- to 120-hr fecal sample of the tolerant dog.

Disposition of ^{3}H-Norcyclazocine in Biologic Tissues of the Nontolerant and Tolerant Dog

^{3}H-Norcyclazocine was not found in cerebral cortex gray or white matter at various time intervals (1 to 6 hr) in nontolerant or tolerant dogs (1 to 24 hr). Table 7 summarizes the data concerning the levels of ^{3}H-norcyclazocine in various tissues and bile of nontolerant and tolerant dogs. No norcyclazocine was found in the heart or colon of either nontolerant or tolerant dogs. The level of drug was quite similar in the liver of the nontolerant and tolerant dog, and similar but lower in the duodenum of these dogs. The concentration of ^{3}H-norcyclazocine was quite similar in the kidney of both dogs. In the spleen, pancreas, and lung, norcyclazocine was not detected at the later time intervals.

The bile contained considerable levels of both free and conjugated norcyclazocine. Peak levels of drug occurred at 2 to 4 hr for free and conjugated

TABLE 6. *Percentage of ³H-norcyclazocine recovered from urine and feces of nontolerant, tolerant, and abstinent dogs after a 1.25 mg/kg (free base) s.c. injection of ³H-cyclazocine*[a]

Biologic material	Dog No.[b]	Percentage recovery								
		Free			Conjugated			Total		
		Non-tolerant	Tolerant	Abstinent	Non-tolerant	Tolerant	Abstinent	Non-tolerant	Tolerant	Abstinent
Urine	30	3.3	1.8	4.0	2.9	2.3	1.1	6.1	4.2	5.1
	31	2.6	2.1	2.0	2.8	2.7	3.2	5.4	4.7	5.2
	33	2.4	3.2	1.2	2.8	3.2	3.1	5.3	6.4	4.3
Feces	30	1.2	3.8	2.0	0.2		0.01	1.4	3.6	1.9
	31	1.9	2.2	1.5	0.4		0.04	2.4	2.1	1.5
	33	1.8	1.2	1.1	1.7	0.3		2.0	1.5	1.1
Mean values[c]										
Urine		2.7	2.3	2.4	2.8	2.7	2.4	5.6	5.1	4.8
Feces		1.6	2.4	1.5	0.7	0.1	0.02	1.9	2.4	1.5
Total		4.3	4.7	3.9	3.5	2.8	2.4	7.5	7.5	6.3

[a] Results represent the percentage of administered ³H-cyclazocine recovered as ³H-norcyclazocine from the urine and feces, collected over 120 hr (5 days).

[b] Dogs 30, 31, and 33 were each studied in the nontolerant, tolerant, and abstinent physiologic states.

[c] Mean values obtained from the urine and feces from dogs 30, 31, and 33 over a 5-day period.

513

TABLE 7. Distribution of ³H-norcyclazocine in various tissues of nontolerant and tolerant dogs after a 1.25 mg/kg (free base) s.c. injection of ³H-cyclazocine

	Mean concentration[a]								
	Nontolerant dogs				Tolerant dogs				
Tissue or fluid	1 hr	2 hr	4 hr	6 hr	1 hr	2 hr	4 hr	6 hr	24 hr[b]
	(ng/g or ng/ml)								
Cerebral cortex gray									
Cerebral cortex white									
Heart									
Liver	445	535	158	237	475	427	262	426	78
Duodenum		108	242	57	106	99	31		48
Colon									
Spleen	136	109			175	136			
Kidney	243	189	51		239	156	93	77	
Pancreas	324	290			763	583	114	173	
Lung	340	101			137	70	24		
Bile	779	4,980	4,823	—[c]	3178	2847	788	9,163	3,255
Bile (conjugated)	3540	16,323	18,904		2494	4476	2412	10,233	42,230

[a] Duplicate determinations were performed on the individual tissues of each animal and the results averaged. The values represent the quantity of ³H-cyclazocine metabolized to ³H-norcyclazocine. Three dogs were sacrificed at 1 and 4 hr, two at 2 hr, and one at 6 hr. The individual values seldom deviated by more than ±27% from the mean.
[b] A single tolerant dog received a 1.25 mg/kg (free base) s.c. injection of ³H-cyclazocine, was abruptly withdrawn from cyclazocine, and was sacrificed 24 hr later.
[c] No sample.

norcyclazocine in the nontolerant dogs. In the tolerant dogs peak level of free drug occurred at 6 hr and at 24 hr for the conjugated drug.

Plasma Levels of ³H-Norcyclazocine in the Nontolerant Dogs

After a 1.25 mg/kg s.c. injection of ³H-cyclazocine in nontolerant dogs, plasma samples were taken at 15, 30, and 60 min and then every hour through 8 hr. No free ³H-norcyclazocine was detected in the plasma samples through 8 hr. This indicated that any ³H-norcyclazocine present in the plasma was below the sensitivity limits of the method after a necessary 1:4 dilution of the available plasma for the analysis. Conjugated norcyclazocine was obtained at each time interval. The levels of conjugated drug ranged between 8 and 25 ng/ml during the first 3 hr, peaking at 118 ng/ml at 4 hr, and at 8 hr a value of 11 ng/ml was observed.

Chromatographic Identification of ³H-Cyclazocine Metabolites

Unhydrolyzed urine studies.

Figure 1 shows the chromatographic scans obtained with unhydrolyzed urine from nontolerant and tolerant dogs. The R_f values for labeled nor-cyclazocine and cyclazocine corresponded to the R_f values of the non-labeled drugs on silicic acid-impregnated paper for both the nontolerant and tolerant dogs (Fig. 1, A and B). On these chromatograms radioactivity also appeared at the origin (R_f, 0.03) and at R_f 0.28 and 0.31 (metabolite 1). It is quite possible that the radioactive compounds present near the origin of the chromatogram represent conjugated norcyclazocine and conjugated cyclazocine. Figure 1, C and D, shows the scans obtained by using 0.1 M phosphate-buffered paper, pH 7.0, in which labeled norcyclazocine, R_f 0.21 to 0.23, and labeled cyclazocine, R_f 0.80, corresponded to the R_f values observed with the nonlabeled compounds. Radioactivity also appeared near the origin (R_f, 0.03) on these chromatograms, but there was no evidence for metabolite 1. Urine from nontolerant and tolerant dogs was also directly applied to 0.1 M phosphate-buffered chromatograms, pH 7.9, along with nonlabeled norcyclazocine and cyclazocine. The chromatograms were developed with tertiary-amyl alcohol-n-butyl ether-water (80:7:13, v/v). The R_f values of the labeled compounds agreed with those of the non-labeled drugs as reported previously (10).

Hydrolyzed urine studies.

Figure 2 represents the chromatographic scans of the radioactivity obtained from hydrolyzed urine of nontolerant and tolerant dogs. In Figure

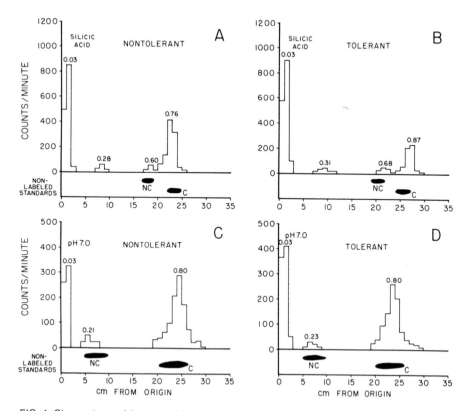

FIG. 1. Chromatographic scan of the radioactivity in unhydrolyzed urine from nontolerant and tolerant dogs applied directly to the paper. *A*. Urine from a nontolerant dog was applied to silicic acid-impregnated paper and developed with ethyl acetate-methanol-NH₄OH (85:10:5, v/v). *B*. Same as *A* except that urine from a tolerant dog was applied. *C*. Urine from a nontolerant dog was applied to 0.1M phosphate-buffered paper (pH 7.0) and developed with tertiary-amyl alcohol-*n*-butyl ether-water (80:7:13, v/v). *D*. Same as *C* except that urine from a tolerant dog was applied. The numbers above the radioactive peaks represent the R_f values and the nonlabeled standards norcyclazocine (NC) and cyclazocine (C) as detected by the iodoplatinate reagent appear below the radioactive scan. (Mulé et al., J. Pharmacol. Exp. Ther. *160*:387, 1968.)

2, *A* and *B*, there appeared to be a good correlation between the radioactive peak for cyclazocine and the R_f of nonlabeled cyclazocine on the buffered chromatograms. However, only a slight indication of radioactivity was present on the chromatogram which corresponded to norcyclazocine. The radioactivity near the origin (R_f, 0.03) was considerably reduced in comparison with the unhydrolyzed urine, which may indicate the absence or reduction of conjugated drugs after acid hydrolysis of the urine. Cyclazocine was easily identified on silicic acid-impregnated paper (Fig. 2*C*), but again

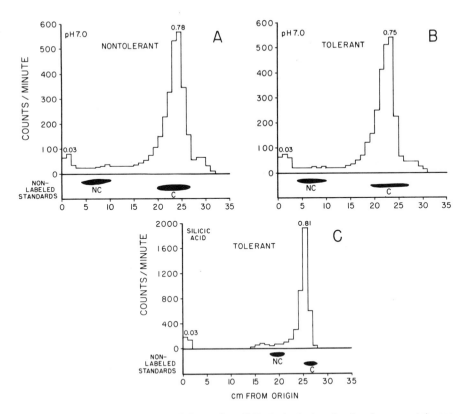

FIG. 2. Chromatographic scan of the radioactivity in hydrolyzed urine from nontolerant and tolerant dogs applied directly to the paper. *A*. Urine from a nontolerant dog was hydrolyzed, neutralized, and applied directly to 0.1 M phosphate-buffered paper (pH 7.0) and developed with tertiary-amyl alcohol-*n*-butyl ether-water (80:7:13, v/v). *B*. Same as *A* except that urine from a tolerant dog was applied. *C*. Urine from a tolerant dog was hydrolyzed, neutralized, and applied to silicic acid-impregnated paper and developed with ethyl acetate-methanol-NH₄OH (85:10:5, v/v). The number above the radioactive peaks represents the R_f values and the nonlabeled standards norcyclazocine (NC) and cyclazocine (C) as detected by the iodoplatinate reagent appear below the radioactive scan. (Mulé et al., J. Pharmacol. Exp. Ther. *160*:387, 1968.)

norcyclazocine did not appear as a significant peak but rather as a tail effect of the labeled cyclazocine scan. Radioactivity was present near the origin of the chromatogram but, again, considerably less than that which was observed with the unhydrolyzed urine.

Physiologic Studies with Cyclazocine and Norcyclazocine

The time-action curves for the mean effects of saline, cyclazocine, and norcyclazocine on the ipsilateral flexor reflex and the mean areas under the curves expressed as percentage depression from control appear in Fig. 3. Cyclazocine produced a 77 to 90% depression, with the greater effect appearing at the lower stimulus strength (0.8 kg). This effect was significantly different from that for both saline and norcyclazocine at the $p < .01$ level. Norcyclazocine (1.0 mg/kg) caused a mean stimulation of the flexor reflex at the lowest stimulus strength and a slight depression with stronger stimuli. However, these effects were not significantly different from those of saline at the $p < .05$ level. Lower doses of norcyclazocine (0.1 and 0.5 mg/kg) had no consistent effect on the flexor reflex. At 2.0 mg/kg of norcyclazocine, a 30 to 35% depression was obtained with all stimuli.

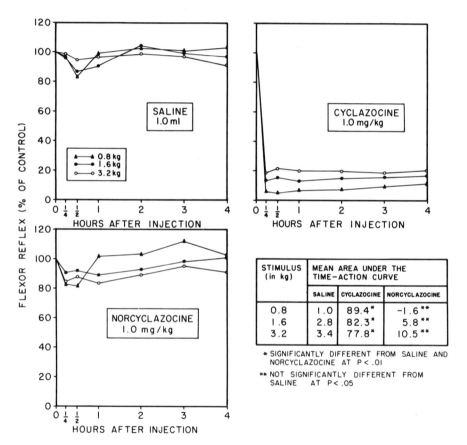

FIG. 3. Time-action curves for the mean effects of saline, cyclazocine, and norcyclazocine on the ipsilateral flexor reflex at three stimulus strengths and the values for the mean area under the time-action curves. (Mulé et al., J. Pharmacol. Exp. Ther. *160*:387, 1968.)

DISCUSSION

A method was developed for the estimation of ³H-cyclazocine and ³H-norcyclazocine in various biological tissues and fluids with a minimal sensitivity of about 3 ng/ml of biological material. The method was sufficiently sensitive to allow the injection of small doses of cyclazocine and subsequent analysis of small samples of biological material.

The purposes of this study were to attempt to correlate the physiological disposition of ³H-cyclazocine with (1) its potent agonist properties; (2) tolerance development and the cyclazocine abstinence syndrome; and (3) to obtain basic data on the distribution and metabolism of cyclazocine, a potent member of the benzomorphan narcotic antagonist class of drugs.

Lasagna et al. (6) have shown cyclazocine to be a potent analgesic in man (mg potency of five to 40 times morphine). The potency data obtained by Martin et al. (1) for cyclazocine in comparison to morphine with reference to miosis, opiate signs, opiate symptoms, and "liking" scores ranged between 10 and 20 (mg potency). The CNS levels of ³H-cyclazocine were six to 10 times higher than C¹⁴-morphine (11) in nontolerant dogs at approximately 1 hr after drug, thus lending support to the increased potency of cyclazocine in comparison to morphine.

The disposition of ³H-cyclazocine in the CNS was quite different in comparison to morphine, but very similar to that reported for nalorphine (12). Therefore, these studies add additional evidence to the hypothesis (1, 8) that cyclazocine is not a morphine-like drug, but closely resembles the narcotic antagonist nalorphine.

It has been demonstrated (1, 4) that patients receiving cyclazocine chronically developed a definite abstinence syndrome when abruptly withdrawn. The abstinence syndrome had a long latency, first manifesting itself on the third or fourth day of abstinence, peaking on the seventh day and was not associated with drug-seeking behavior. Spearman rank order coefficients for the point scores of the cyclazocine and morphine abstinence syndrome were not correlated, but the cyclazocine point scores were correlated with the point scores for the nalorphine abstinence syndrome (8). Thus, the cyclazocine abstinence syndrome was qualitatively different from the morphine abstinence syndrome.

The studies herein reported show that ³H-cyclazocine was not detected in the CNS of an abstinent dog 24 hr after the last dose of the drug, but was still detectable in certain body tissues (i.e., liver, colon, kidney, pancreas) and bile. About 0.06 to 0.13% of the injected ³H-cyclazocine was found in the 120-hr (5 day) urine samples and 0.03 to 0.07% in the 120-hr fecal material of abstinent dogs. Total radioactivity data accounted for about

59% of the administered cyclazocine in abstinent dogs over a 5-day period. These data, therefore, suggest with reference to the cyclazocine abstinence syndrome the following: (1) less than 0.055 nmoles (3.3×10^{13} molecules/g) of cyclazocine/g of brain was present during the 24- to 96-hr abstinent period to prevent signs of abstinence. Higher molecular levels of drug would have been detected. (2) Cyclazocine is metabolized to a less lipid soluble and more polar compound (e.g., norcyclazocine), which slowly gains entrance to the CNS and slowly egresses from the CNS but substitutes satisfactorily for cyclazocine. The data concerning ³H-norcyclazocine negates this hypothesis. (3) The biochemical changes induced at the cellular level were such that neither the presence of cyclazocine nor a metabolite was required to maintain the physically dependent cell over a period of 72 to 96 hr.

The mean total urinary recovery data for cyclazocine collected over a 5-day period showed little difference between the nontolerant, tolerant, and abstinent dogs. In contrast, the mean total fecal recovery of the tolerant dogs was about threefold higher than that of either the nontolerant or abstinent dogs. The higher value was due to the increased excretion of free cyclazocine in the feces of the tolerant dogs. In this regard it is interesting to note the low fecal excretion of free cyclazocine in tolerant dog No. 33, which was associated with a marked increase in the urinary excretion of the free drug. Therefore, the largest percentage recovery (58.5%) of administered ³H-cyclazocine was obtained with the tolerant dogs.

A small percentage of cyclazocine was metabolized to free and conjugated norcyclazocine. The total percentage of the injected dose for urine and feces did not exceed 7.8%. There was little difference between nontolerant and tolerant dogs.

A comparison of the cerebral cortex and subcortical levels of the nontolerant dogs with the tolerant dogs shows a slower egression of free cyclazocine from the CNS of the tolerant dogs. This is in contrast to the faster egression of morphine (11) from the CNS of chronically morphinized dogs.

The observed differences in the gray and white matter of the nontolerant dogs appear to resemble those reported for ³H-nalorphine (12). The gray/white ratios of the cyclazocine-tolerant dogs appeared to remain at a level of one at each time interval, in contrast to the rapid fall observed with time in the morphine-tolerant dogs (11).

The rapid absorption of ³H-cyclazocine into the CNS and egression from the CNS followed quite closely the rise and fall of the drug in plasma of the nontolerant and tolerant dogs. Mean cerebral cortex gray tissue to plasma ratios for free cyclazocine at 60 min were 9.3 and 10.4 for nontolerant and tolerant dogs, respectively. At 6 hr the ratios were 3.3 for the nontolerant dogs and 10.6 for the tolerant. The latter ratio reflects the slower comparative egression of free cyclazocine from the cerebrum of the tolerant dogs. These studies certainly indicate that any binding of cyclazocine by cellular constituents must be freely reversible.

One of the purposes of this study was to obtain data concerning the metabolism of cyclazocine which might help to explain the latency of abstinence observed in man after abrupt withdrawal of cyclazocine (1). The absence of norcyclazocine in the CNS of the dog after each time interval tends to eliminate the possibility that this metabolite might substitute satisfactorily for cyclazocine during abstinence. However, the metabolic fate of cyclazocine in the human may be different from that observed in the dog. Certainly the duration of action of cyclazocine in the human (3) appears to be much greater than that observed in the chronic spinal dog (13). The CNS levels of cyclazocine in the dog also suggest a short duration of action in this species.

The studies on the chronic spinal dog with norcyclazocine indicate that this compound is not very active pharmacologically. Therefore, it might not suppress the abstinence syndrome even if present in the CNS of man as a metabolite of cyclazocine.

Cyclazocine and norcyclazocine were identified chromatographically in different solvent systems as well as at different pH's of buffered paper, either as the extracted drug or by direct application of the hydrolyzed or unhydrolyzed urine. On silicic acid-impregnated paper, an unknown metabolite 1 of the unhydrolyzed urine appeared in both the nontolerant and tolerant dog. This unknown compound was not observed on the pH buffered paper of the unhydrolyzed dog urine or the hydrolyzed dog urine nor on the silicic acid-impregnated chromatograms of the hydrolyzed tolerant dog urine. It is difficult to understand why the metabolite was not present on the chromatogram (silicic acid) of the hydrolyzed dog urine, unless the metabolite was labile under the conditions of acid hydrolysis.

Figure 4 shows schematically the metabolic products of cyclazocine and the mean percentage of the individual compounds excreted in both urine and feces. The total percentage recovery (urine plus feces) of all known metabolites of ³H-cyclazocine was 51.4, 66.0, and 47.0% for the nontolerant, tolerant, and abstinent dogs, as determined over a 5-day period. Thus, some 34 to 53% of ³H-cyclazocine was still unaccounted for. It therefore seems that a significant percentage of ³H-cyclazocine or metabolites remains sequestered within the animal for a longer period than 5 days or is largely metabolized to compounds excreted primarily in the feces. Total radioactivity studies on the urine and feces certainly indicate the presence of

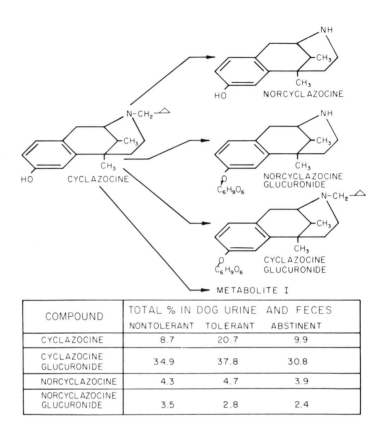

COMPOUND	TOTAL % IN DOG URINE AND FECES		
	NONTOLERANT	TOLERANT	ABSTINENT
CYCLAZOCINE	8.7	20.7	9.9
CYCLAZOCINE GLUCURONIDE	34.9	37.8	30.8
NORCYCLAZOCINE	4.3	4.7	3.9
NORCYCLAZOCINE GLUCURONIDE	3.5	2.8	2.4

FIG. 4. Metabolic products of ³H-cyclazocine after a 1.25 mg/kg (free base) s.c. injection of drug in dogs and the total mean percentage excreted in urine and feces. (Mulé et al., J. Pharmacol. Exp. Ther. *160*:387, 1968.)

nonextractable ³H-compounds of ³H-cyclazocine. However, even the total radioactivity values did not account for 100% of the administered ³H-cyclazocine 5 days after drug administration.

CONCLUSIONS

This investigation allows for the following conclusions: (1) the increased potency of cyclazocine in comparison to morphine may be related to the relatively higher CNS levels of cyclazocine; (2) latency associated with cyclazocine abstinence was apparently not due to residual quantities of cyclazocine in the CNS; (3) the egression of cyclazocine from the CNS and other tissues was significantly slower in the tolerant dogs as compared to the nontolerant; (4) ³H-cyclazocine was excreted in the dog as free and conjugated drug, as free and conjugated norcyclazocine, and as an unknown metabolite 1; (5) an alteration in the physiologic state of the dog did not appear to change the percentage excretion of norcyclazocine (free or conjugated); (6) the absence of norcyclazocine in the CNS indicated that the latency of abstinence from cyclazocine was not due to substitution of cyclazocine with norcyclazocine; (7) norcyclazocine does not appear to be a pharmacologically active metabolite of cyclazocine; (8) total percentage recovery of ³H-cyclazocine and all known metabolites of ³H-cyclazocine ranged between 47 and 66% in the nontolerant, tolerant, and abstinent dogs, as determined over a 5-day period.

REFERENCES

1. Martin, W. R., Fraser, H. F., Gorodetzky, C. W., and Rosenberg, D. E.: Studies of the addiction potential of the narcotic antagonist 2-cyclo-propylmethyl-2'-hydroxy-5,9-dimethyl-6,7-benzomorphan (Cyclazocine, Win 20,740, ARC II-C-3). J. Pharmacol. Exp. Ther. *150*:426–436, 1965b.

2. Fraser, H. F., and Rosenberg, D. E.: Comparative effects of (1) chronic administration of cyclazocine (ARC II-C-3), (2) substitution of nalorphine for cyclazocine and (3) chronic administration of morphine. Pilot cross-over study. Int. J. Addict. *1*:86–98, 1966.

3. Martin, W. R., Gorodetzky, C. W., and McClane, T. K.: An experimental study in the treatment of narcotic addicts with cyclazocine. Clin. Pharmacol. Ther. 7:455–465, 1966.

4. Fraser, H. F., Van Horn, G. D., Martin, W. R., Wolbach, A. B., and Isbell, H.: Methods for evaluating addiction liability. (A) "Attitude" of opiate addicts toward opiate-like drugs, (b) A short-term "direct" addiction test. J. Pharmacol. Exp. Ther. *133*:371–387, 1961.

5. Kolb, L., and Himmelsbach, C. K.: Clinical studies of drug addiction. III. A critical review of the withdrawal treatments with method of evaluating abstinence syndromes. Am. J. Psychol. *94*:759–797, 1938.

6. Lasagna, L., De Kornfeld, T. J., and Pearson, J. W.: The analgesic efficacy and respiratory effects in man of a benzomorphan "narcotic antagonist." J. Pharmacol. Exp. Ther. *144*:12–16, 1964.

7. Jaffe, J. H., and Brill, L. B.: Cyclazocine, a long acting narcotic antagonist: Its voluntary acceptance as a treatment modality by narcotics abusers. Int. J. Addict. *1*:99–123, 1966.

8. Martin, W. R., Gorodetzky, C. W., and McClane, T. K.: Demonstration of antagonism of morphine's (M) dependence producing properties with chronically administered cyclazocine (C). Pharmacologist 7:163, 1965a.

9. Mulé, S. J., and Gorodetzky, C. W.: Physiologic disposition of ³H-cyclazocine in nontolerant, tolerant, and abstinent dogs. J. Pharmacol. Exp. Ther. *154*:632–645, 1966.

10. Mulé, S. J., Clements, T. H., and Gorodetzky, C. W.: The metabolic fate of ³H-cyclazocine in dogs. J. Pharmacol. Exp. Ther. *160*:387–396, 1968.

11. Mulé, S. J., and Woods, L. A.: Distribution of N-C¹⁴-methyl labeled morphine: 1. In central nervous system of nontolerant and tolerant dogs. J. Pharmacol. Exp. Ther. *136*:232–241, 1962.

12. Hug, C. C., and Woods, L. A.: Tritium labeled nalorphine: Its CNS distribution and biological fate in dogs. J. Pharmacol. Exp. Ther. *142*:248–256, 1963.

13. McClane, T. K., and Martin, W. R.: Effects of morphine, nalorphine, cyclazocine, and naloxone on the flexor reflex. Int. J. Neuropharmacol. 6:89–98, 1967.

Narcotic Antagonists, edited by M. C. Braude, L. S. Harris, E. L. May, J. P. Smith, and J. E. Villarreal. *Advances in Biochemical Psychopharmacology, Vol. 8.* Raven Press, New York © 1974.

Metabolism and Pharmacokinetics of Naloxone

Stephen H. Weinstein, Morris Pfeffer, and Joseph M. Schor

Endo Laboratories, Inc., Department of Biochemistry, Garden City, New York 11530

Naloxone (N-allyl-7,8-dihydro-14-hydroxynormorphinone), 7,8-dihydro-14-hydroxynormorphinone, and N-allyl-7,8-dihydro-14-hydroxynormorphine have been identified in human urine after naloxone administration. The metabolites were isolated, after hydrolysis with glusulase, by column chromatography and identified by thin-layer chromatography and spectrofluorometry. These findings indicate that both N-dealkylation and reduction of the 6-oxo group of naloxone as well as glucuronide formation occur in man. Evidence is also presented indicating that N-allyl-7,8-dihydro-14-hydroxynormorphine formation occurs in rabbits as well as in man and chickens. Plasma levels of naloxone in rats were determined by a gas-chromatographic method. Five min after i.v. administration of 1 mg/kg the plasma concentration was 258 ng/ml. Low oral doses could not be detected in the plasma, but after 100 mg/kg the peak level of unchanged drug was almost 5,000 ng/ml. Pharmacokinetic parameters were generated with a computer program, and the constructed models are of a rapidly absorbed and rapidly excreted and/or metabolized drug.

INTRODUCTION

The metabolic fate of naloxone (N-allyl-7,8-dihydro-14-hydroxynormorphinone), a potent opiate antagonist in animals (2, 3) and in man (4, 5), has been studied by Fujimoto (6, 7) and Weinstein et al. (12). Fujimoto (6) initially isolated the glucuronide metabolites of naloxone from rabbits and chickens. The metabolite from rabbits was naloxone-3-glucuronide and that from chicken was N-allyl-14-hydroxy-7,8-dihydronormorphine-3-glucuronide. This meant that in the chicken metabolite the 6-oxo group of naloxone is reduced to an hydroxyl group.

In a later study Fujimoto (7) isolated naloxone-3-glucuronide from human urine. Although Fujimoto did not rule out the formation of the reduced metabolite of naloxone in man, he reported detecting nothing corresponding to N-allyl-14-hydroxy-7,8-dihydromorphine Structure I, Fig. 1, (EN-2265) after thin-layer chromatography of human urine extracts. However, Weinstein et al. (12) identified I in human urine extracts, as well as in the glu-

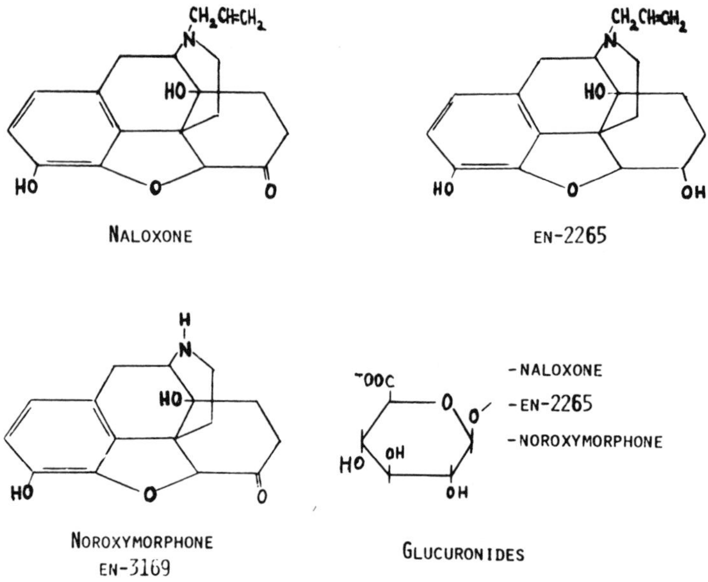

FIG. 1. Naloxone and its metabolites.

curonide isolated from rabbits by Fujimoto. More recent findings concerning naloxone metabolism will be discussed in this chapter.

In addition to metabolic studies, plasma levels of naloxone in rats dosed intravenously (i.v.) and orally (p.o.) with the drug have been determined. Absorption and elimination rate constants, as well as other pharmacokinetic parameters, were generated with the use of a computer program (11), in order to gain insight into the pharmacodynamics of naloxone.

METHODS

Urine obtained from a patient participating in a study of naloxone in the treatment of opiate dependence was extracted and chromatographed as described by Weinstein et al. (12). Glusulase[1] was used to hydrolyze the glucuronides.

A spectrophotofluorometer was used to obtain the fluorescence excitation and emission spectra of I after reaction with ferri-ferrocyanide reagent (8, 9). Pure I was oxidized to "pseudo-I," 2,2'-bi(N-allyl-7,8-dihydro-14-

---

[1] Glusulase (Endo Laboratories) is an enzymatic preparation from *Helix pomatia,* which contains sulfatase and glucuronidase.

hydroxynormorphine), with ferri-ferrocyanide reagent, and the spectra were obtained for comparison with material eluted from thin-layer chromatography plates after spraying with ferri-ferrocyanide spray reagent. The eluting agent was 1 ml of 0.1 M sodium pyrophosphate adjusted to pH 8.5 with 1 N hydrochloric acid. The eluate was transferred to a microcell for fluorometric scanning.

To correlate data from our laboratory with his, Fujimoto supplied the glucuronides isolated from the urine of rabbits and chickens which had been treated orally with naloxone. These glucuronides were hydrolyzed with glusulase, and subjected to column (12) and gas-liquid chromatography.

Gas-liquid chromatography of the urine extracts was performed on a 4% XE-60 column at 240°C. The silyl derivatives were formed on a column by injecting N,O-*bis*-(trimethylsilyl)-trifluoroacetamide with 1% trimethylchlorosilane (BSTFA/TMCS) into the gas chromatograph together with the concentrated urine extract.

Extraction of naloxone from rat plasma was performed as described by Mulé (10), except that chloroform containing 1% isopropanol was used as the solvent and this was back-extracted with 1.3 ml of 0.1 N HCl. A 1-ml portion of the final HCl extract was evaporated to dryness. An internal standard, 500 ng of tetraphenylethylene (25 μl of a 20 ug/ml methanol solution), was then added. The samples were again evaporated to dryness, and 25 μl of *bis*(trimethylsilyl)trifluoroacetamide containing 1% trimethylchlorosilane (BSTFA/TMCS) was added. Wilkinson and Way (13) have demonstrated the efficacy of BSTFA/TMCS as a silylating agent for morphine. We have found it equally useful for naloxone. The tubes were flushed with dry nitrogen, closed with ground glass stoppers and the silylation reaction was carried out for 30 min at 60°C to 65°C in a dry heating block. One-μl aliquots of the silylated samples were injected into a gas chromatograph with carbon tetrachloride as a solvent flush. Naloxone was measured by comparing the peak height ratio of naloxone/tetraphenylethylene in the experimental samples to the peak height ratio obtained from standards extracted from plasma.

The gas chromatograph was equipped with a flame ionization detector. The column was 3.8% UC-W98 on Hi-EFF Chromosorb W, 80/100 mesh. Conditions used were: oven, 245°C; detector, 310°C; flash heater, 300°C; H_2 flow rate, 37 ml/min; He, 75 ml/min; air, 350 ml/min.

Three to five fasted, male, CFN rats (average weight, 397 g) were used for each time interval of the i.v. study. Naloxone·HCl (1 mg/ml, aqueous solution) was administered via the tail vein at a dose of 1 mg/kg while the rats were under light ether anesthesia. Five, 10, 15, 22, 30, 38, 45, 50, and 60 min after dosing, blood was obtained by cardiac puncture with heparinized syringes. The plasma was separated by centrifugation at $3,000 \times g$ for 20 min.

For the oral studies, naloxone·HCl was administered to fasted rats (average weight, 375 g) in aqueous solution (100 mg/ml) via stomach tube at a dose of 100 mg/kg. Two, 3.5, 5, 15, 22, 30, 35, 45, 50, and 60 min after dosing, blood was obtained as described above. Four to 11 rats were used for each time interval.

A computer program (COMPT) for optimizing the solution of integral nonlinear compartmental models of drug distribution written in extended BASIC for use in time-sharing computer systems was used to generate pharmacokinetic parameters (11).

RESULTS

The thin-layer chromatographs of the human urine extracts are shown in Figs. 3 and 4. The alkaloid bases identified after hydrolysis are naloxone, EN-2265 (the reduced naloxone), and the 7,8-dihydro-14-hydroxynormorphinone Structure II, Fig. 1, (EN-3169). Figure 2 is the fluorescence excitation and emission spectra confirming the identity of EN-2265. The gas chromatographic results obtained after hydrolysis of the rabbit and chicken glucuronides are shown in Figs. 5–8. I and naloxone are present.

In the experiments in which plasma levels of naloxone were determined after dosing by different routes it was found that low oral doses of naloxone (10 mg/kg) could not be detected in plasma; however, 100 mg/kg resulted in a peak level of almost 5,000 ng/ml. Five min after i.v. administration of 1 mg/kg of naloxone the plasma level was 258 ng/ml.

Plasma levels of naloxone, after i.v. and p.o. administration, are shown in Figs. 9 and 10. The curves drawn are the best fit computed by the COMPT program. The pharmacokinetic models and parameters are given in Figs. 11 and 12.

Under the described chromatographic conditions tetraphenylethylene had a retention time of 2.2 min and the trimethylsilyl naloxone had a retention time of 4.5 min.

The use of parallel extraction standards as controls was necessary because the recovery of naloxone from plasma was 50 to 60%. There was a linear, reproducible relationship between gas chromatographic response and plasma concentration of naloxone.

DISCUSSION

Naloxone, 7,8-dihydro-14-hydroxynormorphinone, II, and N-allyl-7,8-dihydro-14-hydroxynormorphine, I, have been identified in the urine of a

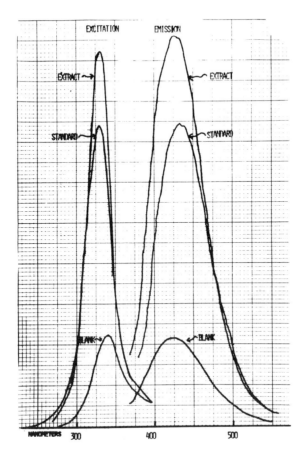

FIG. 2. Fluorescence excitation and emission spectra of EN-2265 eluted from thin-layer chromatography plates.

human subject receiving large oral doses of naloxone. After hydrolysis and extraction of the urine, the three bases were identified by thin-layer chromatography in two systems. The presence of I was confirmed by its fluorescence excitation and emission spectra. Neither naloxone nor II is detectably fluorescent, even after oxidation. The spectra of the metabolite were identical to those of pure I, which has an excitation maximum of 330 nm and an emission maximum of 430 nm (both maxima uncorrected).

Traces of all three bases can be seen on the thin-layer plates prior to hydrolysis, indicating that N-dealkylation and reduction of the 6-oxo group may occur before glucuronidation. Formation of the glucuronide followed

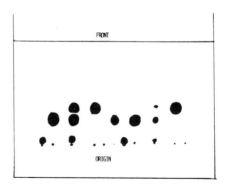

FIG. 3. Thin-layer chromatogram of human urine extract. Solvent — chloroform, dioxane, ethylacetate, conc. ammonia (25:60:10:2.5 v/v). Sample order, left to right: control urine + EN-3169 + glusulase, control urine + EN-2265 + glusulase, patient's urine + glusulase, control urine + naloxone + glusulase, control urine + glusulase, EN-2265 standard, control urine + EN-3169, control urine + EN-2265, patient's urine, control urine + naloxone, control urine.

by N-dealkylation and reduction of the base moiety, followed by hydrolysis, *in vivo*, seems unlikely. It is possible that processing of the urine may result in some hydrolysis without addition of glusulase, but glucuronides are known to be resistant to nonspecific hydrolysis (1).

A small quantity of I was detectable in the rabbit glucuronide fraction by gas chromatography, although a much larger amount of naloxone was present. The opposite was found in the chicken glucuronide fraction, in which I was the predominant base.

The plasma level studies of naloxone after dosing by the i.v. route yielded a pharmacokinetic model (Fig. 12), which gave a rapid elimination rate ($t_{1/2} = 16$ min). The relatively large volume of distribution in compartment 1 could indicate either extensive plasma protein binding or rapid metabolism,

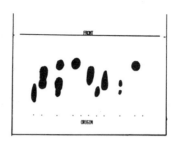

FIG. 4. Thin-layer chromatogram of human urine extract. Solvent — chloroform, methanol, conc. acetic acid (100:60:2, v/v). Sample order: see Fig. 3.

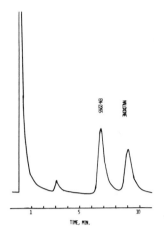

FIG. 5. Gas-liquid chromatogram of standard mixture of EN-2265 and naloxone.

since the model is simply attempting to account for the absence of a large fraction of the administered dose as unchanged drug in plasma. The small values of K_{12} and V_2 and large K_{21} indicate slow entry into, little binding in, and rapid removal from a peripheral compartment.

The one compartment model (Fig. 11) which the naloxone plasma levels conform to after oral administration satisfies the data obtained with this route of administration. If a more sensitive analytical method were available, a leveling off of the plasma concentrations probably would have been ob-

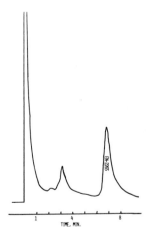

FIG. 6. Gas-liquid chromatogram of EN-2265.

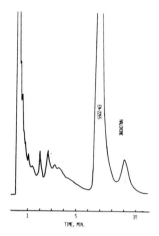

FIG. 7. Gas-liquid chromatogram of glusulase-hydrolyzed chick glucuronide extract.

served after 45 min, and the use of a two compartment model would be indicated.

The observed terminal straight line portion of the curve (Fig. 9) is probably really the distributive phase. The computer-fitted curve does, however, show a very rapid absorption rate ($t_{1/2} = 0.72$ min) for naloxone. The large volume of distribution may indicate either extensive binding or rapid metabolism. The elevated plasma levels observed between 38 and 52 min are due to biliary recycling.

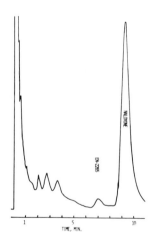

FIG. 8. Gas-liquid chromatogram of glusulase-hydrolyzed rabbit glucuronide extract.

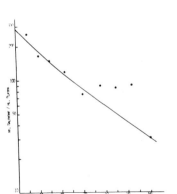

FIG. 9. Naloxone plasma concentrations in rats following 1 mg/kg administered intravenously. Semi-log plot.

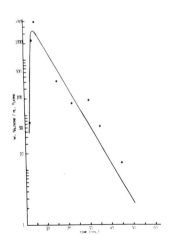

FIG. 10. Naloxone plasma concentrations in rats following 100 mg/kg administered orally. Semi-log plot.

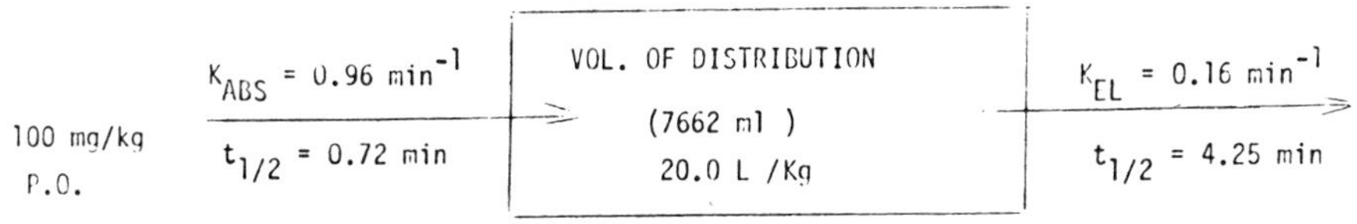

100 mg/kg P.O.	$K_{ABS} = 0.96\ min^{-1}$ $t_{1/2} = 0.72\ min$	VOL. OF DISTRIBUTION (7662 ml) 20.0 L /Kg	$K_{EL} = 0.16\ min^{-1}$ $t_{1/2} = 4.25\ min$

FIG. 11. One compartment open pharmacokinetic model for orally administered naloxone.

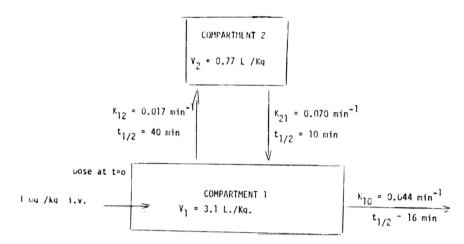

FIG. 12. Two compartment open pharmacokinetic model for intravenous naloxone.

SUMMARY

Evidence has been presented for the occurrence of several conjugated metabolites of naloxone in the urine of a human subject. The substances were isolated from urine after hydrolysis with glusulase, and identified by thin-layer chromatography as naloxone, 7,8-dihydro-14-hydroxynormorphinone, II, and N-allyl-7,8-dihydro-14-hydroxynormorphine, I. The identification of the latter was verified by its fluorescence excitation and emission spectra. The presence of detectable amounts of the free bases prior to hydrolysis indicates that N-dealkylation and reduction of the 6-oxo group probably precedes glucuronidation of the metabolites.

I was also identified as a metabolite of naloxone in rabbits. However, chickens appear to be the only species thus far studied that produces this metabolite in appreciable amounts. Humans and rabbits produce naloxone glucuronide, predominantly, with barely detectable amounts of the other metabolites.

Plasma levels in rats of orally and intravenously administered naloxone yield pharmacokinetic models of a rapidly absorbed and rapidly excreted drug. The pharmacokinetic parameters give some insight into the pharmacodynamics of naloxone. The short duration of action is reflected in the rapid elimination rate. However, the diminution of potency on oral administration cannot be accounted for by poor absorption, since the first order absorption rate of orally administered naloxone is quite rapid. It is more likely, in view of the rapid elimination rate, that the lower oral potency is due to rapid first pass liver metabolism.

ACKNOWLEDGMENTS

The authors are grateful to Mrs. Laura Franklin, Mrs. Miriam Mintz, and Miss Elaine R. Tutko for their excellent technical assistance. We are also grateful to Dr. Arthur Zaks of the Metropolitan Hospital, New York, New York, for obtaining urine from naloxone-treated patients.

REFERENCES

1. Bernheim, F., and Bernheim, M. L. C.: Note on the *in vitro* inactivation of morphine by liver. J. Pharmacol. Exp. Ther. *83*:85, 1945.
2. Blumberg, H., Dayton, H. B., and Wolf, P. S.: Narcotic antagonist activity of naloxone. Fed. Proc. *24*:676, 1968.
3. Blumberg, H., Wolf, P. S., and Dayton, H. B.: Use of writhing test for evaluating analgesic activity of narcotic antagonists. Proc. Soc. Exp. Biol. Med. *118*:763–766, 1965.
4. Fink, M., Zaks, A., Sharoff, R., Mora, A., Bruner, A., Levit, S., and Freedman, A. M.: Naloxone in heroin dependence. Clin. Pharmacol. Ther. *9*:568–577, 1968.
5. Foldes, F. F., Lunn, J. N., Moore, J., and Brown, I. M.: N-Allylnoroxymorphone: A new potent narcotic antagonist. Am. J. Med. Sci. *245*:57–64, 1963.
6. Fujimoto, J. M.: Isolation of two different glucuronide metabolites of naloxone from the urine of rabbit and chicken. J. Pharmacol. Exp. Ther. *168*:180–186, 1969.
7. Fujimoto, J. M.: Isolation of naloxone-3-glucuronide from human urine. Proc. Soc. Exp. Biol. Med. *133*:317–319, 1970.
8. Kupferberg, H., Burkhalter, A., and Way, E. L.: Fluorometric identification of submicrogram amounts of morphine and related compounds on thin-layer chromatograms. J. Chromatogr. *16*:558–559, 1964.
9. Kupferberg, H., Burkhalter, A., and Way, E. L.: A sensitive fluorometric assay for morphine in plasma and brain. J. Pharmacol. Exp. Ther. *145*:247–251, 1964.
10. Mulé, S. J.: Determination of narcotic analgesics in human biological material. Anal. Chem. *36*:1907–1917, 1964.
11. Pfeffer, M.: COMPT, a time sharing program for nonlinear regression analysis of compartmental models of drug distribution. J. Pharmacokin. Biopharm. 1:137–163, 1973.
12. Weinstein, S. H., Pfeffer, M., Schor, J. M., Indindoli, L., and Mintz, M.: Metabolites of naloxone in human urine. J. Pharm. Sci. *60*:1567–1568, 1971.
13. Wilkinson, G. R., and Way, E. L.: Sub-microgram estimation of morphine in biological fluids by gas-liquid chromatography. Biochem. Pharmacol *18*:1435–1439, 1969.

Narcotic Antagonists, edited by M. C. Braude, L. S. Harris, E. L.
May, J. P. Smith, and J. E. Villarreal. *Advances in Biochemical
Psychopharmacology, Vol. 8.* Raven Press, New York © 1974.

Cellular Transport of CNS Drugs in Leukocytes

Fedor Medzihradsky, Michael J. Marks, and Joan I. Metcalfe

*Department of Biological Chemistry and Upjohn Center for Clinical Pharmacology,
University of Michigan Medical Center, Ann Arbor, Michigan 48104*

Using leukocytes as model mammalian cells, the cellular transport of
various CNS drugs was studied. Morphologically intact and metabolically
active rat leukocytes rapidly accumulated pentazocine against a concentration gradient by a process which fulfills the criteria for an active transport.
The energy for the transport is derived from anaerobic metabolism of glucose. The kinetics of the process are characterized by a rapid initial uptake:
5 sec after addition of the drug 60% of the final cellular drug concentration
was reached; saturation was usually obtained between 2 and 3 min. When
pentazocine was present in the medium at micromolar concentrations, the
cellular accumulation of the drug was fivefold. The maximum velocity of
the uptake was 0.12 μmoles/g cells/5 sec and the concentration of drug
necessary to achieve half-maximum velocity (K_m) was 40 μM. The temperature coefficient of the transport process was constant at four drug concentrations and three temperatures: a temperature change of 10°C affected the
uptake by a factor of two. The transport of pentazocine was competitively
inhibited by analogue benzomorphans and its cellular uptake was blocked
by inhibitors of anaerobic glycolysis. The active transport of pentazocine
was independent of the presence of sodium and not affected by ouabain. In
addition to pentazocine, methadone and morphine were also accumulated at a rapid rate into leukocytes. The cells showed marked selectivity
in their uptake of these compounds. The highest affinity for the cellular accumulation, characterized by a K_m of 10 μM, was observed with methadone,
whereas morphine was actively transported into leukocytes with a much
lower affinity: its K_m was 4 mM. Ouabain had no effect upon the uptake of
morphine and methadone. The results suggest the existence in the plasma
membrane of leukocytes of transport systems responsible for the cellular
accumulation of various CNS drugs.

INTRODUCTION

Assuming intracellular sites of action, drugs have to reach a definite
concentration within the cell in order to produce pharmacologic effects.
Various processes which influence cellular drug levels, e.g., absorption,
distribution, binding, and metabolism, represent well-investigated areas of

drug research. Surprisingly little is known, however, about the mechanisms by which drugs enter cells and the biological role of these processes.

There is a considerable amount of information available on the uptake of various compounds, including drugs, into tissue slices, e.g., the uptake of selected CNS drugs into slices from brain was investigated (2, 5, 11, 13). More recently, synaptosomes (3, 4), as well as neuron- and glia-enriched fractions from brain (4), have been used to study the uptake of neurotransmitters. In addition, the human blood platelet was reported to accumulate and store organic bases, including CNS drugs (1, 12, 16, 17). However, no systematic study was undertaken to investigate the processes by which drugs are transported *across* the plasma membrane of cells. The potential importance of these processes led us to investigate the cellular transport of various CNS drugs.

In addition to cellular preparations from nervous tissue, we have utilized rat leukocytes to investigate the feasibility of using these readily available mammalian cells as a model to study the mechanisms of drug transport. If results with rat leukocytes can be shown to correlate with those obtained by using brain slices, synaptosomes, and bulk-isolated fractions of brain cells, it is possible that human leukocytes could be used as a valuable model to gain information on biochemical processes localized in cell tissue which is not readily accessible in man.

In initial experiments we observed the rapid uptake of pentazocine into brain of rats after intraperitoneal administration, indicating the easy transfer of the drug across biological membranes (9). This finding led us to investigate the cellular uptake of pentazocine. Recently we described the accumulation of benzomorphans against their concentration gradient in rat leukocytes (10). The uptake was characterized by its rapid rate and by its dependency on the presence of glucose. The present study concerns the further investigation of this uptake, particularly its characterization as an active transport process, and the evaluation of its structural specificity. Furthermore it was of interest to study the cellular uptake of additional CNS drugs.

MATERIALS AND METHODS

The unlabeled drugs used in this study were kindly provided by Drs. J. E. Villarreal and J. H. Woods (Department of Pharmacology, University of Michigan). Pentazocine-^{3}H (U) was a generous gift obtained from the Sterling-Winthrop Research Institute (Rensselaer, N.Y.). Morphine-(N-methyl-^{14}C)·HCl and methadone-(heptanone-2-^{14}C)·HCl were obtained from Mallinckrodt Chemical Works (St. Louis, Mo.). Protosol, a tissue solubilizer, as well as the scintillators PPO and dimethyl-POPOP were purchased from New England Nuclear (Boston, Mass.). Ouabain, iodoaceta-mide, 2,4-dinitrophenol, sodium azide, and Plasmagel, a modified gelatin solution, were obtained from Sigma Chemical Co. (St. Louis, Mo.) and HTI-Corporation (Buffalo, N.Y.), respectively. All other chemicals used were of reagent grade. The glass fiber filters, Reeve Angel No. 934 AH, 24 mm diameter, were purchased from Sargent-Welch Scientific Co. (Detroit, Mich.).

Male, Sprague-Dawley rats weighing 300 g were used. The collection of blood, its handling, and the separation of leukocytes were described previously (10) with the exception that the centrifugation was done at $80 \times g$, the initially obtained leukocyte pellet was washed by resuspension and that a different basic incubation medium was used. The latter contained a final millimolar concentration of: Na^+, 154; K^+, 4.8; Mg^{2+}, 1.2; Cl^-, 128; SO_4^{--}, 1.2; PO_4^{3}, 16; and glucose, 5.5. The pH of the medium was 7.4.

In a typical experiment, washed leukocytes were suspended in the basic incubation medium to give a concentration of 10^7 cells/ml. This suspension was preincubated for 60 min at 37°C at which time a solution of the drug under investigation was rapidly added in a ratio of 1:1 (vol/vol). The latter solution was made to contain "double strength" concentration of the drug, using the standard incubation medium. In addition, the added solution contained 0.1 to 0.2 μC of the radiolabeled drug.

At given times, which varied from 5 sec to 60 min, the suspension of cells was filtered quickly on a Millipore setup using glass fiber filters. To reduce the retention of radioactivity, the filters were presoaked thoroughly in 0.9% NaCl saturated with amyl alcohol. The cells on the filter were washed rapidly with 20 ml of ice-cold 0.9% NaCl which was squirted onto the filter by means of a syringe. The filters were then laid onto the bottom of standard counting vials and covered with 0.3 ml of Protosol. The vials were capped and incubated at 55°C for 2 hr to complete the digestion of the biological material. After the vials were cooled to room temperature, 10 ml of a scintillation medium (5 g POPOP and 0.3 g dimethyl-POPOP/l of toluene) was added. The radioactivity was measured in a scintillation spectrometer Packard, model 3320. The average counting efficiencies for ^{3}H- and ^{14}C-labeled compounds were 45% and 80%, respectively, as determined by the method of internal standardization. Appropriate blanks were run through the whole procedure. Even in experiments in which low uptakes were observed, the blank did not exceed 50% of the measured net counts.

RESULTS AND DISCUSSION

Although the data reported here were obtained using leukocytes separated from rat blood, preliminary investigations showed that human leukocytes are also capable of selectively transporting various compounds of pharmacological interest (6).

The morphological integrity and viability of the used rat leukocytes were thoroughly investigated and asserted in a preceding study (10).

In previous work on the uptake of benzomorphans by leukocytes the drug concentrations have been estimated by a procedure which involved extraction with an organic solvent and the quantitation of the drug by gas-liquid chromatography (10). The uptake reported here of pentazocine into rat leukocytes (Fig. 1) was investigated using the radiolabeled drug. The necessity for this methodology arose due to the extremely rapid uptake rates (Figs. 1 and 2). As shown in Fig. 2, the V_{max} for the uptake of pentazocine was 125 nmoles/g cells/5 sec. In order to study the uptake in its linear region, it was necessary to develop a procedure which allowed the termination of the uptake a few seconds after the addition of the drug. The adopted procedure is described in the experimental section. In order to eliminate a possible misinterpretation of the results obtained by radioactive measurements, experiments were carried out in which the uptake of pentazocine was determined using both the radioactive methodology and the estimation of pentazocine by gas-liquid chromatography. These experiments gave identical information on the uptake, which was investigated up to 60 min. It was

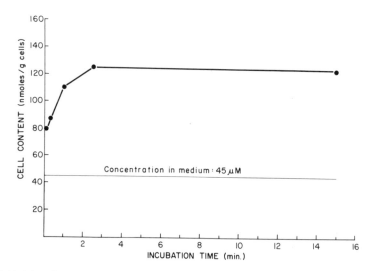

FIG. 1. Uptake of pentazocine by rat leukocytes. The experimental conditions for the uptake were as described in the text. The incubation medium contained an initial concentration of 45 μM DL- pentazocine. One g (wet weight) of leukocytes corresponded to approximately 10⁹ cells. Results of a representative experiment are shown.

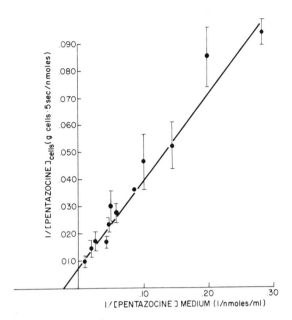

FIG. 2. Kinetics of the uptake of pentazocine by rat leukocytes. Abscissa: reciprocal initial concentrations of pentazocine in the incubation medium; ordinate: reciprocal cellular concentrations of pentazocine at 5 sec. The K_m for the uptake (intercept at the abscissa) is defined as the concentration of pentazocine in the medium necessary to achieve 50% of the V_{max} (intercept at the ordinate). Plotted are the mean values ± S.D. of 12 experiments in which different preparations of leukocytes were used.

of special importance to ascertain the absence of an interference by metabolism in experiments in which the uptake of pentazocine was investigated for longer time periods.

The results of the experiments described in this chapter demonstrate that pentazocine is accumulated in rat leukocytes by an active transport process. The following basic criteria for an uphill transport dependent on metabolic energy were fulfilled: (a) the uptake showed saturation kinetics (Fig. 1); (b) pentazocine is accumulated in leukocytes against its concentration gradient (Fig. 1); (c) a temperature change of 10°C affected the uptake rate by a factor of two (Fig. 3); (d) the uptake was dependent on the presence of glucose in the incubation medium (Fig. 4) and was markedly affected by metabolic inhibitors (Fig. 5); (e) the uptake of pentazocine was competitively inhibited by analogue benzomorphan derivatives (Fig. 6).

These relationships, particularly the dependency of the uptake on metabolic energy as well as the described effects of temperature and chemical analogues, make nonspecific protein binding unlikely as the underlying

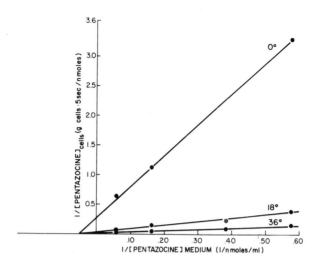

FIG. 3. Double reciprocal plot of the uptake of pentazocine into rat leukocytes at different temperatures. Shown are results of a representative experiment in which the same preparation of leukocytes was used.

phenomenon of our observations. Additional evidence was obtained against protein binding as a major participating mechanism by results of experiments on the uptake of pentazocine by leukocytes which were previously heated at 100°C for up to 5 min or repeatedly frozen (−70°C) and thawed. In addition, the uptake of pentazocine was investigated using red blood cells in suspensions which contained the same protein concentration as present in the standard procedure for leukocytes. In all these control experiments no accumulation of pentazocine in biological material was observed (6, 7).

The markedly strong effects on the pentazocine uptake displayed by inhibitors of anaerobic glycolysis (Fig. 5 and Table 1) are in agreement with the role of this pathway as a major energy yielding (ATP synthetizing) process in leukocytes (14). The findings shown in Fig. 5 were further substantiated by experiments in which the uptake of pentazocine was investigated under anaerobic condition. The results showed no significant change in the cellular accumulation of the drug (6). In recent experiments we were able to correlate the transport of pentazocine into leukocytes with the cellular concentrations of adenosinetriphosphate (ATP), phosphocreatine, and glucose (6). Additional investigations on the interrelationships of the transport processes for drugs with cellular metabolism are in progress.

As Figs. 7 and 8 show, rat leukocytes accumulated other CNS drugs also, in addition to benzomorphans. The common characteristic of these uptakes

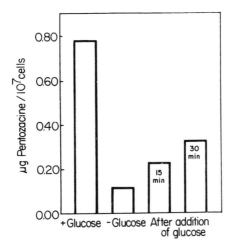

FIG. 4. Glucose dependency of the uptake of pentazocine by rat leukocytes. The first bar (+ *Glucose*) shows the uptake of pentazocine by leukocytes which were incubated at 37°C for 30 min in the incubation medium (pH 7.4) described in the text. The medium contained glucose (5.55 mM) and pentazocine (35 μM). The second bar (− *Glucose*) represents experiments in which leukocytes were preincubated at 37°C for 2 hr in a glucose-free medium, and then pentazocine (35 μM) was added. After reincubation for 30 min, the cellular uptake of the drug was determined as described. The last two bars (*After addition of glucose*) represent the uptake of pentazocine by leukocytes at various times after the addition of glucose (5.55 mM) to the initially preincubated cellular preparation in a glucose-free medium. The additional steps were as described. The results of a representative experiment are given. The values represent averages of results obtained from three individual incubations using the same preparation of leukocytes. The standard deviation about these averages did not exceed 5% of the mean value. The standard deviation for three experiments was 14.5%. [Reproduced by permission from Medzihradsky, F., Marks, M. J., and Carr, E. A., Jr.: Biochem. Pharmacol. 21:1625–1632, 1972 (10).]

was that they fulfilled the criteria for active transport, as described above, which is illustrated by their sensitivity toward metabolic inhibitors (Table 1). However, simultaneously with this similarity, these uptake processes differ considerably in their affinity toward the transported compounds as shown by the markedly different K_m values, which ranged from 10 μM for methadone to 4 mM for morphine (Table 1). As Table 1 shows, ouabain, a potent inhibitor of Na,K-ATPase, the enzyme postulated to be involved in the cellular transport of monovalent cations (15), had no effect on the uptake of either pentazocine, morphine, or methadone. In previous work, the independence of pentazocine accumulation in rat leukocytes from sodium concentrations in the incubating medium was established (10). Whether the uptakes of pentazocine, morphine, and methadone represent one or more transport systems requires additional investigations. There is experimental

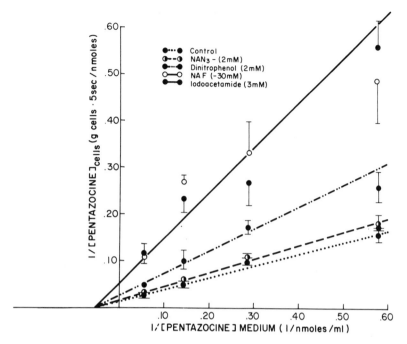

FIG. 5. Pentazocine uptake into rat leukocytes in the presence of metabolic inhibitors. Prior to the addition of pentazocine at initial concentrations as indicated, leukocytes were preincubated for 60 min at 37°C with the inhibitors present at concentrations as indicated. Plotted are the mean values ± S.D. of six separate measurements in which two preparations of leukocytes were used.

evidence, however (6), suggesting the existence, in addition to the transport system for benzomorphans (K_m for pentazocine: 40 μM), of a low-affinity process, which is responsible for the cellular uptake of morphine and is characterized by a K_m in the millimolar range (Table 1). This interpretation is further supported by observations that pentazocine in concentrations near its K_m does not affect the uptake of morphine, whereas at millimolar concentrations of the benzomorphan, the cellular accumulation of morphine is inhibited. On the other hand, morphine at K_m concentrations (4 mM) has no inhibitory effect on the transport of pentazocine. In addition, the transport of morphine was inhibited to a lesser degree by the metabolic poison sodium fluoride (Table 1). The further characterization of the structural specificity of the transport processes described here is in progress. In view of the selective biological actions of various isomers of CNS drugs (8), it is of special interest to investigate the role of isomerism in the cellular transport of these compounds.

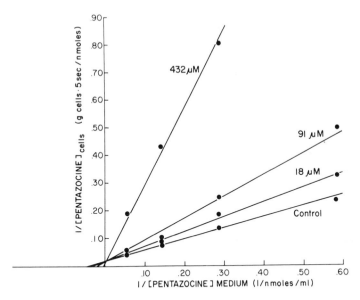

FIG. 6. Uptake of pentazocine into rat leukocytes in the presence of cyclazocine, a benzo-morphan analogue. Leukocytes were incubated simultaneously with pentazocine and cyclazocine at concentrations as indicated. The results of a representative experiment are shown in which the same preparation of leukocytes was used.

The information available on the uptake into other biological preparations of compounds investigated in the present study is not unequivocal. The uptake of morphine and methadone into brain slices was studied by several investigators (2, 5, 11, 13). However, no agreement seems to emerge from

TABLE 1. *Inhibition of drug uptake in rat leukocytes*[a]

	Inhibition (in %) of the uptake of		
Inhibitor	pentazocine (K_m: 40 μM)	methadone (K_m: 10 μM)	morphine (K_m: 4 mM)
Iodoacetamide	80	80	—
Sodium fluoride	55	50	25
Ouabain	0	0	0

[a] The experimental conditions for the uptake are described in the text. Prior to the addition of the investigated drug, leukocytes were preincubated for 60 min at 37°C with either 3 mM iodoacetamide, 30 mM sodium fluoride, or 0.4 mM ouabain. The uptake of the investigated drugs in the presence of inhibitors was compared to controls in which the same preparation of leukocytes was used.

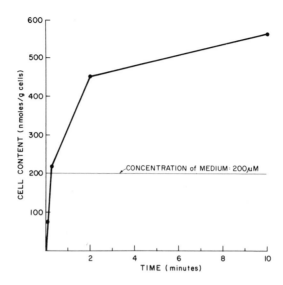

FIG. 7. Uptake of morphine by rat leukocytes. The incubation medium contained an initial concentration of 200 μM morphine. Results of a representative experiment are shown.

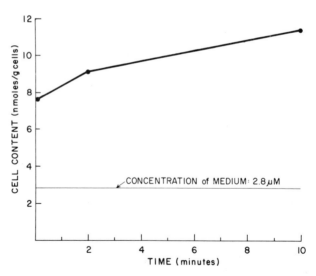

FIG. 8. Uptake of methadone by rat leukocytes. The incubation medium contained an initial concentration of 2.8 μM DL-methadone. Results of a representative experiment are shown.

these reports on the nature of the uptake of these compounds. The process described in the human platelet, which accumulated organic bases, including various drugs, was characterized by its lack of specificity (1, 12, 16, 17). The uptake of these compounds was affected by metabolic inhibitors and ouabain and was dependent on sodium concentrations in the incubation medium. These characteristics emphasize the difference between this nonspecific "amine pump" and the transport processes for CNS drugs existent in leukocytes.

The results of our study showed that the plasma membrane of leukocytes possesses marked activity and selectivity in transporting various CNS drugs. The existence of these processes in a blood cell is of great interest, especially in regard to the possible use of leukocytes as conveniently available models to study the mechanisms of cellular drug transport. However, there still remains the task of establishing the feasibility of using leukocytes to model the cellular transport of CNS drugs in the target tissue (e.g., brain). The correlation of data from leukocytes with those obtained using cellular preparations from nervous tissue is in progress. Nevertheless, all our accumulated evidence strongly suggests a need to revise the widely held assumption that most drugs enter cells by passive diffusion.

CONCLUSIONS

Rat leukocytes exhibited pronounced activity and selectivity in the uptake of various CNS drugs.

The cellular uptakes of benzomorphans, methadone, and morphine fulfilled the criteria for active transport processes.

These transport systems were characterized by rapid initial uptake rates (V_{max} for pentazocine: 125 nmoles/g cells/5 sec) and a wide range of affinities toward the transported compounds. The K_m's for the accumulation in leukocytes of pentazocine, methadone, and morphine were 40 μM, 10 μM, and 4 mM, respectively.

Ouabain had no effect on the accumulation of pentazocine, methadone, and morphine in leukocytes.

Experimental evidence suggests the existence of at least two ouabain-insensitive transport systems, characterized by markedly different affinities for the transported compounds.

ACKNOWLEDGMENT

This work was supported in part by U.S. Public Health Service grants 2 P11 GM15559, RO1-DA-00254, and RR 05383.

REFERENCES

1. Abrams, W. B.: The uptake and release of norepinephrine by the human platelet. Fed. Proc. *28*:544, 1969.
2. Bell, J. L.: Concentration of some analgesic compounds and their analogues in tissue surviving *in vitro:* Relation to *in vitro* metabolism and *in vivo* effects. J. Neurochem. *2*:265–282, 1958.
3. Bogdanski, D. F., Tissari, A., and Brodie, B. B.: Role of sodium, potassium, ouabain and reserpine in uptake, storage and metabolism of biogenic amines in synaptosomes. Life Sci. *7*:419–428, 1968.
4. Henn, F. A., and Hamberger, A.: Glial cell function: Uptake of transmitter substances. Proc. Nat. Acad. Sci. *68*:2686–2690, 1971.
5. Kayan, S., Misra, A. L., and Woods, L. A.: Uptake of [7,8-^{3}H] dihidromorphine by rat cerebral cortical slices and eye tissue. J. Pharm. Pharmacol. *22*:941–943, 1970.
6. Marks, M. J., and Medzihradsky, F.: *Unpublished observations.*
7. Marks, M. J., and Medzihradsky, F.: Characterization of the active transport of benzomorphans in leukocytes. Abstracts, 5. Int. Cong. Pharmacol. p. 149, 1972.
8. Martin, W. R.: Opioid antagonists. Pharmacol. Rev. *19*:463–521, 1967.
9. Medzihradsky, F., and Ahmad, K.: The uptake of pentazocine into brain. Life Sci. *10*:711–720, 1971.
10. Medzihradsky, F., Marks, M. J., and Carr, E. A., Jr.: Energy-dependent uptake of benzomorphans by leukocytes. Biochem. Pharmacol. *21*:1625–1632, 1972.
11. Miller, J. W., and Elliott, H. W.: *In vitro* studies on the diphasic action of methadone. J. Pharmacol. Exp. Ther. *110*:106–114, 1954.
12. Pocelinko, R., and Solomon, H. M.: Accumulation of debrisoquin-^{14}C by the human platelet. Biochem. Pharmacol. *19*:697–703, 1970.
13. Scrafani, J. T., and Hug, C. C., Jr.: Active uptake of dihydromorphine and other narcotic analgesics by cerebral cortical slices. Biochem. Pharmacol. *17*:1557–1566, 1968.
14. Seitz, J. F.: The biochemistry of the cells of blood and bone marrow. pp. 38–62, Charles C. Thomas Publisher, Springfield, Ill., 1969.
15. Skou, J. C.: Enzymatic basis for active transport of Na^+ and K^+ across cell membrane. Physiol. Rev. *45*:596–617, 1965.
16. Solomon, H. M., Ashley, C., Spirt, N., and Abrams, W. B.: The influence of debrisoquin on the accumulation and metabolism of biogenic amines by the human platelet, *in vivo* and *in vitro.* Clin. Pharmacol. Ther. *10*:229–238, 1969.
17. Solomon, H. M., and Zieve, P. D.: The accumulation of organic bases by the human platelet. J. Pharmacol. Exp. Ther. *155*:112–116, 1967.

Narcotic Antagonists, edited by M. C. Braude, L. S. Harris, E. L. May, J. P. Smith, and J. E. Villarreal. *Advances in Biochemical Psychopharmacology, Vol. 8.* Raven Press, New York © 1974.

Design Consideration for Long-Acting Antagonists

Sydney Archer

Rensselaer Polytechnic Institute, Sterling-Winthrop Research Institute, Rensselaer, New York 12144

It is generally agreed that the duration of action of presently known narcotic antagonists is too short for use in the management of opiate addicts. It is well known that incorporation of drugs in sustained-release delivery systems can markedly increase the duration of action. The pharmacokinetic properties of delivery systems and the pharmacological properties of narcotic antagonists which are relevant to the problem will be discussed. Methods for measuring blood levels of drugs over a long period of time will also be considered with special reference to immunoassay procedures.

There seems to be some difference of opinion as to how long acting an ideal narcotic antagonist should be. Some investigators believe that a day or two is long enough whereas others feel that a duration of 20 months or more would be better. However, there is no disagreement that it would be desirable to have available a narcotic antagonist with a long duration of action.

Very few clinically useful drugs have a long biological half-life. The structural requirements necessary for the preparation of a long-acting narcotic antagonist are not known so that, at present, there is no rational way to solve this problem chemically. However, technological developments have progressed far enough to permit us to devise a delivery system which would prolong the useful pharmacological effects of a narcotic antagonist for weeks, if not months.

It is obvious that to be useful a delivery system must be small and convenient to administer. Because of the size limitation, it is essential that the drug be a powerful antagonist.

In order to maintain a constant pharmacological effect over the entire period of drug action, it is important that the rate of release from the delivery system obey zero-order kinetics (3). Consider the model:

$$D_0 \xrightarrow{K_0} D_B \, , \, D_B \xrightarrow{K}$$

where D_0 is the concentration of injected drug, and D_B is the total concentration of the drug in the body. The change in concentration with time is equal to the difference between the rate of entry from the delivery system and the elimination rate as shown in equation (1).

$$\frac{dD_B}{dt} = K_0 - KD_B \tag{1}$$

D_B can be expressed in terms of the concentration of the drug in the sampling compartment C_D if a volume term is introduced to account for all the drug. This term, V_D, is called the "volume of distribution" but has no physiological meaning. Thus,

$$D_B = V_D \cdot C_D$$

Substituting $V_D C_D$ for D_B in equation (1) and integrating gives equation (2).

$$C_D = \frac{K_0}{V_D K}(1 - e^{-Kt}) \tag{2}$$

Note that the D_0 term does not appear in equation (2). The concentration of the drug in the sampling compartment C_D and thus D_B itself are independent of the amount of drug present in the delivery system. Note also that K, the rate constant for the disappearance of the drug, appears both in the exponential term and in the denominator. If the half-life is short, i.e., K is large, then for a given C_D, K_0, the rate constant for the release of the drug must be large. Other things being equal, it is preferable to have a drug with a long half-life. At some time after drug administration when the exponential e^{-Kt} is approaching zero, a plateau concentration of drug, C_D, is reached and maintained as long as the drug is being released from the delivery system. This drug concentration is directly proportioned to the drug release rate which can be controlled. It is also indirectly proportional to the product of the constants V_D and K.

If the release rate obeys first-order kinetics, then

$$\frac{dD_B}{dt} = K_A D_0 - KD_B$$

K_A is the rate constant for the reaction $D_0 \rightarrow D_B$.

Again, substituting $V_D C_D$ for D_B and solving for C_D, equation (3) results:

$$C_D = \frac{K_A D_0 (e^{-Kt} - e^{-K_a t})}{V_D(K_A - K)} \tag{3}$$

Here C_D is dependent on D_0 and as this decreases, C_D becomes smaller. As t increases, the exponential term decreases also. This pharmacokinetic model states not only that C_D is a function of D_0, the injection dose, but also predicts that C_D must decrease with time.

From this brief pharmacokinetic analysis, it may be concluded that a delivery system which obeys zero-order kinetics and employs a drug having a long half-life is preferable to a system which does not have these features.

Since cyclazocine is a potent antagonist with a long half-life in man, it seems to be a good candidate for incorporation in experimental delivery systems. To this end, experiments were initiated using a polyhydroxyalkyl acrylate as the delivery agent. After some experimentation, it was found that a closed hollow cylinder of the polymer filled with cyclazocine base (C) gave the most promising results. In Fig. 1 the amount of C released per day in a pH 7.2 buffer solution is plotted against time. The preparation was fabricated to deliver 2 mg of C/day (*top curve*). After the first day or two, this rate was reached and was more or less maintained at that level for 75 days. A slightly modified polymer was used to deliver approximately 0.25 mg of C/day (*bottom curve*). These preliminary results suggest that this system follows zero-order kinetics.

For *in vivo* studies of any delivery system, it is essential to be able to monitor the blood levels of the antagonist continually. If the drug is highly active pharmacologically, then C_D should be quite low. This situation requires that a highly sensitive assay method be available for the determination of blood levels of the antagonist. For a variety of reasons it is undesirable to incorporate a radiolabeled sample of the drug as a marker. One of the most sensitive ways to monitor drug levels is by immunoassay. Such a method is usually quite specific and relatively easy to carry out after the preliminary work is completed successfully.

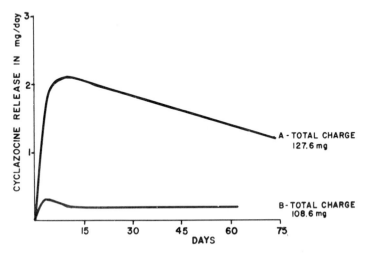

FIG. 1. Release of cyclazocine from HMS-2514-161, a polyhydroxyalkyl acrylate complex, in a pH 7.2 buffer system.

The steps in the development of a radioimmunoassay are: (1) The antagonist or haptene must be converted to an antigen by coupling to a suitable protein or polypeptide. The antigen is injected into animals to produce an antibody which is then isolated. (2) A sample of radiolabeled haptene is prepared and the antibody is mixed with an excess of the labeled haptene. The bound haptene (B) is separated from free haptene (F) and the B/F ratio determined. (3) A known quantity of unlabeled haptene is mixed with the same ratio of labeled antibody-haptene. The competition between the labeled and unlabeled haptene causes a decrease in B and an increase in F. Plotting known concentrations of unlabeled haptene versus the change in B/F ratio furnishes a standard curve which can be used for the assay of unknown samples.

The success of an immunoassay method depends on the preparation of a suitable antibody. Methods are available to convert simple haptenes to antigens. The sensitivity of the method is a function of the specific activity of the radiolabeled haptene. Recently, Spector (4) has succeeded in preparing an antibody to morphine. Preliminary experiments in our laboratory indicate that the preparation of an antibody for cyclazocine is feasible (5).

Recently, Leute, Ullman, and Goldstein (2, 3) reported on the use of a spin immunoassay for opiates, with special reference to the detection of morphine and related compounds. This method is similar in many respects to the radioimmunoassay but appears to be much easier to carry out. After the antibody is prepared a spin-labeled analogue of the haptene used to prepare the antibody is synthesized by coupling a stable free radical at the same position of the haptene used in making the antibody. The spin-labeled haptene is combined with the antibody and the resultant ESR spectrum appears as a broad envelope rather than sharp signals. The structure of spin-labeled morphine is shown below.

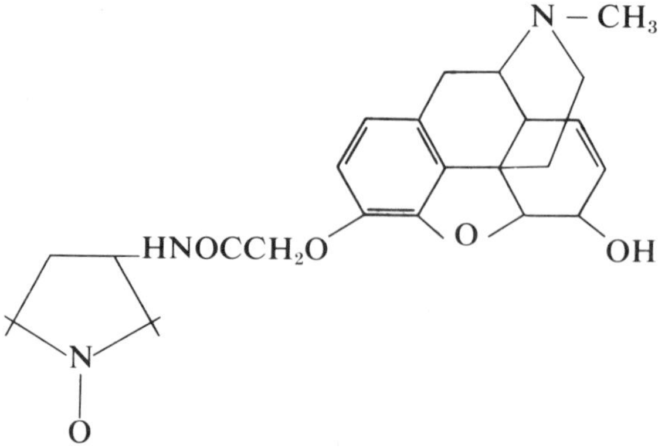

When a free haptene is added, it displaces the spin-labeled haptene, and the latter is recorded in an ESR spectrum as very sharp peaks, which quantitatively measure the number of free radicals in solution. The advantages of this method are: the extreme simplicity of operation, the extreme sensitivity (in the case of morphine 0.285 μg/ml), and the small sample size required (20 μl).

A word or two should be said about the biological character of the delivery system. Ideally such a system should be nontoxic, nonirritating, relatively easy to insert but difficult for the postaddict to remove, and preferably be biologically degradable so that the necessity for its removal from the implant site is obviated. If the device is not degradable, then it ought to be easily removed by the physician or one of his surrogates.

The state of the art has advanced far enough that it is probable that with a sufficient expenditure of effort, the problem of preparing suitable long-acting delivery systems can be solved.

REFERENCES

1. Leute, R. K., Ullman, E. F., and Goldstein, A.: J.A.M.A., *221*:1231, 1972.
2. Leute, R. K., Ullman, E. F., and Goldstein, A.: Nature, New Biology, *236*:93, 1972.
3. Portmann, G. A.: Biopharmaceutics, edited by J. Swarbrick, p. 15. Lea and Febiger, Philadelphia, 1970.
4. Spector, S., and Parker, C.: Science, *168*:1347, 1970.
5. *Unpublished work.* Private communication from Dr. K. Pittman.

Narcotic Antagonists, edited by M. C. Braude, L. S. Harris, E. L.
May, J. P. Smith, and J. E. Villarreal. Advances in Biochemical
Psychopharmacology, Vol. 8. Raven Press, New York © 1974.

Insoluble Salts and Salt Complexes of Cyclazocine and Naloxone[1]

Allan P. Gray* and Donald S. Robinson

Department of Pharmacology, University of Vermont, Burlington, Vermont 05401

The ultimate objective of this research is the development of long-acting narcotic antagonist preparations for intramuscular administration in the treatment of narcotic dependence. To this end, we have thus far prepared 23 salts of cyclazocine and 11 salts of naloxone with various mono- and polybasic organic acids. In general, salts of methadone were more soluble than those of cyclazocine which were more soluble than those of naloxone. From study of a large number of organic acids, a rather complete picture has been deduced of the structural features which need to be present in the acid if it is to yield a water-insoluble salt with an antagonist base. Various methods were explored to incorporate metal ions into complexes with drug and organic acid. Generally, complexes were less soluble than corresponding simple salts. Twelve complexes of cyclazocine and seven of naloxone have been prepared to date. As a guide to the selection of preparations for study in animals, the percent dissociation of our salts and complexes was determined *in vitro* in a simulated physiological medium. Duration of narcotic antagonist activity of selected salts and complexes administered intramuscularly to mice was determined by a modification of the tail-flick test for analgesia, essentially according to Harris et al. (5). Eighteen preparations of cyclazocine and six of naloxone have thus far been evaluated for duration of antagonist activity. A suggestion of a correlation has been observed between duration of activity *in vivo* and percent dissociation *in vitro*. Several of our preparations have significantly increased duration of narcotic antagonist activity in mice. These are being studied further.

Antagonists present a potentially useful alternative to methadone for the treatment of narcotic addiction but, since (unlike methadone) they provide little incentive to the subject to return frequently for maintenance doses, they suffer from the drawback of being too short-acting (8, 10). Our ob-

---

[1] Supported by a contract from the City of New York, Health Services Administration, and by grant MH 21361 from the National Institute of Mental Health.

* Current Address: Chemistry Research Division, IIT Research Institute, 10 West 35 St., Chicago, Illinois 60616.

jective is to overcome this shortcoming. Our approach involves preparation and study of water-insoluble salts and salt complexes of narcotic antagonist drugs since there are ample precedents in other therapeutic areas showing that an intramuscular injection of such dosage forms can provide slow release of drug and a useful prolongation of action (3, 4, 9). Intramuscular injection is considered to be the preferred route of administration of narcotic antagonists for the treatment of drug abuse (8). Oral administration would be ruled out in any event since the ultimate aim is to provide durations of action of the order of months.

In this chapter we describe our experience with certain of our preparations of cyclazocine and naloxone. Several of these, most notably cyclazocine zinc tannate and naloxone zinc tannate, have shown a significant prolongation of antagonist activity when tested in mice.

MATERIALS AND METHODS

DL-Cyclazocine (base),[2] naloxone hydrochloride,[3] methadone hydrochloride,[4] and morphine sulfate[5] were used as received. Various organic acids and/or their alkali metal salts were obtained commercially[6] and were generally used as received.

Preparation of Salts

Because methadone was more readily available to us than the narcotic antagonist drugs, we used methadone as a preliminary guide to the selection of acids potentially useful for the preparation of water-insoluble salts of cyclazocine and naloxone. A large number of acids have been evaluated, and approximately 40 such salts of methadone with mono- and polybasic organic acids were prepared.

To prepare the salts, a stirred aqueous solution of methadone hydrochloride was treated with an aqueous solution containing an equivalent amount of an alkali metal salt of the acid, or of the acid just neutralized with 0.2 N NaOH. In the case of gallotannic acid (tannic acid, Eastman), the equivalent weight was assumed to be $\frac{1}{5}$ of an approximate molecular

---

[2] We thank Drs. S. Archer and F. C. Nachod of the Sterling-Winthrop Research Institute for a generous supply of this material.

[3] Kindly supplied by Endo Laboratories, Inc.

[4] We thank Drs. G. B. Hoey and P. E. Wiegert of Mallinckrodt Chemical Works for a generous supply.

[5] S. B. Penick & Co.

[6] Aldrich Chemical Co. and Eastman Organic Chemicals.

weight of 1,700 (2). The reaction mixture was stirred for 30 min and allowed to stand for 1 hr at room temperature. The precipitated salt was collected, washed with water, and dried *in vacuo* over P_2O_5.

Salts of naloxone were similarly prepared. To prepare salts of cyclazocine, the base was dissolved in an equivalent amount of 0.1 N HCl. We have prepared 23 insoluble salts of cyclazocine and 11 of naloxone.

Preparation of Zinc Complexes

Various methods were explored to incorporate ionic zinc into insoluble complexes with drug and the organic acids which had themselves yielded insoluble salts. To date we have prepared 13 zinc complexes containing methadone, 12 with cyclazocine, and seven with naloxone using essentially the following methods.

1. A stirred aqueous solution of the alkali metal salt of the appropriate organic acid was treated with 0.25 equivalent of $ZnSO_4$ in a 1 M solution, followed in 10 min by one equivalent of an aqueous solution of drug hydrochloride. The reaction mixture was stirred for 1 hr and allowed to stand for 24 hr at room temperature. The precipitate was collected, washed with water, and dried to constant weight *in vacuo* over P_2O_5.

2. One equivalent of a 1 M solution of $ZnSO_4$ was added to a stirred aqueous suspension of preformed water-insoluble drug salt. The reaction mixture was stirred for 1 hr, allowed to stand for 24 hr, and worked up as before.

3. This was the same as Method 1, except that one equivalent of 1 M $ZnSO_4$ was used.

Analysis of Salts and Complexes for Drug

All analyses were run in duplicate. To analyze for methadone or cyclazocine content, an aqueous suspension of a weighed amount of salt or complex was brought to pH > 10 with 20% NaOH, a small amount of Na_2SO_4 was added, and the mixture was extracted with ether. The ether extract was water washed and extracted with 0.1 N HCl. The acid extract was diluted to standard volume with 0.1 N HCl, the absorbance of the solution at 292 nm (methadone) or 280 nm (cyclazocine) was measured with a Beckman Model DU-2 ultraviolet spectrophotometer, and drug content was read off a standard curve.

To analyze for naloxone, an extraction procedure patterned after that of Mulé (7) was used. The suspension of salt or complex was treated with a pH 10.4 phosphate buffer and NaCl was added (final pH 9.5). (When tannate salts and complexes were determined, it was necessary to readjust the pH to approximately 10 with 20% NaOH in order to avoid extraction of weakly acidic, interfering materials.) The aqueous solution was extracted with methylene chloride:butanol (3:1). The organic extract was shaken with 0.1 N HCl, the acid solution was diluted to standard volume, and the absorbance at 280 nm was determined.

Analysis of Complexes for Zinc

A suspension of a weighed amount of complex in 1 N HCl was allowed to stand for 2 hr with occasional shaking; it was then centrifuged, and an aliquot of the supernatant solution was serially diluted with distilled water and 0.1 N HCl. Zinc content was determined by measurement of the responses of a Jarrell-Ash Model No. 82–270 atomic-absorption, flame-emission spectrophotometer in comparison with the dose-response of standard zinc solutions (Fisher standard reference solution of zinc oxide in dilute HNO_3, serially diluted with 0.1 N HCl).

Dissociation of Salts and Complexes

A weighed amount of salt or complex calculated to contain 15 mg of drug was suspended in 10 ml of isotonic phosphate buffer, pH 7.3 (125 ml of 0.2 M KH_2PO_4, 85 ml of 0.2 N NaOH plus 2 g of NaCl, diluted with distilled water and pH adjusted to 7.3 with additional 0.2 N NaOH, final volume 500 ml). The suspension was stirred (magnetic stirrer) for 1 hr in a bath maintained at 37.0 ± 0.1°C and then centrifuged; the supernatant liquor was filtered through a glass wool plug.

For determination of percent dissociation of methadone and cyclazocine, the filtrate was brought to pH > 10 with 20% NaOH and extracted as described above under Analysis.

To determine percent dissociation of naloxone, the filtrate was extracted directly with the methylene chloride:butanol solvent. [When naloxone salts or complexes of certain weak acids (e.g., tannic) were determined, it was necessary to adjust the pH to approximately 10 prior to extraction.]

Drug content was determined spectrophotometrically as described under Analysis.

Measurement of Duration of Pharmacological Activity in Mice

Drug preparations were administered to mice by intramuscular injection, originally in both saline and peanut oil suspensions but later, because differences did not appear significant, only in peanut oil suspension. Peanut oil formed more satisfactory suspensions and would be expected to have any added advantage there was in influencing duration of action.

Analgesic activity of methadone salts and complexes was determined by the mouse tail-flick method of Harris et al. (5). Dose-response curves and ED_{80} values were obtained based on reaction time 30 min after administration of drug preparation.

Duration of analgesic activity was evaluated by testing groups of mice at periodic intervals after administration of the predetermined ED_{80} dose. At least 12 mice were used for every determination (at each dose level and at each time interval).

Antagonism of analgesia by cyclazocine and naloxone salts and complexes was determined similarly by adaptation to the mouse tail-flick procedure (5) of the method of Harris and Pierson (6). Dose-response curves and ED_{80} (antagonism) values were obtained based on measurement of reaction time 40 min after intramuscular administration of drug preparation and 30 min after intraperitoneal administration of a dose of 20 mg/kg of morphine sulfate, which was the ED_{80} (analgesia) dose under normal conditions.

Duration of antagonist activity was evaluated by dosing mice with the drug preparation, and by taking groups of the mice at periodic intervals, challenging these with a 20 mg/kg intraperitoneal dose of morphine sulfate, and testing their reaction time in the tail-flick test 30 min thereafter. Duration of activity was determined both at the ED_{80} (antagonism) dose level and at the high dose level of drug preparation calculated to contain 4.0 mg/kg of drug base. At least 12 mice were used for each individual determination.

The methadone salts were tested primarily to gain experience with the methodology; emphasis has now been shifted entirely over to the evaluation of antagonists. Thus far, nine methadone preparations have been evaluated for duration of analgesic activity, and 18 preparations of cyclazocine and six of naloxone have been evaluated for duration of antagonist activity.

RESULTS AND DISCUSSION

This discussion will primarily be restricted to our findings with preparations of the narcotic antagonists cyclazocine and naloxone. Analytical data and percent dissociation values (in isotonic, pH 7.3 buffer at 37°C) for representative salts of cyclazocine and naloxone are given in Table 1 and for representative zinc complexes in Table 2. Most of the salts and complexes prepared contained 40 to 60% drug, and none was submitted to animal test unless it contained at least 25%.

TABLE 1. *Analytical data on representative water-insoluble salts*

Salt Acid	Melting point (°C)	Mole ratio drug/acid	% Drug[a] Calcd.	% Drug[a] Found	% Dissociation at 37°C[b]
Cyclazocine					
Base[c]	201–204	–	100	–	35.4[d]
I Tannic	182–186	5	44.4	41.1	10.7
II Pamoic	201–205	2	58.3	57.5	10.3
III 3-Hydroxy-2-methyl-					
cinchoninic	198–199.5	1	59.1	60.5	33.3
IV 3,5-Di-*t*-butyl-2,6-					
dihydroxybenzoic	237–238	1	50.5	52.0	<0.8
V 5-*t*-Octylsalicylic	108–115	1	52.0	49.8	11.2
Naloxone					
Hydrochloric[e]	223–229	1	90.0	–	100
VI Tannic	186–190	5	49.0	46.2	53.3
VII Pamoic[f]	198–205	2	62.8	63.8	74.1
VIII 3,5-Di-*t*-butyl-2,6-					
dihydroxybenzoic	168–172	1	54.7	55.3	6.0
IX 5-*t*-Octylsalicylic	118–122	1	56.7	57.5	62.5

[a] See Methods for analytical procedures
[b] Percent of drug dissociating from salt or complex stirred at 37°C in isotonic phosphate buffer, pH 7.3. See Methods for details.
[c] From Sterling-Winthrop.
[d] In this case, % of base dissolving.
[e] From Endo Laboratories.
[f] Independently prepared at Endo Laboratories. H. Blumberg, 13th National Medicinal Chemistry Symposium, The University of Iowa, Iowa City, Iowa, June 18–22, 1972.

In general, percent dissociation of corresponding salts increased in the order methadone < cyclazocine < naloxone. Incorporation of zinc generally reduced dissociation. Percent dissociation ranged from a low of less than 0.8% to 100%.

Rather intriguing relationships were noted in regard to the structural features of the organic acids that formed water-insoluble salts with these drugs. Thus, a variety of aromatic acids yielded insoluble salts whereas the salts of aliphatic acids were almost invariably water soluble. Salts of sulfonic acids were more soluble than those of corresponding aromatic carboxylic acids. Polyphenolic compounds possessing electron-withdrawing substituents frequently provided salts showing low dissociation. In fact, the lowest percent dissociations were observed with aromatic carboxylic acids also bearing phenolic hydroxyl groups.

In addition to the appropriate acidic groups, a sufficient degree of counter-balancing lipophilic bulk was required. Thus, salicylic acid (formula **1** in Fig. 1) did not form water-insoluble salts with any of the drugs; its

TABLE 2. Analytical data on representative zinc complexes

Complex	Acid	Melting point (°C)	Preparative method[a]	Found[a]		Equivalents Ratios[b]		% Dissociation at 37°C[c]
				% Drug	% Zn	Drug/Acid	Zn/Acid	
Cyclazocine								
IA	Tannic	210–215	2	29.6	3.00	0.54	0.48	6.5
IB	Tannic	223–227	3	22.7	4.97	0.39	0.71	4.7
IIA	Pamoic	230–234	3	46.6	2.17	0.65	0.25	6.3
IIIA	3-Hydroxy-2-methyl-cinchoninic	182–183	1	45.2	2.28	0.65	0.27	30.1
IIIB	"	196–197	2	51.2	1.88	0.82	0.25	28.8
VA	5-t-Octylsalicylic	128–130	3	39.7	2.69	0.64	0.36	8.0
Naloxone								
VIA	Tannic	>250	2	26.2	4.36	0.39	0.66	14.3
VIB	Tannic	>250	3	24.2	5.60	0.36	0.84	13.6
VIIA	Pamoic	211–216	2	57.4	0.86	0.81	0.12	70.3
VIIB	Pamoic	255–260	3	47.1	3.70	0.57	0.45	71.0
IXA	5-t-Octylsalicylic	134–137	3	32.7	4.54	0.40	0.56	37.2

[a] See Methods for preparative and analytical procedures.
[b] Equivalents per equivalent of acid; amount of acid assumed by difference. Sum of equivalents ratios of drug and zinc should equal 1.
[c] See footnote b, Table 1.

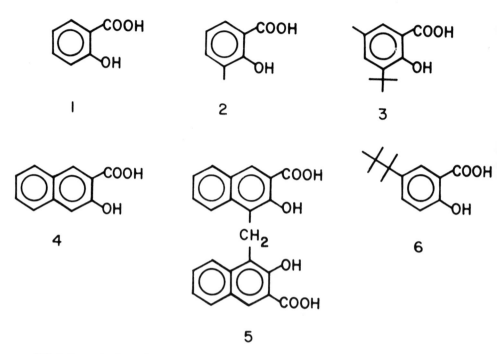

FIG. 1. Formulas for salicylic acid (1), 3-methylsalicylic acid (2), 3-t-butyl-5-methylsalicylic acid (3), 3-hydroxy-2-naphthoic acid (4), pamoic acid (5), 5-t-octylsalicylic acid (6).

3-methyl derivative (formula 2) formed one with methadone only; the 3-t-butyl-5-methyl analogue (formula 3) and the benzo derivative (formula 4) formed insoluble salts with methadone and cyclazocine but not with naloxone; pamoic (formula 5) and 5-t-octylsalicyclic acid (formula 6) formed salts with all three drugs.

Interestingly, one acid, 3,5,-di-t-butyl-2,6-dihydroxybenzoic acid (formula 7 in Fig. 2), provided salts with all three drugs showing the lowest percent dissociations observed, lower than the corresponding tannic acid [approximately penta-(digalloyl)-glucose, formula 8] salts or, indeed, any of the zinc complexes. In fact, presumably owing to the extremely low solubility of the salts of the di-t-butyldihydroxybenzoic acid, attempts to incorporate zinc into them have thus far been abortive.

Data on the narcotic antagonist activity in the mouse tail-flick test of representative salts and zinc complexes of cyclazocine are given in Table 3 and of naloxone in Table 4. Approximate ED_{80} values, based on measurement of reaction time 40 min after intramuscular administration of a suspension of test preparation in peanut oil, are indicated as well as duration of

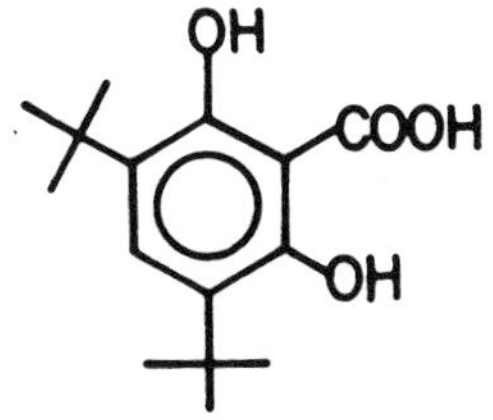

FIG. 2. Formulas for 3,5-di-*t*-butyl-2,6-dihydroxybenzoic acid **(7)**, primary component of gallotannic acid (tannic acid, Eastman) **(8)**.

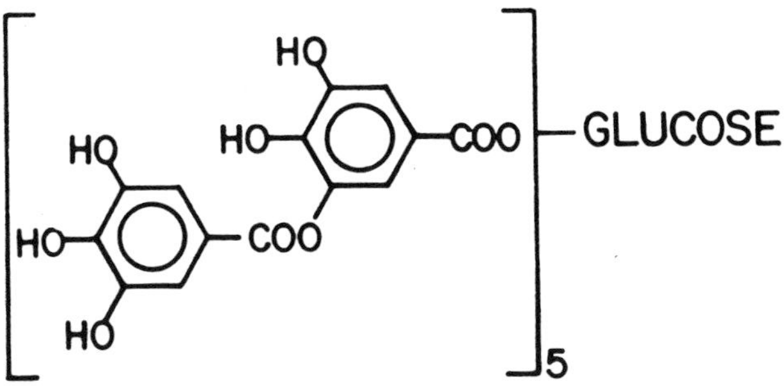

antagonist activity at the ED_{80} dose level and at the high (4 mg/kg) dose level.

Percent dissociation values were used as a rough guide to our selection of salts and complexes for study in mice. At least a hint of a correlation could be discerned between percent dissociation and duration of antagonist activity; i.e., preparations showing lower percent dissociations *in vitro* were more likely to provide longer durations of activity *in vivo*. Data on percent antagonism were somewhat difficult to reproduce, and it was necessary on occasion to test as many as four groups of six mice to obtain valid results. ED_{80} values are only approximate since the dose-response curves tended to flatten as this response level was approached. Nevertheless, it was surprising that alteration of percent dissociation had little, and certainly no consistent, effect on ED_{80}.

Neither cyclazocine base nor its tannate salt **(I)** showed significant antagonist activity beyond 8 hr, even at the 4 mg/kg dose level. The zinc tannate complex **(IA)**, however, which showed a lower percent dissociation *in vitro*, evidenced at least a threefold increase in duration of activity; it was active at 24 hr even at the low dose level but showed essentially no activity at 48 hr.

At 4 mg/kg, cyclazocine pamoate **(II)** had activity at 16 hr; incorporation of zinc **(IIA)** extended some activity (at the 4 mg/kg dose level only) to 24 hr. Similarly, a 4 mg/kg dose of the 5-*t*-octylsalicylate **(V)** was active at 16 hr; duration of activity was not prolonged with the zinc complex **(VA)**.

The cyclazocine salt showing the least dissociation *in vitro*, the 3,5-di-*t*-butyl-2,6-dihydroxybenzoate **(IV)**, showed activity to 24 hr at the 4 mg/kg

TABLE 3. *Duration of narcotic antagonism activity of cyclazocine salts and zinc complexes*

Salt or complex	Dose[b] (mg/kg)	% Antagonism[a]					
		40 min	4 hr	8 hr	16 hr	24 hr	48 hr
Base	0.8	74	64	19	0	0	—
	4.0	90	78	44	0	0	—
I Tannate	0.64	80	28	10	4	2	—
	4.0	87	86	53	0	0	—
IA Zinc tannate	0.8	81	79	70	32	45	0
	4.0	77	88	79	49	32	13
II Pamoate	0.64	81	71	60	8	0	—
	4.0	88	94	61	36	0	—
IIA Zinc pamoate	0.64	73	81	44	0	0	—
	4.0	87	76	74	43	25	5
III 3-Hydroxy-2-methylcinchoninate	0.24	81	52	23	0	0	—
	4.0	88	73	51	0	14	—
IIIB Zinc 3-hydroxy-2-methylcinchoninate	0.72	74	71	27	0	0	—
	4.0	90	86	54	0	0	—
IV 3,5-Di-*t*-butyl-2,6-dihydroxybenzoate	0.8	74	86	13	14	0	—
	4.0	89	82	82	24	25	0
V 5-*t*-Octylsalicylate	0.48	78	26	35	5	0	—
	4.0	87	94	62	41	0	—
VA Zinc 5-*t*-octylsal-icylate	0.48	85	26	41	8	3	—
	4.0	72	99	33	24	0	—

[a] Percent antagonism to a standard morphine sulfate dose of 20 mg/kg administered intraperitoneally 30 min before testing. Time indicates interval between intramuscular administration of test compound in peanut oil and analgesia testing. Each value represents the mean of at least 12 mice.

[b] Expressed as milligrams of cyclazocine base equivalent. The low dose is the approximate ED_{80} dose at 40-min test interval.

dose level only and thus did not live up to its promise. A possible explanation of this might be metabolic destruction of the acid *in vivo* with consequent release of drug. We are looking into the possibility of increasing the stability of the acid while retaining the solubility characteristics of its salts by investigating its relatives with only one hydroxyl group.

Naloxone hydrochloride, even at the very high dose of 4 mg/kg, showed significant activity only to 4 hr. At 4 mg/kg, activity was prolonged to 8 hr with the tannate salt (**VI**), and to at least 24 and possibly to 48 hr with the zinc tannate complex (**VIA**). No activity remained at 72 hr.

Naloxone pamoate (**VII**), which has been reported to show an increased duration of activity in dogs (11)[7] and to have activity lasting for 72 hr at three times the therapeutic dose in man (11), showed no significant activity

[7] W. R. Martin, *personal communication.*

TABLE 4. *Duration of narcotic antagonism activity of naloxone salts and zinc complexes*

Salt or complex	Dose[b] (mg/kg)	% Antagonism[a]					
		40 min	4 hr	8 hr	16 hr	24 hr	48 hr
Hydrochloride	0.064	70	22	10	10	0	—
	4.0	99	79	16	3	10	—
VI Tannate	0.072	88	24	28	17	0	—
	4.0	99	87	66	6	3	—
VIA Zinc tannate	0.064	84	64	11	0	0	—
	4.0	95	99	90	41	42	23
VII Pamoate	0.080	87	39	7	0	0	—
	4.0	100	100	94	11	1	—
VIIB Zinc pamoate	0.076	80	47	39	0	0	—
	4.0	100	100	86	9	0	—
VIII 3,5-Di-t-butyl-2,6-dihydroxybenzoate	0.068	82	3	7	16	0	—
	4.0	100	95	47	7	0	—
IX 5-t-Octylsalicylate	0.064	79	65	31	9	0	—
	4.0	100	78	58	43	18	17
IXA Zinc 5-t-octylsalicylate	0.040	77	50	40	40	0	—
	4.0	99	96	29	57	25	14

[a] Percent antagonism to a standard morphine sulfate dose of 20 mg/kg administered intraperitoneally 30 min before testing. Time indicates interval between intramuscular administration of test compound in peanut oil and analgesia testing. Each value represents the mean of at least 12 mice.

[b] Expressed as milligrams of naloxone base equivalent. The low dose is the approximate ED_{80} dose at 40-min test interval.

beyond 8 hr in our mice administered the high dose, 50 times the ED_{80}. Activity was not prolonged by incorporation of zinc (**VIIB**).

Both the 5-t-octylsalicylate (**IX**) and the corresponding zinc complex (**IXA**) showed significant activity at 16 hr and, at the high dose, some residual activity at least to 24 hr. Again, the 3,5-di-t-butyl-2,6-dihydroxybenzoate (**VIII**) was disappointing, showing definite activity only to 8 hr. None of the salts or complexes showed significant activity at 72 hr.

To date, our most interesting preparations, showing the most significant prolongation of antagonist action, are the zinc tannate complexes **IA** and **VIA**. It may be useful to consider the nature of the contribution of the zinc ion to this effect. We envisage the zinc as bonding, quite possibly covalently, to one or more acid functions while leaving others free to form ionic bonds with drug. Thus the solubility of the salt would be altered. This picture implies that only acids with more than one acid function per molecule could form zinc complexes with modified properties. Monobasic acids would simply form mixtures of zinc salts and drug salts.

We had hoped that acids having a phenolic hydroxyl group and a carboxyl group, e.g., a salicylic acid derivative, could bond to zinc through the former function while leaving the latter free to interact ionically with drug. Alternatively, or additionally, zinc could bond to the phenolic hydroxyl group present in the drug molecule, either cyclazocine or naloxone. Unfortunately, the zinc did not seem to act in this fashion, at least to any major extent, since introduction of zinc invariably displaced drug from the complex and since the sum of the equivalents of zinc plus drug in the complex always approximated the number of equivalents of drug in the simple salt.

Attempts to alter the nature of the zinc complexes by modifying the method of preparation were not very successful. Originally it was felt that treating preformed drug salts with zinc might yield the most useful complexes since the zinc might then interact with free, less acidic functions (i.e., phenolic) and/or displace more readily displaceable drug—that is, if there were any differences in drug binding. In practice, relatively few zinc complexes, most notably the zinc tannate complexes, could be prepared in this way. For most salts, such as the pamoates, it was found very difficult to displace drug by zinc treatment. Usually, therefore, complexes were prepared by treatment of an alkali metal salt of the acid first with zinc and then with drug. The ease of incorporation of zinc depended directly on the solubility of the salt. Naloxone was more readily displaced by zinc than cyclazocine. The preparative method could be tailored to suit the particular drug-acid combination and the amount of zinc desired to be introduced.

Generally, the relative percent dissociation *in vitro* of salts versus corresponding complexes depended more on the relative percent drug in the preparation than on the method of preparation. In certain cases, however, percent dissociation was not significantly reduced by incorporation of zinc (*cf.* **III** vs. **IIIA** and **IIIB**; **VII** vs. **VIIA** and **VIIB**).

Incorporation of zinc had the most significant effect on the duration of antagonist activity *in vivo* with the tannate preparations (*cf.* **I** vs. **IA**, **VI** vs. **VIA**). It is therefore worth speculating as to how this complex might be formulated. Since the sum of the number of equivalents of zinc plus drug per mole of acid in the complex is the same (five) as the number of equivalents of drug in the salt, we can tentatively picture our zinc tannate complexes more or less as shown in formula **9** (Fig. 3). Such a complex might be expected to have altered drug-release properties *in vivo* as well as *in vitro*.

If this picture has any validity, two primary zinc-drug complexes involving only one molecule of tannic acid are possible: one having a ratio of one zinc ion to three drug molecules and the other with two zinc ions to one molecule of drug. Although the amount of zinc can be varied, the zinc:drug ratios in the particular zinc tannate complexes which have been most thoroughly studied to date, **IA** and **VIA**, are 1.2:2.7 and 1.65:1.95, re-

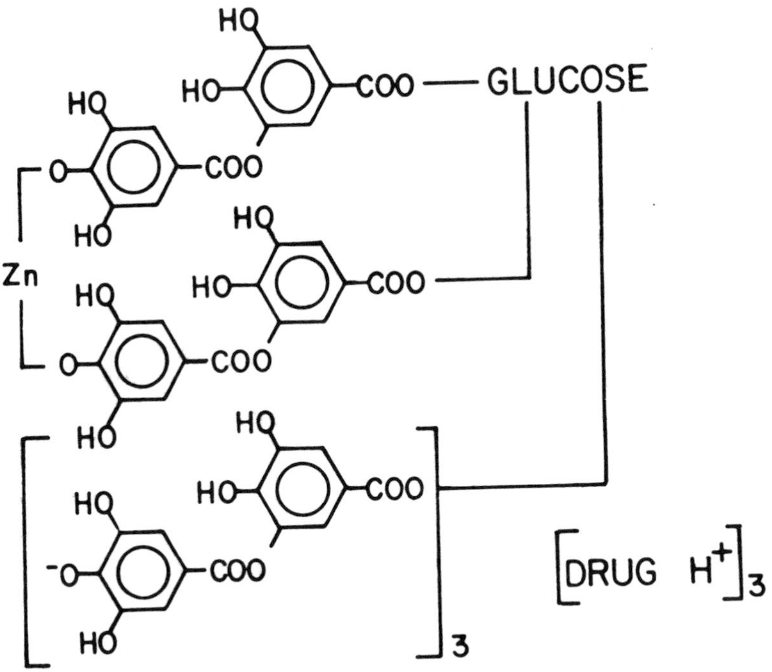

FIG. 3. Speculative formulation of structure of drug zinc tannate complex.

spectively. Thus, it is conceivable that these could essentially be mixtures of the two primary complexes.

Further studies are in progress, on the zinc tannate complexes especially. Drs. Dewey and Harris have confirmed our results in mice with cyclazocine zinc tannate (**IA**) and are studying the preparation in dogs.[8] We have also submitted this complex to Dr. W. R. Martin who has kindly offered to examine its effects on dogs. We plan to submit the naloxone complex **VIA** to these investigators as well. It is particularly important to study these complexes in other species since the mouse, with its high metabolic rate, may be a poor indicator of duration of activity in man. Note that naloxone pamoate showed little increase in duration in our mouse test in comparison with its reported duration in dog and man.

---

[8] W. L. Dewey and L. S. Harris, *personal communication*. We thank Dr. Dewey for this information.

We are examining the effect of varying the dose level on duration, and we plan to study the relation between blood levels, or rate of release *in vivo*, and duration of antagonist activity. Of course we are continuing to screen other salts and complexes, and are particularly interested in incorporating inherently more potent and longer lasting narcotic antagonist drugs into our complexes.

CONCLUSIONS

A number of mono- and polybasic organic acids, especially aromatic carboxylic acids also having phenolic hydroxyl groups, have been found to give water-insoluble salts with cyclazocine and naloxone. Salts of cyclazocine were less soluble than those of naloxone. Incorporation of zinc into complexes with these narcotic antagonist salts generally reduced percent dissociation in simulated physiological fluid *in vitro*.

Several of the salts and complexes showed increased duration of narcotic antagonist activity, as measured by the mouse tail-flick test after intramuscular injection. Those showing the most significantly increased durations of activity *in vivo* were cyclazocine zinc tannate (**IA**) and naloxone zinc tannate (**VIA**). These are being further investigated.

The nature of the zinc tannate complexes is discussed.

ACKNOWLEDGMENTS

We thank Mrs. Brenda A. Ley and Mrs. Marilyn R. Cater for truly outstanding technical assistance. We thank Drs. L. S. Harris, W. L. Dewey, and W. R. Martin for advice and many helpful suggestions.

REFERENCES

1. Blumberg, H.: Thirteenth National Medicinal Chemistry Symposium, A.C.S. Division of Medicinal Chemistry, The University of Iowa, Iowa City: June 18–22, 1972.
2. Cavallito, C. J., and Jewell, R.: J. Amer. Pharm. Ass., Sci. Ed. *47*:166, 1958.
3. Elslager, E. F.: Ann. Reports Med. Chem. 137, 1965.
4. Harper, N. J.: Prog. Drug Res. *4*:221, 247–248, 1962.
5. Harris, L. S., Dewey, W. L., Howes, J. F., Kennedy, J. S., and Pars, H.: J. Pharmacol. Exp. Ther. *169*:17, 1969.
6. Harris, L. S., and Pierson, A. K.: J. Pharmacol. Exp. Ther. *143*:141, 1964.
7. Mulé, S. J.: Anal. Chem. *36*:1907, 1964.
8. Report of the City of New York Health Services Administration, Narcotics Antagonists Research Program, "The Current State of Knowledge of Drug Antagonists for Heroin Addiction," 1971.
9. Wagner, J. G.: J. Pharm. Sci. *50*:383–384, 1961.
10. Zaks, A., Jones, T., Fink, M., and Freedman, A. M.: J.A.M.A. *215*:2108, 1971.

Narcotic Antagonists, edited by M. C. Braude, L. S. Harris, E. L. May, J. P. Smith, and J. E. Villarreal. *Advances in Biochemical Psychopharmacology, Vol. 8.* Raven Press, New York © 1974.

Injection Method for Delivery of Long-Acting Narcotic Antagonists

* Thomas D. Leafe, * Stanley F. Sarner, * James H. R. Woodland, *Seymour Yolles, ** David A. Blake, and ** Francis J. Meyer

* Department of Chemistry, University of Delaware, Newark, Delaware 19711, and ** University of Maryland, College Park, Maryland 20740

Cyclazocine-poly(lactic acid) composites in small particle form were implanted as well as injected into rats and the amounts of cyclazocine released were determined at various intervals of time. The results obtained by the injection method are comparable to those given by implantation. The former method is preferable because it makes surgical incision unnecessary. Particle size, within the dimensions investigated, appears to show small differences on the release rate of cyclazocine.

INTRODUCTION

Previously reported experiments (1, 3, 4) have demonstrated the feasibility of delivering narcotic antagonists over a period longer than 1 month by implanting composites of cyclazocine-poly(lactic acid) in film form. However, the use of a film has the disadvantage of requiring an incision of the body tissue. A considerable advantage would be obtained if the composite could be hypodermically injected rather than surgically implanted.

In this chapter we report the results of comparative tests conducted on rats by injecting as well as by implanting composites in small particles falling within Nos. 25/35 and within Nos. 35/70 sieves. In these tests the composite was hypodermically injected as a suspension in carboxymethylcellulose into the body tissue of rats, and the excreted radioactivity measured at various intervals of time. In order to compare this method with the implantation method, a composite of the same composition and particle size as above was implanted into rats by surgery.

Paralleling this *in vivo* investigation, tests *in vitro* were conducted by extracting the composite with tepid water at various time intervals and determining the release of cyclazocine by monitoring the extracted solutions.

569

METHODS

Preparation of Poly(lactic Acid)

A 1,000-ml resin kettle, oven-dried overnight, cooled to room temperature under nitrogen, was charged under nitrogen with 400 g of L(-)lactide (C. H. Boehringer und Sohn, Ingelheim am Rhein, West Germany). The kettle was then placed in an oil bath at 135°C and stirred until the lactide melted. Diethylzinc (16 ml of 25% heptane solution) was rapidly introduced into the stirred melt. The light-yellow solid that formed within 2 min was taken up in dichloromethane (2,000 ml) after cooling to room temperature and reprecipitated in a blender by adding hexane (v/v ratio: 5 hexane to 1.5 dichloromethane). The fine white powder that formed was then taken up again in dichloromethane (1,000 ml), precipitated as above, and dried. The molecular weight of the polymer obtained, calculated from viscosity measurements, was 45,000.

The results obtained from C and H analyses were within $\pm 0.4\%$ of the theoretical values. The COOH group content, expressed as mg KOH per g of polymer, varied between 2 and 10. The metal content was less than 0.5%.

Preparation of Cyclazocine-Poly(lactic Acid) Composites Coded A and B

A benzene solution of tritiated cyclazocine (New England Nuclear Corp., Boston, Mass.) of specific activity 82.36×10^6 dpm/ml (1.8 ml) was evaporated to dryness. To the residue was first added a solution of unlabeled cyclazocine (Sterling Winthrop Co., 1.0 g) and tributyl citrate (0.25 g) in dichloromethane (50 ml) and then poly(lactic acid) (3.75 g). The solvent was flashed off under reduced pressure, and the residue was wrapped in aluminum foil and melt-pressed (Carver Laboratory Press, Mod. Co.) at 145°C under total load of 1 metric ton for 10 sec (shims 0.91 mm thick were used), to produce films of uniform thickness in which no imperfection due to air or gas was observed. The test samples were obtained by grinding these films into small rectangular particles. The specific radioactivities of these samples were determined by combustion of the polymer matrix, and measurement of the radioactivities in the water trapped in a Tricarb Oxidizer System.

Preparation of Cyclazocine-Poly(lactic Acid) Composites Coded C and D

The above procedure was repeated using 30 ml of a methanolic solution of tritiated cyclazocine of specific activity 2.66×10^9 dpm/ml in place of the benzene solution of tritiated cyclazocine. The characteristics of the test samples are listed in Table 1.

TABLE 1. *Characteristics of the test samples of cyclazocine-poly(lactic acid) used*

Test samples	Particle size falling within sieves nos.	Weight (mg) used		Specific radioactivity (dpm/g)
		in vivo	*in vitro*	
A	25 and 35	400	1040	18.4×10^6
B	35 and 70	—	777	18.4×10^6
C	25 and 35	300	384	$125 \quad \times 10^6$
D	35 and 70	300	—	$125 \quad \times 10^6$

Experiments *in vivo*

These experiments were conducted on groups of three male Sprague-Dawley rats weighing between 550 and 600 g.

A. *Implantation of Test Samples*

A small incision was made through the skin on the dorsal surface of the rats; test sample A was inserted subcutaneously and pushed away from the incision area. The incisions were sutured and the animal immediately placed into an individual metabolism cage designed for the collection of urine and feces. The collected urine and cage washings were combined and counted on a daily basis for the first 10 days and then every 4 days for the duration of the experiment. The excreta samples were diluted to 100 ml with water. Samples of 1 ml were pipetted into 15 ml of scintillation solution and radioassayed by liquid scintillation counting techniques. Internal standardization was used for the calculation of counting efficiency. The values of the cyclazocine delivered in each interval of time are reported as percent of implanted dose calculated on the basis of disintegration per min.

B. *Injection of Test Samples*

The opening at the tip of a 5-ml plastic syringe was enlarged with a 0.081-inch drill. With the tip of the syringe plugged, 210 mg of CMC 7 LF was mixed with a composite (samples A, C, or D) until uniform. One-half ml of normal saline was added and stirred with a small spatula. One-half ml portions of normal saline were added until the total volume was 3 ml. The time of mixing and stirring was approximately 1 min. An intimate mixture of particles in nearly clear, viscous CMC resulted. The plug at the tip of the barrel was replaced with a 15 gauge, thin-wall needle (for test samples coded A and C) or 18 gauge needle (for test sample coded D). The injection site on the rat was shaved, the area having been selected by measuring the length of the needle from the nape of the neck to a lower section of the back. The animal was preferably anesthetized to avoid excessive movement. The time required was approximately 15 sec for injection. On removing the needle the opening, which was pressed and supported with the finger, was painted with Isodine®, and immediately closed with a clip or adhesive tape. The animals were then placed in an individual metabolism cage designed for the collection of urine and feces. The excreta samples were collected and radioassayed as described above.

Experiments *in vitro*

A sample of a composite (sample A or B or C)(0.5 to 1 g) was sewn into a cheesecloth sack and anchored under the water level of the sample holder (1, Fig. 1) of a 300-ml modified Raab extractor. The cyclazocine was extracted with (20° ± 3°C) water as the solvent. At intervals of 6, 24, and 48 hr and then every 6 days the aqueous solution (ave. 150 ml) in the boiler (2) was collected and the volume recorded. The collected solutions were replaced at every sampling with distilled water. A sample of the aqueous solutions (1 ml) was pipetted into 15 ml of scintillation solution and the

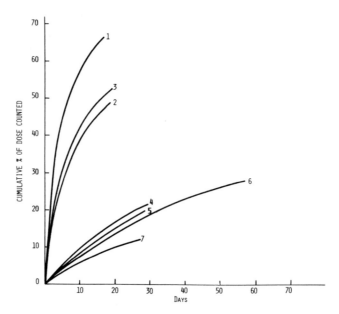

FIG. 1. Modified Raab extractor: (1) sample holder; (2) boiler; (3) condenser; (4) drain; (5) bubbler; (6) thermometer.

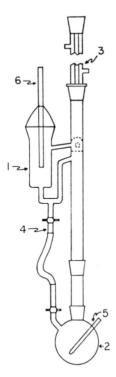

FIG. 2. Cumulative amount of cyclazocine released as a function of time. 1 = C, *in vitro;* 2 = B, *in vitro;* 3 = A, *in vitro;* 4 = C, injected; 5 = D, injected; 6 = A, implanted; 7 = A, injected.

radioactivity measured. The values of cyclazocine extracted in each interval of time are reported as percent of dose initially present in the sample, calculated on the basis of disintegration per minute (Fig. 2).

At the end of the experiment, the sample of composite left in the extractor was dissolved in dichloromethane and the radioactivity of the obtained solution measured. The total radioactivity of the extracted aqueous solution plus the radioactivity found in the sample after extraction checked with that present in the sample before extraction.

RESULTS AND DISCUSSIONS

The values of the cumulative amounts of cyclazocine excreted as well as extracted, expressed as percent of the original dose, are plotted in Fig. 1 as a function of time. The results obtained by injecting suspensions of small particles of cyclazocine-poly(lactic acid) composite are comparable to those obtained by implanting the same composite having the same particle size. Within the first 26 days, 16% of the original dose of cyclazocine was released in the implanation test and an average of 15% in the injection tests.

The release rate of cyclazocine *in vitro* is considerably faster than *in vivo*. However, there is an agreement with respect to order between the results of the two methods.

In the investigation of the influence of the particle size of the composite on the release rate of cyclazocine it was found that the release rate is not very sensitive to variations in particle size (compare curve A with B *in vitro* and curve C with D *in vivo*).

At present we are also investigating the delivery of other narcotic antagonists, e.g., naloxone, by injecting suspensions of small particles of antagonist-poly(lactic acid) composites.

Samples of our composites are under study in dogs at ARC in Lexington and in mice at the University of North Carolina.

CONCLUSIONS

We have demonstrated in animals that sustained release of narcotic antagonists can be achieved over an extended period of time (approximately 30 days) from suspensions of small particles. Further we developed a method for injecting hypodermically these particles which gave results comparable with those obtained by surgical implantation.

ACKNOWLEDGMENTS

This work has been supported by National Institute of Mental Health contract No. HSM 42–72–97.

REFERENCES

1. Blake, D. A., Yolles, S., Helrich, M., Cascorbi, H. F., and Eagan, M. J.: Release of Cyclazocine from Subcutaneously Implanted Polymeric Matrices. Abstract, Academy of Pharmaceutical Sciences, San Francisco, March 30, 1971.
2. Martin, W. R., and Sandquist, Virginia L.: Long-Acting Narcotic Antagonists. Report 34th Annual Meeting Committee on Problems of Drug Dependence, Ann Arbor, Michigan, 1972.
3. Yolles, S.: Development of a Long-Acting Dosage Form for Narcotic Antagonists. 13th National Medicinal Chemistry Symposium. University of Iowa, Iowa City, Iowa, June 18–22, 1972.
4. Yolles, S. et al.: Long-acting delivery system for narcotic antagonists. J. Med. Chem., *16*:897–901, 1973.
5. All countings were performed with a Packard Tri-Carb Model liquid scintillation spectrometer in the *in vivo* experiments and with a Beckman LS-100 spectrometer in the *in vitro*

experiments. The counting solution consisted of a mixture of 2,5-diphenyloxazole (PPO, 22.0g), 1,4-bis [2-(4-methyl-5-phenyl-oxazolyl)] benzene (dimethyl POPOP, 0.4g) and Triton x-100 (1,000 ml) diluted to 4,000 ml with toluene, in the *in vivo* experiments. Aquasol solution (New England Nuclear Corp., Boston, Mass.) was used in the *in vitro* experiments.

The materials on the following pages were submitted after the book was in page proof.

THE ROLE OF THE FEDERAL GOVERNMENT
IN THE DEVELOPMENT OF NARCOTIC ANTAGONISTS

Alan I. Green

Special Action Office for Drug Abuse Prevention, Washington, D.C.

The federal government's program for drug abuse activities in the areas of treatment, education, prevention, rehabilitation, and research is coordinated by the Special Action Office for Drug Abuse Prevention. This office is housed in the Executive Office of the President and was created in mid-1971 by Executive Order of the President. It was given statutory authority in March, 1972, when a bill creating the Special Action Office for Drug Abuse Prevention was signed by the President. One section of the bill that established the Special Action Office specified the need to develop new pharmacological approaches for treatment and prevention of drug-dependent individuals. The office has viewed this task as one of very high priority.

At the present time, there are more than 60,000 people being treated in methadone maintenance programs throughout the country. While the use of methadone is certainly beneficial to thousands of people, it is still the only accepted pharmacological tool for the treatment of heroin-dependent individuals, and other agents are definitely needed. The use of narcotic antagonists is one new treatment approach for opiate-dependent individuals now being developed by the Federal Government.

Theoretically, narcotic antagonists might be useful in a number of different ways. Their use following withdrawal from methadone might prevent relapse to narcotic use. They might be helpful in treating narcotic experimenters or early users. And, they might provide an alternative treatment for individuals who might otherwise be treated with methadone maintenance.

The government interest in the development of these compounds resulted in a meeting of representatives of the pharmaceutical industry, the research community, and the Federal Government that was held in September, 1971, at the Special Action Office. At that meeting, the discussion focused on the narcotic antagonists that were then available, and on new promising antagonists that were in the process of development. The consensus of the meeting was that the development of these agents had not been proceeding at an optimal rate for a number of reasons. First, it was thought that there were inadequate supplies of many of the compounds. Second, there were inadequate preclinical and clinical facilities for the testing of those compounds that had been identified and produced. And, third, it was thought that government funding would be necessary to underwrite the developmental costs of many of these compounds since a profitable market for them was not a likely possibility.

In response to these problems, a number of new efforts have been undertaken over the past year, all aimed at accelerating the development of clinically useful narcotic antagonists. It should be noted that many different groups have participated in these efforts. The pharmaceutical industry has provided information to the government concerning new compounds, and has tested and developed a number of these, as demonstrated at this conference. The Pharmaceutical Manufacturers Association has been helpful as a coordinating mechanism to insure useful government and industry interchange. The Research Community has developed an increased interest in this field, and many of its members have given advice and direction to the Federal effort. Within the Government itself, the National Institute of Mental Health, the Veterans Administration, the Department of Defense, and the Food and Drug Administration have collaborated with the Special Action Office to launch a more than $3,000,000 program for the synthesis of new compounds and the creation of new preclinical and clinical facilities for their meeting.

This government program has resulted in the development and testing of a number of new compounds over the past year. EN-1639A, in addition to the work done on it by Endo, has been purchased by government contract, has undergone early Phase I studies at the Addiction Research Center, and will soon undergo further Phase I and Phase II studies in government-funded facilities. EC-2605 has been developed by Bristol and has been tested in government-funded facilities. M-5050 has been purchased by the government and will be tested in government-funded facilities as soon as the toxicological studies are completed. Naloxone pamoate was produced by Endo and tested in government-funded facilities. Cyclazocine has been made available to the government by Sterling-Winthrop and is being evaluated in Phase II and Phase III studies in government-funded facilities. Naloxone has been produced by Endo and is continuing to be evaluated in Phase III studies in government-funded progress. A number of long-acting preparations are being created and studied in government-funded facilities.

A few of the new narcotic antagonists now available appear to last at least 24 hours and to be side-effect free. These compounds will be tested in large-scale clinical studies to determine their safety and efficacy as treatment or prevention agents. Simultaneously, the search for even longer acting narcotic antagonists will continue. This may require the development of a few of the more potent compounds discussed at this conference, as well as their manipulation by chemical or physical means.

As Dr. Jaffe, Dr. Bunney, and I have all emphasized, the development of narcotic antagonists for clinical use in heroin addicts, while still in its infancy, has proceeded quite rapidly over the past year. The Federal Government is prepared to continue to stimulate the development of these compounds and to provide for their complete evaluation as new treatment or prevention agents for heroin addiction.

Chemistry of Narcotic Antagonists of the Morphine Analogues and Morphinan Types: An Overview
Jack Fishman, Albert Einstein College of Medicine, New York, N. Y.

The progress in the preparation of new narcotic antagonists reported in this session needs to be considered in light of the biological requirements of an antagonist for the treatment of post-narcotic addicts. It has been considered desirable that such an antagonist in addition to being free of deleterious side effects in chronic use be also devoid of agonist activity since the latter is so frequently associated with dependence and other long term CNS effects. If this view prevails, then none of the new compounds, with the possible exception of naltrexone (EN 1639), offers much promise for eventual clinical use since they all possess significant agonist activity and none attains the "pure" antagonist character of naloxone. It is, however, likely that the presence of some agonist activity in conjunction with high antagonist potency may still be consistent with an effective and useful compound. This is possible, because, as is apparently the case with cyclazocine, tolerance to the agonist but not the antagonist activity develops with continued use. Until this tolerance is attained the initial undesirable effects can be blocked by the coadministration of naloxone in the early part of the treatment. If this coexistence of agonist and antagonist activity proves acceptable, then several of the new compounds reported offer considerable hope for the development of a practical antagonist treatment of post-addicts.

The structures which have been obtained by modification of natural products are represented by the nalorphine and naloxone analogues. None of the nalorphine derivatives possesses particularly desirable antagonist activity free of side effects and therefore they do not appear promising, although the structure-activity relationships reported can be useful when applied to another series. The naloxone analogue, naltrexone, on the other hand, contains considerable and immediate promise. It has some agonist activity but offers considerable advantages over naloxone in potency, duration of action, and oral effectiveness. Also, in view of its close similarity to the intensively studied naloxone, it may be expected to produce few unpleasant surprises in clinical trials and use.

The clear desirability of avoiding opium-derived starting materials focuses attention on the totally synthetic antagonists. Among the levellorphan analogues reported, one particularly interesting compound is the 2-hydroxy-N cyclopropylmethylmorphinan, not because of its own pharmacology, but as an indication that the placement of the phenolic hydroxyl at C-2 instead of C-3 can lead to antagonist activity. This modification when applied to other series could produce valuable antagonists. A similar innovative lead is offered in isocyclorphan, which has high antagonist and little or no agonist activity. The "unnatural" configuration of this compound at C-14 suggests that this feature may convey similar antagonist properties when introduced into other potent agonist structures. The discussion of the various synthetic approaches to the isocyclorphan structure demonstrates the progressive evolution of better methods and promises that the material can be made available more readily if it becomes necessary.

The effect of the 14-hydroxy group in potentiating both agonist and antagonist activity depending on the nitrogen substituent has been used by the Bristol group as a guide in the synthesis of 14-hydroxy morphinans. Several of these compounds particularly L-BC 2605 demonstrate outstanding antagonist activity accompanied by a lesser degree of agonist action and by an apparent resistance to metabolic inactivation leading to a long effective biologic life. This series when further modified by a keto group at C-6 provides a compound whose preliminary pharmacology makes it of particular interest for clinical evaluation.

In conclusion, if some agonist activity is acceptable in the antagonist, several of the above approaches offer great promise of arriving at the drug of choice. If, however, no agonist activity should be present at all, then further efforts must be directed to the synthesis of other pure antagonists and concurrently toward methods of extending the duration of action of naloxone, presently the only known "pure" antagonist.

Chemistry of Narcotic Antagonists of the Benzomorphan and Thebaine Types: An Overview

Maxwell Gordon, Bristol Laboratories, Syracuse, New York

Albertson reported on a systematic examination of structure activity relationships in the cyclazocine series, including data on more than 100 new compounds. However, no marked improvement in cyclazocine's antagonist potency was seen with any of the analogues. Inasmuch as no agonist data are reported for these compounds, it is not yet possible to judge whether any of them will have fewer hallucinogenic or other "agonist" effects than seen with cyclazocine. Surprisingly, considering the scope of the program, no 9, 9-disubstitution (substitution on the endomethano group, numbered the 11-position in Albertson's chapter) was reported, since this type of substitution has been found to be interesting by P. A. J. Janssen, E. L. May, and Bristol Laboratories.

Clarke described the search for antagonists among the 5-phenylbenzomorphans. This series continues to be interesting from a structure-activity relationship point of view, yet disappointing from a clinical standpoint. The only "pure" antagonist in the series was the N-propargyl derivative, but its potency of 1/2 to 1/10th that of nalorphine did not encourage further investigation. Other antagonists in this series have either had unacceptable agonist effects in animals or have shown dependence liability in man or in test animals.

Merz described the novel furylmethyl side chain on the benzomorphan nitrogen, in which the classical allyl group is incorporated into a ring. More than 1,500 compounds were prepated in this series and by appropriate methyl substitution of the furyl group "pure" antagonists, agonist-antagonists, and potent agonists could be prepared. Antagonist activities in the nalorphine range were reported, and agonists with the potency of morphine were found in this series, all without physical dependence capacity in the monkey. No data on clinical activity were presented.

A report by Janssen disclosed 9, 9-dimethyl analogues of cyclazocine with five times the potency of cyclazocine and greater duration. However, there was no indication of the degree of agonist effects in animals and no suggestion that the compounds would not be hallucinogenic in man.

Takeda described his homobenzomorphans and one of them was a relatively "pure" antagonist but only had nalorphine potency.

A further report on Reckitt's large series of Diels-Alder adducts of thebaine was given by Lewis, but there is no indication yet that nonhallucinogenic antagonists will be obtained from this series. The "cleanest" candidate, diprenorphine (M-5050), is scheduled for clinical trial.

In summary, naloxone still seems the best model for a "pure" potent antagonist if its duration can be materially extended.

Chemistry of New Classes of Narcotic Antagonists: An Overview

Everette L. May, National Institute of Arthritis & Metabolic Diseases, National Institutes of Health, Bethesda, Maryland, 20014

A series of bridged 2-aminotetralins displayed a mixture of very strong to weak analgesic and antagonist properties in rats and monkeys. With one exception the analgesic effect was greater than the antagonistic effect. Hydroxy substitution on the benzene rings conferred greater analgesic potency than methoxy (M. I. Gluckman).

The chapter by D. A. McCarthy on 3-arylpyrrolidines is mainly historical with respect to the analgesic activity of profadol types. However, the recent discovery of weak properties of antagonism for two N-analogues of profadol, *m*-(1-allyl-3-methyl-3-pyrrolidinyl) phenol and the N-cyclopropyl analogues, appears to provide the basis for developing a strategy for the exploration of the pyrrolidine ring as a framework for compounds having a high degree of selectivity as morphine antagonists.

As discussed by A. Langbein, narcotic antagonists of the 4-phenylpiperidine type can be obtained if essential structural elements (e.g., a *m*-phenolic hydroxyl and N-substituents such as 1-chloroallyl or cyclopropylmethyl) are provided. The synthesis and pharmacological properties of representative compounds are discussed.

7-Hydroxy-1, 2, 4, 5-3H-3-benzazepines with dimethallyl or allyl substituents on the nitrogen exhibit narcotic antagonist action intermediate to or less than nalorphine and naloxone depending upon the test method and route of administration. Duration of antagonism was approximately equivalent to that of naloxone. They did not exhibit analgesic activity. The synthesis of these tetrahydro-3H-benzazepines (which may be viewed as simplified benzamorphans) by two different methods was described by J. E. Giering.

Pharmacological Assay Procedures: An Overview

H. W. Kosterlitz, Department of Pharmacology, University of Aberdeen, Aberdeen, AB9 2ZD Scotland

The most important findings of this session may be summarized as follows. (1) Potent narcotic analgesic drugs: There was general agreement regarding the assessment of these drugs in tests on rodents and other animals. These tests and the assay by the guinea pig ileum method are good predictors of the analgesic potencies in man. (2) Antagonists with no or little agonist activity: The evaluation of the antagonist potencies of these drugs in different species, rodents, dogs, morphine-dependent monkeys and in the guinea pig isolated ileum, gave satisfactory prediction of their antagonist action in man. (3) Antagonists with significant agonist activity: This group of drugs still presents difficulties with regard to the assessment of their agonist and antagonist properties. There is a certain amount of disagreement between the results obtained by the various methods. Several reasons may be adduced for this situation. In whole animals and probably in isolated tissues, the previous history will influence the assay: (a) in an animal which has not been exposed to a narcotic analgesic drug, the agonist potency of a drug with dual action is marked; (b) in an animal pretreated with an agonist, the response to administration of such a drug is a preponderance of the antagonist over the agonist effect, and (c) the morphine dependent animal is particularly sensitive to the antagonist effect.

One of the findings which appears to be of importance for the assessment by the writhing test of the agonist effects of drugs with dual action is the rapid decline of the apparent agonist action after injection of the drug. The agonist potency must therefore be tested when its effect is at its peak. The rapid decline in effectiveness is possibly due to formation of less active metabolites.

For the estimation of antagonist potency, four tests are most commonly used. (1) The tail-flick test which is not sensitive to the agonist activity of drugs with dual actions; interaction between agonist and antagonist activity cannot be tested. (2) The reversal of respiratory depression in animals pretreated with narcotic analgesic drugs. Such a test is more sensitive to the antagonist than to the agonist effects of a drug. (3) The morphine-dependent monkey. This animal is highly sensitive to the antagonist effect of a drug with dual actions. (4) The assessment of agonist and antagonist potencies on the guinea pig ileum. In this test, agonist and antagonist properties are assessed simultaneously and the peak agonist and peak antagonist effect are determined. The assessment of antagonist potencies are in good agreement with other tests but the agonist potencies are usually to be found higher than in other tests, with the possible exception of man. It would appear that, in tests of rodents, the maximum antagonist effect should be related to the maximum agonist effect. At present this would probably relate the results obtained in the rat tail-flick test with those obtained in the mouse writing test.

Another possible difficulty is variability between laboratories. Standardization is essential within a laboratory and highly desirable between laboratories. It has been suggested that reference compounds should always be used in assays.

Tolerance and Physical Dependence to Antagonist Analgesic: An Overview
Monique C. Braude, Center for Studies of Narcotic Drug Abuse, National Institute of Mental Health, Rockville, Maryland

The chapters in this session emphasized the importance of testing compounds for their tolerance or physical dependence producing capacities. Using a pellet implantation method which, for the first time, allowed maintenance of high levels of narcotic antagonists, Nuite showed that, in mice, the pharmacologic profile of these compounds was very dissimilar from that of morphine and that tolerance or physical dependence did not develop after their chronic administration.

Cowan pointed out the need for primate dependence studies rather than single dose suppression studies to evaluate the physical dependence capacities of mixed agonist-antagonists of the oripavine-thebaine type. Mice primary dependence tests, while allowing confident predictions for strong agonist analgesics, do not seem to have as good a predictive value for the abuse potential liability in man of compounds of this series.

Frazer outlined the difficulties in extrapolating the data from animals to man, as well as the differences between species in respect to determination of the abuse potential of agonists and antagonists. He also suggested that a euphoric type antagonist with restricted toxicity and limited physical dependence producing liability may find best acceptance by the addict population.

The Metabolism of Narcotic Antagonists: An Overview
William L. Dewey, Department of Pharmacology, Medical College of Virginia, Richmond, Virginia 23219

Evidence has been presented in the preceding chapters which indicates that the narcotic antagonists naloxone, cyclazocine, and pentazocine are each rapidly taken up following oral and other parenteral routes of administration, readily get into the brain, and then are excreted quite rapidly. The compounds are metabolized to a great extent as demonstrated by the small quantities which are excreted as unchanged material. Narcotic antagonist activity has not been demonstrated for the majority of the metabolites of these compounds. This is at least in part due to the small quantities of metabolites which have been isolated and the fact that the majority of the metabolites are conjugates. The observations suggest that one would prolong the duration of action of a narcotic antagonist by interfering with its metabolism. The non-specificity of the enzymes involved in the metabolism of these drugs indicates that this is not a feasible approach. The effort to date to prolong the action of the narcotic antagonists has been directed toward preparing a formula that would prolong absorption.

Dr. Weinstein has demonstrated that a large number of metabolites are excreted following the administration of naloxone. The structural similarities among the narcotic antagonists suggest that with minor modifications the techniques used in these studies would be useful in studying the metabolism of the other antagonists. Obviously, these techniques would be useful in studying the pharmacokinetics and metabolic fate of naloxone given in various preparations which are intended to prolong its absorption. The techniques used by Dr. Mule in his extensive study into the pharmacokinetics of cyclazocine in tolerant, nontolerant, and abstinent dogs will be useful in studying the purporated slow release preparations of this potent antagonist. The finding by Dr. Mule that levels of cyclazocine and metabolites are below detectable levels for sometime prior to the appearance of the abstinence syndrome suggests that the possibility that chronic cyclazocine treatment produces an effect in the brain which lasts beyond the presence of the compound but is not irreversible.

The radioimmunoassay technique discussed by Dr. Berkowitz holds considerable promise for the detection of pharmacologically active doses of narcotics and their antagonists in laboratory animals. The additional sensitivity provided by the radioimmunoassay technique allows for the detection of plasma and tissue levels for a longer period of time. It is possible that when perfected for cyclazocine, this technique may be sensitive enough to demonstrate that some cyclazocine does exist in the brain prior to the appearance of the abstinence syndrome.

Data have been presented that suggest that the analgesic potency of cyclazocine may at least in part be due to its higher distribution to the brain than is observed with morphine. However, pentazocine, which gives brain concentrations in rodents five times greater than those observed with morphine at equivalent plasma concentrations, is a much less potent analgesic. This indicates a pronounced difference in the "unknown" analgesic potency at the molecular level for these benzomorphans. Dr. Medzihradsky has demonstrated that pentazocine is actively transported into the rat leukocytes. The results of these studies using cellular preparations from nervous tissue should be enlightening concerning the neuronal concentration and distribution of the antagonists.

Development of Long-Acting Preparations: An Overview
Sydney Archer, Rensselaer Polytechnic Institute, Rensselaer, New York

Three different approaches to the problem of developing long-acting preparations of cyclazocine and naloxone were presented. Gray discussed insoluble complexes of these antagonists, Yolles described his work on biodegradable implants, and I gave results from preliminary experiments on the *in vitro* release of cyclazocine from polyhydroxyalkyl methacrylate polymers. Although none of the work has progressed to the stage of clinical trial, it was clear that further research on these delivery systems is warranted.

The application of immunoassay methods for the detection of narcotic antagonists in body fluids was discussed. A radioimmunoassay, a spin immunoassay, and a newly developed enzyme immunoassay have been worked out for morphine. In principle these methods should be applicable to the assay of narcotic antagonists as well. In fact, an antibody to cyclazocine has been prepared and the final steps in the development of a very sensitive radioimmunoassay method await the preparation of a radio-labeled sample of the antagonist with a high specific activity.

Attention was drawn to the possible toxic effects of the vehicles used in the preparation of the long-acting antagonists. The discussants and speakers agreed that appropriate toxicological studies must be carried out before human trials are initiated. Such studies will be required by the Food and Drug Administration.

SUBJECT INDEX

---

* *An asterisk assigned to a page number indicates that numerical data appears on that page.*

---

* *An asterisk assigned to a page number indicates that numerical data appears on that
   page.*

* An asterisk assigned to a page number indicates that numerical data appears on that
   page.

* An asterisk assigned to a page number indicates that numerical data appears on that
   page.

* An asterisk assigned to a page number indicates that numerical data appears on that
   page.

* *An asterisk assigned to a page number indicates that numerical data appears on that page.*

---

* *An asterisk assigned to a page number indicates that numerical data appears on that page.*

*   *An asterisk assigned to a page number indicates that numerical data appears on that page.*

---

*   *An asterisk assigned to a page number indicates that numerical data appears on that page.*

---

* An asterisk assigned to a page number indicates that numerical data appears on that
 page.

*   *An asterisk assigned to a page number indicates that numerical data appears on that page.*